KU-735-224

High Altitude Medicine and Physiology

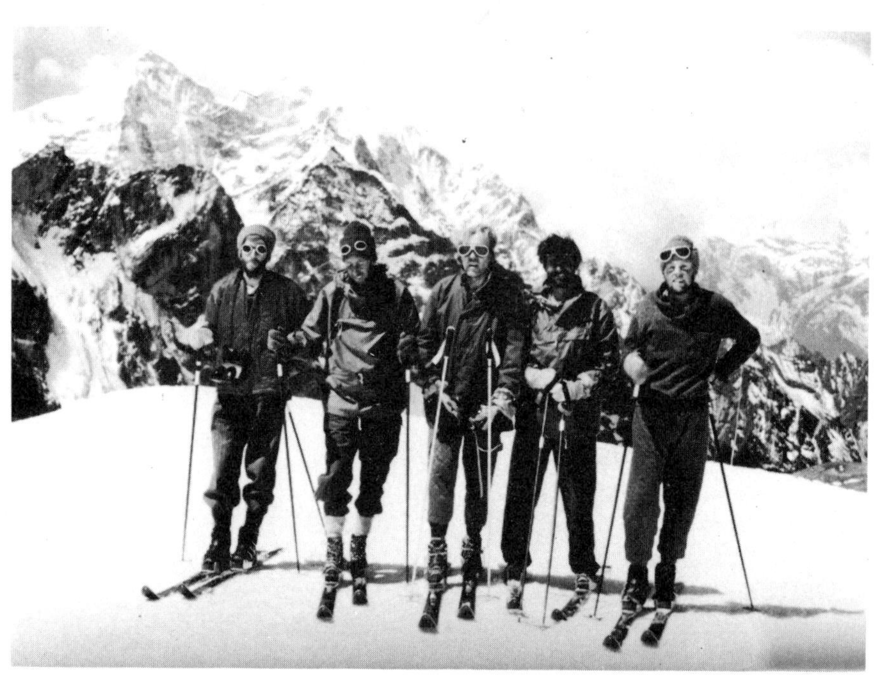

The authors, with two other colleagues, outside the Silver Hut at 5800 m in the Everest region during the Himalayan Scientific and Mountaineering Expedition, 1960–61. Left to right: Dr J.S. Milledge, Professor J.B. West, Dr L.G.C.E. Pugh, Mr M.P. Ward and Dr M.B. Gill.

High Altitude Medicine and Physiology

Second edition

Michael P. Ward CBE, MD, FRCS

Master, Society of Apothecaries of London, Formerly Consultant Surgeon and Lecturer in Clinical Surgery, London Hospital Medical College, London, UK

James S. Milledge MD, FRCP

Consultant Respiratory Physician and Medical Director at Northwick Park Hospital, Harrow, UK

John B. West MD, PhD, DSc, FRCP, FRACP

Professor of Medicine and Physiology at the School of Medicine, University of California, San Diego, USA

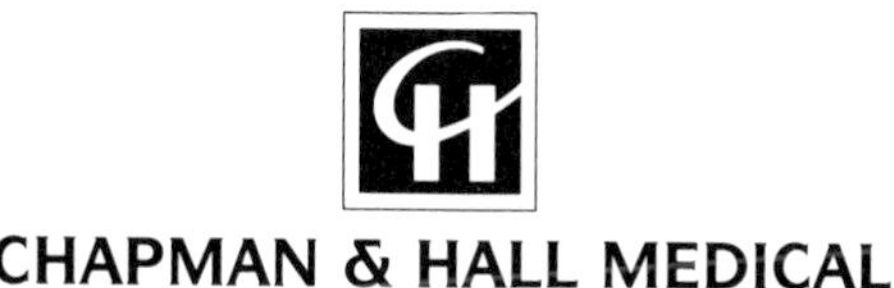

CHAPMAN & HALL MEDICAL

London · Glasgow · Weinheim · New York · Tokyo · Melbourne · Madras

Published by Chapman & Hall, 2–6 Boundary Row, London SE1 8HN, UK

Chapman & Hall, 2–6 Boundary Row, London SE1 8HN, UK

Blackie Academic & Professional, Wester Cleddens Road, Bishopbriggs, Glasgow G64 2NZ, UK

Chapman & Hall GmbH, Pappelallee 3, 69469 Weinheim, Germany

Chapman & Hall USA, One Penn Plaza, 41st Floor, New York NY 10119, USA

Chapman & Hall Japan, ITP-Japan, Kyowa Building, 3F, 2-2-1 Hirakawacho, Chiyoda-Ku, Tokyo 102, Japan

Chapman & Hall Australia, Thomas Nelson Australia, 102 Dodds Street, South Melbourne, Victoria 3205, Australia

Chapman & Hall India, R. Seshadri, 32 Second Main Road, CIT East, Madras 600 035, India

First edition 1989

Second edition 1995

© 1989, 1995 Michael P. Ward, James S. Milledge and John B. West

Typeset in 10/12 pt Palatino by Best-set Typesetter Ltd., Hong Kong
Printed in Great Britain by University Press, Cambridge

ISBN 0 412 54610 8

Apart from any fair dealing for the purposes of research or private study, or criticism or review, as permitted under the UK Copyright Designs and Patents Act, 1988, this publication may not be reproduced, stored, or transmitted, in any form or by any means, without the prior permission in writing of the publishers, or in the case of reprographic reproduction only in accordance with the terms of the licences issued by the Copyright Licensing Agency in the UK, or in accordance with the terms of licences issued by the appropriate Reproduction Rights Organization outside the UK. Enquiries concerning reproduction outside the terms stated here should be sent to the publishers at the London address printed on this page.

The publisher makes no representation, express or implied, with regard to the accuracy of the information contained in this book and cannot accept any legal responsibility or liability for any errors or omissions that may be made.

A catalogue record for this book is available from the British Library

Library of Congress Catalog Card Number: 94-71202

∞ Printed on acid-free text paper, manufactured in accordance with ANSI/NISO Z39.48-1992 (Permanence of Paper).

Contents

Preface

The first edition of this book was very well received and, because of the rapid progress in knowledge about high altitude medicine and physiology during the last five years, we thought it important to bring the text up to date. Some idea of the pace of new work can be obtained by looking at the *Bibliography of High Altitude Medicine and Physiology* prepared by the Colorado Altitude Research Institute, USA. They list no fewer than 1369 articles, and abstracts dated 1987–1993. The number of people who go to high altitude for skiing, trekking or climbing continues to increase and now many millions are involved. Just as important is the great increase in commercial activities at high altitude, particularly in the South American Andes. For example, there are now a substantial number of mines at altitudes exceeding 4000 m in Chile, Peru and Bolivia.

All the chapters in the second edition have been extensively revised and brought up to date. In addition, there are new chapters on high altitude populations and on medical and surgical emergencies, and the ordering of the chapters has been rearranged on what we consider to be a more logical basis. This new edition has enabled us to respond to a number of the comments and criticisms generated by the first edition. We have tried to strike a balance between being too academic on the one hand, and producing a *vade mecum* for doctors accompanying trekking groups. Our objective has been to provide a rigorous scientific basis for the main topics in high altitude medicine and physiology, including the management of common medical and surgical conditions in the mountains, but not necessarily to deal with all the practical details of climbing and skiing accidents or trekking illnesses. Other wilderness handbooks do this well.

One or two reviewers of the first edition commented that there was undue repetition of material, particularly in the historical introductions. The reason for this is that we have tried to make each chapter readable in its own right, because no one reads a book like this from cover to cover. We hope that any irritation caused by occasional duplication of information will be more than offset by having each chapter provide a comprehensive coverage of each topic.

Finally, we very much appreciate comments and constructive criticisms of the book, particularly identification of any factual errors. As with the first edition, we hope that this book will make the high places of the world safer, and thus increase the pleasure to be gained by those who visit these regions of outstanding natural beauty.

Michael P. Ward
James S. Milledge
John B. West

Acknowledgements

We wish to acknowledge help from many friends and colleagues who have read and commented helpfully on parts of the text, especially Michael J. Ball FRCS, F.E. Gallas, Eugene Gippenreiter, Surg. Rear-Adm., Frank Golden OBE, RN, Steven C. Hempleman PhD, Michael C. Hogan PhD, Professor W.R. Keatinge, Sukhamay Lahiri PhD, Robert Mahler FRCP, Betty A. Milledge MB, ChB, Odile Mathieu-Costello PhD, H.G. Nicol MB, John F. Nunn FFARCS, David C. Poole PhD, Frank L. Powell PhD, Dr S.P.L. Travis DPhil, MRCP, Peter D. Wagner MD, E.J.M. Weaver FRCS, David C. Willford PhD, Edward S. Williams FRCP, and Sarah Wells of the Department of Medical Illustration, Clinical Research Centre, Harrow. We also gratefully acknowledge the invaluable help of our secretaries, Mrs Norma Saunders and Amy Clay and the staff of our publishers at Chapman & Hall including Peter Altman and all the editorial and production staff involved in producing this book.

We would like to thank all those who have contributed to the original work on which much of this book is based. These include Sherpas, climbers and scientists, subjects and supporters who made the projects possible.

Conversion tables

Table F.1 Conversion of pressure units mmHg (millimetres of mercury) or Torr to kPa (kilopascal)

mmHg or Torr	*kPa*
1	0.133
10	1.33
20	2.67
30	4.00
40	5.33
50	6.67
60	8.00
80	10.7
100	13.3
200	26.7
300	40.0
500	66.7
700	93.3
760	101.3

Table F.2 Conversion of height units and barometric pressure according to the ICAO Standard Atmosphere. Note that in the great mountain ranges the actual pressure will usually be higher than given by the table (Chapter 2)

Altitude		*Pressure*
m	*ft*	*mmHg or Torr*
0	0	760
1000	3 281	674
2000	6 562	596
3000	9 843	526
4000	13 123	462
5000	16 404	405
6000	19 685	354
7000	22 966	308
8000	26 247	267
9000	29 528	231

Table F.3 Coversion of temperature units, °C (degrees Centigrade) to °F (degrees Fahrenheit)

°C	°F
−40	−40
−30	−20
−25	−13
−20	−4
−15	5
−10	14
−5	23
0	32
5	41
10	50
15	59
20	68
25	77
30	86
35	95
40	104

Table F.4 Conversion of energy units, kcal (kilocalories) to kJ (kiloJoules)

kcal	*kJ*
50	209.4
100	418.8
250	1047
500	2094
1000	4188
2000	8375
3000	12563
4000	16750
5000	20938
6000	25126

1

History

1.1 INTRODUCTION

The story of our attempts to climb higher and higher by our own unaided efforts is one of the most colourful and exciting in medicine and physiology, if only because scientists have been repeatedly astonished by mountaineers' ability to ascend higher than their confident predictions.

Over the centuries investigation into the effects of human hypoxia and the exploration of the world's highest mountain ranges have run a parallel and often overlapping course (Table 1.1).

Numerous clinical and physiological lessons have been learnt from altitude studies, which share a number of features found in the chronically hypoxic patient with cardiovascular and respiratory disorders (Chapter 30). The physiological problems of altitude are due in the main to hypoxia and cold: hypoxia because with gain in altitude there is reduction in atmospheric and hence oxygen pressure (Chapter 2); cold because of the temperature lapse with altitude and wind-chill (Chapter 22).

Frost-bite is mentioned in a Tibetan medical text named the *Blue Beryl*, published in 1688. However, it seems possible that the text may have originated much earlier, and a date of 889 BC has been suggested (Parfionovitch *et al.*, 1992).

Early mountain travellers, like Xenophon, who crossed the mountains of Armenia following the battle of Cunaxa (401 BC) were more concerned with cold than altitude. Similarly Plutarch (45–120 AD) tells us that Alexander's army crossing the Hindu Kush to India in 326 BC, suffered severely from the 'state of the weather'. One of the earliest European accounts of the rarefied air of high altitude was given by the Greeks who, on their yearly ceremonial visit to the summit of Mt Olympus (2911 m) were not able to survive, we are told, unless they applied moist sponges to their noses (possibly soaked in vinegar) (Burnett, 1983).

Table 1.1 Chronology of some principal events in the development of high altitude medicine and physiology

Year	*Event*
c. 30 BC	Reference to the Great Headache Mountain and Little Headache Mountain in the Tseen Han Shoo (classical Chinese history)
1590	Publication of the first edition (Spanish) of *Naturall and morall historie of the East and West Indies* by Joseph de Acosta with an account of mountain sickness
1644	First description of mercury barometer by Torricelli
1648	Demonstration of fall in barometric pressure at high altitude in an experiment devised by Pascal
1777	Clear description of oxygen and the other respiratory gases by Lavoisier
1783	Montgolfier brothers introduce balloon ascents
1786	First ascent of Mt Blanc by Balmat and Paccard
1878	Publication of *La Pression Barométrique* by Paul Bert
1890	Viault describes high altitude polycythemia
1890	Joseph Vallot builds high altitude laboratory at 4350 m on Mt Blanc
1891	Christian Bohr publishes *Uber die Lungenathmung*, giving evidence for both O_2 and CO_2 secretion by the lung
1893	Angelo Mosso completes the high altitude station, Capanna Regina, Margherita, on a summit of Monte Rosa at 4559 m
1906	Publication of *Hohenklima und Bergwanderungen* . . . by Zuntz *et al*.
1909	The Duke of Abruzzi reaches 7500 m in the Karakoram without supplementary oxygen
1910	Zuntz organizes an international high altitude expedition to Tenerife; members included C.G. Douglas and Joseph Barcroft
1910	August Krogh publishes *On the Mechanism of Gas-Exchange in the Lungs*, disproving the secretion theory of gas exchange
1911	Anglo–American Pikes Peak expedition (4300 m); participants C.G. Douglas, J.S. Haldane, Y. Henderson and E.C. Schneider
1913	T.H. Ravenhill publishes *Some experiences of mountain sickness in the Andes*, describing puna of the normal, cardiac, and nervous types
1920	Barcroft *et al*. publish the results of the experiment carried out in a glass chamber in which he lived in a hypoxic atmosphere for six days
1921	A.M. Kellas publishes *Sur les Possibilites de Faire l'Ascension du Mount Everest*, (Congrès de l'Alpinisme, Monaco, 1920)
1921–1922	International High Altitude Expedition to Cerro de Pasco Peru, led by Joseph Barcroft
1924	E.F. Norton ascends to 8500 m on Mt Everest without supplementary oxygen
1925	Barcroft publishes *Lessons from High Altitude*

Table 1.1 Continued

Year	*Event*
1935	International High Altitude Expedition to Chile, D.B. Dill Scientific Leader
1946	Operation Everest I carried out by C.S. Houston and R.L. Riley
1948	Monge, C. publishes *Acclimatization in the Andes*, describing the permanent residents of the Peruvian Andes
1949	H. Rahn and A.B. Otis publish *Man's Respiratory Response During and After Acclimatization to High Altitude*
1952	L.G.C.E. Pugh and colleagues carry out experiments on Cho Oyu near Mt Everest in preparation for the 1953 expedition
1953	First ascent of Mt Everest by Hillary and Tensing (with supplementary oxygen)
1960–1961	Himalayan Scientific and Mountaineering Expedition in the Everest region, Scientific Leader L.G.C.E. Pugh. Laboratory at 5800 m, measurements up to 7440 m
1968–1979	High altitude studies on Mt Logan (5334 m), Scientific Director C.S. Houston
1973	Italian Mt Everest Expedition with laboratory at 5350 m, Scientific Leader P. Cerretelli
1978	First ascent of Everest without supplementary oxygen by Reinhold Messner and Peter Habeler
1981	American Medical Research Expedition to Everest, Scientific Leader J.B. West
1981–1991	French Scientific expeditions to Numbur (6956 m), Annapurna IV (7525 m) and Mt Sajama (6542 m)
1985	Operation Everest II, Scientific Leaders C.S. Houston and J.R. Sutton
1983 to present	Research at Capanna Regina Margherita (4559 m) by Professor O. Oelz, P. Bärtsch and co-workers from Zurich, Berne and Heidelberg
1984 to present	Studies at Observatoire Vallot (4350 m) on Mt Blanc by Professor J.-P. Richalet and co-workers

1.2 THE CHINESE HEADACHE MOUNTAIN STORY

The first documented description of mountain sickness comes from Chinese sources:

> In the time of the Emperor Ching-Te (32–7 BC) Ke-pin (possibly Afghanistan) again sent an envoy with offerings and an acknowledgement of guilt. The supreme board wished to send an envoy with a reply to escort the Ke-pin envoy home. Tookim (a Chinese official) addressed the Generalissimo Wang Fung to the follow-

> ing effect . . . 'From Pe-shan southwards there are four to five kingdoms not attached to China. The Chinese Commission will in such circumstances be left to starve among the hills and valleys . . . Again on passing the Great Headache Mountain, the Little Headache Mountain, the Red Land, and the Fever Slope, men's bodies become feverish, they lose colour and are attacked with headache and vomiting; the asses and cattle being all in like condition.'
>
> *(Wylie, 1881)*

Gilbert (1983a) considers that either the Kilik Pass or the Mintaka Pass across the Karakoram are possible candidates for the Greater Headache Mountain, but a pass is not a peak, and the Chinese are meticulous observers. Pi-shan, 37.6°N 78.2°S (Mountains of Central Asia, 1987), mentioned as the starting place, is situated South East of Shache (Yarkand) and West of Hotien (Khotan). From here to Afghanistan there are a great number of routes across the mountains, and the one followed has yet to be identified.

Gilbert also draws attention to a case of acute mountain sickness that was reported by Fa-Hsien (399–414 AD) who in 403 AD travelled in Kashmir and Afghanistan. He noted that his companion foamed at the mouth and later died as they were ascending a mountain pass. This was possibly a case of high-altitude pulmonary edema, as the clinical description is classic.

It has been suggested too that the occurrence of mountain sickness and its complications may have been taken by the Chinese as a sign for them not to transgress their natural boundaries. (Needham, 1954).

1.3 CENTRAL AND SOUTH AMERICA: DE ACOSTA

In each inhabited mountain region whether it is in Asia, Europe or the Americas (Figure 1.1) there is a vast depository of legend and folklore. The peaks, passes and glaciers are deemed to have been created by a series of gods, Titans and tribal heroes, and individual peaks have been enshrined with virtues and defects, like any human. For instance, in South America there is the legend of the trauco found in Southern Chile and Argentina, a mythical animal who feeds on the blood of animals and human beings which is very similar to the yeti legend, found in the Himalayas and mountains of Central Asia (Reinhard, 1983; Napier, 1972).

Well built, pre-Columbian structures too have been found near the summit of Llullaillaco (6721 m) and are probably associated with mountain worship. Human sacrifice was carried out on these peaks and an Inca body has been found at 6300 m on El Toro. The summits of a number of volcanos, up to 6425 m and easily accessible from

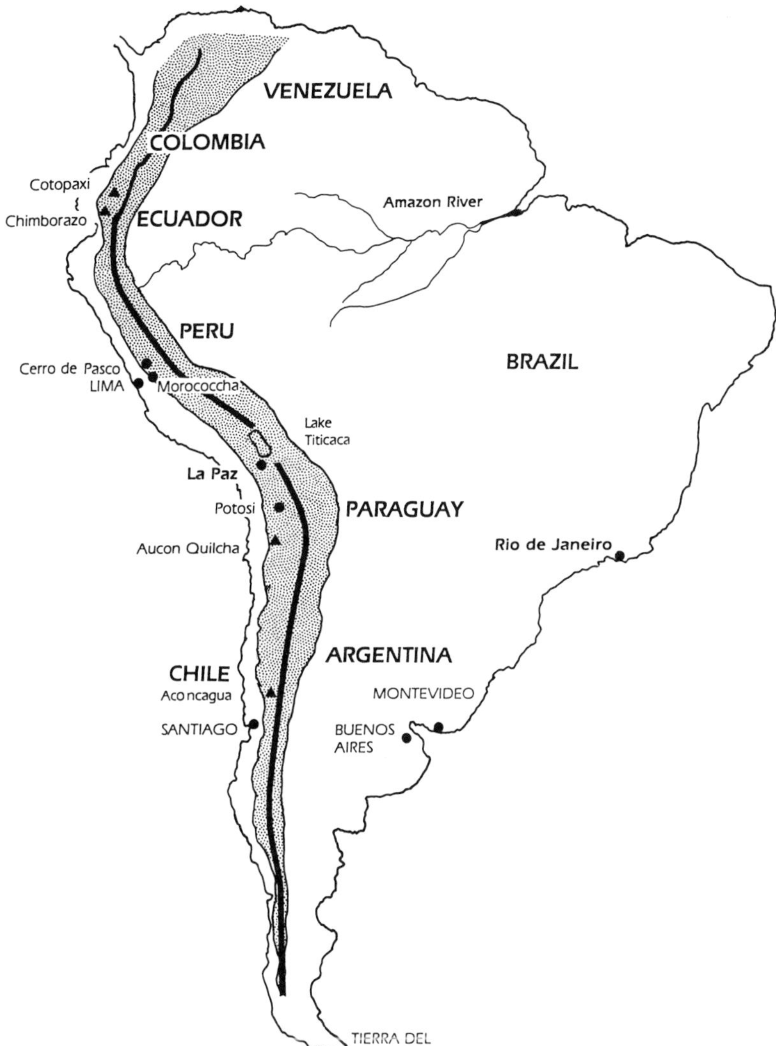

Figure 1.1 South America.

Arequipa, may have been used as the altars of sacrificial shrines. These peaks, with few glaciers and easy rounded slopes, present little technical difficulty other than altitude and South American highlanders were used to ascending to great heights for worship in the late fifteenth century. Altitudes in excess of 6000 m were probably not reached on foot in Asia until the later part of the nineteenth century (Echevarria, 1968, 1979, 1983).

In Central America the Spanish Conquistadores were active in the sixteenth century and in 1519 Cortes sent Diego Ordaz to attempt the ascent of Mt Popacatepetl. They remarked, 'To increase their distress, respiration in these aerial regions became so difficult that every effort was attended with sharp pain in the head and limbs'. Two years later Francisco Montana and four Spaniards reached the summit and obtained sulphur from the crater for the manufacture of gun powder (Prescott, 1891).

Symptoms of mountain sickness were not described in any detail by these explorers and it was left to a Jesuit priest, Joseph de Acosta, to give the first classical account. The local names were puna, soroche, mareo and veta, and the cause thought to be emanating from the metal antimony. In other regions the vapours from rhubarb, primroses and roses were said to make men and animals ill. The government of the Incas clearly understood the effects of climate on health and it was known, for instance, that people who lived by the sea died in great numbers if transported to the mines at 3000–4000 m. The cause is unknown but it is likely to have been a combination of malnutrition, disease, altitude and cold.

The account of mountain sickness given by Joseph de Acosta in *The Naturall and Morall Historie of the East and West Indies* first published in 1590 in Seville (Figure 1.2) is worth quoting at length for his accuracy of description, feelings and cause of the symptoms:

> There is in Peru a high mountaine which they call Pariacaca . . . When I came to mount the degrees, as they call them, which is the top of this mountaine, I was suddenly surprised with so mortall and strange a pang, that I was ready to fall from the top to the ground and although we were many in company, yet everyone made haste (without any tarrying for his companion) to free himself speedily from this ill passage . . . I was surprised with such pangs of straining and casting as I thought to cast up my heart too: for having cast up meate, fleugme and choller both yellow and greene, in the end I cast up blood with the straining of my stomach. To conclude, if this had continued I should undoubtedly have died. *(de Acosta, 1604)*

de Acosta's route across the Andes has been investigated by Gilbert (1983b) and, of a number of alternatives, he considers that the pass of the Escaleras de Pariacaca (4800 m) is the most likely candidate. Recently Bonavia *et al.* (1985) have made an on site inspection of the Pariacaca area and corrected a number of topographical misconceptions. Gilbert (1988) reported information from mountaineers who had climbed in the region that, where as the peak Pariacaca is known by this name to inhabitants to the south-west (the direction from which de Acosta

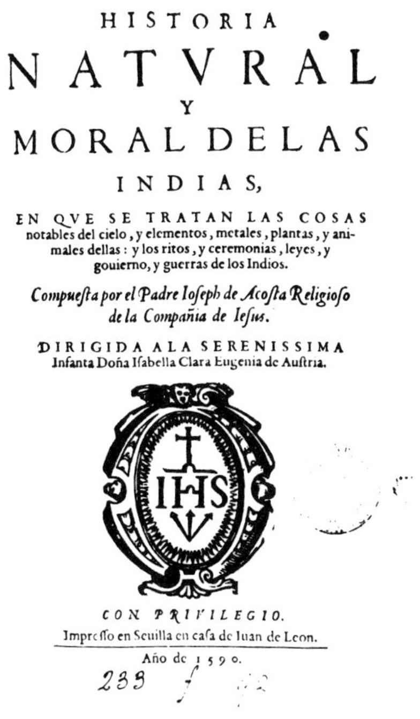

HISTORIA

NATVRAL

Y

MORAL DELAS

INDIAS,

EN QVE SE TRATAN LAS COSAS notables del cielo, y elementos, metales, plantas, y animales dellas: y los ritos, y ceremonias, leyes, y gouierno, y guerras de los Indios.

Compueſta por el Padre Ioſeph de Acoſta Religioſo de la Compañia de Ieſus.

DIRIGIDA ALA SERENISSIMA Infanta Doña Iſabella Clara Eugenia de Auſtria.

CON PRIVILEGIO.

Impreſſo en Seuilla en caſa de Iuan de Leon.

Año de 1590.

Figure 1.2 Title page of first edition of Joseph de Acosta's book published in Spanish in 1590 in Seville. (Reproduced with permission of the Bodleian Library.)

made his approach), it is also known as Tullujuto to those living to the north-east. The peak is named Tullujuto on the few maps on which it is marked. It is not unusual for a peak to have more than one name but this does give rise to confusion.

1.4 CENTRAL ASIA: MOGHULS AND THE JESUITS (Figure 1.3)

In 1531, the Moghuls invaded Ladakh and western Tibet and described mountain sickness which they called 'yas', and which the Tibetans called 'damgiri' or 'dam' (breath seizing), or 'dugri' (poison of the mountain). The clinical features were vomiting, exhaustion, difficulty in sleeping, aphasia and swelling of the hands and feet. Death often occurred unless descent was rapid, and the moghul sultan, Said Khan, died of damgiri on the Suget Pass on his way from Ladakh to Kashgar. This illness was made worse by cold, and horses also were severely affected. The moghuls recorded other central Asian names for mountain sickness: 'tunk' (wakhi and badakhshi), 'esh' (turki) and 'bish-ka-hawa'

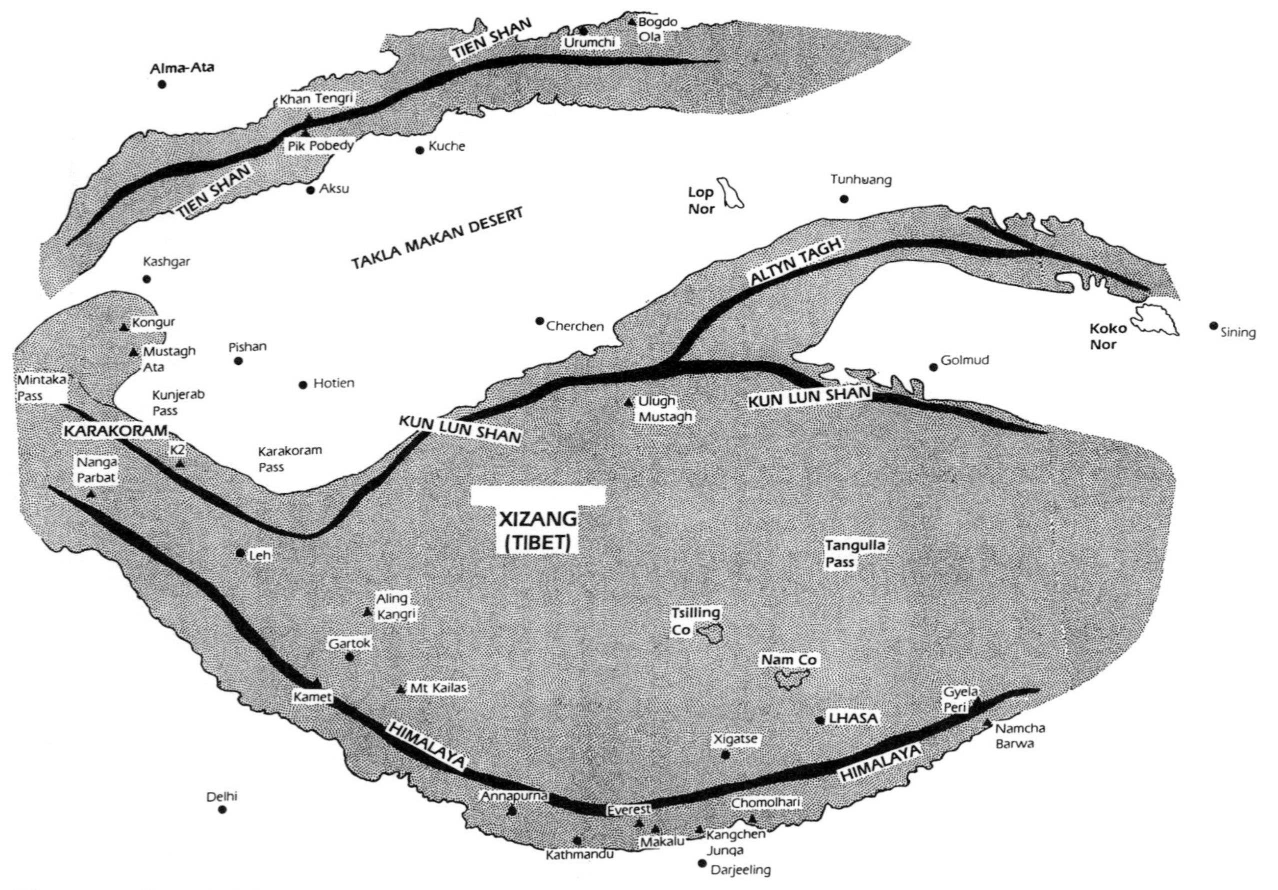

Figure 1.3 Central Asia.

(a term used by some Indian populations of the Himalayas) (Elias and Ross, 1898).

In the middle of the seventeenth century there were rumours of Nestorian Christian colonies living in Central Asia and a number of missionaries from Rome were sent out to contact them. These remarkable men established missions in Tibet and they were among the first Europeans to bring back detailed information about this mysterious land from first hand knowledge. Inevitably they suffered from acute mountain sickness and had views on its cause.

The Jesuit, Father Andrade, was the first European to enter Tibet. He crossed the Himalayas by the Mana pass (5450 m) in 1624 and was more concerned with hypothermia than with hypoxia.

> Many people die on account of the noxious vapours that arise, for it is a fact that people in good health are suddenly taken ill and die within a quarter of an hour, but I think it is rather owing to the intense cold and want of heat, which reduces the heat of the body.
> *(Wessels, 1924)*

In 1661, two Jesuit fathers, Grüber and D'Orville, left Peking, and crossed the Tibetan plateau to Lhasa. Staying a month in the capital they then crossed the Himalayas by the Thung La, arriving in Kathmandu several months after leaving Peking. Grüber called the Himalayas the Langur mountains and comments that, 'man cannot breathe in the Langur mountains because the air is so subtile'. He adds that 'in summer certain poisonous weeds grow there which extrude such a bad smell and dangerous odour that one cannot stay up there without losing one's life'. It seems likely that he was applying Joseph de Acosta's experience to Central Asia. Father Desiderei, another Jesuit who founded a mission in Lhasa in 1716, also comments on the 'reek of certain materials' but goes on to say that he believes that the unpleasant symptoms 'are due to sharp thin air'. He also suffered from excruciating headaches.

In 1739 Father Belligatti alludes to the 'singular influence which mountains exercise over both men and animals whether this arises from the rarefaction of the atmosphere or from deleterious exhalations' (Hedin, 1913). This may have been a reference to 'la-drak' as the 'poison of the pass' which was considered by the Tibetans to be the exhalation of mischievous gods who caused earthquakes and avalanches (Landon, 1905). Rockhill (1891) describes how mountain sickness was called 'yen-chang' by the inhabitants of the Koko Nor and 'chang-chi' in Szechuan. Both expressions mean a 'pestilential vapour' thought to be given off by the large quantities of rhubarb which grew in the mountains. Eating garlic and smoking tobacco was held to be an antidote. 'Tutek' is another term used by Central Asians for acute mountain sickness (Hedin, 1903a). He also describes chronic mountain sickness occurring in gold miners in north Tibet which may be fatal (Hedin, 1903b). The Tibetan remedy for mountain sickness in ponies was to slit their noses (Bower, 1893). In men an incision was made in the forehead at the hairline (Bonavalot, 1891).

Other clinical features ascribed to mountain sickness were described by Humboldt (1769–1859), who in 1802 climbed to 5500 m on Mt Chimborazo in the Andes of Ecuador (Maggilivary, 1853). He and his companion suffered from bleeding of the lips and gums as well as malaise and nausea, thought to be due to low barometric pressure. De Saussure (Mathews, 1898) on the third ascent of Mt Blanc in 1787 also suffered very considerably from fatigue, thought at the time to be the cause of mountain sickness.

The exploration of the Himalayas began in the early part of the nineteenth century and symptoms of mountain sickness were noted by many travellers including the Schlagintweit brothers, who, in 1855, climbed to 22 260 ft on Mt Ibi Gamin in the Garwhal Himal, a record that stood for 30 years (Von Schlagintweit and Von Schlagintweit, 1862).

1.5 PAUL BERT

During this period in Europe considerable interest in experimental physiology was being generated by Claude Bernard. Paul Bert, a pupil of his, was born in 1833 and the study of the medical aspects of low barometric pressure and resulting hypoxia became his life's work; he is recognized as the father of altitude physiology. He was the first to conduct experiments in a decompression chamber where he studied the effects of both reduced and increased barometric pressure in small animals and man. He showed that breathing air under conditions of reduced barometric pressure, as at altitude, was dangerous because of oxygen lack, whereas breathing oxygen even under reduced pressure restored function.

Bert collected accounts from travellers and scientists from all over the world and, in addition to his work in steel decompression chambers given by his patron Dr Jourdanet, he became interested in the opportunities that balloon flights offered for the study of altitude physiology.

The first 350 or so pages of his classic work *La Pression Barométrique* are considered to be the most authoritative early account of the history of the physiological effects of decreased atmospheric pressure (Bert, 1878).

His work did not go uncriticized, particularly by Mosso and Kronecker (Kellogg, 1978). Kellogg also points out that Kronecker reviewed various case histories including one diagnosed as pulmonary edema at autopsy. Mosso (1898), who was Professor of Physiology at Turin,

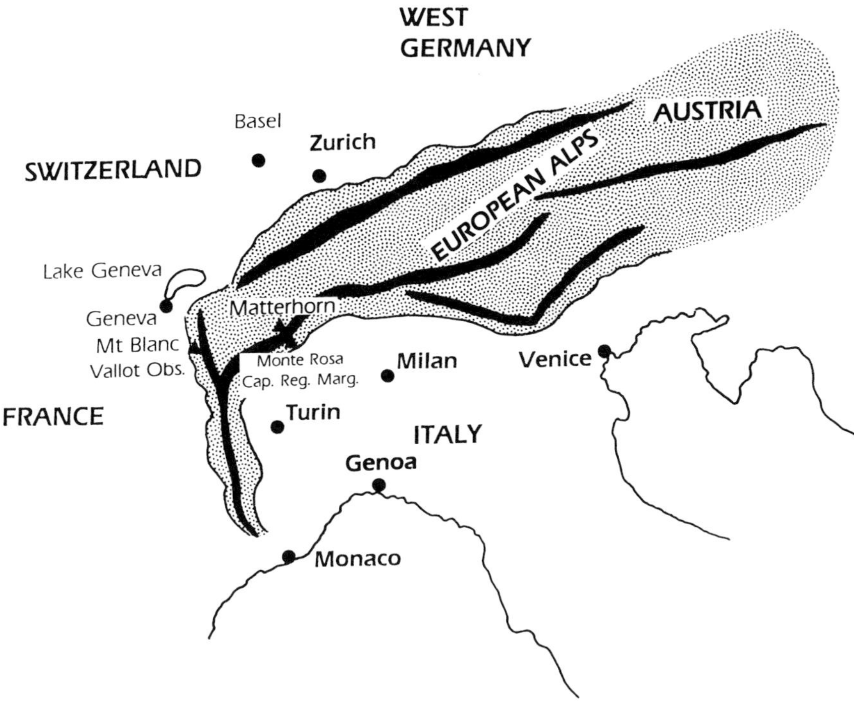

Figure 1.4 European Alps.

was responsible for the construction of the Capanna Regina Margharita on the Punta Gniffeti (4560 m), one of the summits of Monte Rosa (Figure 1.4). He did not believe that mountain sickness was due to oxygen lack but thought it was due to lack of carbon dioxide. He was a major figure in altitude physiology, tracing the breathing pattern of periodic respiration; he also published the first clinical report of pulmonary oedema.

1.6 ALPINE CLUB

In the middle of the nineteenth century mountain travel was becoming increasingly popular and the Alpine Club was founded in the UK in 1857. The Alpine Journal, 'a record of mountain adventure and scientific observation' contained a number of articles on mountain sickness in its early issues. Count Henry Russel (Russel, 1871) comments that mountain sickness was 'known all over the world (though less in the tropics) . . . and in the Himalaya where the silly natives attribute it to the exhalations of a venomous plant'. Spinal anaemia, the result of diminished atmospheric pressure, was suggested as a cause of the weakness of the lower limb 'which was so prominent a feature of mountain sickness' (Monro, 1893).

A year later Thomas (1894) thought that the very dry air of Tibet and the Karakoram might be a factor, as the overall effect of altitude was felt there at a lower level than in damper Sikkim. A review of the eighteenth and nineteenth century theories on mountain sickness and its cause is given by Hepburn (1901, 1902). He suggests that following certain training, dietary and breathing routines, a man could climb to 30 000 ft (9144 m). He concludes: 'but even so we have yet to prove that dyspnoea and fatigue are dependant on lack of oxygen at any level either directly or indirectly, though the probabilities are in favour of such a theory'.

In a salutary article on alcohol and climbing, Marcet (1886–1888b) writes that mountain sickness 'is certainly neither provided against nor relieved by the use of alcoholic beverages'. He ends by saying that, 'strong drinks do not give strength, and as a means of keeping the body warm they go in the opposite tack doing away with the natural powers that man possesses of resisting cold and thus acting as a "delusion and snare"'. Albutt (1876) in fact considered that the use of alcohol predisposed to frostbite. Earlier, Albutt (1870) had observed that the hard exercise of climbing accelerated the 'morning rise in temperature' (taken sublingually). However, rectal temperatures in two guides taken during the ascent of Monte Rosa showed a rise in one and a fall in the other (Payot, 1881). Payot also considered that the increased respiration of climbing was associated with an increase in water loss from the lungs and poor urine output, a fact confirmed by Pugh in 1952.

Marcet (1886–1888a) suggested that potassium chlorate be taken, as when it is heated it gives off oxygen and would combat the effects of altitude. He observed that it been used by Sir Douglas Forsyth in the 'Cashmere mountains on the way to Kashgar' and by Whymper on the first ascent of Chimborazo. It is clear from Bellew (1875) that the salt was eaten!

In 1879 Edward Whymper, the conqueror of the Matterhorn, mounted an expedition to the Andes of South America specifically to study mountain sickness. He divided the clinical effects into permanent (which included poor appetite, fatigue and increased respiration) and transient (increase in blood pressure, temperature and heart rate) (Whymper, 1892).

1.7 BALLOONISTS

Whilst observations on mountain sickness were being made by mountain travellers, more dramatic episodes were occurring to balloonists.

The Montgolfier brothers, Etienne and Joseph, the most famous pioneers of early ballooning, made the first ascent in a hot air balloon in November 1783, and, in the same month, De Rezier, a French apothecary, and the Marquis d'Arlandes, crossed Paris in a 'Montgolfier'. In the same year the physicist, Charles, who had invented the hydrogen balloon, left the Tuileries and landed 2 h 45 min later in the plain of Nesles. Roberts, his companion, disembarked here and the lightened balloon rose to over 1500 fathoms. Later Gay-Lussac ascended to over 7000 m, noticing that both his pulse and respiration were much increased.

Nearly a century later in September 1862, Coxwell and Glaisher, two English meteorologists were carried to 8800 m, escaping death only because Coxwell managed to pull the release valve with his teeth. Glaisher (Glaisher *et al.*, 1871) made a number of further flights and considered that he had developed a tolerance to altitude. Though both a decrease in barometric, and therefore oxygen, pressure had been demonstrated on these ascents, the early balloonists had still not fully grasped that the dangers at altitude were due to hypoxia.

In March 1874 Croce-Spinelli and Sivel came to Paul Bert's laboratory prior to an attempt on the balloon altitude record. Following decompression chamber experiments the balloonists were convinced of the effectiveness of oxygen but planned to carry too little for safety. Bert was alarmed and wrote indicating it was not enough but the letter arrived too late. On 15 April 1875, the balloon named Zenith rose to around 8000 m; Tissandier the survivor, described in detail the features of hypoxia which killed his two companions and would have killed him if he had not vented some hydrogen which caused Zenith to descend (Tissandier, 1875) (Chapter 15).

1.8 LATE NINETEENTH AND EARLY TWENTIETH CENTURY EXPLORERS AND PHYSIOLOGISTS

In the late nineteenth and early twentieth centuries there was increasing medical scientific interest in both the oxygen transport system and altitude adaptation, and many discoveries were made. Viault (1890) recorded the best known physiological response to altitude, namely an increase in the number of red cells. He found a rise from 5.0 million at sea level to between 7.5 to 8.0 million at Morococha (4540 m) and observed that this change took place over a short period. By contrast, Bert had thought that it took place gradually over generations at altitude (Chapter 7). Later, Hingston (1914) considered that the symptoms of mountain sickness were due to failure to increase the number of red blood cells on ascent to high altitude.

Disorders of respiration that had the 'Stokes character' were also described at 4400 m (Egli-Sinclair, 1891–1892, 1894). A similar episode had been noted by Hirst in 1857 when he made an ascent of Mt Blanc with the well known physicist and mountaineer Professor J. Tyndall. Tyndall fell asleep on the summit and Hirst roused him saying 'I have listened for some minutes and have not heard you breathe once' (Tyndall, 1860). Periodic respiration had, in fact, been described by the surgeon John Hunter in his case records in 1781 (Ward, 1973) over 30 years prior to Cheyne's paper (Cheyne, 1818) (Chapter 12).

Though a case of pulmonary oedema due to altitude had been recorded by Kronecker at autopsy (Kellogg, 1978), it is likely that the first full clinical description occurs in Mosso's book *Life of Man on the High Alps* (Mosso, 1898). The victim, Dr Jacottet, died on Mt Blanc at 4300 m, and the autopsy report attributed the waterlogged lungs to pneumonia. Later, Ravenhill (1913), a doctor in a mining town in South America, differentiated between a cerebral and a cardiac form of mountain sickness, the latter being now regarded as pulmonary oedema. Twenty years later Hurtado (1937) suggested that the pneumonia or pulmonary oedema of altitude was not due to infection but altitude *per se* and Lundberg (1952) presented six cases of acute pulmonary oedema to the Asociacion Medica de Yauli. Houston (1960) 're-discovered' the condition, since when it has become widely recognized (Chapter 18).

Commercial groups were starting to build railways into the mountains to improve access and boost tourism and plans were discussed for a railway to the top of the Jungfrau, in Switzerland. The scientific investigations were carried out on the Theodule Pass (3500 m) between Zermatt and Cervinia in 1894 (Kronecker, 1903). Eventually this railway was built as far as the Jungfraujoch. The dangers, to elderly travellers and those with angina pectoris, of ascent by railway to even moderate altitude was discussed by Zangger (1899, 1903).

Though minor vascular disorders were often reported at altitude, the first major vascular accident to be reported occurred to a Russian traveller Roborovsky (1896), whilst crossing the Mangur Pass (4270 m) in east Tibet. He suffered a transient stroke and it was eight days before he could move (Chapter 21).

The tempo of Himalayan exploration accelerated in this period and Conway on Pioneer Peak (7000 m) in 1892 described the debilitating effects of long periods at high altitude. He also took sphygmograph pulse records at intervals up to and including the summit (Figure 1.5). Whilst his resting pulse remained between 90–100/min there is one reading at 6100 m when it was 48. Could this have been an incident of transient 2:1 heart block? (Roy, 1894).

By contrast, the Duke of Abruzzi's expedition to the Karakoram in 1909 climbed to 7500 m with few of the symptoms due to altitude. Interestingly, however, Filippi (1912) also reports 'the atmosphere of

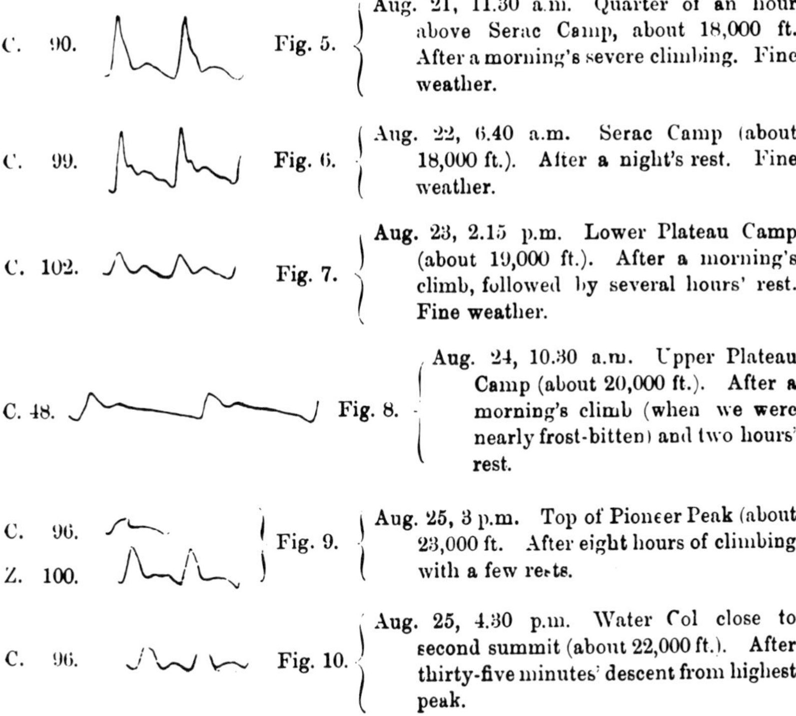

Figure 1.5 Pulse sphygmograph records on Pioneer Peak (7000 m) taken by Conway in 1892 (from Roy, 1894). Note resting pulse of 48 beats per minute in Figure 8, possibly due to 2:1 heart block. (Reproduced with permission of the Library of the Royal Geographical Society.)

the expedition did work some evil effect revealing itself only gradually after several weeks of life above 17 500 ft', and he goes on to give a description of high altitude deterioration (section 3.8.2).

Anticipating the modern trend, some amazingly fast ascents were made, particularly by Longstaff, a British physician, who ascended 2000 m to 7180 m in ten hours on Mt Trisul (section 1.10). He was also one of the first to recognize that sugar was of great importance in the diet at high altitude (Longstaff, 1906, 1908).

An amusing vignette is supplied by Waddell, Medical Officer on the British Expedition to Lhasa 1903–1904:

> 'A peculiarity of the language of the Tibetans in common with the Russians and most arctic nations is the remarkably few vowels in their words and the extraordinarily large number of consonants. Indeed so full of consonants are Tibetan words that most of them

could be articulated with an almost semi-closed mouth, evidently from the enforced necessity to keep the lips closed as far as possible against the cutting cold when speaking.' *(Waddell, 1905)*

1.9 THE OXYGEN SECRETION CONTROVERSY

The ascent to 7500 m by the Duke of Abruzzi's party amazed many physiologists for it was thought that lung diffusion was inadequate for extreme exercise at low oxygen pressure. However, it was becoming apparent that in some organs 'chemicals' could move against the concentration gradient. If the lungs could secrete oxygen this might explain both the variability with which individuals reacted to altitude and also their ability to ascend so high.

The arguments deployed for and against this theory are reviewed in Chapter 5. Initially, in favour of secretion was the theoretical impossibility for the diffusion of 5–6 l of oxygen across the lung each minute during extreme exercise. However, at the turn of the century, Marie Krogh measured the diffusing capacity of the lung to carbon monoxide from which the diffusing capacity of oxygen could be inferred. She showed that the lung was a very good diffuser of oxygen partly because of its enormous surface area and partly because of the affinity of haemoglobin for oxygen. However, her work was ignored, being rediscovered in the 1930s.

Haldane and Barcroft, both distinguished respiratory physiologists, held opposing views, but after a number of investigations, including the Cambridge 'glass box' experiment of Barcroft, and expeditions to high altitude by groups led by both workers, it was finally shown by Barcroft that the arterial PO_2 was always lower than the alveolar PO_2. The diffusion theory was correct and Barcroft's book, *Lessons from High Altitudes*, became a classic work on the subject (Barcroft, 1925; Milledge, 1985).

1.10 THE EVEREST STORY

In 1921, after years of prevarication, the government of Tibet gave permission for a British party to attempt Mt Everest from the northern Tibetan side.

The individual who knew most about the physical and physiological problems that would be encountered was Alexander Kellas, a lecturer in chemistry at the Middlesex Hospital Medical School. He had made a number of expeditions to the Sikkim Himal and the Tibetan border before World War I and had become increasingly interested in the problems of altitude (Kellas, 1917).

Before he went on the first Everest reconnaissance expedition in

1921, Kellas wrote a paper entitled 'A consideration of the possibility of ascending Mt Everest'. Unfortunately he died on the approach march at Kampa Dzong on the Tibetan plateau, within sight of the mountain, and this paper was never published, though copies of the manuscript were lodged in the archives of the Royal Geographical Society and the Alpine Club (West, 1987). In it he considers both the difficulties of access and the physiological problems.

The section of the 1921 manuscript entitled 'The process of acclimatisation to altitude' is of great interest because although there are many factual errors his insight in asking the correct questions was uncanny.

As Kellas saw it, the main issue was whether sufficient adaptation could occur to allow a climber to ascend from a camp at about 7700 m to the summit (8848 m) in one day without supplementary oxygen. His conclusion was that this was possible and, in fact, the first such ascent by Habler and Messner in 1978 started from a camp at 7950 m. He calculated too that the barometric pressure on the summit would be 251 mmHg, a more accurate figure than estimates based on the 'standard atmosphere' (Chapter 2). The current value of 253 mmHg was measured on the summit by the American Medical Research Expedition in 1981. Kellas estimated the maximum oxygen uptake on the summit to be 970 ml min^{-1} and the current value is thought to be about 1070 ml min^{-1}. As far as climbing rate near the summit, his estimate of 100–120 m h^{-1} closely parallels the rate of Habler and Messner: 'The last 100 m took us more than one hour to climb.' Finally he thought that man could live indefinitely at 6100 m.

Some of the few values for which his figures were too low were alveolar P_{O_2}, oxygen saturation and arterial pH; this was because he underestimated the degree of hyperventilation and assumed a normal arterial pH.

It is difficult to assess the probable effects of this paper had it been published but at least it might have encouraged subsequent expeditions to consider more fully the scientific aspects of the ascent.

The series of expeditions between 1921 and 1953, the year of the first ascent, give a fascinating insight into the effects of altitude and cold and the attitude of mountaineers towards climbing the highest mountain in the world. It soon became obvious that the main obstacles to the ascent were altitude and weather, and not technical difficulty. The main controversy was whether supplementary oxygen should be used and this was compounded by personality clashes. The medical preparations for the first Everest expeditions in 1921, 1922, and 1924 were very thorough.

In 1920, Kellas and Morshead of the Survey of India went to Kamet, a peak of over 7000 m in the western Himalayas, on behalf of the Everest Committee of the Alpine club and Royal Geographical Society, to test primus stoves and oxygen equipment. At the suggestion of Professor Leonard Hill of Oxford, Oxylite bags containing sodium peroxide which when mixed with water gave off oxygen were also taken (Morshead, 1921; Kellas, 1921).

Because neither the primus stoves nor the oxygen cylinders worked satisfactorily the stoves were tested in the decompression chamber at the laboratory of Professor Dryer at Oxford University, in 1921. Dryer had strong views on the use of supplementary oxygen on Everest: 'I do not think that you will get up without, but if you do you might not get down again.' In March 1921, before the first reconnaissance of Everest left for India, Finch, a possible member of the party and later professor of physical chemistry at Imperial College London, and two members of the committee witnessed the stoves being tested in the decompression chamber. Dryer easily convinced Finch that supplementary oxygen should be used on Everest, and persuaded him to stay overnight. Next day he was decompressed to 6400 m and exercised both with and without supplementary oxygen. Not surprisingly, without the benefit of acclimatization, Finch was convinced of the benefit of supplementary oxygen at altitude.

As the 1921 expedition was for reconnaissance only, supplementary oxygen was not taken, but, in preparation for the 1922 attempt on the summit, Finch returned to Oxford in January 1922 with another party member, Somervell, a surgeon, and took part in further experiments, being decompressed to 7010 m. It was because of these experiments that supplementary oxygen was used in 1922. In 1922 four men ascended to 8250 m without supplementary oxygen and two men reached a similar height using it. Many clinical features of chronic hypoxia were recognized: poor appetite, loss of weight, dehydration, exhaustion and failure to recover from fatigue being the most obvious (Unna, 1922).

The beneficial effects of using oxygen were noted by Finch, confirming the observations of Paul Bert. However, in 1924 Odell spent 11 days above 7000 m, climbing on two occasions to 8300 m without supplementary oxygen (Bruce, 1923; Norton, 1925). His performances were equal to those using supplementary oxygen; when he used supplementary oxygen at $1\,l\,min^{-1}$ there was no improvement, and this observation clouded the clinical picture. Also, as Sherpa porters carrying loads without supplementary oxygen ascended as fast as those with it, an element of uncertainty was introduced which was not resolved until the work of Pugh in 1952 on the Menlung La (5800 m) in the Everest region (see below). Another feature of high altitude was emphasized by Mathews who considered that loss of heat could occur through increased respiration (Mathews, 1932). However, it is now apparent that the upper respiratory tract acts as a very efficient heat exchanger.

Successive expeditions in 1933, 1935, 1936 and 1938 failed to ascend higher than 8500 m, mainly because supplementary oxygen at 2 l min^{-1} only was used and this failed to increase climbing rate.

After World War II the Nepalese side of Everest was visited in 1950 by an Anglo–American party that included Houston and Tilman, and in 1951 a British party led by Shipton revealed a possible route. In 1951 investigations into the scientific problems posed by Everest were started in London by Pugh of the Medical Research Council under the general guidance of Professor Sir Bryan Mathews. The following year, 1952, a Sherpa, Tensing and Lambert, on a Swiss attempt, reached 8500 m using oxygen intermittently but, not only was their flow rate of oxygen inadequate to compensate for the weight of the sets, they were also grossly dehydrated (Dittert *et al.*, 1954). In the same year a British mountaineering and scientific party visited a neighbouring peak Cho Oyu (8153 m) and Pugh carried out scientific work in a tented laboratory at 5800 m on the Menlung La which was vital to the subsequent ascent of Everest in 1953.

The most important outcome was the development of a reliable and not too heavy open-circuit oxygen apparatus which delivered oxygen at 4 l min^{-1}, twice the flow rate used on all previous expeditions. This compensated for the weight of the set and increased climbing rate sufficiently so that the mountaineer could ascend to the summit from a high camp and descend safely within the hours of daylight. In addition, the marked dehydration of altitude was shown to be due partly to respiratory water loss through increased respiration, and adequate levels of food intake and clothing insulation were identified (Pugh, 1952; Ward, 1993; Milledge, 1993).

The consecutive expeditions in 1951, 1952 and 1953 also enabled the basic clinical features of altitude exposure up to 8848 m to be established (Pugh and Ward, 1956). On the first successful ascent of Everest, Hillary and Tensing removed their oxygen masks on the summit. Hillary (1954) remarks: 'I had now had my oxygen mask off for nearly eight minutes and was becoming rather clumsy fingered . . . We put on our oxygen masks and set off from the top down the way we had come.'

In 1978, Everest was climbed for the first time without using supplementary oxygen by Habeler and Messner (Messner, 1979). They had little in reserve: 'After every few steps we huddled over our ice axes mouths agape struggling for sufficient breath', and the last 100 m took more than one hour. Over 50 of such ascents have now been made without supplementary oxygen both by sea-level visitors and high altitude residents, though the mortality rate is significant.

A Sherpa, Angrita, has reached the summit on seven occasions and made the first winter ascent in December 1987, without supplementary

Table 1.2 Everest 1921 – end of 1992

Total Ascents – 485 by 425 climbers, including 16 women
Ascents without supplementary oxygen – 51
Oldest – 60 years (1993)
Youngest – 17 years
Fastest – 22.5 h from base camp to summit
Most times – 7 by Sherpa Ang Rita without supplementary oxygen
Deaths – 115

oxygen (*Mountain*, 1988). By the end of 1992, 425 individuals had climbed Everest (Gillman, 1993) (Table 1.2).

Following the example of Longstaff, some very rapid ascents and descents of Everest have been made. In 1986 two mountaineers climbed the North Face by the Hornbein Conloir without supplementary oxygen. They started from the West Rongbuk glacier (5800 m) at 22.00 h and in 12 h, overnight, reached a bivouac at 7800 m. Here they rested, then they ascended to the summit (8848 m) arriving at 14.30 h. After spending 1 h 30 min on the top they descended to their bivouac in 3 h. From there to the glacier (5800 m) took only 2 h (Everest, 1987). The fastest Everest ascent took 22.5 h from base camp to summit (Gillman, 1993).

1.11 MEDICAL AND PHYSIOLOGICAL EXPEDITIONS

Although medical and physiological observations have been made on expeditions from the earliest times, probably the first series of investigations mounted primarily to study the physiology of high altitude were those of Angelo Mosso at the end of the nineteenth century. In the early years of this century Barcroft and Haldane, with their co-workers, were also involved in a series of research programmes in Tenerife, the European Alps, Pikes Peak, and Cerro de Pasco.

In 1935 the International High Altitude Expedition went to the Andes. They spent several months in Chile studying many aspects of acclimatization to altitude including lactacidosis on exercise, the acid–base status of the blood and arterial blood gases, both in members of the expedition and in local residents at various altitudes (Dill, 1938).

In 1946 'Operation Everest' was carried out at Pensacola Naval Air Station in Florida. Four volunteers lived in a decompression chamber for 34 days, reaching 6600 m on the 27th day after gradual decompression. On day 30 the chamber was decompressed to 235 mmHg – equivalent to 8850 m on the standard atmosphere scale (Chapter 2).

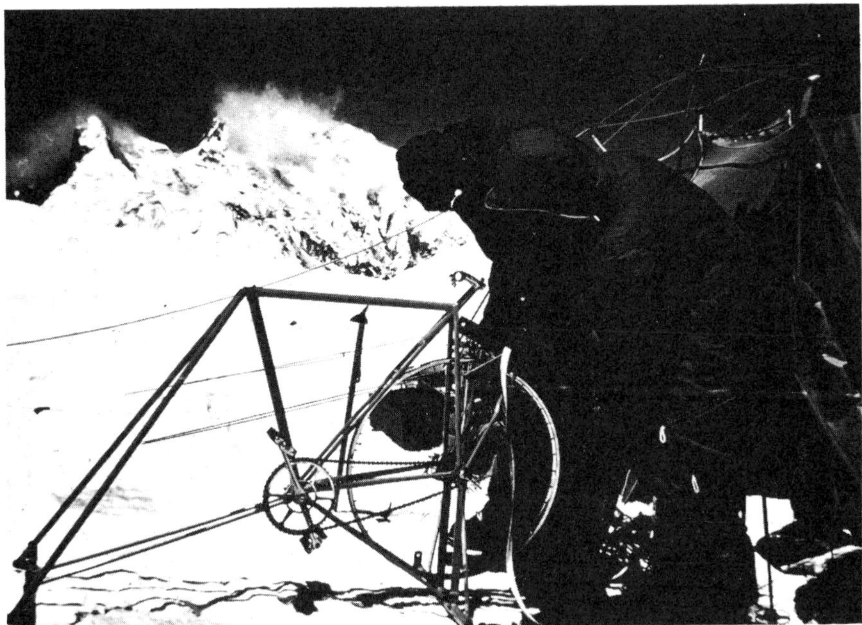

Figure 1.6 Bicycle ergometer being assembled at 7400 m on the Makalu Col by Ward and West, 1961.

Two men were able to tolerate this altitude for 30 min 'on the top of Everest'. The results strongly suggested a diffusion limitation of oxygen transfer during exercise (Houston and Riley, 1947). A similar investigation, 'Operation Everest II' was completed in 1985 at the US Army Institute of Environmental Medicine at Natick, Massachusetts (Houston *et al.*, 1987).

Although important physiological observations were made on Cho Oyu in 1952, and on Everest in 1953 by Pugh, the next expedition devoted to high-altitude physiology was in 1960–1961, which was led by Hillary with Pugh as scientific leader. A fully equipped physiological laboratory, the Silver Hut, was installed at 5800 m in the Everest region. The results from this expedition have formed the basis for much subsequent investigation into extreme altitude, and the expedition was an important landmark in high altitude studies. The Silver Hut was occupied for six months between November 1960 and May 1961, and an attempt on Mt Makalu (8481 m) was also made when maximum work studies were completed at 7440 m by West and Ward (Figure 1.6). This still remains the highest altitude at which such studies have been made.

Projects included studies on exercise, lung diffusion, changes in the control of breathing, ECG changes, basal metabolic rate, blood volume and haemoglobin changes, and psychomotor function. Two vascular accidents occurred – one cerebral, the other pulmonary; there was ample evidence to suggest that despite good living conditions all deteriorated during long-term residence at 5800 m (Pugh, 1962).

The next 20 years saw a number of field investigations into the physiology and medicine of high altitude and an increasing number of people – skiers, trekkers and tourists, as well as mountaineers – were going to high altitude all over the world.

In 1962 the Indian Defence Authorities arranged a 'symposium on the problems of high altitude' at Darjeeling (Symposium (Indian), 1962). This was during the period when China was threatening the northern Himalayan border of India. The Indians appreciated that the Chinese, who had acclimatized for long periods on the Tibetan plateau, would be at an advantage in any conflict in the Himalayas, as Indian soldiers, who lived at low altitude, would not have had time to acclimatize.

In 1964 China did invade India; their soldiers suffered considerably from acute mountain sickness and high-altitude pulmonary oedema. The work of Inder Singh and his colleagues dates from this period (Singh *et al.*, 1969). Since then the clash between India and Pakistan on the Siachen glacier of the Karakoram has provided an added stimulus to high-altitude studies in both countries.

In 1967 a permanent laboratory was placed at 5300 m on Mt Logan in Alaska (Figure 1.7) and this was visited regularly by medical scientists until 1979. During these years, studies included retinal blood flow, the incidence of retinal haemorrhage and the value of acetazolamide in preventing acute mountain sickness. Evidence of subclinical pulmonary oedema on ascending to the laboratory was found in many subjects (Houston, 1980).

Studies on acute mountain sickness and the use of acetazolamide have also been carried out by groups from Birmingham, UK (Acute mountain sickness, 1979, 1987).

On the successful Italian expedition to Everest in 1973, Cerretelli made an extensive series of measurements at 5350 m on climbers who had been to 8000 m. One of the many interesting observations was the failure of maximum oxygen uptake of subjects acclimatized to 5350 m to return to sea-level values when pure oxygen was breathed. Noted also by Pugh and others, this finding has never been satisfactorily explained (Cerretelli, 1976).

In 1980–1981 a Sino–British team explored the Kongur Massif in Southern Xinjiang, Chinese Central Asia, climbing Kongur (7719 m), the highest peak in the Kun Lun range which runs along the northern edge of the Tibetan plateau (Ward, 1983). Half the team were medical

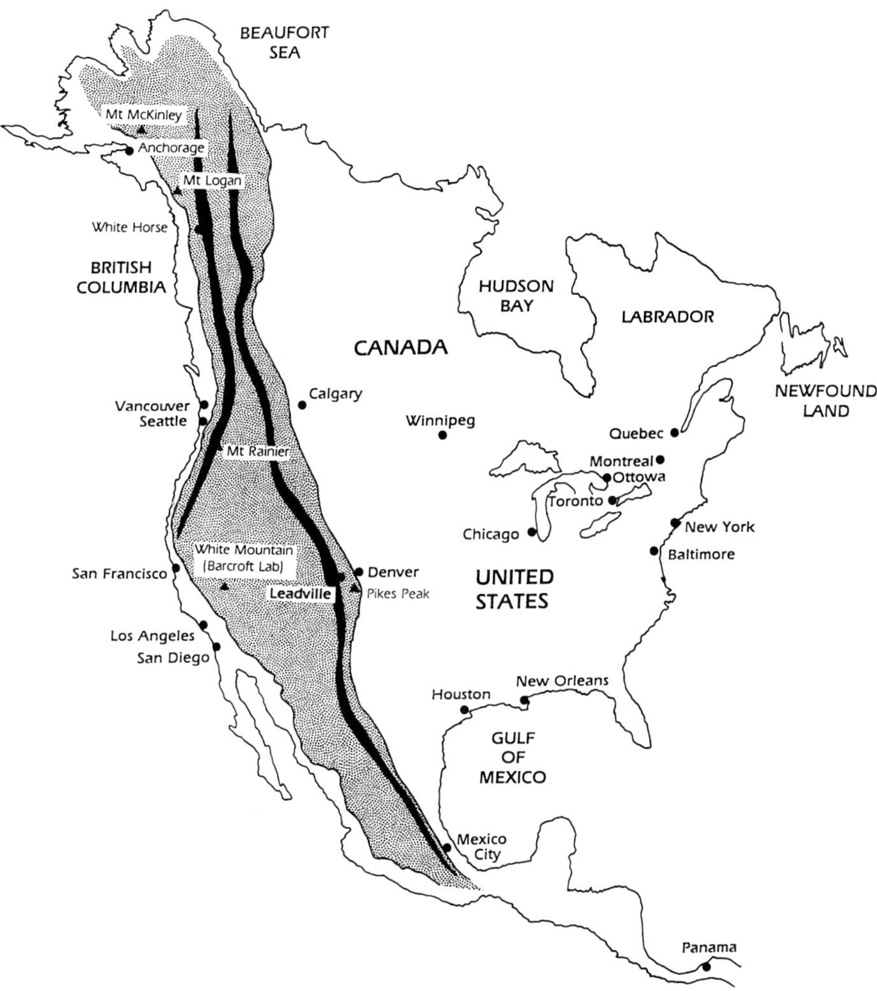

Figure 1.7 North America.

scientists and work was done on the cardiorespiratory response in elite mountaineers, on erythropoietin changes with ascent to altitude (Milledge and Cotes, 1985), and on the renin/aldosterone system (Milledge, 1984).

In 1981 the American Medical Research Expedition to Everest was led by West. The barometric pressure, measured for the first time on the summit was found to be 253 mmHg. This was higher than predicted by some authorities (Chapter 2). Alveolar gas samples were taken on the summit of Everest for the first time by Pizzo and very low P_{CO_2}

values were observed indicating extremely high ventilation rates at rest. Pizzo and Hacket also obtained blood samples on the South Col from which it was deduced that there would have been extreme alkalosis on the summit (Chapter 11). In the Western Cwm a fully equipped laboratory was set up and important observations made on exercise, sleep, metabolism, nutrition, hormones and psychomotor function (West, 1982, 1985).

In the last 25 years too, numerous expeditions have been made on the Tibetan plateau by the Academia Sinica, including a traverse of the plateau by a Royal Society/Academica Sinica party in 1985 (Dong-Sheng, 1981; Chang *et al.*, 1986). In the course of these expeditions a number of peaks, including Everest, have been climbed and high altitude work carried out by members of the Shanghai Institute of Physiology led by Professor Hu Hsu-Tsu and other groups. During the Chinese ascent of Everest in 1975 telemetry of the heart was carried out and a number of other studies made (Shi *et al.*, 1980; Hu, 1983).

Russian contributions have been considerable. The most important early work on the effects of rarefied air on man came from I.M. Sechenov after the deaths in the balloon, Zenith, in 1875. He studied the oxygen transport system which formed the basis of later work on high altitude and in aviation.

At the end of the nineteenth century, P. Gorbachev, N. Tretiakov and O. Shlomm studied the effects of adaptation to altitude on soldiers in the Pamir and Tien Shan, probably in association with the 'Great Game' or rivalry with the UK for influence in Central Asia.

The year 1923 saw the birth of Soviet mountaineering with the ascent of Mt Elbruz in the Caucasus. The first scientific expedition took place in 1926 and, between then and the outbreak of war with Germany in 1950, 25 expeditions from three main centres, Leningrad Military Medical Academy, Moscow and Kiev, took place to the Caucasus, Pamir, Altai and Tien Shan.

The father of Russian high altitude physiology is considered to be Nicolai Sirotinon (1897–1977), who built up the Institute of Physiology in Kiev, mainly to study the effects of hypoxia. His primary interest was in acid–base balance and he attributed the symptoms of mountain sickness to lack of carbon dioxide as did Angelo Mosso. Between 1930 and 1940 he organized and took part in nine high-altitude expeditions. Another very important physiologist was Z.I. Barbashova (1910–1980) who studied the effects of hypoxia on the cells and peripheral tissues, and showed tissue adaptation to be present.

Post-war studies were stimulated by populations living at altitude for commercial reasons and the growth of space science. Good tolerance to hypoxic stress was considered an indication of the ability to combat the generalized stress of space flight.

In 1973 a permanent medical and biological station was opened in Terskol at the foot of Elbruz, at about 2000 m, whilst research expeditions have taken place in Tadzhikistan and Kirghizia, where M.M. Mubrakhimov has studied indigenous populations.

In 1983 rigorous exercise tests on potential Everest climbers revealed unsuspected cardiac abnormalities (Gippenreiter, 1983, 1993 (personal communication); Gazenko, 1987).

Many workers world-wide are now active in this field, including Japanese, French, German and Scandinavian workers as well as those from South America, India and Pakistan (Rivolier, 1959, 1976; Brendel and Zink, 1982; Richalet, 1984; Richalet *et al.*, 1992; Ueda *et al.*, 1992).

1.12 PERMANENT HIGH-ALTITUDE LABORATORIES

In 1890 Joseph Vallot built the Observatoire Vallot on Mt Blanc (4350 m) where studies on astronomy, glaciology and, later, physiology were carried out. The first high altitude laboratory dedicated to physiological studies was built by Angelo Mosso on Monte Rosa (4560 m) in 1893. Since then other laboratories have been constructed. These include one on Pikes Peak (4300 m), although initially work was carried out in the railway station building, on Mt Evans (4348 m) and the Barcroft Laboratory (3800 m) on White Mountain in North America. Facilities also exist at Morococha (4540 m) and Cerro de Pasco (4300 m) in Peru. In La Paz (3500 m) is the Instituto Boliviano de Biologia de Altura. A centre for further study of cold and high altitude is situated at Anchorage, Alaska and a Medical Research Centre was opened at Xining on the north-east edge of the Tibet plateau in 1984. Studies are also being carried out in Lhasa (3568 m) and in Leh (3500 m) in Ladakh, India. In Shanghai a decompression chamber dedicated to long-term studies has been constructed. In the Sola-Khumbu, Nepal the 'Ev-K2-CNR' pyramid laboratory was built at just over 5000 m at Lobuche in 1990. In order to study large numbers of people at moderate altitude, the Colorado Altitude Research Institute was established in 1988 at 2500 m.

1.13 STUDIES OF INDIGENOUS HIGH-ALTITUDE DWELLERS

The extraordinary high work output of high-altitude residents was emphasized by Barcroft (1925) when describing native miners at Cerro de Pasco (4328 m) in the Andes: 'Every few minutes like a bee out of some hive . . . someone would appear from the mouth of the mine. He would be much out of breath, he would take frequent pauses on the way up, but the weight on his back would be one hundred pounds.'

Possibly with his tongue in his cheek, Barcroft commented that, 'All dwellers at altitude are persons of impaired physical and mental

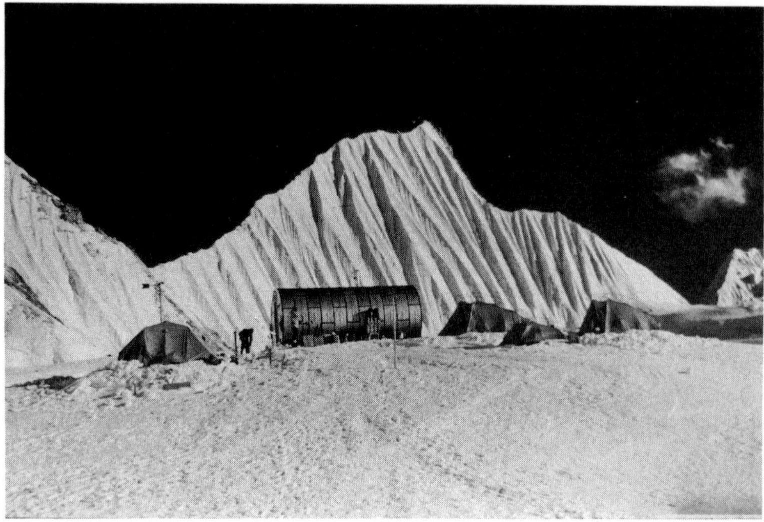

Figure 1.8 The Silver Hut with Rakpa Peak in the background (taken at 5800 m during the Himalayan Scientific and Mountaineering Expedition in the Everest region 1960–61).

powers.' This drew an immediate and indignant response from Carlos Monge, a Peruvian physician: 'Andean man must be physically distinct from sea-level man, requiring much further research before one may define let alone apply the terms inferior and superior.' He and his associates were stimulated to a study of Andean high-altitude populations (Monge, 1948; Hurtado, 1964) and studies have also been carried out in Ethiopia, the Himalayan valleys of Bhutan, and Nepal, as part of the International Biological Programme (Baker, 1978), on the Tibetan plateau (Sun, 1986) and in Lhasa. Work has also been done on Caucasian subjects in Leadville (3100 m) especially by a group from the University of Colorado, Denver (Winslow and Monge, 1987).

REFERENCES

Acosta, J. de (1590) *The Naturall and Morall Historie of the East and West Indies.* English translation by E.G. (1604) Edward Blount and William Aspley, London, p. 146.

Acute mountain sickness. (1979) *Postgrad. Med. J.*, **55**, 445–512.

Acute mountain sickness. (1987) *Postgrad. Med. J.*, **63**, 163–93.

Albutt, T.C. (1870) On the effect of exercise upon the body temperature. *Alpine J.*, **5**, 212–18.

Albutt, T.C. (1876) On the health and training of mountaineers. *Alpine J.*, **8**, 30–40.

Baker, P.T. (ed.) (1978) *The Biology of High Altitude Peoples*, Cambridge University Press, Cambridge.

Barcroft, J. (1925) Lessons from high altitudes. In *The Respiratory Function of the Blood*, Cambridge University Press, Cambridge.

Bellew, H.W. (1875) *Kashmir and Kashgar*, Trubner, London, pp. 163–4.

Bert, P. (1878) *Barometric Pressure: Researches in Experimental Physiology*. Translated by M.A. Hitchcock and R.A. Hitchcock (1943), College Book Co., Columbus, Ohio.

Bonavalot, G. (1891) *Across Thibet*, Cassell, London, p. 166.

Bonavia, D., Leon-Velarde, F., Monge, C.C., *et al.* (1985) Acute mountain sickness: critical appraisal of the Pariacaca story and on-site study. *Respir. Physiol.*, **62**, 125–34.

Bower, H. (1893) *Diary of a Journey across Tibet*, Office of the Superintendent of Government Printing, Calcutta, India, p. 5.

Brendel, W. and Zink, R.A. (eds) (1982) *High Altitude Physiology and Medicine*, Springer-Verlag, New York.

Bruce, C.G. (1923) *The Assault on Mount Everest*, Arnold, London, p. 237.

Burnett, C.S.F. (1983) High altitude mountaineering 1600 years ago. *Alpine J.*, **88**, 127.

Cerretelli, P. (1976) Limiting factors to oxygen transport on Mount Everest. *J. Appl. Physiol.*, **40**, 658–67.

Chang, C., Chen, N., Coward, M.P., *et al.* (1986) Preliminary conclusions of the Royal Society and Academia Sinica 1985 Geotraverse of Tibet. *Nature*, **323**, 501–7.

Cheyne, J. (1818) A case of apoplexy in which the fleshy part of the heart was converted into fat. *Dublin Hosp. Rep.*, **2**, 216–23.

Dill, D.B. (1938) *Life, Heat and Altitude*, Harvard University Press, Cambridge, Mass., pp. 144–74.

Dittert, R., Chevalley, G. and Lambert, R. (1954) *Forerunners to Everest*, Allen and Unwin, London, pp. 141–53.

Dong-Sheng, L. (ed.) *Proceedings of Symposium on Qinghai-Xizang (Tibet) Plateau*, vols 1 and 2. (1981) Beijing Science Press, Gordon and Breach, New York.

Echevarria, E. (1968) The South American Indian as a pioneer alpinist. *Alpine J.*, **73**, 81–8.

Echevarria, E. (1979) Note on objects found on Andean summits. *Am. Alpine J.*, **23**, 588.

Echevarria, E. (1983) Legends of the high Andes. *Alpine J.*, **88**, 85–91.

Egli-Sinclair. (1891–1892) Ueber die Bergkrankheit. *Jahrbuch des Schweizer Alpen Klub.*, **27**, 308–26.

Egli-Sinclair. (1894) Le mal de montagne. *Rev. Sci.* (*Rev. Rose*), Series 4, **1**, 172–80.

Elias, N. and Ross, E.D. (1898) *A History of the Moghuls of Central Asia, Being the Tarikh-I-Rashidi of Mirza Muhammed Haidar, Dughlat*, Sampson, Low & Co., London, pp. 412–3.

Everest: the Hornbein Couloir direct from Tibet. (1987) *Am. Alpine J.*, **29**, 302–4.

Fa-Hsien. (399–414) *A Record of Buddhistic Kingdoms Being an Account by the Chinese Monk Fa-Hsien of His Travels in India and Ceylon* (AD *399–414) in Search of the Buddhist Books of Discipline*. Translated and annotated with a Corean recension of the Chinese text by J. Legge, Dover Publications, New York, (1965) pp. 40–41, (p. 12 of the Korean text).

Filippi, F. de (1912) *Karakoram and Western Himalaya, 1909*, Constable, London, p. 364.

Gazenko, O.G. (1987) *Physiology of Man at High Altitude*, Nauka (Science) Publishing, Moscow (in Russian).

Gilbert, D.L. (1983a) The first documented report of mountain sickness: the China or Headache Mountain story. *Respir. Physiol.*, **52**, 315–26.

Gilbert, D.L. (1983b) The first documented description of mountain sickness: the Andean or Pariacaca story. *Respir. Physiol.*, **52**, 327–47.

Gilbert, D.L. (1988) Mountain sickness at Pariacaca: What's in a name (abst). FASEB meeting, April 1988.

Gillman, P. (1993) *Everest*, Little Brown, Boston.

Gippenreiter, E. (1983) Biomedical experiences on the first Soviet expedition to Mount Everest, in *Hypoxia, Exercise and Altitude*, (eds J.R. Sutton, C.S. Houston and N.L. Jones), Proceedings of the Third Banff Symposium, Liss, New York, pp. 183–7.

Glaisher, J., Flammarion, C., De Fonvielle, E. and Tissandier, G. (1871) Ascents from Wolverhampton, in *Travels in the Air*, (ed. J. Glaisher), Lippincott, Philadelphia, pp. 50–8.

Hedin, S. (1903a) *Central Asia and Tibet*, Hurst and Blackett, London, vol. 1, p. 25.

Hedin, S. (1903b) *Central Asia and Tibet*, Hurst and Blackett, London, vol. 2, p. 20.

Hedin, S. (1913) *Trans-Himalaya*, Macmillan, London, vol. 3, pp. 123–8.

Hepburn, M.L. (1901) The influence of high altitude in mountaineering. *Alpine J.*, **20**, 368–93.

Hepburn, M.L. (1902) Some reasons why the science of altitude illness is still in its infancy. *Alpine J.*, **21**, 161–79.

Hillary, E.P. (1954) Everest 1953: (4) The last lap. *Alpine J.*, **59**, 235–8.

Hingston, R.W.G. (1914) Blood observations at high altitude and some conclusions drawn from this enquiry in relation to mountain distress, records of the Survey of India, completion of the link connecting the triangulations of India and Russia, 1913. Trigonometrical survey. *Dehra Dun*, **6**, 88–91.

Houston, C.S. and Riley, R.L. (1947) Respiratory and circulatory changes during acclimatisation to high altitude. *Am. J. Physiol.*, **149**, 565–88.

Houston, C.S. (1960) Acute pulmonary edema of high altitude. *N. Engl. J. Med.*, **263**, 478–80.

Houston, C.S. (ed.) (1980) *High Altitude Physiology Study*, Collected Papers, Arctic Institute of North America, Arlington, Virginia/Calgary, Alberta.

Houston, C.S., Sutton, J.R., Cymerman, A. and Reeves, J.T. (1987) Operation Everest II: Man at extreme altitude. *J. Appl. Physiol.*, **63**, 877–82.

Hu, S.T. (1983) Hypoxia research in China: An overview, in *Hypoxia, Exercise and Altitude*, (eds J.R. Sutton, C.S. Houston and N.L. Jones), Proceedings of the Third Banff Symposium, Liss, New York, pp. 157–71.

Hurtado, A. (1937) *Aspectos fisiologicos y patologicos de lavida en la altura*, Imp. Edit Rimas, S.A. Lima.

Hurtado, A. (1964) Animals in high altitudes: resident man, in *Handbook of Physiology, Section 4*, American Physiological Society, Washington, DC, pp. 843–60.

Kellas, A.M. (1917) A consideration of the possibility of ascending the loftier Himalaya. *Geogr. J.*, **49**, 26–48.

Kellas A.M. (1921) Expedition to Kamet, in 1920. *Alpine J.*, **33**, 313–19.

Kellogg, R.H. (1978) La pression barometrique: Paul Bert's hypoxia theory and its critics. *Respir. Physiol.*, **34**, 1–28.

Kronecker, C. (1903) *Die Bergkrankheit*, Berlin und Wien.

Landon, P. (1905) *Lhasa*, vol. 2, Hurst and Blackett, London, p. 39.
Longstaff, T.G. (1906) *Mountain Sickness and its Probable Causes*, Spottiswode, London, p. 54.
Longstaff, T.G. (1908) A mountaineering expedition to the Himalaya of Garhwal. *Geogr. J.*, **31**, 361–95.
Lundberg, E. (1952) Edema agudo del pulmon en el soroche. Conferencia sustentada en la ascociacion medica de Yauli, Oroya. (Quoted in Hultgren, H.N., Spickard, W.B., Hellriegel, K. and Houston, C.S. (1961) High altitude pulmonary edema. *Medicine*, **40**, 289–313).
Maggilivary, N. (1853) *The Travels and Researches of Alexander Von Humboldt*, Nelson, London, p. 285.
Marcet, W. (1886–1888a) Climbing and breathing at high altitude. *Alpine J.*, **13**, 1–13.
Marcet, W. (1886–1888b) On the use of alcoholic stimulants in mountaineering. *Alpine J.*, **13**, 319–27.
Mathews, C.E. (1898) *Annals of Mont Blanc*, T. Fisher Unwin, London, p. 82.
Mathews, B. (1932) Loss of heat at high altitudes. *J. Physiol.*, **77**, 28–29P.
Messner, R. (1979) *Everest: Expedition to the Ultimate*, Kaye and Ward, London, pp. 174–80.
Milledge, J.S. (1984) Renin aldosterone system, in *High Altitude and Man*, (eds J.B. West and S. Lahiri), American Physiological Society, Bethesda, Maryland.
Milledge, J.S. (1985) The great oxygen secretion controversy. *Lancet*, **2**, 1408–11.
Milledge, J.S. and Cotes, P.M. (1985) Serum erythropoietin in humans at high altitude and its relation to plasma renin. *J. Appl. Physiol.*, **59**, 360–4.
Milledge, J.S. (1993) Respiratory water loss at altitude. *ISSM Newsletter*, **2**, 5–7.
Monge, C. (1948) *Acclimatization in the Andes*, Johns Hopkins Press, Baltimore.
Morshead, H.T. (1921) Report of the expedition to Kamet, 1920. *Geogr. J.*, **57**, 213–19.
Mosso, A. (1898) *Life of Man on the High Alps*, T. Fisher Unwin, London, pp. 289–92.
Mountain (1988) 121, 11.
Mountains of Central Asia (1987) Compiled by the Royal Geographical Society and Mount Everest Foundation, London.
Monro, C.G. (1893) Mountain sickness. *Alpine J.*, **16**, 446–55.
Napier, J. (1972) *Big Foot: The Yeti and Sasquatch in Myth and Reality*, Cape, London.
Needham, J. (1954) *Science and Civilisation in China*, Cambridge, p. 195.
Norton, E.F. (1925) *The Fight for Everest, 1924*, Arnold, London, pp. 120–43.
Parfionovitch, Y., Dorge, G. and Meyer, F. (1992) *Tibetan Medical Paintings: Illustrations to the* Blue Beryl *Treatise of Sangye Gyamtso (1653–1705)*, Serindia, London, p. 103.
Payot, A. (1881) *Du mal des Montagnes*, Thése pour le Doctorat en Medicine, Alphonse Derenne, Paris.
Plutarch (46–120) Alexander and Caesar. *Loeb Classics*, Vol. 7. (1971) Heinemann, London, p. 389.
Prescott, W.H. (1891) *History of Mexico*, Swan Sonnerschein & Son, London, p. 253.
Pugh, L.G.C.E. (1952) *Report on Cho Oyu Expedition*, Medical Research Council, London.
Pugh, L.G.C.E. and Ward, M.P. (1956) Some effects of high altitude on man. *Lancet*, **2**, 1115–21.

Pugh, L.G.C.E. (1962) Physiological and medical aspects of the Himalayan Scientific and Mountaineering Expedition 1960–61. *Br. Med. J.*, **2**, 621–7.

Ravenhill, T. (1913) Some experiences of mountain sickness in the Andes. *J. Trop. Med. Hyg.*, **16**, 314–20.

Reinhard, J. (1983) High altitude archaeology and Andean mountain gods. *Am. Alpine J.*, **25**, 54–67.

Richalet, J.-P. (1984) *Medicine de l'Alpinisme*, Masson, Paris.

Richalet, J.P., Bittel, J., Merry, J.P., *et al.* (1992) Pre-acclimatization to high altitude in a hypobaric chamber: Everest turbo, in *Hypoxia and Mountain Medicine*, (eds J.R. Sutton, J. Coates and C.S. Houston), Queen City Printers, Vermont, USA.

Rivolier, J. (1959) *Expéditions Francaises à l'Himalaya: Aspect Médical*. Hermann, Paris.

Rivolier, J. (ed.) (1976) *Colloque Médicine et Haute Montagne*. Fédération Francaise et de la montagne, Grenoble, Juin 11–12.

Roborovsky (1896) The Central Asian expedition of Capt. Roborovsky and Lt. Kozloff. *Geogr. J.*, **8**, 161.

Rockhill, W.W. (1891) *The Land of the Lamas*, Longmans Green, London, p. 149.

Roy, C.S. (1894) Mountain sickness: maps and scientific reports, in *Climbing and Exploration in the Karakoram Himalayas*, (ed. W.M. Conway), T. Fisher Unwin, London, pp. 117–27.

Russel, H. (1871) On mountains and mountaineering in general. *Alpine J.*, **5**, 241–8.

Shi, Z.Y., Ning, X.H., Zhu, S.C., *et al.* (1980) Electrocardiogram made on ascending the Mount Everest from 50 m a.s.l. *Sci. Sin.*, **23**, 1316–25.

Singh, I., Khanna, P.K., Srivastava, M.C., *et al.* (1969) Acute mountain sickness. *N. Engl. J. Med.*, **280**, 175–84.

Sui, G.T., Lui, Y.H., Cheng, X.S., *et al.* (1988) Sub-acute infantile mountain sickness. *J. Pathol.*, **155**, 161–70.

Sun, S.F. (1986) Epidemiology of hypertension on the Tibetan plateau. *Hum. Biol.*, **58**, 507–15.

Symposium (Indian). (1962) *International Symposium on Problems of High Altitude at Darjeeling*, Armed Forces Medical Services: Gulabons Offset Works. Delhi.

Thomas, P.W. (1894) Rocky mountain sickness. *Alpine J.*, **17**, 140, 149.

Tissandier, G. (1875) Le Voyage a grande hauteur du ballon 'Le Zenith'. *Le Nature (Paris)*, **3**, 337–44.

Tyndall, J. (1860) *Glaciers of the Alps*, Murray, London, p. 80.

Ueda, G., Reeves, J.T. and Sekiguchi, M. (1992) High altitude Medicine. Shinshu University, Matsumoto, Japan.

Unna, P.J.H. (1922) The oxygen equipment of the 1922 Everest expedition. *Alpine J.*, **34**, 235–50.

Viault, E. (1890) Sur l'augmentation considérable des globules rouge dans le sang chez les habitants des haut plateau de l'Amérique du sud. *Compte Rendu Hebdomaire des Séances de l'Académie des Sciences (Paris)*, **111**, 917–18.

Von Schlagintweit, A.H. and Von Schlagintweit, R. (1862) *Results of a Scientific Mission to India and High Asia, vol. I*, Trubner, London, p. 18.

Waddell, L.A. (1905) *Lhasa and its Mysteries*, Murray, London, p. 144.

Ward, M.P. (1973) Periodic respiration. *Ann. R. Coll. Surg. Engl.*, **52**, 330–4.

Ward, M.P. (1983) The Kongur Massif in Southern Xinjiang. *Geogr. J.*, **149**, 137–52.

Ward, M.P. (1993) The first ascent of Mount Everest. *Br. Med. J.*, **306**, 1455–8.

Wessels, C. (1924) *Early Jesuit Travellers in Central Asia, 1603–1721*, Nijhoff, The Hague, p. 54.

West, J.B. (1982) American Medical Research Expedition to Everest. *Physiologist*, **25**, 36–8.
West, J.B. (1985) *Everest: The Testing Place*, McGraw-Hill, New York.
West, J.B. (1987) Alexander M. Kellas and the physiological challenge of Mount Everest. *J. Appl. Physiol.*, **63**, 3–11.
Whymper, E. (1892) *Travels Among the Great Andes of the Equator*, Murray, London, pp. 366–84.
Winslow, R.M. and Monge, C.C. (1987) Hypoxia, polycythemia and chronic mountain sickness. Johns Hopkins University Press, Baltimore, pp. 15–16.
Wylie, A. (1881) Notes on the Western Regions. Translated from the *Tseen Han Shoo Book 96, Part 1*, *J. R. Anthropol. Inst.*, **10**, 20–73.
Zangger, T. (1899) On the danger of high altitudes for patients with arteriosclerosis. *Lancet*, **1**, 1628–9.
Zangger, T. (1903) On the danger of railway trips to high altitudes especially for elderly patients. *Lancet*, **1**, 1730–5.

2

The atmosphere

2.1 INTRODUCTION

It has been known since the time of Paul Bert and the publication of *La Pression Barométrique* (Bert, 1878) that most of the deleterious effects of high altitude on man are caused by hypoxia. This in turn is a direct result of the reduction in atmospheric pressure. Yet in spite of the fact that we celebrated the centennial of Bert's book several years ago, there is still confusion in the minds of some physicians and physiologists about the relationship between barometric pressure and altitude, particularly at extreme heights. For example, some environmental physiologists are still surprised to learn that the barometric pressure at the summit of Mt Everest is considerably higher than that predicted by the standard pressure–altitude tables used by the aviation industry, and that humans can only reach the summit without supplementary oxygen because the tables are inapplicable.

Although most of the undesirable effects of high altitude are due to hypoxia, under some circumstances additional deterioration results from cold, dehydration, solar, and even ionizing radiation. However most of these hazards of the environment can be avoided by proper clothing or shelter. Only hypoxia is unavoidable unless, of course, supplementary oxygen is available. The low barometric pressure in itself has no physiological sequelae unless the decompression is rapid, for example, in the case of explosive decompression which occurs when a window fails in a pressurized aircraft. Rapid decompression causes so-called barotrauma as a result of the very rapid enlargement of airspaces within the body including the lungs and middle ear cavity. Such accidents can also occur in ascent from deep diving but are not considered here.

That low pressure *per se* is innocuous was not always realized. Indeed, early theories of mountain sickness included a number of exotic explanations based on the reduced pressure itself (Bert, 1878, pp. 342–7 in 1943 translation). One was weakening of the coxo-femoral articulation; it was thought that barometric pressure was an important factor in pressing the head of the femur into its socket and that, at high altitudes, the necessary increase in action of the neighbouring muscles resulted in fatigue. Another hypothesis was that superficial blood vessels would dilate and rupture if the barometric pressure which normally supported them was reduced. Indeed modern day medical students occasionally raise issues of this kind when they are first introduced to high altitude physiology. A further theory was that distension of intestinal gas would interfere with the action of the diaphragm and also impede venous return to the heart. All these theories neglect the fact that, when humans ascend to high altitude, all the hydrostatic pressures in the body fall together. In other words, although the pressure outside the superficial blood vessels falls, the pressure inside the vessels falls to the same extent and therefore the pressure differences across the vessels are unchanged.

2.2 BAROMETRIC PRESSURE AND ALTITUDE

2.2.1 Historical

The notion that air has weight and therefore exerts a pressure at the surface of the earth evaded the ancient Greeks and had to wait until the Renaissance. Galileo (1638) was well aware of the force associated with a vacuum and therefore the effort required to 'break' it, but he thought of this in the context of a force required to break a copper wire by stretching it, that is, the cohesive forces within the substance of the wire. In 1647, Otto von Guericke provided a graphic demonstration of the forces associated with a vacuum when he showed that teams of horses could not separate two carefully fitting hemispheres from which the air had been pumped. But it was left to Galileo's pupil Torricelli to realize that the force of a vacuum is due to the weight of the atmosphere. In his memorable letter addressed to Michelangelo Ricci in 1644, he wrote, 'We live submerged at the bottom of an ocean of the element air, which by unquestioned experiments is known to have weight' (Torricelli, 1644). How simple and striking this is. Moreover, Torricelli wondered whether the air pressure became less on the tops of high mountains where the air 'begins to be distinctly rare . . .'as he put it. Torricelli is credited with making the first mercury barometer, though barometers filled with other liquids had apparently been constructed previously, for example by Gaspar Berti. These were unsatisfactory because of the effect of the vapour pressure of the liquid.

The Jesuit priest, Joseph de Acosta, who accompanied the early Spanish explorers in Peru, gave his dramatic description of acute mountain sickness as early as 1590 (de Acosta, 1590). This included the inspired guess that the deleterious effects of high altitude were caused by the thinness of the air. However the landmark experiment took place in 1648 when the French philosopher and mathematician, Blaise Pascal, suggested that his brother-in-law, F. Périer take a barometer to the top of the Puy de Dôme (1463 m) in central France to see whether the pressure fell (Pascal, 1648). The results were communicated to Pascal in a delightful letter by Périer in which he described how the level of the mercury barometer fell some three pouces (about three inches) during the ascent of '500 fathoms' of altitude. The experiment had elaborate controls. For example, the Reverend Father Chastin, 'a man as pious as he is capable', stood guard over one barometer in the town of Clermont while Périer and a number of observers (including clerics, counsellors, and a doctor of medicine) took another to the top of the mountain. On returning, it was found that the first barometer had not changed, and Périer even checked it again by filling it with the same mercury that he had taken up the mountain. Another observation was made the next day on the top of a high church tower in Clermont, and this also showed a fall in pressure, though of much smaller extent.

A few years later, Robert Boyle carried out experiments with the newly invented air pump and wrote his influential book *New experiments physico-mechanical touching the spring of the air, and its effects*. In the second edition of this book published in 1662 he formulated his famous law, which states that gas volume and pressure are inversely related (at constant temperature) (Boyle, 1662).

An influential analysis of the relationships between altitude and barometric pressure was made by Zuntz *et al.*, in 1906. They pointed out the important effect of temperature on the altitude–pressure relationship noting that, on a fine warm day, the up-currents carry air to high altitudes and thus increase the sea-level barometric pressure. Indeed this is the basis for weather prediction based on barometric pressure.

Zuntz *et al.* (1906) gave the following logarithmic relationship for determining barometric pressure at any altitude:

$$\log b = \log B - \frac{h}{72(256.4 + t)}$$

where h is the altitude difference in metres, t is the mean temperature (°C) of the air column of height h, B is the barometric pressure (mmHg) at the lower altitude, and b is the barometric pressure at the higher altitude. Note that this expression implies that the higher the mean temperature, the less rapidly would barometric pressure decrease with altitude. In addition, if temperature were constant, $\log b$ would be proportional to negative altitude, that is the pressure would decrease exponentially as altitude increased. Zuntz *et al.* cite Hann's *Lehrbuch der Meteorologie* where the pressure–altitude relationship is given in a slightly different form (Hann, 1901).

Zuntz *et al.*'s expression was used by FitzGerald (1913) in her study of alveolar P_{CO_2} and haemoglobin concentration in residents of various altitudes in the Colorado mountains during the Anglo–American Pikes Peak expedition of 1911. She showed that barometric pressures calculated from the Zuntz formula agreed closely with pressures observed in the mountains when a sea-level pressure of 760 mmHg and a mean temperature of the air column of +15°C were assumed. Kellas (1917) used the same expression to predict barometric pressures in the Himalayan ranges obtaining a value of 251 mmHg for the summit of Mt Everest, assuming a mean temperature of 0°C. This was almost the same as the pressure of 248 mmHg given by Bert (1878, Appendix I) in contrast to the erroneously low values used 70 years after Bert because of the inappropriate application of the Standard Atmosphere (section 2.2.3). However a major difficulty with the use of the Zuntz formula is the sensitivity of the calculated pressure to temperature and the fact that the mean temperature of the air column is not accurately known. For example, the barometric pressure on the summit of Mt Everest was calculated by Kellas to be 267 mmHg for a mean temperature of +15°C, but only 251 mmHg for a mean temperature of 0°C.

2.2.2 Physical principles

Barometric pressure decreases with altitude because the higher we go, the less atmosphere there is above us pressing down by virtue of its weight. If the atmosphere were incompressible, as is very nearly the case in a liquid, barometric pressure would decrease linearly with altitude, just as it does in a liquid. However, because the weight of the upper atmosphere compresses the lower gas, barometric pressure decreases more rapidly with height near the earth's surface. If temperature were constant, the decrease in pressure would be exponential with respect to altitude, but because the temperature decreases as we go higher (at least, in the troposphere), the pressure falls more rapidly than the exponential law predicts.

The relationships between pressure, volume and temperature in a gas are governed by simple laws. These derive from the kinetic theory of gases which states that the molecules of a gas are in continuous random motion, and are only deflected from their course by collision with other molecules, or with the walls of a container. When they strike the walls and rebound, the resulting bombardment results in a pressure. The magnitude of the pressure depends on the number of molecules present, their mass and their speed.

Boyle's law states that, at constant temperature, the pressure (P) of a given mass of gas is inversely proportional to its volume (V), or

$$PV = \text{constant (temperature constant)}$$

This can be explained by the fact that as the molecules are brought closer together (smaller volume), the rate of bombardment on a unit surface increases (greater pressure).

Charles' law states that at constant pressure, the volume of a gas is proportional to its absolute temperature (T), or

$$\frac{V}{T} = \text{constant (pressure constant)}$$

The explanation is that a rise in temperature increases the speed and momentum of the molecules thus increasing their force of bombardment on the container. Another form of Charles' law states that at constant volume, the pressure is proportional to absolute temperature. (Note that absolute temperature is obtained by adding 273 to the centigrade temperature. Thus 37°C = 310° Kelvin.)

The **ideal gas law** combines the above laws thus:

$$PV = nRT$$

where n is the number of gram molecules of the gas and R is the 'gas constant'. When the units employed are mmHg, litres, and degrees Kelvin, then $R = 62.4$. Real gases deviate from ideal gas behaviour to some extent under certain conditions because of intermolecular forces.

Dalton's law states that each gas in a mixture exerts a pressure according to its own concentration, independently of the other gases present. That is, each component behaves as though it were present alone. The pressure of each gas is referred to as its partial pressure or tension (now obsolete). The total pressure is the sum of the partial pressures of all gases present. In symbols:

$$P_x = PF_x$$

where P_x is the partial pressure of gas x, P is the total pressure and F_x is the fractional concentration of gas x. For example, if half the gas is oxygen, $F_{O_2} = 0.5$. Conventionally the fractional concentration always refers to dry gas.

The kinetic theory of gases explains their diffusion in the gas phase. Because of their random motion, gas molecules tend to distribute themselves uniformly throughout any available space until the partial pressure is the same everywhere. Light gases diffuse faster than heavy gases because the mean velocity of the molecules is higher. The kinetic theory of gases states that the kinetic energy ($0.5\,mv^2$) of all gases is the same at a given temperature and pressure. From this it follows that the rate of diffusion of a gas is inversely proportional to the square root of its density (**Graham's law**).

On the basis of different diffusion rates, one might expect that very light gases such as helium would separate and be lost from the upper atmosphere. This does happen to some extent at extreme altitudes. However at the altitudes of interest to us, say up to 10 km, convective mixing maintains the composition of the atmosphere constant.

Vertically, the atmosphere can be divided on the basis of temperature variations into the troposphere, stratosphere, and regions above that. The troposphere is the region where all the weather phenomena take place and is the only region of interest to high altitude medicine. Here, the temperature decreases approximately linearly with altitude until a low of about − 60°C is reached. The troposphere extends to an altitude of about 19 km at the equator but only to about 9 km at the poles. The average upper limit is about 10 km.

Above the troposphere is the stratosphere where the temperature remains nearly constant at about −60°C for some 10–12 km of altitude. The interface between the troposphere and stratosphere is known as the tropopause.

Beyond the stratosphere, temperatures again vary with altitude. One of the important components of this region is the ionosphere where the degree of ionization of the molecules makes short wave radio propagation possible.

2.2.3 Standard Atmosphere

With the development of the aviation industry in the 1920s it became necessary to develop a barometric pressure–altitude relationship which could be universally accepted for calibrating altimeters, low-pressure chambers and other devices. Although it had been recognized for many years that the relationship between pressure and altitude was temperature-dependent and, as a result, latitude-dependent, there were clear advantages in having a model atmosphere which applied approximately to mean conditions over the surface of the earth. This is often referred to as the ICAO standard atmosphere (1964) or the US standard atmosphere (NOAA, 1976). These two are identical up to altitudes of interest to us.

The assumptions of the standard atmosphere are a sea-level pressure of 760 mmHg (1013 millibars), sea-level temperature of +15°C and a linear decrease in temperature with altitude (lapse rate) of 6.5°C per kilometre up to an altitude of 11 km (Table 2.1). Haldane and Priestley (1935) gave the following expression for the pressure–altitude relation-

Table 2.1 Standard atmosphere (ICAO, 1964)

Altitude		*Pressure* (P_B)		P_{O_2}*		*Temperature*	*Density*
m	*ft*	*torr (mmHg)*	*millibars*	*dry, torr*	*moist, torr*	°C	$kg\,m^{-3}$
0	0	760	1013.3	159.2	149.3	15	1.225
1000	3281	674.1	898.8	141.2	131.4	8.50	1.112
2000	6562	596.3	795.0	124.9	115.1	2.00	1.007
3000	9843	526.0	701.2	110.2	100.3	−4.49	0.909
4000	13123	462.5	616.6	96.9	87.0	−10.94	0.819
5000	16404	405.4	540.5	84.9	75.1	−17.47	0.736
6000	19685	354.2	472.2	74.2	64.3	−23.96	0.660
7000	22966	308.3	411.1	64.6	54.7	−30.45	0.590
8000	26247	267.4	356.5	56.0	46.2	−36.94	0.526
9000	29528	231.0	308.0	48.4	38.5	−43.42	0.467

* P_{O_2} of moist inspired gas is 0.2094 (P_B − 47)

ship of the standard atmosphere in the second editon of their textbook *Respiration*:

$$P_O/P = \left(\frac{288}{288 - 1.98H}\right)^{5.256}$$

where P_O and P are the pressures in mmHg at sea level and high altitude respectively, and H is the height in thousands of feet. A more rigorous description is given in the Manual of the ICAO standard atmosphere (1964).

It should be emphasized that this model atmosphere was never meant to be used to predict the actual barometric pressure at a particular location. Rather it was developed as a model of more or less average conditions within the troposphere with full recognition that there would be local variations caused by latitude and other factors. Nevertheless the standard atmosphere has assumed some importance in respiratory physiology because it is universally used as the standard for altimeter calibrations, and it has frequently been inappropriately used to predict the pressure at various specific points of the earth's surface, particularly on high mountains.

Haldane and Priestley (1935) clearly understood that the standard atmosphere predicted barometric pressures considerably lower than those given by the expression of Zuntz *et al.* (1906) which had been shown by FitzGerald to predict accurately pressures in the Colorado mountains when a mean air column temperature of +15°C was assumed.

Nevertheless, some physiologists have used the standard atmosphere for predicting the pressure at great altitudes, for example on Mt Everest (Houston and Riley, 1947; Houston *et al.*, 1987; Riley and Houston, 1951; Rahn and Fenn, 1955). The barometric pressure calculated in this way for the Everest summit (altitude 8848 m) is 236 mmHg which is far too low. In retrospect, one of the reasons for the indiscriminate use of the standard atmosphere was undoubtedly its very frequent employment in low-pressure chambers during the very fertile period of research on respiratory physiology during World War II.

2.2.4 Barometric pressures in the Himalayan and Andean ranges

When expeditions to high altitude resumed after World War II, it soon became apparent that barometric pressures in the Himalayas and Andes exceeded those predicted from the standard atmosphere. A particularly important study was carried out by Pugh (1957) who took part in British Himalayan expeditions to Cho Oyu (8153 m) in 1952 and Mt Everest (8848 m) in 1953. He clearly showed that barometric pressures measured in the pre-monsoon season up to altitudes of about 7300 m followed the curve of Zuntz *et al.* (mean air temperature 15°C) better than the standard atmosphere (Figure 2.1). He went on to calculate the pressure on the Everest summit using the measured pressure of 308 mmHg at an altitude of approximately 7315 m. A mean temperature of −26°C between that altitude and the summit was assumed based on temperature measurements up to an altitude of 8500 m.

These calculations gave a pressure on the Everest summit of 250 mmHg which was remarkably accurate in the light of present day knowledge. However in the same article Pugh also calculated the summit pressure from measurements made by Greene in 1934 and obtained a value of 269 mmHg. This was clearly an overestimate. Further measurements were obtained on the Himalayan Scientific and Mountaineering Expedition of 1960–1961 when a barometric pressure of 300 mmHg was measured on the Makalu Col at an altitude of 7440 m (Pugh *et al.*, 1964). Again this pressure was considerably higher than that given by the standard atmosphere.

The first direct measurement of barometric pressure on the Everest summit was obtained by Pizzo in 1981 during the course of the American Medical Research Expedition (West *et al.*, 1983b). The value of 253 mmHg together with other measurements of barometric pressure at points where the altitude was accurately known allowed the pressure–altitude relationship on the world's highest mountain to be accurately defined (Figure 2.2). Note that the pressure on the summit was 17 mmHg higher than predicted from the standard atmosphere.

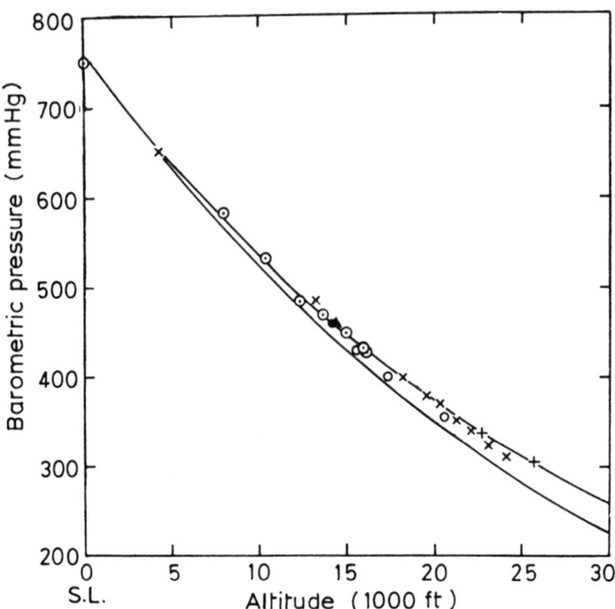

Figure 2.1 Relationship between barometric pressure and altitude. The upper curve is calculated from the formula of Zuntz *et al.* (1906) using a mean air column temperature of 15°C. The lower curve follows the Standard Atmosphere (ICAO, 1964). The plotted points represent observations made on Mt Everest and elsewhere, mainly in the Andes. They clearly fit the upper curve better than the lower. (From Pugh, 1957.) (1000 ft = 304.8 m)

2.2.5 Variation of barometric pressure with latitude

The limited applicability of the standard atmosphere is further clarified when we look at the relationship between barometric pressure and altitude for different latitudes (Figure 2.3). This shows that the barometric pressure at the earth's surface and at an altitude of 24 km is essentially independent of latitude. However, in the altitude range of about 6–16 km, there is a pronounced bulge in the barometric pressure near the equator both in winter and summer. Since the latitude of Mt Everest is 28°N, the pressure at its summit (8848 m) is considerably higher than would be the case for a hypothetical mountain of the same altitude near one of the poles.

The cause of the bulge in barometric pressure near the equator is a very large mass of very cold air in the stratosphere above the equator (Brunt, 1952). In fact, paradoxically, the coldest air in the atmosphere is above the equator. This is brought about by a combination of complex

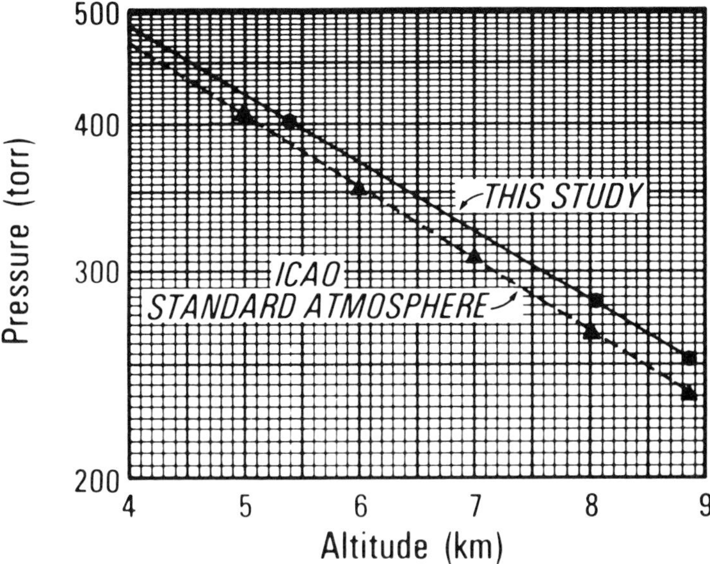

Figure 2.2 Upper line (●): barometric pressure–altitude relationship measured on Mt Everest during the American Medical Research Expedition to Everest, 1981. The three data points are for altitudes that are accurately known, the right lower point being the summit. Broken line (▲): relationship for the standard atmosphere (ICAO, 1964). (From West *et al.*, 1983b.) (1 torr = 1 mmHg)

radiation and convective phenomena. Another corollary of the same phenomenon is that the height of the tropopause is much greater near the equator than near the poles. These latitude-dependent variations of pressure are of great physiological significance for anyone attempting to climb Mt Everest without supplementary oxygen because they result in a barometric pressure on the Everest summit which is considerably higher than that predicted from the model atmosphere.

2.2.6 Variation of barometric pressure with season

Not only does barometric pressure alter with latitude, but there are marked variations according to the month of the year. For example, Figure 2.4 shows the mean monthly pressures for an altitude of 8848 m as obtained from radio-sonde balloons released from New Delhi, India over a period of 15 years. Delhi has about the same latitude as Everest. Note that the mean pressures were lowest in the winter months of January and February (243.0 and 243.7 mmHg, respectively) and highest in the summer months of July and August (254.5 mmHg for both months). The monthly standard deviation showed a range of

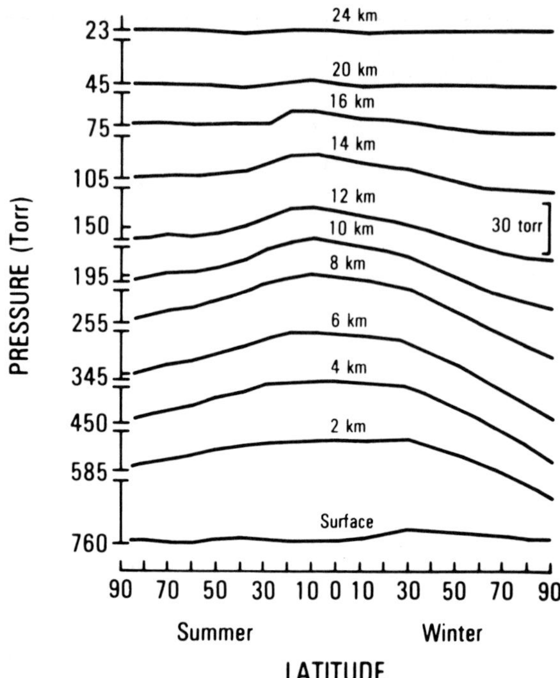

Figure 2.3 Increase of barometric pressure near the equator at various altitudes in both summer and winter. Vertical axis shows the pressure increasing upwards according to the scale on the right. The numbers on the left show the barometric pressures at the poles for various altitudes; the altitude of Mt Everest is 8848 km. (From Brunt, 1952.) (1 torr = 1 mmHg)

0.65 mmHg (July) to 1.66 mmHg (December). The daily standard deviation was as low as 1.54 in the summer and as high as 2.92 in the winter. The standard deviation shown on Figure 2.4 is the mean of the monthly standard deviation for the 12 months of the year.

The single measurement of barometric pressure (253.0 mmHg) made by Pizzo on October 24, 1981 is also shown on Figure 2.4. This was 4.3 mmHg higher than that predicted from the date shown in Figure 2.3, which is twice the daily standard deviation of barometric pressure for the month of October. It should be added that Pizzo had an exceptionally fine day for his summit climb, the temperature on the summit being measured as −9°C, much higher than expected for that altitude (section 2.3.1).

Figure 2.5 combines the effects of latitude and month of the year on the barometric pressure at an altitude of 8848 m. The data are for the northern hemisphere, and the pressures for the months of January

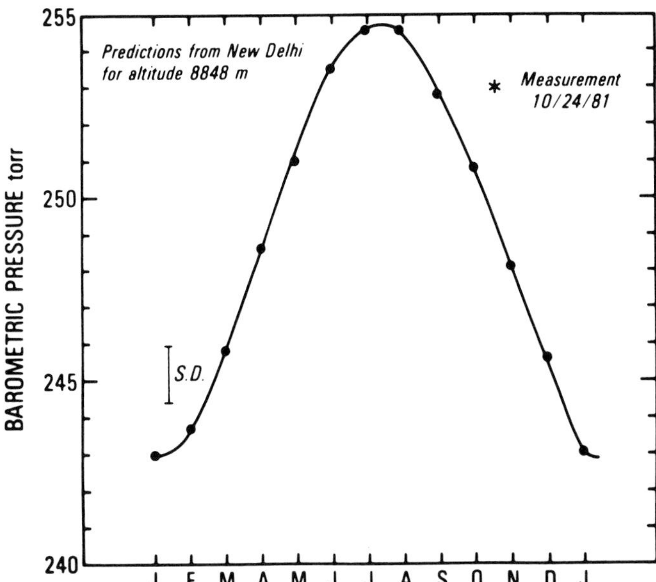

Figure 2.4 Mean monthly pressures for 8848 m altitude as obtained from weather balloons released from New Delhi, India. Note the increase during the summer months. The mean monthly standard deviation (SD) is also shown. The barometric pressure measured on the Everest summit on 24 October, 1981(*) was unusually high for that month. (From West *et al.*, 1983b.) (1 torr = 1 mmHg)

(midwinter), July (midsummer), and October (preferred month for climbing in the post-monsoon period) are compared. The profile for the month of May, which is the usual month for reaching the summit in the pre-monsoon season, is almost the same as that for October. The data are the means from all longitudes (Oort and Rasmusson, 1971). The data clearly show the marked effects of both latitude and season on barometric pressure. It is interesting that in midsummer the pressure reaches a maximum near the latitude of Mt Everest (28°35′N).

Radio-sonde balloons are released from meteorological stations all over the world twice a day, and the resulting data on the relationship between barometric pressure and altitude are available from constant-pressure charts. Details on how to obtain these are given in West (1993). Using these data it can be shown that the barometric pressure on the Everest summit was 251 mmHg when Messner and Habeler made their first ascent without supplementary oxygen in 1978. In August 1980, Messner made the first solo ascent without supplementary oxygen and he was fortunate that the barometric pressure was un-

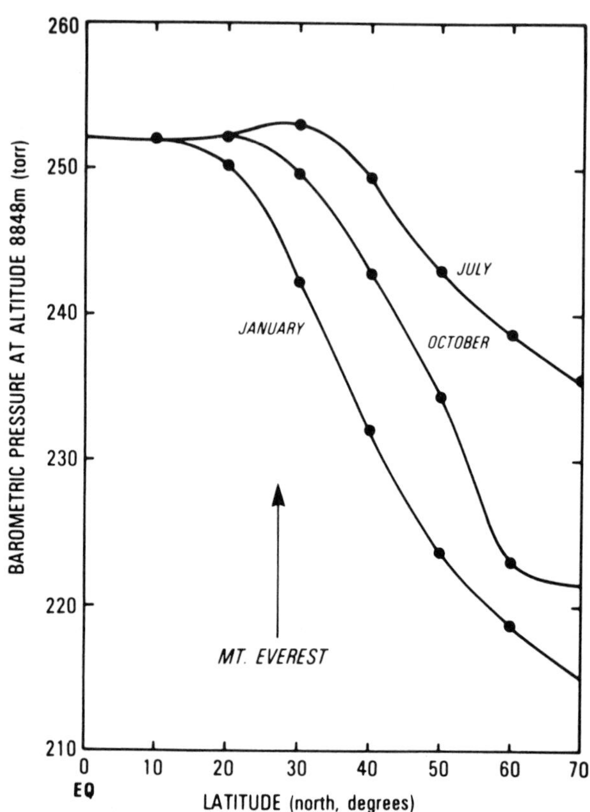

Figure 2.5 Barometric pressure at the altitude of Mt Everest plotted against latitude in the northern hemisphere for midsummer, midwinter, and the preferred month for climbing in the post-monsoon period (October). Note the considerably lower pressures in the winter. The arrow shows the latitude of Mt Everest. (From West *et al.*, 1983b.) (1 torr = 1 mmHg)

usually high at 256 mmHg; when Sherpa Ang Rita made the first winter ascent on 22 December 1987, the barometric pressure was only 247 mmHg.

2.2.7 Barometric pressure and inspired P_{O_2}

As we have seen, the composition of the atmosphere is constant up to altitudes well above those of medical interest so it is safe to assume that the concentration of oxygen in dry air is approximately 20.94%. However the effects of water vapour on the inspired P_{O_2} become increasingly important at higher altitudes.

When air is inhaled into the upper bronchial tree, it is warmed and moistened and becomes saturated with vapour at the prevailing temperature. The water vapour pressure at 37°C is 47 mmHg and this, of course, is independent of altitude. Thus the P_{O_2} of moist inspired gas is given by the expression:

$$PI_{O_2} = 0.2094(P_B - 47)$$

where P_B is barometric pressure.

This equation shows how much more important water vapour pressure becomes at very high altitudes. For example, at sea-level, the water vapour pressure at 37°C is only 6% of the total barometric pressure. However on the summit of Mt Everest, where the barometric pressure is about 250 mmHg, the water vapour pressure is nearly 19% of the total pressure, and the inspired P_{O_2} is correspondingly further reduced (Table 2.1).

It has been pointed out from time to time that a relatively small reduction in body temperature at extreme altitude would confer a substantial increase in inspired P_{O_2}. For example if the body temperature fell to 35°C where the water vapour is 42 mmHg, the P_{O_2} of moist inspired gas would be increased from 42.5 to 43.5 mmHg. This increase of 1 mmHg would be beneficial because the arterial P_{O_2} would increase by approximately the same extent, and since the oxygen dissociation curve is very steep at this point, there would be an appreciable gain in arterial oxygen concentration. However there is no evidence that body temperature falls at extreme altitude. Nor is it reasonable to assume that the temperature in the alveoli where gas exchange takes place would be significantly less than that of the body core temperature.

2.2.8 Physiological significance of barometric pressure at high altitude

Since the barometric pressure directly determines the inspired P_{O_2}, it is clear that the variations of barometric pressure with latitude and season as described in sections 2.2.5 and 2.2.6 will affect the degree of hypoxaemia in the body. For example, a climber on Mt McKinley in Alaska, which is situated at a latitude of 63°N, will be exposed to a considerably lower barometric pressure on the summit than would be the case for a mountain of the same height located in the tropics.

The variations of barometric pressure with latitude and season become particularly significant from a physiological point of view at extreme altitudes such as near the summit of Mt Everest. For example, it has been shown that if the pressure on the Everest summit conformed to the Standard Atmosphere, it would be impossible to climb the mountain without supplementary oxygen (West, 1983). In addition, the variation of barometric pressure with month of the year shown in Figure 2.4 indicates that it would be considerably more difficult to reach the summit without supplementary oxygen in the winter as a result of the reduced inspired P_{O_2}, quite apart from the obvious difficulties of lower temperatures and high winds. Although there have now been many ascents of Everest without supplementary oxygen in the pre-monsoon and post-monsoon seasons, only one person has made a winter ascent without supplementary oxygen. This was Sherpa Ang Rita on 22 December 1987. This topic is considered in more detail in Chapter 11.

2.3 FACTORS OTHER THAN BAROMETRIC PRESSURE AT HIGH ALTITUDE

2.3.1 Temperature

Temperature falls with increasing altitude at the rate of about 1°C for every 150 m. This lapse rate is essentially independent of latitude. The consequence is that on a very high mountain, such as Mt Everest, the average temperature near the summit is predicted to be about −40°C. Most climbers choose the warmer months of the year. In May, a temperature of −27°C was measured at an altitude of 8500 m on Everest (Pugh, 1957) while Pizzo obtained a temperature of −9°C on the summit in October (West *et al.*, 1983a). In the winter the temperatures are much lower. However even then they do not approach the extremely low temperatures seen in northern Canada or Siberia during midwinter.

More important than temperature *per se* is the wind-chill factor. Wind velocities on Himalayan peaks have often been estimated to be in excess of 150 km h^{-1} though few measurements have been made. Such high winds result in extremely severe chill factors at low temperatures and can make climbing impossible. Cold injury is common in the mountains and is discussed in Chapters 24 and 25.

2.3.2 Humidity

Absolute humidity is the amount of water vapour per unit volume of gas at the prevailing temperature. This value is extremely low at high altitude because the water vapour pressure is so depressed at the reduced temperature. Thus even if the air is fully saturated with water vapour, the actual amount will be very small. For example, the water vapour pressure at +20°C is 17 mmHg but only 1 mmHg at −20°C.

Relative humidity is a measure of the amount of water vapour in the air as a percentage of the amount which could be contained at the prevailing temperature. This value may be low, normal or high at altitude. The disparity between absolute and relative humidities is explained by the fact that even saturated air is unable to contain much water vapour because of the very low temperature. If this air is warmed without allowing additional water vapour to form, its relative humidity falls.

The very low absolute humidity at high altitude frequently causes dehydration. First, the insensible water loss caused by ventilation is great because of the dryness of the inspired air. In addition, the levels of ventilation may be extremely high, especially on exercise (Chapter 10), and this increases water loss. For example, near the summit of Mt Everest, the total ventilation is increased some five-fold compared with sea-level for the same level of activity. Water loss through sweating is also increased during work because the air is so dry. It is unusual to see sweat forming at high altitude but this is simply because it is rapidly removed by evaporation as it is formed. Pugh (1964) found that during exercise at 5500 m altitude, the rate of fluid loss from the lungs alone was about 2.9 g water per 100 l of ventilation (BTPS). This is equivalent to about 200 ml of water per hour for moderate exercise.

There is evidence that the dehydration resulting from these rapid fluid losses does not produce as strong a sensation of thirst as at sea-level. As a result, climbers find it is necessary to drink large quantities of fluids at high altitude to remain hydrated even though they have little desire to do so. For men climbing seven hours a day at altitudes over 6000 m, three to four litres of fluid are required in order to maintain a urine output of 1.5 l day^{-1} (Pugh, 1964). Even so it appears that people living at very high altitude are in a state of chronic volume depletion. In a group of subjects living at an altitude of 6300 m during the American Medical Research Expedition to Everest, serum osmolality was significantly increased compared with sea-level in spite of the fact that ample fluids were available and the lifestyle in terms of exercise and diet was not exceptional (Blume *et al.*, 1984).

2.3.3 Solar radiation

The intensity of solar radiation increases markedly at high altitude for two reasons. First the much thinner atmosphere absorbs less of the sun's rays, especially those of short wavelength in the near ultraviolet region of the spectrum. Second, reflection of the sun from snow greatly increases radiation exposure.

The reduced density of the air causes an increase in incident solar radiation of up to 100% at an altitude of 4000 m compared with sea-level (Elterman, 1964). The fact that mountain air is so dry is another important factor because water vapour in the atmosphere absorbs substantial amounts of solar radiation.

The efficiency with which the ground reflects solar radiation is known as its albedo. This varies from less than 20% at sea-level to up to 90% in the presence of snow at great altitudes (Buettner, 1969). Mountaineers are familiar with the extreme intensity of solar radiation especially on a glacier in a valley between two mountains. Here the sunlight is reflected from both sides as well as from the snow or ice on the glacier and the heat can be very oppressive in spite of the great altitude. A consequence of this is the extreme variation in temperature which has been noted in camps under these conditions.

2.3.4 Ionizing radiation

The intensity of cosmic radiation increases at high altitude because there is less of the earth's atmosphere to absorb the rays as they enter from space. This is the reason why cosmic radiation laboratories are often located on high mountains. It has been shown that at an altitude of 3000 m, the increased cosmic radiation results in an increased radiation dose to a human being of approximately 70 m rads (0.0007 Gy) per year. This should be considered in relation to the normal background radiation dose from all sources of 50–200 m rads (0.005–0.002 Gy) per year. The increased ionizing radiation of high altitude has been cited as one of the factors causing acute mountain sickness (Bert, 1878). However there is no scientific basis for this assertion.

REFERENCES

Acosta, J. de (1590) Historia Natural y Moral de las Indias. Iuan de Leon, Lib 3, Cap. 9. Seville. Section of English translation of 1604. Reprinted in *High Altitude Physiology*, (ed. J.B. West), Hutchinson Ross Publishing Company, Stroudsburg, Pennsylvania, 1981.

Bert, P. (1878) *La Pression Barométrique*. Masson, Paris, English translation by M.A. Hitchcock and F.A. Hitchcock. College Book Company, Columbus, Ohio, 1943.

Blume, F.D., Boyer, S.J., Braverman, L.E., *et al.* (1984) Impaired osmoregulation at high altitude. *J. Am. Med. Assoc.*, **252**, 524–6.

Boyle, R. (1662) *New Experiments Physico-Mechanical, Touching the Air*, 2nd edn, Thomas Robinson, Oxford. Relevant pages reprinted in *High Altitude Physiology*, (ed. J.B. West), Hutchinson Ross Publishing Company, Stroudsburg, Pennsylvania, 1981.

Brunt, D. (1952) *Physical and Dynamical Meteorology*, 2nd edn, Cambridge University Press, Cambridge, p. 379.

Buettner, K.J.K. (1969) The effects of natural sunlight on human skin, in *The Biologic Effects of Ultraviolet Radiation with Special Emphasis on the Skin*, (ed. F. Urbach), Pergamon Press, Oxford.

Elterman, L. (1964) *Atmospheric Attenuation Model 1964 in the Ultraviolet Visible and Infrared Regions for Altitudes to 50 km*. US Air Force Cambridge Research Laboratories. Environmental research paper No. 46. AFCRL-64-740.

FitzGerald, M.P. (1913) The changes in the breathing and the blood of various altitudes. *Philos. Trans. R. Soc. London Ser. B.*, **203**, 351–71.

Galileo, G. (1638) *Dialogues Concerning Two New Sciences*. English translation of relevant pages in *High Altitude Physiology*, (ed. J.B. West), Hutchinson Ross Publishing Company, Stroudsburg, Pennsylvania, 1981.

Haldane, J.S. and Priestley, J.G. (1935) *Respiration*, 2nd edn, Yale University Press, New Haven, Connecticut, p. 323.

Hann, J. (1901) *Lehrbuch der Meteorologie*, C. Tauchnitz, Leipzig. English translation by R.D.C. Ward, New York. MacMillan, 1903, p. 222.

Houston, C.S. and Riley, R.L. (1947) Respiratory and circulatory changes during acclimatization to high altitude. *Am. J. Physiol.*, **149**, 565–88.

Houston, C.S., Sutton, J.R., Cymerman, A. and Reeves, J.T. (1987) Operation Everest II: man at extreme altitude. *J. Appl. Physiol.*, **63**, 877–82.

International Civil Aviation Organization (1964) *Manual of the ICAO Standard Atmosphere*, 2nd edn, Int. Civil Aviation Org., Montreal, Quebec.

Kellas, A.M. (1917) A consideration of the possibility of ascending the loftier Himalaya. *Geogr. J.*, **49**, 26–47.

National Oceanic and Atmospheric Administration (1976) *US Standard Atmosphere, 1976*. NOAA, Washington, DC.

Oort, A.H. and Rasmusson, E.M. (1971) *Atmospheric Circulation Statistics*, US Dept. of Commerce, NOAA, Rockville, Maryland, pp. 84–5.

Pascal, B. (1648) *Story of the great experiment on the equilibrium of fluids*. English translation of relevant pages in *High Altitude Physiology*, (ed. J.B. West), Hutchinson Ross Publishing Company, Stroudsburg, Pennsylvania, 1981.

Pugh, L.G.C.E. (1957) Resting ventilation and alveolar air on Mount Everest: with remarks on the relation of barometric pressure to altitude in mountains. *J. Physiol. London*, **135**, 590–610.

Pugh, L.G.C.E. (1964) Animals in high altitude: man above 5000 meters – mountain exploration, in *Handbook of Physiology. Adaptation to the Environment*. Am. Physiol. Soc., Washington DC, sect. 4, pp. 861–8.

Pugh, L.G.C.E., Gill, M.B., Lahiri, S., *et al.* (1964) Muscular exercise at great altitude. *J. Appl. Physiol.*, **19**, 431–40.

Rahn, H. and Fenn, W.O. (1955) *A Graphical Analysis of the Respiratory Gas Exchange*. Am. Physiol. Soc., Washington, DC.

Riley, R.L. and Houston, C.S. (1950–1) Composition of alveolar air and volume of pulmonary ventilation during long exposure to high altitude. *J. Appl. Physiol.*, **3**, 526–34.

Torricelli, E. (1644) Letter of Torricelli to Michelangelo Ricci. English translation of relevant pages in *High Altitude Physiology*, (ed. J.B. West), Hutchinson Ross Publishing Company, Stroudsburg, Pennsylvania, 1981.

West, J.B. (1983) Climbing Mt Everest without supplementary oxygen: an analysis of maximal exercise during extreme hypoxia. *Respir. Physiol.*, **52**, 265–79.

West J.B. (1993) Acctimatization and tolerance to extreme altitude. *J. Wild. Med.*, **4**, 17–26.

West, J.B., Hackett, P., Maret, K.H., *et al.* (1983a) Pulmonary gas exchange on the summit of Mount Everest. *J. Appl. Physiol.*, **55**, 678–87.

West, J.B., Lahiri, S., Maret, K.H., *et al.* (1983b) Barometric pressures at extreme altitudes on Mt Everest: physiological significance. *J. Appl. Physiol.*, **54**, 1188–94.

Zuntz, N., Loewy, A., Muller, F. and Caspari, W. (1906) Atmospheric pressure at high altitudes. In *Höhenklima und Bergwanderungen in ihrer Wirkung auf den Menschen*, Bong, Berlin, pp. 37–9. Translation of relevant pages in *High Altitude Physiology*, (ed. J.B. West), Hutchinson Ross Publishing Company, Stroudsburg, Pennsylvania, 1981.

3

Geography and the human response to altitude

3.1 INTRODUCTION

Although the expression 'high altitude' has no precise definition, the majority of individuals have certain clinical, physiological, anatomical and biochemical changes which occur at levels above 3000 m. Individual variation is, however, considerable and some people are affected at levels as low as 2000 m. For sea-level visitors, an altitude of 4600–4900 m represents the highest acceptable level for permanent habitation, whilst for high altitude residents 5800–6000 m is the highest so far recorded (West, 1986). At greater altitudes physical and mental deterioration occurs and permanent habitation is not possible (section 3.8.2; Chapter 16). In South America archaeological sites have been found at 6271 m on Llullaillaco, but there is no evidence that these were permanent dwellings.

The main areas of the world above 3000 m are:

- The Tibetan plateau
- The Himalayan range and its valleys
- The Tien Shan and Pamir
- The mountain ranges of east Turkey, Iran, Afghanistan, and Pakistan
- The Rocky mountains and Sierra Nevada of the USA and Canada
- The Sierra Madre of Mexico
- The Andes of South America
- The European Alps
- The Pyrenees between Spain and France
- The Atlas mountains of North Africa
- The Ethiopian highlands
- The mountains of East and South Africa
- The plateau and mountains of Antarctica
- New Guinea and other small regions such as Hawaii, Tenerife, New Zealand.

The three main regions that support large populations are the Tibetan plateau and Himalayan valleys, the Andes of South America, and the Ethiopian highlands. Although the plateau and peaks of Antarctica cover a large area there is no indigenous population.

3.1.1 The Himalayas and Tibetan plateau

The Himalayas form a topographically extremely complex region, extending 1500 miles from Nanga Parbat (8125 m) in the west to Namcha Barwa (7756 m) in the east. At its western extremity it is part of a confused mass of peaks, passes and glaciers where the western Kun Lun, Karakoram, Pir Panjal and Pamirs form an area the size of France. The Himalayas contain the world's highest mountain, Everest (8848 m) and many other peaks over 7500 m. The main range forms the watershed between Central Asia and India, and there are middle ranges at intermediate altitudes. The outer Himalayas (up to 1500 m) form foothills rising from the plains of India.

The Tibetan plateau is an area occupied by Tibetans, who have a well defined culture. It extends in the south, to the Himalayas and high Himalayan valleys. To the west the plateau is demarcated by the northward curve of the Himalayas which continues into Kashmir, Baltistan and then to Gilgit and the Karakoram. To the north the peaks (up to 7700 m) of the Kun Lun range, 1500 miles long, mark off the plateau of Tibet from Xinjiang (Chinese Turkestan), whilst to the east it extends to the Koko Nor or Qinghai lake and, further south, the valleys of Qinghai and Sikiang and the gorge country of southeast Tibet.

The area covers about 1.5 million square miles and is the largest and highest plateau in the world, much of it between 4600–4900 m. It presents an enormous range of climate and topography. 'Every 10 li (3 miles) heaven is different.' The major climatic contrast is between the southern side of the Himalayas and the high valleys exposed to the summer Indian monsoon with very high rainfall, particularly in the east, and the aridity and low rainfall of the Tibetan plateau. The change is so abrupt that in some passes in the eastern Himalayas, vegetation may change from tropical to subarctic within a few yards.

The Tibetans believe that in the prehistoric era their land was a large sea, Tethys, which according to the Theory of Plate Tectonics, is correct. The Royal Society/Chinese Academy of Sciences Tibet Geotraverse in 1985–1986 established that the thickness of the Tibetan plateau crust, which at 70 km is about twice that of normal, is due mainly to folding and thrusting that has occurred as a result of India colliding with Asia, rather than India moving under Asia and elevating to a plateau (Chang *et al.*, 1986). In mythology, Tibetans are descended from the union of a forest monkey and a demoness of the rocks, with the site of the first cultivated field being at Sothang in southeast Tibet but other legends place their origin further east.

The Tibetans have always regarded themselves as living in the northern part of the world; the Indians, however, considered the Himalayas to be the abode of the Gods and inhabited by a race of supermen gifted with special knowledge, particularly of magic, and this probably accounts for the popular European belief of Tibet as a place where the immortal sages dwell, guarding the ultimate secrets. Far from being isolated, however, Tibetans have been subject to influences from China, India, Central Asia and the Middle East for many centuries (Stein, 1972).

There are 2.5–3.0 million people living over 3000 m, and it is estimated that the amount of this land available for agriculture is 5%. In the valleys, fields are terraced, whilst on the plateau, larger fields are found in sheltered areas on valley floors, but all are threatened by snow, hail, wind and erosion. Permanent buildings are found up to 3500 m with nomadic populations at higher levels. Neolithic human remains have been found near Lhasa (Ward, 1990, 1991).

3.1.2 Andes of South America

The highland zone extends from Colombia in the north to Central Chile in the south, and is flanked by an arid desert on its west, with a deeply eroded escarpment to the east which adjoins the Amazon basin.

The central Andean region has three broadly defined areas running parallel with the Pacific Ocean: the Cordillera Occidentale, the Altiplano, a broad undulating plain at 4000 m in the middle, and the Cordillera Orientale in the east.

The earliest archaeological evidence for human occupation dates back 20 000 years (MacNeish, 1971) and has been found at Ayacucho, Peru at 2900 m, whilst other early finds are recorded in central Chile, Venezuela and Argentina. The skeleton of a man who lived 9500 years ago has been found at Lauricocha (4200 m) in Peru (Hurtado, 1971). The pre-Inca civilizations were situated mainly along the Pacific Coast and the population subsisted mainly on seafood. Little is known of the highland population during this period.

The Inca civilization only achieved a position of major importance in the 100 years preceding the Spanish invasion of 1532. Spanish settlement of highland areas was hindered by ecological restraints imposed by altitude and the nature of the terrain, and, after consolidation of Spanish rule, Peru remained under colonial domination for 300 years, achieving independence in 1824.

Both agriculture and stock raising dominate the subsistence economy, with the upper limit of agriculture at 4000 m and the upper limit of vegetation at 4600 m. Mining is carried out at even greater altitudes.

3.1.3 Ethiopian highlands

No well circumscribed highland zone exists. The country is intersected by a number of rift valley systems, establishing a connection between the African rift valley in the south with the Red Sea; this is responsible for the division of the country into three reasonably well defined regions. These are the western highlands, the eastern highlands and the rift valley itself with the lowland area.

The northern part of the western highlands, the Amhara highlands, attain the greatest altitude (2400–3700 m). The highest peak of Ethiopia, Ras Dashau (4620 m) is a volcanic outcrop and Lake Tana, the origin of the Blue Nile, lies at the centre of the region. Much of Ethiopian history centres on this area, which has been settled for many centuries. It is inhabited by the largest of Ethiopia's many population groups, the Amharas and Tigraeans, who are the descendants of people who came from southern Arabia prior to 1000 BC (Sellassie, 1972).

Gondar (3000 m) in the Amhara highlands, with a population of 100 000, became the second largest city in Africa, and it remained the capital of Ethiopia until the middle of the first century, when Addis Ababa was founded.

Much of the population of Ethiopia lives above 2000 m and in the highland area two types of cultivation, by plough and by hoe, predominate. Teff, a type of grass which produces a small seed, is grown up to 3000 m and is the mainstay of the agricultural economy.

3.2 TERRAIN

Although mountain country varies widely, there are two distinct types: the high, flat, plateaux (Tibet and the altiplano of South America) and deep valleys (Himalayas and Andes).

Plateaux can support large populations and large towns but they may be isolated by virtue of distance from lowland cities, which are usually the centre of government, commerce and industry.

In mountain valleys, because flat ground is at a premium, populations tend to be smaller, with groups perched on slopes and ridges far from one another. The placing of houses in sunny positions is more difficult and isolation within the community is common. Communications are easily severed by land slips, avalanches and other natural disasters. The funnelling effect of valleys on wind may increase its velocity with an ensuing stunting effect on vegetation and trees. This also restricts the placing of houses as does the availability of water and the possibility of natural disasters.

3.3 CLIMATE

The climate near the ground at high altitude has several basic features.

At any given latitude, seasonal variation of monthly temperature is less at high altitude than at sea-level and, as the equator is reached, seasonal variation virtually disappears. Diurnal variations are considerable, and can show a range of 30°C. This is because of high levels of long wave radiation that occur in cloudless skies during the day and escape to clear skies at night. In overcast conditions the diurnal variation decreases.

With increasing altitude the temperature falls. There is no uniform value for decline although the figure 1°C for every 150 m is usually given.

Solar radiation is an important factor in maintaining thermal balance in man at extreme altitude.

3.3.1 Rainfall

In Asia, the monsoon flows from east to west across India, cooling as it is forced to ascend by the Himalayas. Water vapour condenses and falls as rain, and as it passes to the west it becomes depleted of water, the eastern Himalayas being very wet, the western dry.

In Darjeeling the annual rainfall is 2000–3000 mm a year; in the central Himalayas at Simla it is 1500 mm, whilst in the west at Ladakh it is 75 mm. The Karakoram is arid whilst the eastern Himalayan region is tropical.

There is also considerable north–south variation with palaearctic species on the Tibetan plateau and tropical species often only a few hundred yards away to the south. This is particularly marked on some passes in the eastern Himalayas. On the plateau, although 'monsoon' clouds are seen on the Tangulla range, about 700 km north of Lhasa precipitation is small. In the deserts of the Tarim basin and Tsaidam to the north of the Tibetan plateau, annual rainfall may be less than 100 mm a year.

In the Andes the Pacific coastal strip is desert. 'It never rains in Lima.' Along the whole length of the coast the cold Humboldt current cools the air above the sea, reducing its capacity to retain moisture which normally falls as rain. Once air passes over the land, it is warmed again and increases its capacity to retain moisture, making rain unlikely.

The western slopes of the Andes are dry, cacti and eucalyptus trees flourish and only a few high mountains are snow covered. The eastern slopes which descend to the Amazon basin become progressively more humid and tree covered.

The rainfall in the UK and Europe is influenced by the gulf stream and records between 1884 and 1901, kept by the observatory on the summit of Ben Nevis, Scotland (1300 mm), the highest peak in the UK, show that the average daily sunshine was only two hours and the annual rainfall was 3500 mm, similar or higher than in Darjeeling (MacPhee, 1936).

3.3.2 Temperature

The fall in temperature globally with altitude has been discussed in Chapter 2, however, the temperature of mountain regions is very variable and records of the observatory on the summit of Ben Nevis (1300 m) between 1884 and 1901 show that the mean temperature over these 17 years was −0.1°C; the lowest temperature was −17°C and the highest +19°C. On the plateau of the Cairngorms in Scotland, which has an average height of around 1000 m, similar temperatures have been recorded with winds gusting to over 160 km hr^{-1} (100 mph).

In North America, Alaska and the Yukon a number of peaks of 6000 m lie within the Arctic circles. Because of their latitude the barometric pressure, and therefore alveolar P_{O_2}, is lower than peaks of a corresponding altitude in the Himalayas, which are at a latitude of 28°N. They therefore appear to be 'higher', with all the corresponding dangers of mountain sickness and altitude deterioration (Chapter 2). Temperatures of −30°C at 5500–6000 m have been recorded, with gale force winds, in the winter (Mills, 1973).

In the European Alps, the average temperature was −13°C during a winter expedition up to 4000 m, carried out over several days, in the Bernese Oberland in Switzerland (Leuthold *et al.*, 1975); gale force winds were not uncommon. Temperatures on the summit of Everest (8848 m) in winter are probably of the order of −60°C, whilst in summer the average temperature would be about −20°C. Hillary recorded a temperature of −27°C at 8500 m on Everest at 3 a.m. on 29 May 1953, the day the first ascent was made (Ward, 1993). On the Changthang (the northern part of the Tibetan plateau) which has an average height of 4900 m, there are few days when the temperature reaches as high as 10°C and −25°C has been recorded.

In Lhasa (3658 m) there are about 100 days a year when the temperatures are around 10°C; in summer it may rise as high as 27°C whilst in the winter it falls to −15°C.

In Antarctica, the lowest recorded temperature is −88.2°C and the highest 15.2°C. The dangers of cold injury, therefore, are likely to complicate accidents or illness in mountain regions.

3.3.3 Humidity

This influences heat loss from the body by evaporation, and, in regions where the humidity is high, heat regulation is more difficult. In arid areas with a low humidity, heat regulation is easier.

3.3.4 Solar radiation

Although temperature falls with altitude there is increased exposure to solar radiation (Chapter 2). The amount absorbed by the body depends on clothing and posture. The clear mountain air permits an increased degree of direct radiation which is enhanced by indirect radiation reflected from the snow. The altitude of the sun is also important (Chrenko and Pugh, 1961). The solar heat absorbed depends on the type of clothing as dark clothing absorbs more than light.

3.3.5 Ultraviolet radiation

There appears to be some increase in the level of ultraviolet radiation at high altitude.

Snow reflects up to 90% of ultraviolet radiation compared with 9–17% reflected from ground covered by grass (Buettner, 1969). Hence in snow covered terrain the combination of direct (incident) and reflected ultraviolet radiation is considerable.

3.4 ECONOMY

Most mountain communities depend on animal husbandry and agriculture; mining is important in some regions whilst more recently tourism is assuming a greater significance.

Animal husbandry predominates in regions above the limit of agriculture. On the Tibetan plateau, or Changtang, which covers two-thirds of Tibet, there are immense herds of yak, sheep and goats herded by nomads. In the bitter climate nomadic pastoralism is the only viable and economic way of life and this may have started between nine and ten thousand years ago. The survival of the animals depends exclusively on natural fodder, which creates problems as the sedges and grasses have only a short growing season between May and September. Because there are no areas on the plateau where grass will grow in the winter they cannot escape the climate and, as extensive migration would weaken the stock, only short distances, up to 40 miles, are traversed. Each family has a 'home base', which is sometimes a house, and migrates to set areas whose boundaries, though not fenced, are all well known. Here, tents made of yak and sheep's wool are used as dwellings. Further north camels are common (Goldstein and Beall, 1989). In the upper Himalayan valleys the pattern is similar, with flocks spending the summer on pastures up to 5000 m, but below the snow-line, whilst in the winter they return to more permanent and protected locations at 4000 m.

The llama (*Lama glama*) and yak (*Bos grunniens*) are extremely important to the economy of the populations of the South American altiplano, and of Tibet and the Himalayan valleys. Both these species show genetic adaptation to high altitude (Chapter 16).

The limiting factor in agriculture is the number of months that the soil remains frozen; a single period of the year only may be available for cultivation. The type of crop may influence the size of population. Potatoes introduced into the high Himalayan valleys of Nepal between 1850 and 1860 increased the population of Sola Khumbu in the Everest region from 169 households in 1836 to 596 in 1957 (Fuhrer-Haimendorf, 1964). Immigrants came from Tibet over the Nangpa La, a glacier pass of 5800 m, and, because food was more abundant, were able to adopt the religious life and built many new monasteries.

Increasing the productivity of the land, as well as the area under cultivation in Tibet, may change the pattern of life near the centres of population under the present Chinese-organized regime. Level land may have to be manufactured in the form of terraces, which range in size from a few square feet to a relatively large area, which is usually too small for pasture. Irrigation may involve ingenious construction of water conduits from surrounding streams. The task of building and maintaining terraces is considerable, especially as manure has to be carried up and placed manually. Despite this, terracing is a marked feature of populated mountain valleys and, as it involves ownership and maintenance by groups rather than individuals, the social implications are important. High grazing pasture (alps) is also communal pasture land and this too has social overtones.

Mining, which is often carried out above the pasture level or in rocky terrain, may involve the building of special towns and roads. Frisancho (1988) suggests that one reason for the relatively high haemoglobin concentration observed in Andean high altitude populations as opposed to the Himalayan is that miners (amongst whom respiratory disease is common) were included in some Andean samples. In Tibet gold mining has been carried on for centuries, often at 5000 m. However, shallow trenches were used and no deep mines were worked. Recently a gold mine in northern Chile has been established at 4500 m.

Tourism, particularly skiing, may involve developing an area which has no natural amenities except good snow fields and glaciers. Sixteen thousand tourists visited the Everest region in 1992 and pollution, often in the form of non-biodegradable rubbish, is a considerable problem.

Isolation, together with unexplained natural catastrophes, will contribute to the undoubted tendency that mountain people have towards the religious life. Once this is established, the disinclination to accept change, so prevalent in religious dominated communities, will prevent the development of such communities and they will then become easy prey to their more technically advanced neighbours.

3.5 HOUSES AND SHELTER

Cultural mechanisms which provide a comfortable microclimate and reduce heat loss have been developed in all high altitude communities. The ideal house should be draught free with a low surface area to volume ratio and well constructed of material which diminishes the daily extremes of temperature. The roof should be well insulated.

In the Andes the adobe (dried mud) building has the first metre or so of the walls made of stone, the roof is of tile, grass or tin and walls are plastered with mud to provide an airtight structure; the roof is tightly fitted and the floor may be wood or dirt. Because of the method of construction the diurnal change is reduced (Baker, 1966). In the Himalayas the thermal protection of stone structures built for semi-nomadic occupation appears to be less. Sherpa houses often have only one storey, with stone walls and wooden roofs held on with stones. The ground floor is without windows and provides quarters for animals; the first floor is for human habitation. Windows usually have no glass, but have wooden shutters, and an open fire is placed in the centre of one side, but this provides only a transient increase in temperature.

In north Bhutan houses are similarly constructed but animals are kept in a yard. Cracks between stones in both Bhutanese and Sherpa houses are filled with earth. Tibetan houses may be of more than one storey and are often in terraces. Glass is rare and they too are heated by an open fire or stove. Nomads have tents with a loose wide weave which enables warm air to be entrapped but allows egress of smoke from open fires and is waterproof. However some semi-nomadic families have a stove with a chimney.

3.6 CLOTHING

Because of the generally low temperature and loss of heat, particularly due to radiation and convection, clothing with good insulation is necessary to provide a warm microclimate. Trapped, still air is the best insulation and wool is the best naturally available insulating material; it resists compacting and loses only 40% of its insulating value when wet. Garments that are loosely woven entrap more air than those that are tightly weaved.

A multiple layered system for garments is preferable to one thick layer because insulation can be varied at will, thus minimizing perspiration. The outer layer should be as impermeable to wind as possible. A sheepskin coat is the best naturally available garment which has many of these characteristics and is usually worn with cotton or wool undergarments.

In general, Andean clothing conforms to the above model and natural clothing is adequate for the conditions encountered. Measurements of insulation of normal clothing without hats, shawls and ponchos showed values for men slightly less than those for women (Little and Hanna, 1978). The greatest increase in surface temperature occurred in the hands and feet. At night, Andean highlanders, who use a bedding of skins, can maintain their metabolic rate by light shivering that does not disturb sleep.

In the high Himalayan valleys and Tibet, clothing assemblies are similar. The main garment is a thick sheepskin 'chupa' with 15 cm (6 inch) sleeves which when extended keep the hands warm; gloves are never used. Normally the garment is gathered around the waist by a belt and hitched up to the knees so that there is a pocket for loose objects in front of the chest. When the belt is loosened the garment extends to the ground and thus can be used as a sleeping robe; often in warm conditions one or both shoulders are left bare. Under this is a woollen shirt and often long woollen, cotton or sheepskin trousers. A soft leather boot with decorative wool leggings extending to the knees is packed with grass, straw or leaves but a Tibetan often may walk in bare feet in the snow or through streams. Some wear a felt hat or balaclava and, to prevent snow blindness, yak hair is put in front of the eyes if goggles are not available (Desideri, 1712–27; Moorcroft and Trebeck, 1841). Other methods used by Tibetans include blackening the eyelids and wearing masks with tiny eye holes, the rims of which were blackened (MacDonald, 1929). Cotton clothing is favoured at high temperatures and low altitudes, whilst nomads wear wool or sheepskin. Many now wear wool sweaters and leather boots. Tibetan nomads sleep whilst resting on their elbows and knees with all their clothes piled on their backs (Holditch, 1907). This 'foetal position' diminishes surface area and therefore heat loss: contact with the ground is also minimal.

Some Tibetan llamas have developed the ability to 'warm without fire'. The central core temperature is kept raised under cold conditions, both by increasing the metabolic rate, probably by continuous light shivering, and also by the practice of g-tum-mo yoga, which appears to involve peripheral vasodilatation (Pugh, 1963; Benson *et al.*, 1982).

Children have oil rubbed over their bodies and adults seldom wash, the natural skin oils forming a protective layer. Very few Tibetans living on the plateau are obese (Bell, 1928).

3.7 POPULATION

Most of the high altitude areas of the world are in the economically least developed regions and for this reason population numbers in relation to altitude are difficult to obtain. Whilst the total population living in mountainous regions is estimated at 400 million, the majority live at low altitude in the valleys. De Jong (1968) 'guessed' that between 13 and 14 million people lived at altitudes above 3000 m.

In South America large populations have lived at high altitude since pre-history and the Andean population at the time of the Spanish conquest was estimated as between 4.5 and 7.5 million. In 1980 it was considered that between 10 and 17 million were living at over 2500 m and in Peru 30–40% of the population of 4 million lived at or above this height, with 1.5% living at over 4000 m.

In Asia and Africa the estimates are less accurate. On the Tibetan plateau, which consists of the autonomous region of Tibet (Xizang) and Qinghai Province, the population is estimated as between 4 and 5 million. Lhasa (3658 m), in 1986, had about 130 000 inhabitants, mainly Tibetan but recent immigration of Han Chinese has increased this number. Relatively small groups, nomads (at up to 5450 m), and miners (at up to 6000 m), live at higher levels. Fairly large numbers live at altitudes exceeding 3000 m in the upper valleys of eastern Tibet, whilst in Nepal about 60 000 live above this level with a number of villages in Dolpo being at 5000 m (Snellgrove, 1961). In Ethiopia about 50% of the total population of 26 million live above 2000 m. Small populations in Mexico, the USA and the former USSR live above the 3000 m level.

In the mainly subsistence economy of high mountain regions survival means the capacity to perform physical work and high altitude natives living at altitude have a capacity similar to that of low-altitude dwellers at low altitude. Many live to over 80 years of age and a Tibetan female hermit is said to have died at the age of 130 years (Taring, 1970) (Section 16.2.1), whilst the founder of traditional Tibetan medicine, Yu-Thog, is considered to have lived to the age of 125 years.

In tropical latitudes permanent settlements are usually placed where both pasture and timber can be used and the upper limit of habitation may fall between the two. Further from the equator the upper limit falls below the timber line and variation in temperature becomes seasonal; the upper pasturelands are thus used for a semi-nomadic economy. Permanently inhabited villages are found at lower levels with isolated groups of buildings or shelters on the pastures occupied for the grazing season and evacuated during the winter. Considerable migration may occur and part of the population may always be on the move. Mines are worked at 5950 m in South America where, although the miners live at rather lower altitudes, the caretakers live there permanently (West, 1986).

Those who spend periods at greater altitude are mountaineers, who have evolved specialized techniques of movement above the snow-line. In winter, movement across snow is essential for the feeding of livestock quartered in isolated shelters. Since pre-historic times boards have been placed on the feet to facilitate movement and the earliest references to primitive skis are found in the Nordic sagas of 3000 BC and, in northern Norway, rock engravings of skiers are dated at around 2500 BC. In the UK skis were used in Cumberland at the start of the eighteenth century. The modern sport dates from 1870. No historical evidence of the use of skis has been found in South American or Tibetan populations.

Highland populations, being strategically placed between prosperous lowland centres, play a vital role in trade. Because they are physiologically well adapted they are capable of crossing high mountain passes with heavy loads and use their animals to carry produce. Major mountain passes have for centuries been arteries for trade, the movement of people and ideas, and the dissemination of disease. The closing of passes such as the Nangpa La between the two different economies of Tibet and Nepal caused a fall in living standards until readjustments had been made.

3.8 HUMAN RESPONSE TO COLD AND ALTITUDE

The main environmental stresses of living in mountain regions are the hypoxia of altitude and cold.

3.8.1 Cold

This is a more important factor than altitude in colonizing high mountainous regions; high-altitude residents seem to withstand cold better than sea-level visitors to altitude.

Most of the process of adaptation to cold consists of the adoption of clothing and housing which reduce cold stress by maintaining a microclimate as close as possible to the preferred temperature. However, some studies have demonstrated different physiological responses in high altitude residents to experimental cold stress compared with low altitude controls. These have been summarized by

Little and Hanna (1978) in drawing from work on Andean and Tibetan high altitude residents.

In response to abrupt exposure to cold, high-altitude residents, when contrasted with sea-level Caucasian control subjects, show the following responses:

- no dramatic fall of core temperature;
- a slightly elevated basal metabolic rate;
- consistently high surface temperatures in extremities;
- a slightly greater loss of body heat.

These changes are probably the result of lifelong intermittent exposure to modest cold stress rather than cold plus altitude. Pugh (1963) found a number of these responses in a Nepalese pilgrim studied at 4500 m, who came from a village at only 1800 m. Benson *et al.* (1982) found similar changes in Tibetans practising g-tum-mo yoga (an advanced form of Tibetan yoga). The elevation of basal metabolic rate may be the effect of hypoxia and cold acting together (Little and Hanna, 1978). Further aspects of cold adaptation are considered in Chapter 19.

3.8.2 Hypoxia

The responses of an animal organism to hypoxia are complex and far reaching. They depend amongst other things upon the severity of and the rate at which hypoxia is imposed. Severe sudden hypoxia as experienced, for instance, by aviators if they lose cabin pressure at altitude, produces an entirely different result to the effect of the same altitude reached by a climber after weeks of acclimatization, whilst people with lifelong exposure to altitude develop further changes in response to hypoxia when compared with even well acclimatized lowlanders. Further adaptations may come about after a species has lived at altitude for generations, due to natural selection of genes advantageous to life in the hypoxic environment.

Broadly, the responses to hypoxia can be divided into four categories according to the duration of hypoxia:

- acute hypoxia, from seconds to an hour or two;
- chronic hypoxia from hours to many years (i.e. sea-level residents going to altitude, subjects of chamber experiments, mountaineers and those who go to live and work in the high mining towns of North and South America and Tibet);
- lifelong hypoxia (i.e. altitude residents who were born, bred and live at altitude);
- species who have lived at altitude for generations.

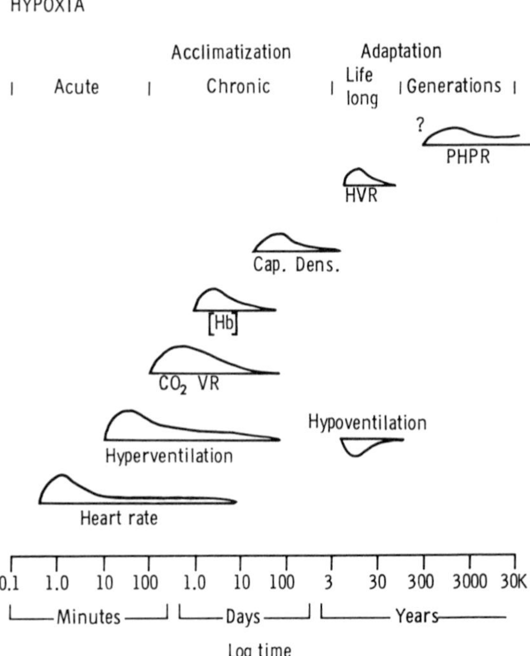

Figure 3.1 Time courses of a number of acclimatization and adaptive changes plotted on a log time scale, the curve of each response denoting the rate of change, which is fast at first then tailing off. Included are: heart rate, hyper- and hypoventilation, the CO_2 ventilatory response (CO_2 VR), haemoglobin concentration ([Hb]), changes in capillary density (Cap. Dens.), hypoxic ventilatory response (HVR) and the pulmonary hypoxic pressor response (PHPR).

Obviously these times are rather arbitrary and the second category, chronic hypoxia, needs subdividing when describing changes in various systems.

Figure 3.1 shows the time course of a number of acclimatization and adaptive changes on a log time scale. The processes are considered in detail in later chapters. This figure shows the impossibility of answering the question commonly asked, 'How long does it take to become acclimatized?'

Acute hypoxia

The effect of acute, often severe, hypoxia has been studied intensively since Paul Bert first pointed out the danger of ascent to high altitude to early balloonists (Chapter 1).

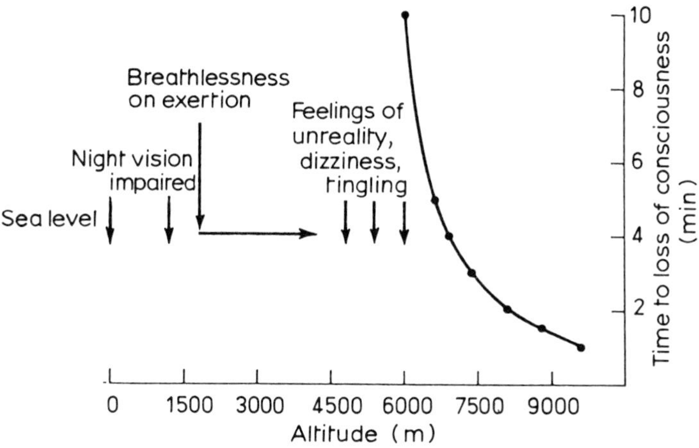

Figure 3.2 The effect of sudden exposure to various altitudes. At extreme altitude consciousness will be lost after an average time indicated by the curve on the right. There is considerable variability in this time. (Data from Sharp, 1978.)

Figure 3.2 shows the effect of sudden exposure to various, increasing altitudes. At modest altitude breathlessness may be felt on exertion and some rise in heart rate noticed but the main effect is on the central nervous system. At levels as low as 1500 m night vision is impaired (Pretorius, 1970). At 4000–5000 m some tingling of the fingers and mouth may be noticed but, although the subject would now definitely be hypoxic, there would be very little subjective sensation to indicate this fact. Above about 5000 m some subjects may become unconscious and above 7000 m most will do so (Sharp, 1978). Figure 3.2 shows the average time to loss of consciousness after sudden exposure to given altitudes. It will be seen that, on acute exposure to the altitude equivalent to the summit of Everest, the unacclimatized subject remains conscious for only about two minutes.

Chronic hypoxia

Acclimatization

The fact that man can not only remain conscious on the summit of Mount Everest (8848 m), but actually climb there without supplementary oxygen, is due to a number of changes that take place over a period of hours to months at altitude. These changes, termed acclimatization, occur in different systems of the body and have different time courses as shown in Figure 3.1.

These time courses are only approximate. In some cases they involve a biphasic response; for instance, the heart rate response to hypoxia shows a rise within minutes followed by a fall over weeks at altitude (Chapter 6). The change measured can include two responses with different time courses (e.g. minute ventilation which involves the rapid hypoxic ventilatory response, within a few minutes, followed by the slow change of the CO_2 response, in 1–20 days (Chapter 4). Similarly, the well known increase in haemoglobin concentration in the blood is due to the rapid decrease in plasma volume followed by the much slower increase in the red cell mass (Chapter 7).

Adaptation

This term is usually used to denote changes which take place over decades or are the result of being born and bred in the mountain environment and which fit the individual for life at altitude. Examples include the increase in the number of branches leaving the main coronary trunks (Chapter 6) and blunting of the hypoxic ventilatory response (Chapter 4).

This term is also used to denote changes observed in high altitude species as a result of evolutionary pressure selecting for genes which give an advantage at altitude. One example of such an adaptation is the high altitude yak which has been shown to have lost its pulmonary artery pressor response in contrast to the low altitude cow. This seems to be due to a single dominant gene (Harris, 1986). Recent work in Tibet suggests that the population there may also have adapted in this way (Section 16.4.5). The time course for these changes is shown in Figure 3.1.

High-altitude deterioration

The term high-altitude deterioration was first used by members of early Everest expeditions to denote a deterioration in human mental and physical condition as a result of prolonged stay at altitude. The condition had been noted by Filippi (1912) during an expedition to the Karakoram. He writes:

> The atmosphere of the expedition did work some evil effect revealing itself only gradually after several weeks of life above 17 500 feet in a slow decrease of appetite and consequent lack of nourishment without, however, any disturbance of digestive function.
> *F. de Filippi (1912)*

On high-altitude expeditions deterioration can frequently be attributed to factors such as dehydration, starvation, physical exhaustion and cold. However, in the absence of such factors it seems that hypoxia *per se* can cause deterioration if sufficiently severe (Pugh, 1962). The altitude at which this becomes manifest is about 5000–6000 m, with considerable individual variation. Highlanders can probably tolerate prolonged periods at a higher altitude better than can most lowlanders (West, 1986).

High-altitude deterioration (in the absence of dehydration, starvation etc.) is characterized by weight loss, poor appetite, slow recovery from fatigue, lethargy, irritability and an increasing lack of will-power to start new tasks (Ward, 1954). The specific mechanisms underlying this deterioration are unknown. An attempt to investigate the mechanism underlying the recovery from fatigue of muscles under hypoxia was made by Milledge *et al.* (1977), who followed the resynthesis of muscle glycogen after depletion by exercise at sea-level under normoxia and hypoxia. They showed that, although the rate of resynthesis was not significantly slowed by hypoxia in the muscle overall, there was an enhancement of the difference between the Type I and Type II fibres. This suggested that hypoxia depresses glycogen synthesis in Type I though not Type II fibres. This might contribute to the slowness of recovery from severe exercise at high altitude.

REFERENCES

Baker, P.T. (1966) Microenvironment cold in a high altitude Peruvian population, in *Human Adaptability and Its Methodology*, (eds H. Yoshimura and J.S. Weiner), Japanese Society for the Promotion of Sciences, Tokyo, pp. 67–77.

Bell, C. (1928) *The People of Tibet*. Oxford University Press, Oxford, p. 197.

Benson, H., Lehmann, J.W., Malhotra, M.S., *et al.* (1982) Body temperature changes during the practice of g-tum-mo yoga. *Nature*, **295**, 234–6.

Buettner, K.J.K. (1969) The effect of natural sunlight on human skin, in *The Biologic Effects of Ultraviolet Radiation with Special Emphasis on the Skin*, (ed. F. Urbach), Pergamon Press, Oxford, pp. 237–49.

Chang, C., Chen, N., Coward, M.P., *et al.* (1986) Preliminary conclusions of the Royal Society and Academia Sinica 1985 Geotraverse of Tibet. *Nature*, **323**, 501–7.

Chrenko, F.A. and Pugh, L.G.C.E. (1961) The contribution of solar radiation to the thermal environment of man in Antarctica. *Proc. R. Soc. Lond. [Biol]*., **155**, 243–65.

De Filippi, F. (1912) *Karakoram and Western Himalaya, 1900*. Constable, London, p. 364.

De Jong, G.F. (ed.) (1968) *Demography of high altitude populations*. WHO/PAHO/IBP Meeting of Investigators on Population Biology of Altitude, Pan American Health Organisation, Washington DC.

Desideri, I. (1712–1727) Journey across the great desert of Nguari Giongar, and assistance reudered by a Tartar princess and her followers, in *An Account of Tibet*, (ed. F. de Filippi), (1932), Routledge, London, p. 87.

Frisancho, A.R. (1988) Origins of differences in hemoglobin concentration between Himalayan and Andean populations. *Respir. Physiol.*, **72**, 13–18.

Fuhrer-Haimendorf, C. von (1964) *The Sherpas of Nepal: Bhuddist Highlanders*, John Murray, London, p. 10.

Goldstein, M.C. and Beall, C.M. (1989) *Nomads of Western Tibet*, Serindia, London.

Harris, P. (1986) Evolution, hypoxia and high altitude, in *Aspects of Hypoxia*, (ed. D. Heath), Liverpool University Press, Liverpool, pp. 207–16.

Holditch, T. (1907) *Tibet the Mysterious*, Alston Rivers, London, pp. 242–3.

Hurtado, A. (1971) The influence of high altitude on physiology, in *High Altitude Physiology*, (eds R. Porter and J. Knight), Ciba Foundation Symposium, Churchill Livingstone, Edinburgh, p. 3.

Leuthold, E., Hartmann, G., Buhlman, R., et al. (1975) Medical and physiological investigations on mountaineers. A field study during a winter climb in the Bernese Oberland, in *Mountain Medicine and Physiology*, (eds C. Clarke, M. Ward and E. Williams), Alpine Club, London, pp. 32–7.

Little, M.A. and Hanna, J.M. (1978) The responses of high altitude populations to cold and other stresses, in *The Biology of High Altitude Peoples*, (ed. P.T. Baker), Cambridge University Press, Cambridge, pp. 251–98.

MacDonald, D. (1929) *The land of the Lama*, Seeley Service, London, p. 182.

MacNeish, R.S. (1971) Early man in the Andes. *Sci. Am.*, **224**, 36–46.

MacPhee, G.G. (1936) *Ben Nevis*, Scottish Mountaineering Club, Edinburgh, pp. 6–9.

Milledge, J.S., Halliday, D., Pope, C., *et al.* (1977). The effects of hypoxia on muscle glycogen resynthesis in man. *Q. J. Exp. Physiol.*, **62**, 237–45.

Mills, W.J. (1973) Frostbite. A discussion of the problem and a review of an Alaskan experience. *Alaska Med.*, **15**, 27–37.

Moorcroft, W. and Trebeck, G. (1841) *Travels in the Himalayan Provinces of Hindustan and the Punjab; in Ladakh and Kashmir; in Peshawar, Kabul, Kuduz and Bokhara*, vol. 1, (ed. H.H. Wilson), John Murray, London, p. 399.

Pretorius, H.A. (1970) Effect of oxygen on night vision. *Aerospace Med.*, **41**, 560–2.

Pugh, L.G.C.E. (1962) Physiological and medical aspects of the Himalayan Scientific and Mountaineering Expedition 1960–61 (Silver Hut). *Br. Med. J.*, **2**, 621–7.

Pugh, L.G.C.E. (1963) Tolerance to extreme cold at altitude in a Nepalese pilgrim. *J. Appl. Physiol.*, **18**, 1234–8.

Sellassie, S.H. (1972) *Ancient and Medieval Ethiopian History to 1270*, United Printers, Addis Ababa, Ethiopia.

Sharp, G.R. (1978) Hypoxia and hyperventilation, in *Aviation Medicine Physiology and Human Factors*, (ed. J. Ernsting), Tir-Med Books, London, p. 78.

Snellgrove, D. (1961) *Himalayan Pilgrimage*, Cassirer, Oxford.

Stein, R.A. (1972) *Tibetan Civilization*, Faber, London, pp. 26–37.

Taring, R.D. (1970) *Daughter of Tibet*, Murray, London, p. 170.

Ward, M.P. (1954) High-altitude deterioration, in *A Discussion on the Physiology of Man at High Altitude, Proc. R. Soc. Lond* [*Biol.*], **143**, 40–2.

Ward, M.P. (1990) Tibet: human and medical geography. *J. Wild. Med.*, **1**, 36–46.

Ward, M.P. (1991) Medicine in Tibet. *J. Wild. Med.*, **2**, 198–205.

Ward, M.P. (1993) The first ascent of Mount Everest, 1993: the solution of the problem of the 'last thousand feet'. *J. Wild. Med.*, **4**, 312–18.

West, J.B. (1986) Highest inhabitants in the world. *Nature*, **324**, 517.

4

The ventilatory response to hypoxia and carbon dioxide

4.1 THE OXYGEN TRANSPORT SYSTEM

4.1.1 Introduction

Figure 4.1 shows the oxygen transport system at sea-level and at high altitude. This diagram can be used as a 'table of contents' of changes due to acclimatization which will be followed in succeeding chapters.

The changes induced by the chronic hypoxia of high altitude are numerous. Many of them can be considered as an attempt on the part of the body to mitigate the effect of low inspired P_{O_2} on the tissues by reducing the loss of P_{O_2} at each stage in the oxygen transport system from ambient (outside) air to tissue cells.

Figure 4.1 shows that the P_{O_2} falls at each stage as oxygen is transported from outside air ambient P_{O_2} to inspired, to alveolar, to arterial, and to mixed venous which approximates to the mean tissue P_{O_2}. This forms a staircase or cascade of P_{O_2}. The process of acclimatization can be thought of as reducing each step in this cascade as far as possible.

4.1.2 Ambient to inspired PI_{O_2} (PI_{O_2})

The ambient P_{O_2} of dry air at sea-level is about 160 mmHg (20.9% of 760 mmHg, the barometric pressure). At an altitude of 5800 m in the example shown in Figure 4.1, the barometric pressure is just half that of sea-level (Chapter 2) so the ambient P_{O_2} is also half the sea-level value, 80 mmHg. The drop seen in the figure from ambient to inspired P_{O_2} of about 10 mmHg is due to the addition of water vapour to the inspired air as it is wetted and warmed to body temperature in the nose, mouth, larynx and trachea. The water vapour pressure at body temperature is 47 mmHg, and this displaces almost 10 mmHg P_{O_2}. This physical cause of P_{O_2} reduction is beyond the control of the body and

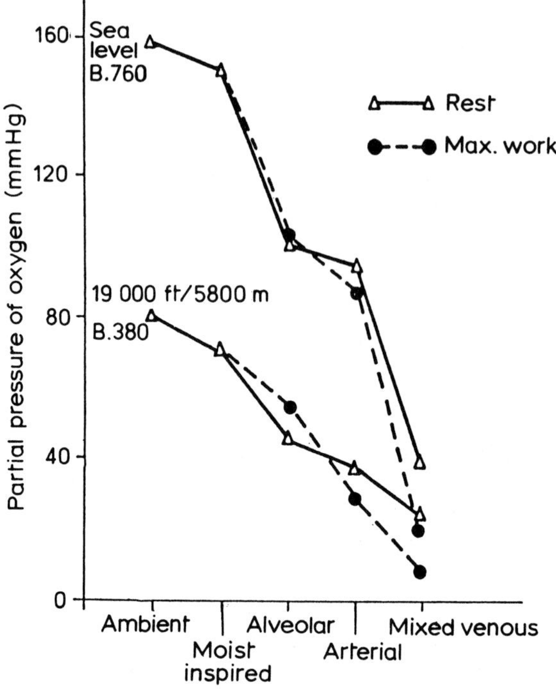

Figure 4.1 The oxygen transport system from outside air through the body at sea-level and at an altitude of 5800 m. (Reproduced with permission from Pugh, 1964.) (B = barometric pressure.)

so applies equally at altitude, where its effect is proportionately more important.

4.1.3 Inspired to alveolar P_{O_2} (PA_{O_2})

At sea-level there is a drop of about 50 mmHg at this point in the oxygen transport system. This drop can be thought of as being due to the addition of carbon dioxide and the uptake of oxygen and so depends, in part, on the metabolic rate; it also depends on minute ventilation and, for a given oxygen uptake and carbon dioxide output, the size of this reduction is entirely due to ventilation. A doubling of ventilation results in a halving of this drop. If ventilation were infinite there would be no reduction and alveolar gas would be fresh air. After acclimatization at 5800 m resting alveolar ventilation is approximately doubled and this step in the system as shown in Figure 4.1 is halved.

This increase in ventilation is one of the most important aspects of acclimatization and the mechanisms underlying it (the changes in control of breathing), are dealt with later in this chapter.

Figure 4.1 shows also the effect of exercise on the oxygen transport system (the dashed lines). At sea level the PA_{O_2} is little changed by exercise but at altitude the increase of ventilation is far greater in response to exercise than at sea-level so that with exercise the PA_{O_2} is increased and PA_{CO_2} decreased (Chapter 10).

4.1.4 Alveolar to arterial P_{O_2} (Pa_{O_2})

Oxygen passes across the alveolar–capillary membrane by diffusion, resulting in a small pressure drop but in the normal lung this accounts for less than 1 mmHg. The total alveolar–arterial (A–a) P_{O_2} gradient at sea-level is about 6–10 mmHg. The major part of this gradient is due to ventilation/perfusion ratio ($\dot{V}/\dot{Q}$) inequalities. Even in the healthy lung the matching of ventilation to blood flow is not perfect. In lung disease such as emphysema or pulmonary embolism this mismatching results in much greater (A–a) oxygen gradients and in significant hypoxaemia. This important topic has been discussed fully by West (1986).

At altitude, at rest there is little change in the (A–a) P_{O_2} gradient. The diffusing capacity of the lung is not increased by acclimatization (West, 1962); the $\dot{V}/\dot{Q}$ ratio inequality is modestly reduced. This is due to the increase in pulmonary artery pressure due to hypoxia (Chapter 6), which reduces the gravitational effect on the distribution of blood flow in the lung.

However on exercise at altitude the A–a P_{O_2} gradient increases significantly and becomes important in limiting exercise performance. This is shown as the dashed line in Figure 4.1. This diffusion limitation, shown by West *et al.* (1962), is explored more fully in Chapters 5, 10 and 11.

4.1.5 Arterial to mixed venous P_{O_2} (Pa_{O_2})

The last drop in P_{O_2} from arterial to mixed venous shown in Figure 4.1 is due to the uptake of oxygen in the systemic capillaries. Its magnitude is influenced by the metabolic rate, the cardiac output and the oxygen carrying capacity of the blood (i.e. the haemoglobin concentration [Hb]). Probably the best known aspect of acclimatization is the increase in [Hb]. A modest increase is beneficial in that it increases the oxygen carrying capacity of the blood and, at altitudes up to about 4000 m, this is sufficient to balance the reduction in oxygen saturation due to reduced Pa_{O_2}. However, the increase in viscosity of the higher [Hb] is the price paid and if this is too great the cardiac output falls and so oxygen delivery is reduced. This aspect of acclimatization is the subject of Chapter 7.

Cardiac output changes with acute and chronic hypoxia as well as other effects on the vascular system are discussed in Chapter 6. Changes in the oxygen dissociation curve at altitude, also important in this section of the oxygen transport system, are reviewed in Chapter 8.

Taking the body as a whole, the mixed venous P_{O_2} can be thought of as reflecting the mean tissue P_{O_2}. It can be seen in Figure 4.1 that the effect of these processes of acclimatization is to maintain this critical P_{O_2} as near as possible to the sea-level value. Beyond this there is the possibility of adaptation at the tissue level involving the microcirculation and then intracellular mechanisms. These form the subject of Chapter 9.

4.2 HYPOXIC VENTILATORY RESPONSE (HVR)

The HVR is the increase in ventilation brought about by acute hypoxia. This is not a simple linear response and the effect of ventilation on P_{CO_2} complicates the response. As ventilation rises in response to hypoxia, P_{CO_2} falls. Thus the CO_2 drive to breathing is reduced and the hypoxic response is masked unless measures are taken to prevent this fall in P_{CO_2}.

If the inspired P_{O_2} is reduced acutely (i.e. over a period of a few minutes, either by breathing a low oxygen mixture or by decompression in a hypobaric chamber), the minute ventilation is increased. However, this increase in ventilation varies greatly from individual to individual and does not usually begin until the inspired P_{O_2} is reduced to approximately 100 mmHg (equivalent to about 3000 m altitude) (Rahn and Otis, 1949). This corresponds to an alveolar P_{O_2} of about 50 mmHg. Thereafter, as inspired P_{O_2} is further reduced, ventilation increases more rapidly.

The relationship of ventilation to P_{O_2} is hyperbolic, as shown in Figure 4.2. However, if arterial saturation is measured by an oxymeter, the relationship between it and ventilation is found to be approximately linear (Figure 4.2). The Pa_{O_2} at which ventilation starts to increase corresponds to the P_{O_2} at which the oxygen dissociation curve begins to steepen.

The actual effect of acute hypoxia on ventilation will depend upon whether P_{CO_2} is allowed to fall or not. Unless the experimental arrangement allows control of PA_{CO_2}, a rise in ventilation will result in a fall of P_{CO_2}. As P_{CO_2} is reduced some drive to breathing will be lost so that the full hypoxic response is not seen.

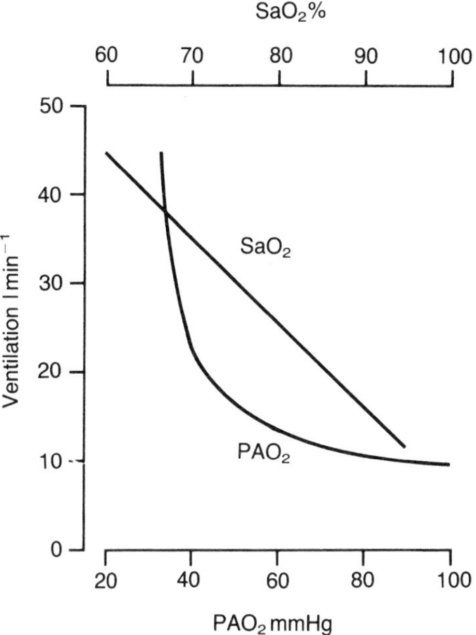

Figure 4.2 Diagrammatic representation of the hypoxic ventilatory response to PA_{O_2} and arterial oxygen saturation (Sa_{O_2}).

4.3 THE CAROTID BODY

Before considering HVR further, the transduction of the hypoxic response will be briefly considered. A transducer effects the conversion of one mode of signal to another, in this case from Pa_{O_2} to a neural signal by the carotid body.

4.3.1 Historical

The stimulating effect of oxygen lack on respiration had been known for many years before it became apparent at the turn of the century that, under normal sea-level conditions, carbon dioxide was the main chemical stimulus to ventilation.

In the late 1920s, the father and son team of Heymans and Heymans in Belgium, using complex cross-circulation experiments in dogs, localized the main sensing organ for hypoxia to the carotid body (Heymans and Heymans, 1927). Not long afterwards Comroe showed that the aortic bodies have a similar function (Comroe, 1938). These bodies are known collectively as the peripheral chemoreceptors. However, in most animals including man, the main organ for transduction of the hypoxic signal is the carotid body and if this is removed or denervated, acute hypoxia actually causes depression of ventilation due to general depression of the central nervous system.

4.3.2 Anatomy and physiology of the carotid body

The carotid body in man weighs about 10 mg and is situated just above the bifurcation of the common carotid artery. It has an extremely rich blood flow for its mass and its oxygen consumption, and thus it is a very low extraction organ (i.e. it extracts only a very small percentage of the oxygen in the blood presented to it). This explains how it is able to respond to arterial P_{O_2} (or saturation) and not to oxygen content. Thus it responds to hypoxaemia but not anaemia or reduced flow. This is appropriate, since an increase in ventilation would not help the organism overcome the tissue hypoxia caused by anaemia or low cardiac output, but does help in a hypoxic environment.

Despite an enormous amount of anatomical, neurophysiological and biochemical research work having been carried out on the carotid body, it is still not clear which cells or nerves actually sense the hypoxaemia or which transmitters are involved. It has been assumed that the glomus cells (Type I), the characteristic cell of the carotid body, are the sites of chemoreception and that modulation of neurotransmitter release from the glomus cells by physiological and chemical stimuli affects the discharge rate of the carotid body afferent fibres. Undoubtedly the signal is modified, enhanced or suppressed by parts of the system not involved with the primary sensing process.

Two key observations need to be explained.

- Carotid body chemoreceptors are excited physiologically by hypoxia, hypercapnia, and acidosis.
- Chemical agents which interfere with mitochondrial oxidative phosphorylation (and therefore reduce the ATP/ADP ratio) stimulate chemoreceptors.

There are two leading hypotheses. One is that hypoxia may slow down mitochondrial electron transport due to the presence of a reduced affinity cytochrome in the oxygen transport chain. This could stimulate neurotransmitter release from glomus cells by progressive breakdown of the mitochondrial electrochemical gradient and release of mitochondrial calcium into the cytoplasm. The elevated intracellular calcium would then cause release of the neurotransmitter. Metabolic blockers which interfere with electron transport and oxidative phosphorylation would have a similar effect (Biscoe and Duchen, 1990).

A second hypothesis is that glomus cells have potassium channels in their cell membranes that are modulated by the partial pressure of oxygen. The probability that the channel is open decreases with hypoxia and acidosis, and the result is a reduction in overall potassium conductance which causes membrane depolarization. This could explain chemotransduction as follows: the membrane depolarizes, voltage sensitive calcium channels open, and these allow extracellular calcium to enter the cell; the elevated intracellular calcium then promotes neurotransmitter release.

The potassium channel has been demonstrated in submicron-sized membrane patches which continue to be modulated by oxygen when removed from the cell. It was recently suggested that the channel itself contains a heme group which may interact with oxygen directly, thus modifying channel confirmation and the probability of its being open (Ganfornina and Lopez-Barneo, 1991).

The glossopharyngeal nerve carries sensory fibres from the carotid to the CNS where the sensory input stimulates the respiratory centre or centres in the pons. Another area of uncertainty is the existence or otherwise of efferent fibres in the glossopharyngeal nerve going to the carotid and modifying its response, and the suggestion that sensory nerves and synapses can work both ways (i.e. as afferent or efferent).

Dopamine is the most abundant transmitter found in the carotid body, followed by noradrenaline and 4-hydroxytryptamine. There are also small quantities of acetylcholine and enkephalin-like peptides in some glomus cells. Hypoxia increases the rate of release of dopamine from glomus cells and so may well be involved in the transmission of the hypoxic signal.

It should be noted that, while the most important function of the peripheral chemoreceptors (carotid and aortic bodies) is to respond to hypoxia, they do also respond to increases in Pa_{CO_2} and decreases in arterial pH. However, the greatest response to P_{CO_2} is via the central chemoreceptors in the brain stem (section 4.13.1).

4.4 HVR AT SEA-LEVEL

4.4.1 Methods for measuring HVR

There have been a number of different methods for measuring HVR; each have their advantages and disadvantages. Probably the most popular method for studies involving large number of subjects is the rebreathing method using an oxymeter to measure oxygen saturation continuously while the P_{CO_2} is held constant (Rebuck and Campbell, 1974).

4.4.2 Variability of HVR

The range of HVR found in healthy sea-level residents is wide. The coefficient of variation varies between 23% and 72% in different studies

(Cunningham *et al.*, 1964; Weil *et al.*, 1970; Rebuck and Campbell, 1974).

Various groups of subjects at sea-level have been shown to have lower HVRs than controls, for instance, endurance athletes (Byrne-Quinn *et al.*, 1971) and swimmers (Bjurstrom and Schoene, 1986). With increasing age HVR becomes lower (Kronenberg and Drage, 1973; Chapman and Cherniack, 1986) and respiratory depressant drugs and anaesthetics inhibit HVR (Davis *et al.*, 1982; Sahn *et al.*, 1974).

4.5 HVR AND MAN AT HIGH ALTITUDE

4.5.1 HVR and acclimatization

During the first few days at altitude, respiratory acclimatization takes place. This is shown by an increase in ventilation and a decrease in PA_{CO_2}. PA_{O_2} falls immediately on exposure to acute altitude and then rises (as PA_{CO_2} falls) over the next few days. The rise in ventilation on acute exposure to hypoxia is mediated by the HVR (by definition) but further increase in ventilation is due to changes in ventilatory control because of changes in the ventilatory response to CO_2 (section 4.12) and the sensitivity of the carotid body.

The peripheral chemoreceptors are essential for normal respiratory acclimatization; animals which have had their carotid bodies denervated fail to acclimatize normally (Lahiri *et al.*, 1981; Forster *et al.*, 1981; Smith *et al.*, 1986). After denervation these animals have a raised Pa_{CO_2}, which rises further with acute hypoxia due to central depression of ventilation. With chronic hypoxia, at least in some cases, there is a small fall in Pa_{CO_2} which has been taken by some workers as evidence of acclimatization (Sorensen and Mines, 1970). This and other evidence suggests that chronic hypoxia produces some effect on ventilation via mechanisms other than the carotid body, possibly via cerebral metabolism. All agree, however, that denervated animals appeared ill at altitude and many die.

It might be expected that exposure to hypoxia over some days or months would result in attenuation or sensitization of the HVR. Michel and Milledge (1963), found increases in the hypoxic parameter A in three out of four subjects after one to three months at 4800 m. Parameter A is the 'shape' parameter of the hyperbola relating PA_{O_2} to ventilation (Figure 4.2). The larger the value, the greater the response. There was no change in the other hypoxic parameter, C (the P_{O_2} at which ventilation theoretically becomes infinite, the P_{O_2} asymptote of the hyperbola). Cruz *et al.* (1980), also found an increase in parameter A after 74 hours of altitude exposure; this was not seen in subjects whose PA_{CO_2} was not allowed to fall.

The question of a change in chemoreceptor responsiveness during acclimatization has been reviewed by Weil (1986), who points out that a number of studies have not found any change in HVR with acclimatization though the presence of hypocapnic alkalosis, which has a depressant effect on HVR at sea-level may have obscured a real change. However, more recent studies have found an increase in responsiveness. Barnard *et al.* (1987) have found neurophysiological evidence of increased sensitivity of the carotid body for hypoxia in cats after chronic hypoxia of 28 days but not after only 2–3 h and Vizek *et al.* (1987), also presented evidence from work in cats of an increase in HVR (parameter A) after 48 hours' hypoxia. Engwall and Bisgard (1990) found an increase in HVR after four hours of hypoxia in awake goats. Yamaguchi *et al.* (1991), Sato *et al.* (1992) and Goldberg *et al.* (1992) found a significant increase in HVR in lowland subjects after acclimatization at 3730–4860 m compared with pre-exposure values. Masuda *et al.* (1992) measured HVR serially in seven lowland subjects after arrival at Lhasa (3700 m) and as they acclimatized over 27 days. They found a biphasic response: a small decrease over the first 3–5 days then a considerable increase from days 5 to 27.

This increase in HVR over the period of a few days to a few weeks could explain the further increase in ventilation over this period of altitude exposure.

The question of the role of HVR in effecting the change in CO_2 response and brain extracellular $[HCO_3^-]$ are considered in section 4.13. In man, after decades at altitude HVR becomes blunted (section 4.5.2). In cats this blunting is seen after 3–4 weeks if the hypoxia is sufficiently severe. Tatsumi *et al.* (1991) showed blunting of HVR after this time at a simulated altitude of 5500 m. They also found that HVR measured by recording from the carotid sinus nerve was blunted. They considered that both central and peripheral parts of the system contributed to the reduction in overall HVR.

4.5.2 HVR and altitude residents

Chiodi (1957) reported that altitude residents in the Andes had higher PA_{CO_2} than acclimatized lowlanders. Severinghaus *et al.* (1966) showed that Andean Indians born and living at altitude had a blunted HVR and similar findings were reported in Sherpas, natives to high altitude in the Himalayas (Lahiri and Milledge, 1967; Milledge and Lahiri, 1967). Steady-state inhalation experiments typical of a lowlander and a Sherpa are shown in Figure 4.3. The 'opened out fan' of the lowlander indicates a brisk HVR whilst the 'closed fan' of the Sherpa shows that changing PA_{O_2} between 200 and 30 mmHg has very little effect on ventilation. These early reports have been confirmed and Lahiri (1977)

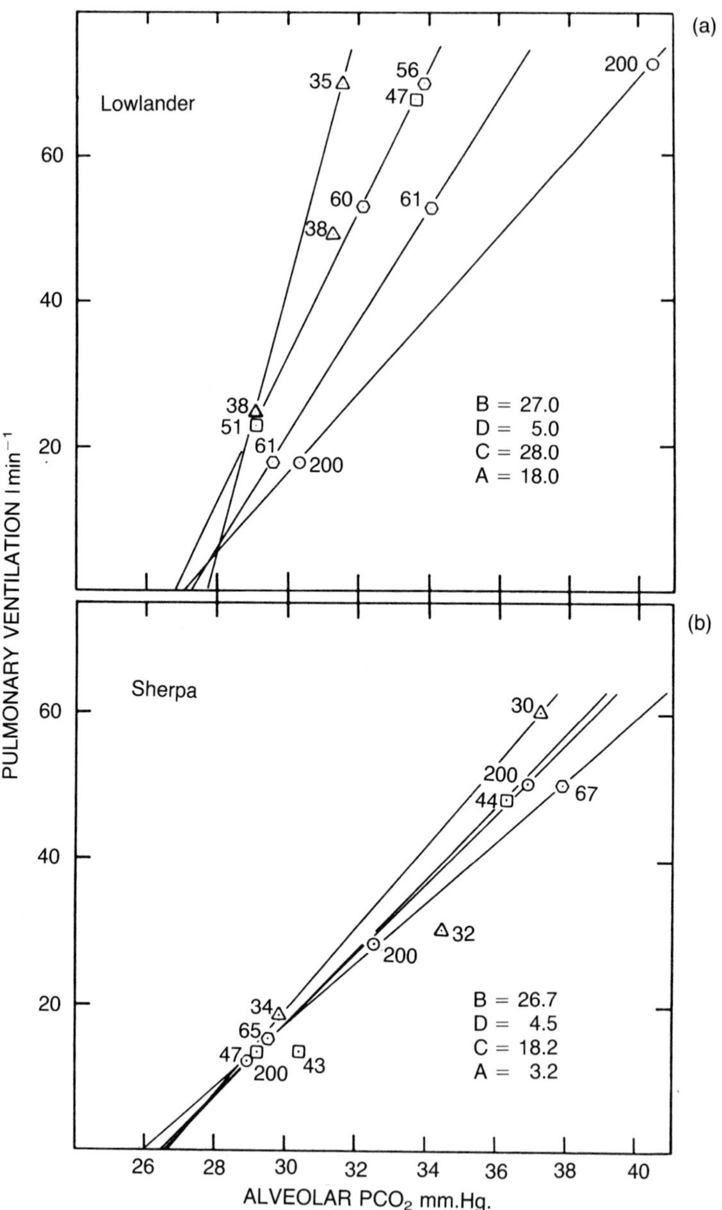

Figure 4.3 Two steady-state inhalation experiments typical of a lowlander (a) and a Sherpa highlander (b). The numbers refer to the P_{O_2} of each point. There is no significant difference in HCVR but the 'closed fan' of the Sherpa indicates very little HVR. The letters A–D refer to the parameters relating to HVR (A and C) and HCVR (B and D). (From Milledge and Lahiri, 1967.)

has reviewed the data from these studies. There is considerable variability amongst these people, the HVR varying from almost zero response to values within the lowlander range. One study (Hackett *et al.*, 1980) claimed that Sherpas did not show this blunted HVR; however, even this study showed that HVR was lower in Sherpas with the longest altitude exposure.

Weil *et al.* (1971) showed blunting of HVR in Caucasian people born and living at Leadville, Colorado (3100 m), HVR being only 10% of that found in the sea-level controls.

4.5.3 Lowlanders resident at high altitude

Early studies of lowland subjects resident for a few years at high altitude suggested that HVR remains unchanged indefinitely (Sorensen and Severinghaus, 1968; Lahiri *et al.*, 1969). However, in a study of lowlanders resident at altitude for decades (Weil *et al.*, 1971) it was shown that blunting did take place slowly.

4.5.4 Highlanders resident at sea-level

The HVR was found not to change in high altitude natives who came down to live at low altitude (Lahiri *et al.*, 1969).

4.5.5 The development of blunted HVR

Lahiri *et al.* (1976) found evidence in Andean Indians that HVR was normal in children and became blunted only as they grew into adulthood at altitude. They suggested the rate of blunting was more rapid the higher the place of residence. Weil *et al.* (1971) showed that in Caucasian subjects blunted HVR also developed only after decades of high altitutde residence. In cats blunting can be induced in 3–4 weeks if the altitude is as high as 5500 m but not below 5000 m (Tatsumi *et al.*, 1991).

These findings prove that the blunting of the HVR takes many years to develop in man and is due to environmental and not genetic factors.

4.6 HVR AND ACUTE MOUNTAIN SICKNESS

Acute mountain sickness (AMS) is a condition affecting otherwise fit people on ascending rapidly to altitude. Details of symptomatology, aetiology and treatment are given in Chapter 17. It would seem axiomatic that a brisk HVR by increasing ventilation reduces the degree of hypoxia and must be protective against AMS. There is some evidence that this may be the case but it is by no means overwhelming.

Hu *et al.* (1982) showed that six good acclimatizers had brisk HVR while four poor acclimatizers had blunted responses. Richalet *et al.*

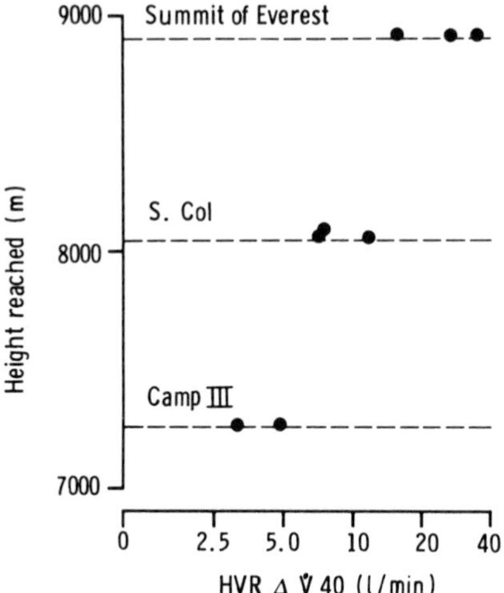

Figure 4.4 HVR and height reached on Mt Everest by eight mountaineers on the American Medical Research Expedition, 1981. (Re-drawn from data of Schoene *et al.*, 1984.)

(1988) found that in 128 climbers going to altitude on various expeditions a measure of HVR carried out before departure indicated that a low response was a risk factor for AMS. Hackett *et al.* (1988) found low HVR, measured at altitude, in subjects with high-altitude pulmonary oedema compared with controls. However, high-altitude residents and peoples native to high altitude have blunted HVR (section 4.5.2) and yet tend to be less subject to AMS than lowlanders. Milledge *et al.* (1988, 1991), in lowland climbers of varying altitude experience, found no correlation between HVR, measured before expeditions to Everest, Mount Kenya and Bolivia, and the symptom score for AMS in the first few days after arrival at altitude.

Masuda *et al.* (1992), who found an initial decrease in HVR 1–5 days after arrival at Lhasa (3700 m) followed by an increase, suggested that this might explain why these first few days are the time of risk for AMS.

4.7 HVR AND ALTITUDE PERFORMANCE

Apart from acute mountain sickness some people 'go well' at altitude while others, just as athletically fit, seem much more affected by the altitude. In general, there is a good correlation between freedom from AMS and good altitude performance. Again, it would seem advantageous for a mountaineer to have a brisk HVR in order to maintain a better oxygen supply to his working muscles. However, the evidence for this is conflicting.

Climbers with a brisk HVR were found to suffer greater impairment of mental performance at altitude (Hornbein *et al.*, 1989) presumably as a result of reduced brain blood flow due to lower Pa_{CO_2} (Chapter 15).

Schoene (1982) showed that 14 high altitude climbers had significantly higher HVR than ten controls. During the 1981 American Medical Research Expedition to Everest, Schoene *et al.* (1984) extended this work, showing again that the HVR measured before and on the expedition correlated well with performance high on the mountain (Figure 4.4). They also showed that, at altitude, the fall in oxygen saturation on exercise is greater in subjects with a low HVR and least in those with a brisk response. Thus, subjects with a blunt HVR are not only more hypoxic at rest but have even greater hypoxia on exercise than brisk responders. This is because there is a correlation between HVR and exercise ventilatory response (Martin *et al.*, 1978).

Matsuyama *et al.* (1986) found that five climbers who reached an altitude of 8000 m on Kangchenjunga (8486 m) had a higher HVR than five climbers who did not.

However the blunted HVR in peoples native to high altitude who perform at least as well as lowlanders argues against the necessity for a brisk HVR. They have probably adapted in other ways at a tissue level (Chapter 9). There is also evidence of a not so brisk HVR in top level climbers. Four elite climbers on the British Mount Kongur Expedition were found to have less HVR than four scientists on the same expedition (Milledge *et al.*, 1983). Schoene *et al.* (1987) studied one of the two climbers to first reach the summit of Mt Everest without supplementary oxygen and found him to have a blunted HVR. Oelz *et al.* (1986) also showed that six elite climbers who had all reached at least 8400 m without supplementary oxygen had HVRs no different from controls. In a prospective study of 128 climbers going on expeditions to the great ranges, Richalet *et al.* (1988) found that a measure of HVR did not correlate with the height reached whereas the sea-level measured $\dot{V}_{O_2}$ max did.

Serebrovskaya and Ivanshkevich (1992) found that subjects with the highest HVR had higher physical capacity at moderate altitude but tolerated extreme hypoxia less well, in that the P_{O_2} at which they had a disturbance of consciousness was higher than subjects with less brisk HVR.

4.8 HVR AND SLEEP

A feature of sleep at high altitude is periodic breathing. This not only disturbs sleep, the subject often waking with a distressing sensation of suffocation, but also results in quite profound hypoxia for short but repeated periods following the apnoeic phase of the periodic breathing (Chapter 12). It may be that these short but repeated periods of profound hypoxia are more detrimental than a steady moderate hypoxia, although the peak and average Sa_{O_2} tend to be higher during periodic breathing. Lahiri *et al.* (1984) have shown that to produce periodic breathing a brisk HVR is needed, so in this respect a brisk HVR may be a disadvantage.

4.9 HVR AT ALTITUDE: CONCLUSIONS

Animals that have had their carotid bodies denervated appear sick on being taken to altitude and have a high mortality; an HVR sufficient to at least counter the central depressant effect of hypoxia is therefore clearly beneficial. Whether a very brisk HVR is more advantageous than a more modest response is questionable on available evidence. Relative hypoventilation at altitude is almost certainly a risk factor for AMS but the sea-level-measured HVR is only one factor in determining the ventilation after a day or two at altitude. The speed of respiratory acclimatization may be more important, depending on the rate of ascent.

In subjects with a brisk HVR it seems likely that periodic breathing will begin at lower altitudes and be present for more of the night than in subjects with a more blunted HVR. Mental performance at altitude, and even after return to sea-level, may be more impaired in subjects with a brisk HVR (Chapter 15).

Possibly lowlanders with little or no altitude experience will acclimatize faster and be more free of acute mountain sickness if they are endowed with a brisk HVR. Highlanders with decades of altitude living probably develop adaptations at the tissue level which allow them to dispense with this 'emergency' response to hypoxia and avoid the need for hyperventilation.

Highly experienced climbers may also have made some progress towards this adaptation and so not require a brisk HVR to avoid mountain sickness and perform well at altitude.

4.10 ALVEOLAR GASES AND ACCLIMATIZATION

It has been pointed out that if PI_{O_2} is progressively reduced over a few minutes there is very little effect on ventilation until PI_{O_2} falls to about 100 mmHg (equivalent to about 3000 m). In residents at altitudes lower than this, ventilation is found to be increased. This effect of chronic hypoxia in increasing ventilation (over and above that due to acute hypoxia) is an important aspect of respiratory acclimatization.

Minute ventilation ($\dot{V}$) at rest is not easy to measure accurately because the actual placing of a mouth piece or a mask on a subject tends to increase ventilation. Therefore it is usual to use the PA_{CO_2} as an index of ventilation since, during steady-state, there is a close (inverse) relationship between PA_{CO_2} and ventilation. Classically, PA_{CO_2} has been measured by the Haldane–Priestley method of delivering a sample of 'alveolar gas'. With acute hypoxia there is no reduction in PA_{CO_2} until the PI_{O_2} is reduced to less than 100 mmHg, whereas with chronic hypoxia PA_{CO_2} is reduced with any reduction in PI_{O_2} below the sea-level value.

The classical description of the effect of altitude on alveolar gases is demonstrated on the O_2/CO_2 diagram by Rahn and Otis (1949) (Figure 4.5) where alveolar gases in subjects acutely exposed to varying PI_{O_2} in a decompression chamber are compared with results from residents at various altitudes culled from the literature.

It will be seen that in chronic hypoxia P_{CO_2} falls in a linear fashion from sea-level up to altitudes of about 5400 m, above which P_{CO_2} falls more rapidly so that the line dips down. These are altitudes above the highest permanent habitation and are from climbers who have been there for some days or weeks. At this altitude complete acclimatization is probably not possible and the physiology of this region is further discussed in Chapter 11.

Figure 4.5 also shows that at about 4000 m the difference in alveolar gases is greatest between the two lines (i.e. acclimatized and unacclimatized subjects). The PA_{CO_2} is 10–12 mmHg lower in acclimatized subjects, indicating an increase in ventilation of over 40% compared with unacclimatized subjects.

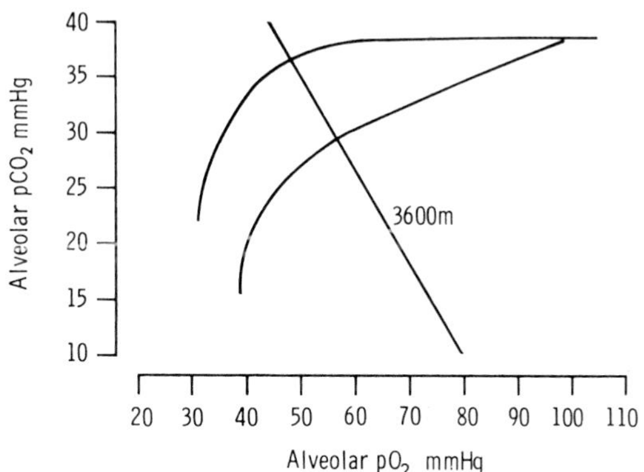

Figure 4.5 Alveolar gas concentrations and altitude. The upper line represents the P_{O_2} and P_{CO_2} found in subjects acutely exposed to increasing hypoxia in a chamber. The lower line is from residents at various altitudes and from acclimatized mountaineers. (After Rahn and Otis, 1949.)

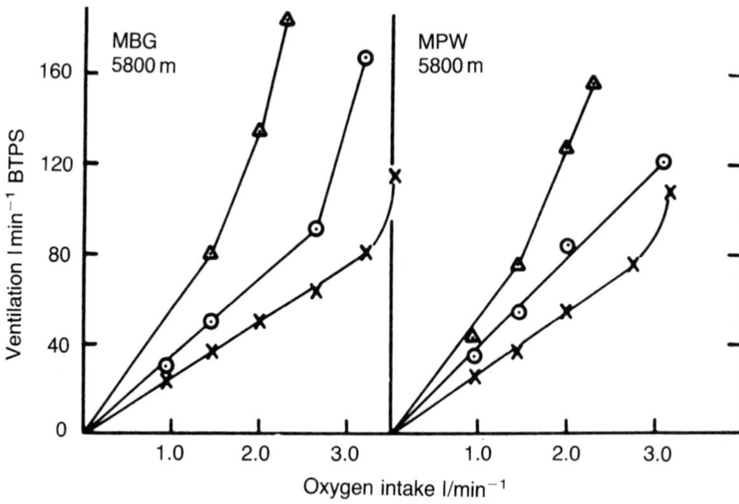

Figure 4.6 The effect of breathing sea-level PI_{O_2} on exercise minute ventilation in two acclimatized subjects (○) compared with their ventilation during air breathing at altitude (△) and at sea-level (×). (Reproduced from Milledge, 1968.)

4.11 ACUTE NORMOXIA IN ACCLIMATIZED SUBJECTS

Respiratory acclimatization can be well demonstrated by returning acclimatized subjects to normal (sea-level) P_{O_2}, either by rapid return to sea-level or by breathing a gas mixture appropriately enriched with oxygen. The ventilation is reduced and the PA_{CO_2} rises but does not return to sea-level values. The remaining elevation of ventilation and depression of PA_{CO_2} indicates the degree of respiratory acclimatization. This is most accurately measured when ventilation is measured during exercise (Figure 4.6). This Figure 4.6 shows results from two typical experiments (Milledge, 1968). It will be seen that by breathing sea-level PI_{O_2} the increase in $\dot{V}$ at altitude compared with sea-level is reduced by about 40% at any given submaximal work rates.

4.12 CO_2 VENTILATORY RESPONSE AND ACCLIMATIZATION

An important aspect of respiratory acclimatization is the change in CO_2 or hypercapneic ventilatory response (HCVR) measured either by the steady state (Lloyd *et al.*, 1958) or by rebreathing method (Reed, 1967). The effect of time at altitude on the HCVR is shown in Figure 4.7 which is taken from the work of Kellogg (1963). The steady-state method was used in three subjects to measure the HCVR before ascent to White Mountain. The measurement was repeated a few hours after

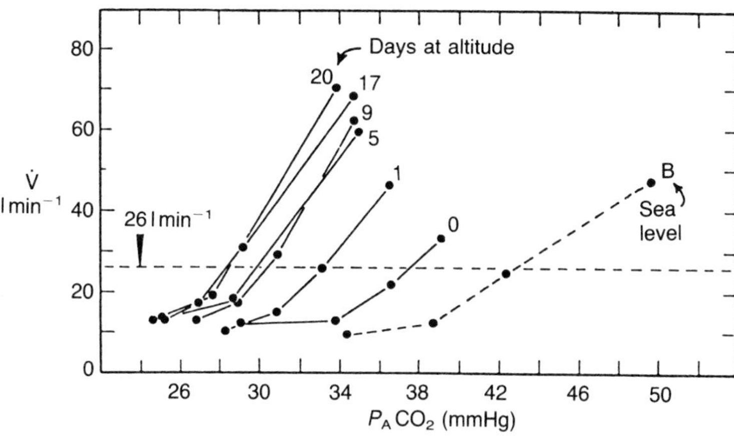

Figure 4.7 Effect of acclimatization on HCVR at an altitude of 4340 m. (Reproduced with permission from Kellogg, 1963.)

arrival by road at 4340 m and thereafter at intervals as indicated on the figure. It will be seen that the HCVR line shifts progressively leftwards and steepens.

4.13 MECHANISM FOR RE-SETTING HCVR

4.13.1 The central chemoreceptors

Although the peripheral chemoreceptors are sensitive to changes in P_{CO_2} and hydrogen ion concentration, the main sensor for changes in P_{CO_2} is the central medullary chemoreceptor. This is a paired region of the central nervous system situated just beneath the surface of the fourth ventricle in the medulla. Work by Mitchell (1963) has shown that this area is sensitive to changes in $[H^+]$ in the brain extracellular fluid. Such changes are brought about primarily by changes in arterial P_{CO_2}.

The blood–brain barrier is readily permeable to dissolved CO_2, less permeable to H^+ and even less to HCO_3^-. Thus, a rise in Pa_{CO_2} is rapidly reflected in CSF P_{CO_2} and causes a rapid increase in CSF $[H^+]$. Increases in $[H^+]$ sensed by the chemoreceptors result in increased stimulation of the respiratory centre and an increase in ventilation.

4.13.2 The importance of CSF bicarbonate

The chemoreceptors sense the $[H^+]$ in the brain extracellular fluid (or possibly some other extra or intracellular compartment) but, since this

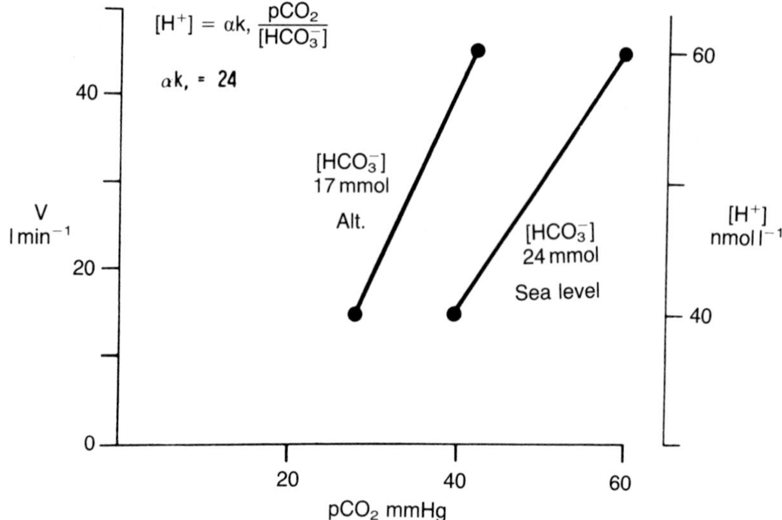

Figure 4.8 The calculated effect of reducing CSF $[HCO_3^-]$ on the HCVR using the Henderson–Hasselbalch equation and assuming CSF pH is held constant by ventilatory induced changes in P_{CO_2}.

cannot be sampled, the following discussion centres on the CSF acid–base changes which can be measured. Further discussion of the differences between these two compartments is given in section 4.15.1.

The Henderson–Hasselbach equation, which defines the relationship between P_{CO_2}, HCO_3^- and pH ($[H^+]$) is shown in Figure 4.8. This indicates that for $[H^+]$ to be held constant a change of bicarbonate concentration must be followed by a change of P_{CO_2} in the same direction. Assuming the sensitivity of the central chemoreceptors to $[H^+]$ remains constant, a reduction in $[HCO_3^-]$ will result in an increase in $[H^+]$ which will stimulate the central chemoreceptor and cause a rise in ventilation. This, in turn, will lower the P_{CO_2} and restore the H^+ concentration to normal, but now with a lower P_{CO_2}. Thus a reduction in CSF $[HCO_3^-]$ has the effect of re-setting the chemoreceptor to start responding at a lower P_{CO_2} (a shift to the left of the HCVR line). A rise in CSF $[HCO_3^-]$ has the opposite effect and is seen in patients with chronic bronchitis and hypercapnia. If the chemoreceptor responds to log $[H^+]$ (i.e. pH), then changes in P_{CO_2} at low values for example at 20–21 mmHg, will have twice the effect as that at normal values (i.e. 40–41 mmHg). This would then explain the steepening of the HCVR seen in acclimatized subjects.

These effects are shown in Figure 4.8. This is a theoretical representation of the effect on HCVR of a reduction in CSF $[HCO_3^-]$. A typical HCVR line at sea-level is shown on the right. The CSF $[HCO_3^-]$

is 24 mmol l^{-1}. If the CSF [HCO_3^-] is reduced to 19 mmol l^{-1} the chemoreceptor now 'sees' an increased [H^+] and ventilation is stimulated until [H^+] is reduced to the previous value. The resulting P_{CO_2} values are plotted and joined by a line giving the new HCVR on the left. This looks very similar to the actual effect of acclimatization on HCVR.

It is suggested that the mechanism of the change in HCVR is a reduction in CSF [HCO_3^-]. Evidence for this is provided by the experiments of Pappenheimer *et al.* (1964) in which they perfused the cerebral ventricles of awake goats with artificial CSF, varying the pH and [HCO_3^-]. They showed that by simply reducing the [HCO_3^-] in the CSF the HCVR was shifted to the left.

Bisgard *et al.*, 1986, found evidence of the importance of CSF [HCO_3^-] in maintaining the residual ventilation of acclimatization on giving normoxia. These workers perfused the carotid body in awake goats with hypoxaemic blood whilst the rest of the animal, including the brain, was normoxic. Carbon dioxide was added to the inspired gas to maintain normocarbia despite hyperventilation. There was a time-dependent increase in $\dot{V}$ over the 4 h of the experiment, but since brain and body were normocapneic and normoxic, there would have been no change in CSF [HCO_3^-]. Full respiratory acclimatization did not take place since, on switching the carotid perfusion to normoxia, ventilation promptly fell to normal.

4.13.3 Reduction in CSF [HCO_3^-] at altitude

In lowlanders going to an altitude of 3800 m the CSF [HCO_3^-] is reduced from a mean sea-level value of 24.7 mmol l^{-1} to 20.4 mmol l^{-1} on the second day at altitude and 20.1 mmol l^{-1} on day 8 (Severinghaus *et al.*, 1963). Similar results (mean 20.1 mmol l^{-1}) were found at 4880 m (Lahiri and Milledge, 1967). Residents at high altitude had similar values, 19.1–21.3 mmol l^{-1} (Lahiri and Milledge, 1967; Severinghaus and Carcelan, 1964; Sorensen and Milledge, 1971). Thus the reduction in CSF [HCO_3^-] of 4–5 mmol l^{-1} measured at altitude sufficiently explains the shift of the HCVR line to the left, though respiratory acclimatization probably also involves contributions from other mechanisms such as changes in the hypoxic ventilatory response (section 4.5.1).

4.14 MECHANISMS FOR REDUCTION IN CSF [HCO_3^-]

4.14.1 Possible mechanisms

Figure 4.9 shows three possible routes by which hypoxia could cause a reduction in CSF [HCO_3^-]. On the left is the 'classical' pathway.

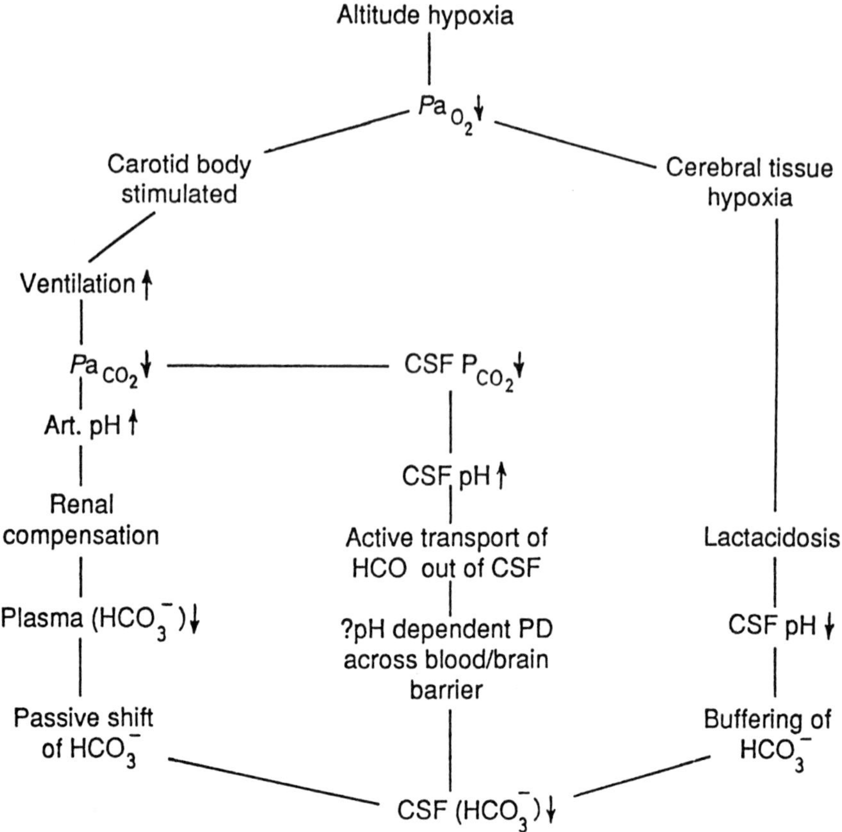

Figure 4.9 Possible mechanisms by which altitude hypoxia could cause a reduction in CSF [HCO_3^-].

Hypoxia stimulates the peripheral chemoreceptors, resulting in increased ventilation, decreased Pa_{CO_2} and hence respiratory alkalosis. The kidneys respond to the increased pH by excreting [HCO_3^-] in the urine and plasma [HCO_3^-] falls. A gradient develops for [HCO_3^-] across the blood–brain barrier and CSF [HCO_3^-] passes out slowly down the concentration gradient.

In 1963 Severinghaus *et al.* reported that early in altitude acclimatization their subjects had less increase in CSF pH and a greater fall in CSF [HCO_3^-] than in the plasma. Thus HCO_3^- appeared to pass out of the CSF against the concentration gradient, suggesting active transport of these ions out of, or H^+ into, the CSF. This mechanism is shown in the centre of the diagram (Figure 4.9).

On the right is the third possible mechanism for CSF [HCO_3^-]

reduction. With hypoxia there is a partial switch in cerebral metabolism of glucose from the aerobic to the anaerobic pathway. This results in formation of lactic and pyruvic acids. The H^+ produced will directly buffer HCO_3^-.

There is now abundant evidence supporting the conclusions of Severinghaus *et al.* (1963) that changes in CSF acid–base balance are faster than renal compensation of plasma acid–base changes, and, though the latter may contribute to the later changes of respiratory acclimatization, the major early changes, largely complete in 24 hours, have little to do with renal compensation.

4.14.2 Active transport of CSF [HCO_3^-]

Severinghaus' postulate that an active transport of HCO_3^- out of the CSF has stimulated a great deal of work aimed at disproving or proving this hypothesis. Fencl *et al.* (1966), using awake goats and ventricular perfusion, also presented data supporting the idea of active transport of HCO_3^- out of the CSF.

However, we must consider not only ionic concentrations in blood and CSF but also the electrical potential difference (PD) across the blood–brain barrier. This PD between CSF and blood, normally about +6.4 mV in dogs and +3 mV in man becomes more positive as blood pH increases (Bledsoe and Hornbein, 1981). The change is of the order of 32–43 mV per pH unit, depending on the type of acid–base change. CSF pH changes do not affect PD. There is also a species difference in the magnitude, and even direction, of change so that extrapolation from experiments on animals to man must be made with caution. To complicate the matter even further, PD is also affected by changes in plasma potassium concentration.

4.14.3 Passive transport of CSF [HCO_3^-]

In 1969 Siesjo and Kjallquist proposed that the apparent disequilibrium of [H^+] and [HCO_3^-] across the blood–brain barrier could be explained by these changes in PD. That is, that shift of these ions across the barrier was by passive transport. Many papers have addressed this problem; these are reviewed by Bledsoe and Hornbein (1981). Their conclusion is that neither the active nor the passive transport hypothesis is proven.

4.14.4 Cerebral tissue hypoxia and lactacidosis

It is well known that hypoxia increases lactate (and pyruvate) levels in the blood and CSF and, in the paper proposing active transport of

HCO_3^- Severinghaus *et al.* (1963), discussed the possibility that increased lactic acid in the CSF might account for the reduction in $[HCO_3^-]$; but the increase in lactate was only about 1 mmol l^{-1} compared with 4–5 mmol l^{-1} reduction in $[HCO_3^-]$. However lactic acid dissociates to lactate and H^+ in the cell. The two species then pass through the cell membrane to the extracellular fluid, to the CSF and across the blood–brain barrier, with probably different rates at each stage. There is no reason therefore to expect a simple one-to-one relationship between their two concentrations in the CSF. In other words, production of H^+ from lactic acid might well be greater than is indicated by the relatively small change in lactate concentration in CSF.

There is evidence that hypoxia produces respiratory acclimatization independent of increased ventilation or decreased Pa_{CO_2}:

- Eger *et al.* (1968) found that the effect of hyperventilation on the position of the CO_2 ventilatory response curve, was greater when subjects breathed a more hypoxic mixture than air. This showed that hypoxia had an effect independent of any change in P_{CO_2}.
- Many high-altitude residents having practically no ventilatory response to acute hypoxia nevertheless at altitude have Pa_{CO_2}, HCVR and CSF $[HCO_3^-]$ very similar to lowlanders with a brisk HVR, indicating similar respiratory acclimatization.
- Sorensen and Mines (1970) showed that goats who had had their carotid bodies denervated, so that acute hypoxia actually depressed their respiration, nevertheless showed a reduction in PA_{CO_2} at altitude compared with sea-level values. In a companion study (Sorensen, 1970) it was shown that rabbits whose peripheral chemoreceptors were denervated had a reduction of CSF $[HCO_3^-]$ similar to that of controls when taken to altitude. Steinbrook *et al.* (1983) also found evidence of good respiratory acclimatization in goats with ablated carotid bodies. However, in other studies in goats (Lahiri *et al.*, 1981; Smith *et al.*, 1986) respiratory acclimatization apparently did not take place in the denervated animals, in that Pa_{CO_2} did not fall significantly. Certainly, animals with denervated or absent carotid bodies fare badly at altitude and most studies have reported a number of deaths in their animals.
- Fencl *et al.* (1979), in the awake goat with perfused ventricles, showed that in the acclimatized animal lactate was higher and $[HCO_3^-]$ lower in the brain extracellular fluid than in the CSF (at sea-level there was no concentration difference).

These lines of evidence suggest that hypoxia *per se* has a role in respiratory acclimatization, presumably by its effect on cerebral metabolism.

4.15 BRAIN ACID–BASE BALANCE

4.15.1 Brain extracellular fluid

In the foregoing sections, CSF pH has been discussed because that was what had been measured in the studies quoted. However, it must remembered that the central chemoreceptor senses the $[H^+]$ in the fluid in its immediate vicinity, the local brain extracellular fluid, or possibly some other intra- or extracellular compartment. It has been calculated from studies in awake goats perfused with artificial CSF (Pappenheimer *et al.*, 1964) that in the steady-state this represents a point about three-quarters of the way along the concentration gradient for H^+ and HCO_3^- between CSF and plasma.

In a situation of changing acid–base balance, as for instance the developing respiratory alkalosis on going to altitude, the local brain extracellular fluid will change more rapidly than the bulk CSF. This is especially the case for respiratory as compared with metabolic changes. Within a few seconds of a fall in brain P_{CO_2}, brain $[HCO_3^-]$ also falls. The buffering capacity of brain extracellular fluid is greater by one-third than the CSF so the compensation for pH change is faster and greater in this compartment than in the CSE (Dempsey and Forster, 1982).

It must also be remembered that the brain extracellular fluid is affected by cerebral blood flow, so that changes in Pa_{O_2} and Pa_{CO_2} will have secondary effects by changing cerebral blood flow. This makes interpretation of studies even more difficult.

4.15.2 The lack of stability of CSF pH

Since the sensitivity to P_{CO_2} is via the pH sensitive central chemoreceptors, and since Pa_{CO_2} is so closely regulated, it seemed reasonable to assume that CSF pH was extremely stable. At sea-level a fall of about 0.03 pH units results in a doubling of the resting ventilation. Even when this is converted to a change of $[H^+]$ concentration it represents an increase of only 7%. Thus we have a negative feedback loop of very high gain, suggesting very tight regulation of pH.

However, during acclimatization the CSF pH rises by about 0.03 to 0.06 units while ventilation goes up. The reverse happens with acute normoxia (Dempsey and Forster, 1982). The change in pH is, of course, much less than would have occurred without the change in $[HCO_3^-]$ as discussed in 4.13.3. There are three possible explanations for this paradoxical change of CSF pH:

- The drive from peripheral chemoreceptors is sufficient to increase ventilation even when the central drive is reduced. In subjects with a brisk HVR this is the most important cause of CSF alkalosis.

- The brain extracellular fluid may well be different from the bulk CSF in respect of $[H^+]$ and $[HCO_3^-]$ (section 4.15.1), so that cerebral lactacidosis causes higher $[H^+]$ in brain extracellular fluid than in CSF. This is suggested by work on awake goats with perfused ventricles at altitude (Fencl *et al.*, 1979).
- The effect of acute hypoxia on cerebral blood flow was studied by Crawford and Severinghaus (1978), who calculated that, at an altitude of 3810 m, hypoxia causes a 30% rise in blood flow to the central chemoreceptor area, resulting in a rise in pH of 0.006 units. Acute normoxia causes a similar, though opposite, change.

These effects would seem to account for most of the 'negative correlation' of $[H^+]$ with $\dot{V}$ pointed out by Dempsey *et al.* (1979). It is not necessary to invoke any change in sensitivity of the central chemoreceptor to $[H^+]$, although this cannot be ruled out.

Thus, it would seem that CSF pH is the result of the combined effects of peripheral and central drive and is not, in fact, very tightly controlled. Where peripheral drive is strong, as in lowlanders at altitude, the CSF pH is increased. Where peripheral drive is low, as at sea-level, highlanders and especially subjects with denervated carotid bodies, CSF pH is reduced.

4.15.3 Brain intracellular pH

Using magnetic resonance spectroscopy on unacclimatized lowland subjects in a hypobaric chamber, Goldberg *et al.* (1992) found that after a week at a simulated altitude of 4267 m, there was no significant change in intracellular pH, although, on return to normobaria, there was a significant intracellular acidosis.

4.16 LONGER TERM ACCLIMATIZATION

4.16.1 Highlanders

People native to high altitude have lower ventilation and higher Pa_{CO_2} than acclimatized newcomers (Chiodi, 1957). This is probably due to their blunted HVR (section 4.5.2). The HCVR of Andean natives (Severinghaus *et al.*, 1966), Sherpas (Milledge and Lahiri, 1967) and Tibetans (Shi *et al.*, 1979) have the same slope as have lowlanders at the same altitude. The position of the CO_2 ventilatory response line may be to the right (Severinghaus *et al.*, 1966) or not significantly different from lowlanders (Milledge and Lahiri, 1967). That is there is little difference between highlanders and lowlanders in their CO_2 ventilatory response.

4.16.2 Lowlanders

Although most of the respiratory acclimatization takes place within the first few hours and days at altitude, there may be further changes over the following weeks. In humans, there is a further increase in ventilation and Pa_{O_2} with a further decrease in Pa_{CO_2} (Forster *et al.*, 1974), though in other animals (e.g. pony and goat), the Pa_{CO_2} reaches the lowest point at 8–12 hours and then rises. The rat responds like man with a continued fall in Pa_{CO_2} up to 14 days (Dempsey and Forster, 1982). There is no significant change in acid–base balance over this period to account for this further ventilatory adaptation. It is possible that there is an increase in sensitivity of the carotid body over this period (section 4.5.1) and it is possible that changes in control from higher centres, such as have been demonstrated in cats by Tenney *et al.* (1977), may be responsible.

REFERENCES

Barnard, P., Andronikou, S., Pokorski, M., *et al.* (1987) Time-dependant effect of hypoxia on carotid body chemosensory function. *J. Appl. Physiol.*, **63**, 684–91.

Biscoe, T.J. and Duchen, M.R. (1990) Cellular basis of transduction in carotid body chemoreceptors. *Am. J. Physiol.*, **258**, L270–8.

Bisgard, G.E., Busch, M.A. and Forster, H.V. (1986) Ventilatory acclimatization to hypoxia is not dependent on cerebral hypocapnic alkalosis. *J. Appl. Physiol.*, **60**, 1011–14.

Bjurstrom, R.L. and Schoene, R.B. (1986) Ventilatory control in elite synchronized swimmers. *Am. Rev. Respir. Dis.*, **133(suppl)**, A134.

Bledsoe, S.W. and Hornbein, T.F. (1981) Central chemosensors and the regulation of their chemical environment, in *Regulation of Breathing, Part I*, (ed. T.F. Hornbein), Marcel Dekker, New York, pp. 347–428.

Byrne-Quinn, E., Weil, J.V., Sodal, I.E., *et al.* (1971) Ventilatory control in the athlete. *J. Appl. Physiol.*, **30**, 91–8.

Chapman, K.R. and Cherniack, N.S. (1986) Aging effects on the interaction of hypercapnia and hypoxia as ventilatory stimuli. *Am. Rev. Respir. Dis.*, **133(suppl)**, A137.

Chiodi, H. (1957) Respiratory adaptations to chronic high altitude hypoxia. *J. Appl. Physiol.*, **10**, 81–7.

Comroe, J.H. (1938) The location and function of the chemoreceptors of the aorta. *Am. J. Physiol.*, **127**, 176–91.

Crawford, R.D. and Severinghaus, J.W. (1978) CSF pH and ventilatory acclimatization to altitude. *J. Appl. Physiol.*, **44**, 274–83.

Cruz, J.C., Reeves, J.T., Grover, R.F., *et al.* (1980) Ventilatory acclimatization to high altitude is prevented by CO_2 breathing. *Respiration*, **39**, 121–30.

Cunningham, D.J.C., Patrick, J.M. and Lloyd, B.B. (1964) The respiratory response of man to hypoxia, in *Oxygen in the Animal Organism*, (eds F. Dickens and E. Niel), Pergamon, Oxford, pp. 277–93.

Davis, R.O., Edwards, M.W. and Lahiri, S. (1982) Halothane depresses the response of carotid body chemoreceptors to hypoxia and hypercapnia in the cat. *Anesthesiology*, **47**, 143–9.

Dempsey, J.A., Forster, H.V., Bisgard, G.E., *et al.* (1979) Role of cerebrospinal fluid [H^+] in ventilatory deacclimatization from chronic hypoxia. *J. Clin. Invest.*, **64**, 199–204.

Dempsey, J.A. and Forster, H.V. (1982) Mediation of ventilatory adaptations. *Physiol. Rev.*, **62**, 262–346.

Eger, E.I., Kellogg, R.H., Mines, A.H., *et al.* (1968) Influence of CO_2 on ventilatory acclimatization to altitude. *J. Appl. Physiol.*, **24**, 607–14.

Engwall, M.J.A. and Bisgard, G.E. (1990) Ventilatory response to chemoreceptor stimulation after hypoxic acclimatization in awake goats. *J. Appl. Physiol.*, **69**, 1236–43.

Fencl, V., Miller, T.B. and Pappenheimer, J.R. (1966) Studies on the respiratory response to disturbance of acid–base balance, with deductions concerning ionic composition of cerebral interstitial fluid. *Am. J. Physiol.*, **210**, 449–72.

Fencl, V., Gabel, R.A. and Wolfe, D. (1979) Composition of cerebral fluids in goats adapted to high altitude. *J. Appl. Physiol.*, **47**, 408–13.

Forster, H.V., Dempsey, J.A. and Chosy, L.W. (1974) Incomplete compensation of CSF [H^+] in man during acclimatization to high altitude (4300 m). *J. Appl. Physiol.*, **38**, 1067–72.

Forster, H.V., Bisgard, G.E. and Klein, J.P. (1981) Effect of peripheral chemoreceptor denervation on acclimatization of goats during hypoxia. *J. Appl. Physiol.*, **40**, 392–8.

Ganfornina, M.D. and Lopez-Barneo, J. (1991) Single K channels in membrane patches of arterial chemoreceptor cells are modulated by O_2 tension. *Proc. Natl Acad. Sci. USA*, **88**, 2927–30.

Goldberg, S.V., Schoene, R.B., Haynor, D., *et al.* (1992) Brain tissue pH and ventilatory acclimatization to high altitude. *J. Appl. Physiol.*, **72**, 58–63.

Hackett, P.H., Reeves, J.T., Reeves, C.D., *et al.* (1980) Control of breathing in Sherpas at low and high altitude. *J. Appl. Physiol.*, **49**, 374–9.

Hackett, P., Roach, R.C., Schoene, R.B., *et al.* (1988) Abnormal control of ventilation in high-altitude pulmonary edema. *J. Appl. Physiol.*, **64**, 1268–72.

Heymans, J.-F. and Heymans, C. (1927) Sur les modifications directes et sur la regulation réflexe de l'activité du centre respiratoire de la tête isolée du chien. *Arch. Intern. Pharmacodyn.*, **33**, 273–370.

Hornbein, T.F., Townes, B.D., Schoene, R.B. *et al.* (1989) The cost to the central nervous system of climbing to extremely high altitude. *N. Engl. J. Med.*, **321**, 1714–19.

Hu, S.T., Huang, W.Y., Chu, S.C. and Pa, F.C. (1982) Chemoreflex ventilatory response at sea level in subjects with past history of good acclimatization and severe mountain sickness, in *High Altitude Physiology and Medicine*, (eds W. Brendel and R.A. Zink), Springer-Verlag, New York, pp. 28–32.

Kellogg, R.H. (1963) The role of CO_2 in altitude acclimatization, in *The Regulation of Human Respiration*, (eds D.J.C. Cunningham and B.B. Lloyd), Blackwell Scientific, Oxford, pp. 379–94.

Kronenberg, R.S. and Drage, C.W. (1973) Attenuation of the ventilatory and heart rate responses to hypoxia and hypercapnia with aging in normal men. *J. Clin. Invest.*, **42**, 1812–19.

Lahiri, S. and Milledge, J.S. (1967) Acid–base in Sherpa altitude residents and lowlanders at 4880 m. *Respir. Physiol.*, **2**, 323–34.

Lahiri, S., Kao, F.F., Velasquez, T., *et al.* (1969) Irreversible blunted sensitivity to hypoxia in high altitude natives. *Respir. Physiol.*, **6**, 360–7.

Lahiri, S., Delaney, R.G., Brody, J.S., *et al.* (1976) Relative role of environmental and genetic factors in respiratory adaptation to high altitude. *Nature*, **261**, 133–4.

Lahiri, S. (1977) Physiological responses and adaptations to high altitude, in *International Review of Physiology: Environmental Physiology II*, Vol. 14, (ed. D. Robertshaw), University Park Press, Baltimore, pp. 217–51.

Lahiri, S., Edelman, N.H., Cherniack, N.S. and Fishman, A.P. (1981) Role of carotid chemoreflex in respiratory acclimatization to hypoxemia in goat and sheep. *Respir. Physiol.*, **46**, 367–82.

Lahiri, S., Maret, K.H., Sherpa, M.G. and Peters, R.M. (1984) Sleep and periodic breathing at high altitude: Sherpa natives versus sojourners, in *High Altitude and Man*, (eds J.B. West and S. Lahiri), American Physiological Society, Bethesda, pp. 73–90.

Lloyd, B.B., Jukes, M.G.M. and Cunningham, D.J.C. (1958) The relation of alveolar oxygen pressure and the respiratory response to carbon dioxide in man. *Q. J. Exp. Physiol.*, **43**, 214–27.

Martin, B.J., Wiel, J.V., Sparks, K.E., *et al.* (1978) Exercise ventilation corresponds positively with ventilatory chemoresponsiveness. *J. Appl. Physiol.*, **44**, 447–84.

Masuda, A., Kobayashi, T., Honda, Y., *et al.* (1992) Effect of high altitude on respiratory chemosensitivity. *Jpn. J. Mount. Med.*, **12**, 177–81.

Matsuyama, S., Kimura, H., Sugita, T., *et al.* (1986) Control of ventilation in extreme altitude climbers. *J. Appl. Physiol.*, **61**, 400–06.

Michel, C.C. and Milledge, J.S. (1963) Respiratory regulation in man during acclimatization to high altitude. *J. Physiol.*, **168**, 631–43.

Milledge, J.S. (1968) *The Control of Breathing at High Altitude*, MD Thesis, University of Birmingham, Birmingham.

Milledge, J.S. and Lahiri, S. (1967) Respiratory control in lowlanders and Sherpa highlanders at altitude. *Respir. Physiol.*, **2**, 310–22.

Milledge, J.S., Ward, M.P., Williams, E.S. and Clarke, C.R.A. (1983) Cardiorespiratory response to exercise in men repeatedly exposed to extreme altitude. *J. Appl. Physiol.*, **44**, 1379–84.

Milledge, J.S., Thomas, P.S., Beeley, J.M. and English, J.S.C. (1988) Hypoxic ventilatory response and acute mountain sickness. *Eur. Respir. J.*, **1** , 948–51.

Milledge, J.S., Beeley, J.M., Broom, J., *et al.* (1991) Acute mountain sickness susceptibility, fitness and hypoxic ventilatory response. *Eur. Respir. J.*, **4**, 1000–03.

Mitchell, R.A. (1963) The role of the medullary chemoreceptors in acclimatization to high altitude, in *Proceedings of the International Symposium on Cardiovascular Respiration*, Karger, Basel, pp. 124–44.

Oelz, O., Howald, H., di Prampero, P.E., *et al.* (1986) Physiological profile of world class high altitude climbers. *J. Appl. Physiol.*, **60**, 1734–42.

Pappenheimer, J.R., Fencl, V., Heisey, S.R. and Held, D. (1964) Role of cerebral fluids in control of respiration as studied in unanesthetized goats. *Am. J. Physiol.*, **208**, 436–40.

Rahn, H. and Otis, A.B. (1949) Man's respiratory response during and after acclimatization to high altitude. *Am. J. Physiol.*, **147**, 444–62.

Rebuck, A.S. and Campbell, E.J.M. (1974) A clinical method for assessing the ventilatory response to hypoxia. *Am. Rev. Respir. Dis.*, **109**, 344–40.

Reed, D.J.C. (1967) A clinical method of assessing the ventilatory response to carbon dioxide. *Australas. Ann. Med.*, **16**, 20–32.

Richalet, J.-P., Keromes, A., Dersch, B., *et al.* (1988) Caractéristiques physiologiques des alpinistes de haute altitude. *Sci. Sports*, **3**, 89–108.

Sahn, S.A., Lakshminarayan, S., Pierson, D.J. and Weil, J.V. (1974) Effect of ethanol on the ventilatory responses to oxygen and carbon dioxide in man. *Clin. Sci. Mol. Med.*, **49**, 33–8.

Sato, M., Severinghaus, J.W., Powell, F.L., *et al.* (1992) Augmented hypoxic ventilatory response in men at altitude. *J. Appl. Physiol.*, **73**, 101–7.

Schoene, R.B. (1982) Control of ventilation in climbers to extreme altitude. *J. Appl. Physiol.*, **43**, 886–90.

Schoene, R.B., Lahiri, S., Hackett, P.H., *et al.* (1984) Relationship of hypoxic ventilatory response to exercise performance on Mount Everest. *J. Appl. Physiol.*, **46**, 1478–83.

Schoene, R.B., Hacket, P.H. and Roach, R.C. (1987) Blunted hypoxic chemosensitivity at altitude and sea level in an elite high altitude climber, in *Hypoxia and Cold*, (eds J.R. Sutton, C.S. Houston and G. Coates), Praeger, New York, p. 432.

Serebrovskaya, T.V. and Ivanshkevich, A.A. (1992) Effects of a 1-yr stay at altitude on ventilation, metabolism and work capacity. *J. Appl. Physiol.*, **73**, 1749–55.

Severinghaus, J.S., Mitchell, R.A., Richardson, B.W. and Singer, M.M. (1963) Respiratory control at high altitude suggesting active transport regulation of CSF pH. *J. Appl. Physiol.*, **18**, 1144–66.

Severinghaus, J.W. and Carcelen, A. (1964) Cerebrospinal fluid in man native to high altitude. *J. Appl. Physiol.*, **19**, 319–21.

Severinghaus, J.W., Bainton, C.R. and Carcelen, A. (1966) Respiratory insensitivity to hypoxia in chronically hypoxic man. *Respir. Physiol.*, **1**, 308–34.

Shi, Z.Y., Ning, X.H., Huang, P.G., *et al.* (1979) Comparison of physiological responses to hypoxia at high altitudes between highlanders and lowlanders. *Sci. Sin.*, **22**, 1446–69.

Siesjo, B.K. and Kjallquist, A. (1969) A new theory for the regulation of extracellular pH in the brain. *Scand. J. Clin. Lab. Invest.*, **24**, 1–9.

Smith, C.A., Bisgard, G.E., Nielsen, A.M., *et al.* (1986) Carotid bodies are required for ventilatory acclimatization to chronic hypoxia. *J. Appl. Physiol.*, **60**, 1003–10.

Sorensen, S.C. and Severinghaus, J.W. (1968) Respiratory sensitivity to acute hypoxia in man at sea level and at high altitude. *J. Appl. Physiol.*, **24**, 211–16.

Sorensen, S.C. (1970) Ventilatory acclimatization to hypoxia in rabbits after denervation of peripheral chemoreceptors. *J. Appl. Physiol.*, **28**, 836–9.

Sorensen, S.C. and Mines, A.H. (1970) Ventilatory responses to acute and chronic hypoxia in goats after sinus nerve section. *J. Appl. Physiol.*, **28**, 832–4.

Sorensen, S.C. and Milledge, J.S. (1971) Cerebrospinal fluid acid–base composition at high altitude. *J. Appl. Physiol.*, **31**, 28–30.

Steinbrook, R.A., Donovan, J.C., Gabel, R.A., *et al.* (1983) Acclimatization to high altitude in goats with ablated carotid bodies. *J. Appl. Physiol.*, **44**, 16–21.

Tatsumi, K., Pickett, C.K. and Weil, J.V. (1991) Attenuated carotid body hypoxic sensitivity after prolonged hypoxic exposure. *J. Appl. Physiol.*, **70**, 748–55.

Tenney, S.M. and Ou, L.C. (1977) Ventilatory response of decorticate and decerebrate cats to hypoxia and CO_2. *Respir. Physiol.*, **29**, 81–2.

Vizek, M., Pickett, C.K. and Weil, J.V. (1987) Increased carotid body sensitivity during acclimatization to hypobaric hypoxia. *J. Appl. Physiol.*, **63**, 2403–10.

West, J.B., Lahiri, S., Gill, M.B., *et al.* (1962) Arterial saturation during exercise at high altitude. *J. Appl. Physiol.*, **17**, 617–21.

West, J.B. (1962) Diffusing capacity of the lung for carbon monoxide at high altitude. *J. Appl. Physiol.*, **17**, 421–6.

West, J.B. (1986) Ventilation/blood flow and gas exchange 4th edition. Blackwell Scientific Publications, Oxford.

Weil, J.V. (1986) Ventilatory control at high altitude, in *Handbook of Physiology*, Section 3, Vol II, (eds N.S. Cherniack and J.G. Widdicome), American Physiological Society, Bethesda, pp. 703–27.

Weil, J.V., Byrne-Quinn, E., Sodal, I.E., *et al.* (1970) Hypoxic ventilatory drive in normal man. *J. Clin. Invest.*, **49**, 1061–72.

Weil, J.V., Byrne-Quinn, E., Sodal, I.E., *et al.* (1971) Acquired attenuation of chemoreceptor function in chronically hypoxic man at high altitude. *J. Clin. Invest.*, **40**, 186–94.

Yamaguchi, S., Matsuzawa, S., Yoshikawa, S., *et al.* (1991) Effect of acclimatization and decacclimatization of hypoxic ventilatory response. *Jpn. J. Mount. Med.*, **11**, 77–84.

5

Lung diffusion

5.1 INTRODUCTION

Diffusion refers to the process by which oxygen moves from the alveolar gas into the pulmonary capillary blood, and carbon dioxide moves in the reverse direction. That this step in the cascade of oxygen transfer from the air to the mitochondria might be a limiting factor at high altitude was suggested near the beginning of this century. However it has only been within the last ten years that the role of diffusion at high altitude has been clearly elucidated.

Diffusion as defined above refers to the movement of oxygen in solution through the issues of the blood–gas barrier, and for convenience we also include the delay caused by the chemical combination of oxygen with haemoglobin in the pulmonary capillary blood (section 5.3.4). The term diffusion is also used in another context in the lung, that is the transport of gas in the small airways by the random movement of molecules in the gas phase. This process plays an important role in the movement of oxygen from the terminal bronchioles to the alveoli. It is unlikely that this process ever limits oxygen transfer in the normal lung at sea-level though the issue cannot be considered completely settled. At high altitude, diffusion in the gas phase becomes even less likely as a potential limiting factor because the mean free path of the molecules is increased as a result of the rarefaction of the gas. Consequently, diffusion in the gas phase will not be considered further.

5.2 HISTORICAL

The role of diffusion in the lungs was a topic of great controversy among respiratory physiologists in the last decade of the last century and the first two decades of this, and the arguments specifically involved the issue of diffusion at high altitude. Paradoxically much of the disagreement was generated by physiologists who contended that passive diffusion was *not* the primary mechanism of oxygen transfer through the blood–gas barrier, but that this process was achieved by active secretion. By this they meant that oxygen could be moved from a region of low partial pressure to one of high partial pressure as a result of some active process in the epithelial cells which required energy.

One of the strongest proponents of the secretion hypothesis was the Danish physiologist Christian Bohr. In a paper published in 1891 he compared the P_{O_2} and P_{CO_2} of alveolar gas with that of gas in a tonometer equilibrated with arterial blood taken at the same time. In some instances the alveolar P_{O_2} was reported to be as much as 30 mmHg below, and the P_{CO_2} as much as 20 mmHg above, the arterial blood values. Bohr's conclusion was, 'In general, my experiments have shown definitely that the lung tissue plays an active part in gas exchange; therefore, the function of the lung can be regarded as analogous to that of the glands' (Bohr, 1891).

Bohr referred to the secretion ability of the lung as its 'specific function.' In 1909 he published a long paper on this topic claiming that the active secretion of oxygen and carbon dioxide could use large amounts of oxygen, up to 60% of the total requirements of the body. If this were true, the Fick principle for deriving cardiac output from the oxygen consumption measured at the mouth would be invalid. Although the first part of his paper was devoted to active secretion, the second analysed the basic principles of oxygen diffusion through the blood–gas barrier. Here Bohr introduced the mathematical process which is now known as the 'Bohr integration.' It forms the basis for modern calculations of the time course of oxygen transfer from the alveolar gas into the blood as it moves along the pulmonary capillary (Bohr, 1909).

August Krogh was one of Bohr's students and assisted him in his experiments on gas secretion from 1899 till 1908. Krogh gradually became persuaded that passive diffusion rather than active secretion could account for the experimental data and in 1910 published a landmark paper on this topic. Since Bohr was his major professor and very jealous of the secretion theory, the introductory section of Krogh's paper required an unusually delicate touch. Part of it reads:

> I shall be obliged in the following pages to combat the views of my teacher Prof. Bohr on certain essential points and also to criticize a few of his experimental results. I wish here not only to acknowledge the debt of gratitude which I, personally, owe to him, but also to emphasize the fact, patent to everybody, who is familiar with the problems here discussed, that the real progress, made during the last twenty years in the knowledge of the processes in the lungs, is mainly due to his labors . . .
>
> *(Krogh, 1910)*

The British physiologist J.S. Haldane visited Bohr in Copenhagen and also became convinced of the secretion theory, at least as far as oxygen was concerned. For example, in 1897 Haldane and Lorraine Smith wrote: 'The absorption of oxygen by the lungs thus cannot be explained by diffusion alone' (Haldane and Smith, 1897). Haldane argued that oxygen secretion would be particularly beneficial at high altitudes, and in order to test the hypothesis, the Anglo–American expedition to Pike's Peak was organized in 1911. Arterial P_{O_2} was calculated by an indirect method following the inhalation of carbon monoxide, and the results appeared strongly to support the secretion hypothesis.

However the theory was also attacked by Marie Krogh (wife of August) when she developed a method for measuring the diffusing capacity of the lung using small concentrations of carbon monoxide (Krogh and Krogh, 1910). Her results indicated that the normal lung was capable of transferring very large amounts of oxygen by passive diffusion even when the inspired P_{O_2} was greatly reduced.

Various measurements in low-pressure chambers and during climbs to great altitudes were used as evidence to support one or other of the two camps. For example, Zuntz and his co-workers made some measurements in the first high altitude research station, the Capanna Regina Margherita on the Monte Rosa in the Italian Alps, and Bohr used the results as evidence for active secretion of oxygen. In this experiment, the oxygen consumption of one subject was $1.52\,l\,min^{-1}$ when alveolar P_{O_2} was only 57 mmHg (Zuntz *et al.*, 1906). Bohr had just described his mathematical integration procedure and he claimed that the experimental data were inconsistent with passive diffusion being the only mode of oxygen transfer (Bohr, 1909).

In the same year that Bohr's paper appeared, the aristocratic Italian climber, the Duke of the Abruzzi, reached the extraordinary altitude of 7500 m in the Karakorum mountains without supplementary oxygen. This was an astonishing climb because only a few years before, experienced alpinists had reported that 21 500 ft (6500 m) was 'near the limit at which man ceases to be capable of the slightest further exertion' (Hinchliff, 1876). Indeed one of the reasons given for the Duke's expedition was 'to see how high man can go' (Filippi, 1912).

Douglas, Haldane and their co-workers were duly impressed by the Duke's achievement and estimated from the reported barometric pressure of 312 mmHg that the alveolar P_{O_2} was only 30 mmHg. They therefore concluded that adequate oxygenation of the arterial blood would be impossible under these conditions without active secretion (Douglas *et al.*, 1913). However, this conclusion was disputed by Marie Krogh (1915) who argued that Douglas and his colleagues had markedly underestimated the diffusing capacity of the lung. Incidentally we now know that Douglas *et al.*'s estimate of an alveolar P_{O_2} of 30 mmHg for a barometric pressure of 312 mmHg was much too low; the actual value is approximately 35 mmHg (Gill *et al.*, 1962) in a region of the oxygen dissociation curve where an increase of 5 mmHg makes a world of difference.

Another physiologist who did not accept the secretion story was Joseph Barcroft. He conducted a heroic experiment on himself by living in a sealed glass chamber filled with hypoxic gas for six days (Barcroft *et al.*, 1920). His left radial artery was exposed 'for an inch-and-a-half' and blood was taken for measurements of oxygen saturation. There was a 'somewhat dramatic moment' when the first blood sample was drawn because it 'looked dark', an observation which was believed to be inconsistent with oxygen secretion. The conclusion was that diffusion was the only mechanism necessary for oxygen transfer across the blood–gas barrier during hypoxia.

Barcroft and his colleagues subsequently tested the secretion hypothesis further on their expedition to Cerro de Pasco in the Peruvian Andes in 1921–1922. The diffusing capacity of the lung for carbon monoxide was measured on five members of the expedition both at sea-level and at Cerro de Pasco and only a small increase was found. Barcroft therefore argued that the tendency for the arterial oxygen saturation to fall during exercise at high altitude could be explained by the failure of equilibration of P_{O_2} between alveolar gas and pulmonary capillary blood (Barcroft *et al.*, 1923). This was one of the first direct demonstrations of diffusion limitation, a finding that has been confirmed many times since.

It is remarkable that J.S. Haldane remained a staunch supporter of oxygen secretion all his life. In the second edition of his book *Respiration* written with J.G. Priestley and published in 1935, a year before Haldane's death, a whole chapter was devoted to evidence for oxygen secretion (Haldane and Priestley, 1935). Haldane gradually shifted his position as evidence mounted against the secretion hypothesis. While he initially thought that oxygen secretion occurred under all conditions, he later argued that it only became significant at high altitude, and later still that it required a period of acclimatization. His obsession with this theory long after seemingly overwhelming evidence had been provided against it was remarkable in this great physiologist.

5.3 PHYSIOLOGY OF DIFFUSION IN THE LUNG

5.3.1 Anatomical basis

The structure of the human lung is well suited to its role of allowing passive diffusion of oxygen from the alveolar gas to the interior of the

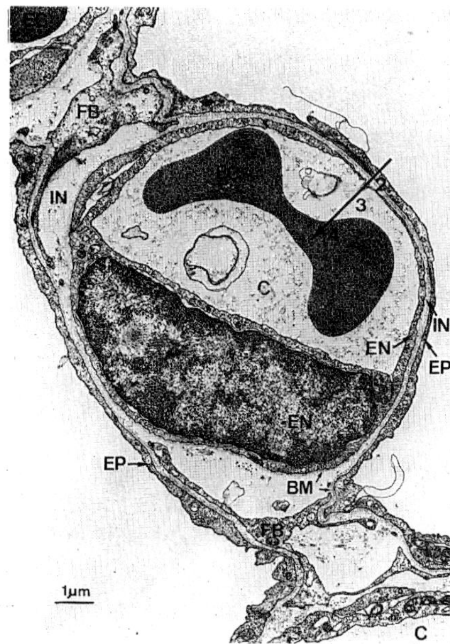

Figure 5.1 Electron micrograph showing a pulmonary capillary (C) in the alveolar wall. Note that in many places, the thickness of the blood–gas barrier is less than 0.5 μm. The large arrow shows the diffusion path from the alveolar gas to the interior of the erythrocyte (EC) and includes the alveolar epithelium (EP), interstitium (IN), and the capillary endothelium (EN), (these are grouped as (2) in the figure), plasma (3) and red blood cell (4). Other labelled structures include fibroblasts (FB) and the basement membrane (BM). (From Weibel, 1970.)

red blood cell. The blood–gas barrier is extremely thin, being only 0.3 μm thick in many places, and the area of the blood–gas barrier available for diffusion is 50–100 m^2.

Figure 5.1 shows an electron micrograph of a pulmonary capillary and emphasizes the short distance over which oxygen diffuses in (or carbon dioxide diffuses out). The various tissues through which oxygen moves are: layer of surfactant (not shown in this preparation because of the method of fixation), Type I alveolar epithelial cell (EP), interstitium (IN) (often much thinner on one side of the capillary than the other), capillary endothelial cell (EN), plasma, red blood cell. Note that the path length through the blood–gas barrier itself is only a small fraction of the total diffusion distance from the alveolar gas to the centre of the red blood cell.

Recently, several morphometric studies have been made of the pulmonary blood–gas barrier in man and other animals. Since the diffusion rate of a gas through a tissue slice is inversely proportional to its thickness, the appropriate variable to be calculated for diffusion resistance is the harmonic mean of the width of the blood–gas barrier. An intriguing feature of these studies is that the calculated pulmonary diffusing capacity for the human lung is apparently higher than that found experimentally. For example, Gehr and his colleagues (1978) calculated a maximum diffusing capacity in the human lung of $263\,\text{ml}\,\text{min}^{-1}\,\text{mmHg}^{-1}$ by morphometry whereas the maximum values found experimentally are generally less than one-half of this (Riley *et al.*, 1954; Shepard *et al.*, 1958; Turino *et al.*, 1963; Haab *et al.*, 1965). The discrepancy may be related to artefacts of the morphometric techniques, for example assuming that all the pulmonary capillaries can take part in gas exchange at any instant of time, whereas in practice some of them may not be recruited even during maximum exercise. However, it should be noted that the measurement of the pulmonary diffusing capacity for oxygen is difficult and indeed some estimates have given values which are closer to the morphometric range (Wagner *et al.*, 1987). Nevertheless there still appears to be a disparity between the anatomical and functional estimates.

5.3.2 Fick's Law of Diffusion

This states the rate of transfer of a gas through a sheet of tissue is proportional to the area of the tissue and to the difference in gas partial pressure between the two sides, and inversely proportional to the tissue thickness. As indicated above, the area of the blood–gas barrier in the human lung is some $50–100\,\text{m}^2$, and the thickness is less than half a micron in many places, so the dimensions of the barrier are well suited to diffusion.

In addition, the rate of gas transfer is proportional to a diffusion constant which depends on the properties of the tissue and the particular gas. The constant is proportional to the solubility of the gas and inversely proportional to the square root of its molecular weight. This means that carbon dioxide diffuses about 20 times more rapidly than oxygen through tissue sheets since its solubility is about 24 times greater at 37°C and the molecular weights of carbon dioxide and oxygen are in the ratio of 1.375 to 1.

Fick's law can be written thus:

$$\dot{V}_{\text{gas}} = \frac{A}{T} D(P_1 - P_2)$$

where $\dot{V}$ means volume per unit time, A is area, T thickness, D is the diffusion constant, and P_1 and P_2 refer to the two partial pressures.

For a complex structure like the blood–gas barrier of the human lung, it is not possible to measure the area and thickness during life. Instead, we combine A, T, D and rewrite the equation as:

$$\dot{V}_{gas} = D_L(P_1 - P_2)$$

where D_L is called the diffusing capacity of the lung.

The gas of choice for measuring the diffusing capacity of the lung is carbon monoxide (at very low concentrations) because the avidity of haemoglobin for this gas is so great that the partial pressure in the capillary blood is extremely small (except in smokers) and thus the uptake of the gas is solely limited by the diffusion properties of the blood–gas barrier. (The complication caused by finite reaction rates is considered below). Thus if we rewrite the above equation as:

$$D_L = \frac{\dot{V}_{CO}}{P_1 - P_2}$$

where P_1 and P_2 are the partial pressures of alveolar gas and capillary blood respectively, we can set P_2 to zero. This leads to the equation for measuring the diffusing capacity of the lung for carbon monoxide:

$$D_L = \frac{\dot{V}_{CO}}{PA_{CO}}$$

In words, the diffusing capacity of the lung for carbon monoxide is the volume of carbon monoxide transferred in $\text{ml}\,\text{min}^{-1}\,\text{mmHg}^{-1}$ of alveolar partial pressure.

5.3.3 Measurement of diffusing capacity

Several techniques can be used for measuring the diffusing capacity of the lung for carbon monoxide. The popular single breath method is essentially a modification of that originally suggested by Marie Krogh (1915). The subject makes a vital capacity inspiration of a very dilute mixture of carbon monoxide, and the rate of its disappearance from alveolar gas during a ten-second breath-hold is calculated. This is often done by measuring the inspired and expired concentrations of carbon monoxide with an infra-red analyser. The alveolar concentration of carbon monoxide is not constant during the breath-holding period but allowance can be made for that; it is assumed that its disappearance is exponential with time. Helium is also added to the inspired gas so that by its dilution the lung volume in which the single breath has mixed can be calculated.

In the steady-state carbon monoxide method, the subject breathes a low concentration of the gas (about 0.1%) for half a minute or so until a steady state of uptake has been reached. The constant rate of disappearance of carbon monoxide from alveolar gas is then measured for a further short period along with the alveolar concentration. The normal value of the diffusing capacity for carbon monoxide at rest is about 25 ml min^{-1} mmHg^{-1}, and it increases to two or three times this value on exercise.

The measurement of the diffusing capacity for oxygen in man is much more difficult. An early method was to measure the alveolar–arterial P_{O_2} difference during severe hypoxia (Riley *et al.*, 1954; Shepard *et al.*, 1958) but it is difficult to remove the contribution caused by ventilation–perfusion inequality. A promising technique is to use an isotope of oxygen, for example oxygen-18 (Hyde *et al.*, 1966). Other measurements have been made in experimental animals during severe hypoxia assuming linearity of the oxygen dissociation curve but this may introduce significant errors.

All methods of measuring pulmonary diffusing capacity are affected by the presence in the lung of ventilation–perfusion and diffusion–perfusion inequalities. No satisfactory way of allowing for these sources of error has yet been devised. However recent studies using the multiple inert gas elimination technique can separate the hypoxaemia caused by diffusion limitation from that due to ventilation–perfusion inequality (section 5.5).

5.3.4 Reaction rates with haemoglobin

Early workers assumed that all of the resistance to the transfer of oxygen from the alveolar gas into the capillary blood could be attributed to the diffusion process within the blood–gas barrier. However, when the rates of reaction of oxygen with haemoglobin were measured using a rapid reaction apparatus, it became clear that the rate of combination with haemoglobin might also be a limiting factor. If oxygen is added to deoxygenated blood, the formation of oxyhaemoglobin is quite fast, being well on the way to completion in 0.2 s. However, oxygenation occurs so rapidly in the pulmonary capillary that even this rapid reaction significantly delays the loading of oxygen by the red cells. Thus the uptake of oxygen can be regarded as occurring in two stages: (1) diffusion of oxygen through the blood–gas barrier (including the plasma and red cell interior); and (2) reaction of the oxygen with haemoglobin (Figure 5.2). In fact it is possible to sum the two resulting resistances to produce an overall resistance (Roughton and Forster, 1957).

We saw above that the diffusing capacity of the lung is defined as:

$$D_L = \frac{\dot{V}_{gas}}{P_1 - P_2}$$

that is, as the flow of gas divided by the pressure difference. It follows that the inverse of D_L is pressure difference divided by flow and is

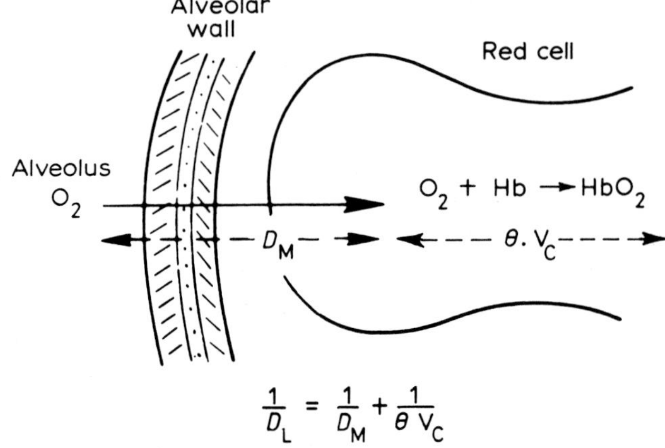

Figure 5.2 Diagram to show how the measured diffusing capacity of the lung (D_L) is made up of two components, one due to the diffusion process itself (D_M) and one attributable to the time taken for oxygen to react with haemoglobin (θV_c).

therefore analogous to electrical resistance. Consequently the resistance of the blood–gas barrier in Figure 5.2 is shown as $1/D_M$ where M means membrane. The rate of reaction of oxygen with haemoglobin can be described by θ, which gives the rate in ml min^{-1} of oxygen which combine with 1 ml blood mmHg^{-1} P_{O_2}. This is analogous to the 'diffusing capacity' of 1 ml of blood and, when multiplied by the volume of capillary blood (V_c), gives the effective 'diffusing capacity' of the rate of reaction of oxygen with haemoglobin. Again its inverse, $1/(\theta V_C)$, describes the resistance of this reaction.

It is possible to add the resistances offered by the membrane and the blood to obtain the total resistance. Thus the complete equation is:

$$\frac{1}{D_L} = \frac{1}{D_M} + \frac{1}{\theta V_c}$$

In practice the resistances offered by the membrane and blood components are approximately equal in the normal lung.

5.3.5 Rate of oxygen uptake along the pulmonary capillary

By using Fick's law of diffusion, and data on reaction rates of oxygen with haemoglobin, it is possible to calculate the time course of P_{O_2} along the pulmonary capillary as the oxygen is loaded by the blood. The application of Fick's law to this situation is not trivial because of the chemical bond which forms between oxygen and haemoglobin.

This means that the relationship between P_{O_2} and oxygen concentration in the blood is non-linear as shown by the oxygen dissociation curve. This problem was first solved by Bohr (1909) and the numerical integration procedure which he developed is known as the 'Bohr integration.'

A further complication occurs because, as oxygen is being taken up, carbon dioxide is given off, and this alters the position of the oxygen dissociation curve. A full treatment of this latter process should take into account not only the rate of diffusion of carbon dioxide through the blood–gas barrier, but also the rates of reaction of carbon dioxide in blood. Since not all the rate constants are known under all the required conditions, some assumptions and simplifications are necessary.

Figure 5.3 shows a typical time course calculated for the lung of a resting subject at sea-level (Wagner and West, 1972; West and Wagner, 1980). The diffusing capacity of the blood–gas barrier itself (D_M) was assumed to be 40 ml min^{-1} mmHg^{-1}, and the time spent by the blood in the pulmonary capillary was taken as 0.75 s (Roughton, 1945). Other

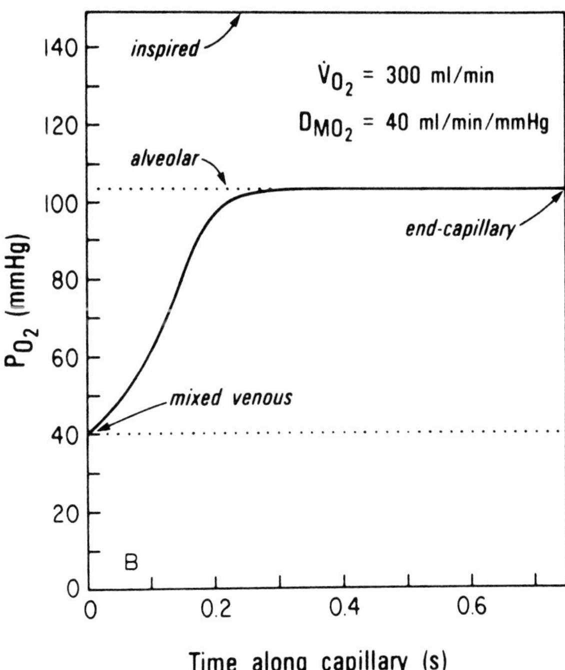

Figure 5.3 Calculated time course for P_{O_2} in the pulmonary capillary at sea level in resting man. Note that there is ample time for equilibration of the P_{O_2} between alveolar gas and end-capillary blood. (From West and Wagner, 1980.)

assumptions include a resting cardiac output of $6\,l\,min^{-1}$ and oxygen uptake of $300\,ml\,min^{-1}$.

Note that the blood comes into the lung with a P_{O_2} of 40 mmHg and the P_{O_2} rapidly rises to almost the alveolar P_{O_2} level by the time the blood has spent only about one-third of its available time in the capillary. The rate of rise of P_{O_2} in the latter two-thirds of the capillary is extremely slow, and there is a negligible P_{O_2} difference between alveolar gas and end-capillary blood.

This time course can be contrasted with that calculated for a resting climber breathing air on the summit of Mt Everest (Figure 5.4). Again, the membrane diffusing capacity of the blood–gas barrier was assumed to be $40\,ml\,min^{-1}\,mmHg^{-1}$ based on measurements made on acclimatized lowlanders at an altitude of 5800 m (West, 1962). The oxygen uptake was taken to be $350\,ml\,min^{-1}$, and other blood and alveolar gas variables were taken from measurements made on the American Medical Research Expedition to Everest (West *et al.*, 1983b). The time spent by the blood in the pulmonary capillary was assumed to be unchanged at 0.75 s because this is determined by the ratio of capillary blood volume to cardiac output (Roughton, 1945). The capillary blood

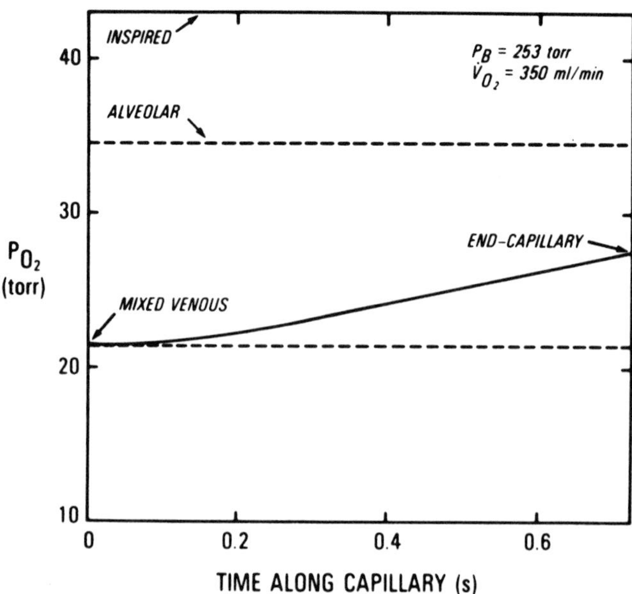

Figure 5.4 Calculated time course of the P_{O_2} along the pulmonary capillary for a climber at rest on the summit of Mt Everest. Note that there is considerable diffusion limitation of oxygen uptake with a large alveolar end-capillary P_{O_2} difference. (From West *et al.*, 1983b.) (1 torr = 1 mmHg)

volume was shown to be unchanged at 5800 m (West, 1962), and the cardiac output is also the same as at sea-level according to the measurements of Pugh (1964) (Chapter 10).

It can be seen that the oxygen profile is very different at this extreme altitude. The blood comes into the lung with a P_{O_2} of only about 21 mmHg, and the P_{O_2} rises very slowly along the pulmonary capillary, reaching a value of only 28 mmHg at the end. Thus there is a large P_{O_2} difference of some 7 mmHg between alveolar gas and capillary blood. This indicates marked diffusion limitation of oxygen transfer. It can be shown that this diffusion limitation becomes more striking as the oxygen consumption is increased by exercise.

The very different time courses for P_{O_2} shown in Figures 5.3 and 5.4 represent the extremes between sea-level and the highest point on earth for resting man. At intermediate altitudes, the difference between alveolar and end-capillary P_{O_2} will be considerably reduced at rest and may be negligibly small. However exercise will always tend to increase the alveolar end-capillary P_{O_2} difference.

Whether carbon dioxide elimination is ever limited by diffusion is still unknown. This is partly because some of the reaction rates of carbon dioxide in blood remain uncertain. Many physiologists believe that some diffusion limitation of carbon dioxide output may occur during heavy exercise.

5.3.6 Diffusion and perfusion limitation of oxygen transfer

It is clear from Figure 5.3 that a resting subject at sea-level has no diffusion limitation of oxygen transfer because there is no P_{O_2} difference between alveolar gas and end-capillary blood. Under these conditions, the amount of oxygen which is taken up by the blood is determined by the pulmonary blood flow. This means that oxygen uptake is perfusion-limited.

By contrast, Figure 5.4 shows a situation where oxygen uptake is, in part, diffusion-limited. This is indicated by the large P_{O_2} difference between alveolar gas and end-capillary blood. However, under these conditions, oxygen uptake is also partly perfusion-limited because increasing pulmonary blood flow will increase oxygen uptake.

The conditions under which diffusion and perfusion limitation occur have been clarified by Piiper and Scheid (1980). They used a simplified model with several assumptions including linearity of the oxygen dissociation curve in the working range. This is approached during conditions of severe hypoxia when the lung is operating very low on the oxygen dissociation curve, though even here it can be shown that the rapid elimination of carbon dioxide in the early part of the capillary substantially increases the slope of the oxygen dissociation curve (West,

1982). This introduces appreciable errors; nevertheless the model is valuable conceptually.

Using this simplified model, Piiper and Scheid showed that the total transfer rate $\dot{M}$ of a gas is given by the expression:

$$\dot{M} = (P_A - P_v)\,\dot{Q}\beta(1 - e^{-D/\dot{Q}\beta})$$

where P_A and P_v are the partial pressures of oxygen in the alveolar gas and venous blood respectively, $\dot{Q}$ is cardiac output, D is the diffusing capacity, and β is the slope of the oxygen dissociation curve (assumed to be linear). The total conductance G for gas exchange between alveolar gas and capillary blood may be defined as the transfer rate divided by the total effective partial pressure difference $(P_A - P_v)$ or:

$$G = \dot{Q}\beta(1 - e^{-D/\dot{Q}\beta})$$

This expression clarifies the factors responsible for diffusion and perfusion limitation. The equation shows that if D is very much larger than $\dot{Q}\beta$, the expression inside the large brackets tends to one, and gas transfer is limited by perfusion only. In this case, the (perfusive) conductance is given by $G = \dot{Q}\beta$. The relative difference between the conductance without diffusion limitation and the actual conductance is an index of diffusion limitation, L_{diff} in Figure 5.5.

By contrast, diffusion limitation occurs if $\dot{Q}\beta$ is so large that is greatly exceeds D, or to put it in another way, D becomes relatively very small. In this case the (diffusive) conductance is given by $G = D$. The relative difference between the conductance without perfusion limitation and the actual conductance is an index of perfusion limitation L_{perf} in Figure 5.5.

Figure 5.5 shows that oxygen uptake is entirely perfusion-limited in hyperoxia (top right of diagram) and that this is also true for the uptake of the inert gases nitrogen and sulphur hexafluoride. However, oxygen transfer during hypoxia becomes perfusion-limited to some extent (middle right) and this is particularly the case during exercise when oxygen consumption is greatly increased. For carbon monoxide, gas transfer is essentially diffusion-limited under all conditions (bottom right).

The above analysis emphasizes that an important factor leading to diffusion limitation is an increase in β, that is the slope of the blood–gas dissociation curve. This is the reason why the uptake of carbon monoxide is entirely diffusion-limited; the slope of its dissociation curve is extremely large. An increased slope of the oxygen dissociation curve tending to diffusion limitation occurs for three reasons at high altitude. First, the lung is working on a low part of the oxygen dissociation curve which is very steep. Secondly, the polycythaemia of high altitude increases the change in blood oxygen concentration per unit change in

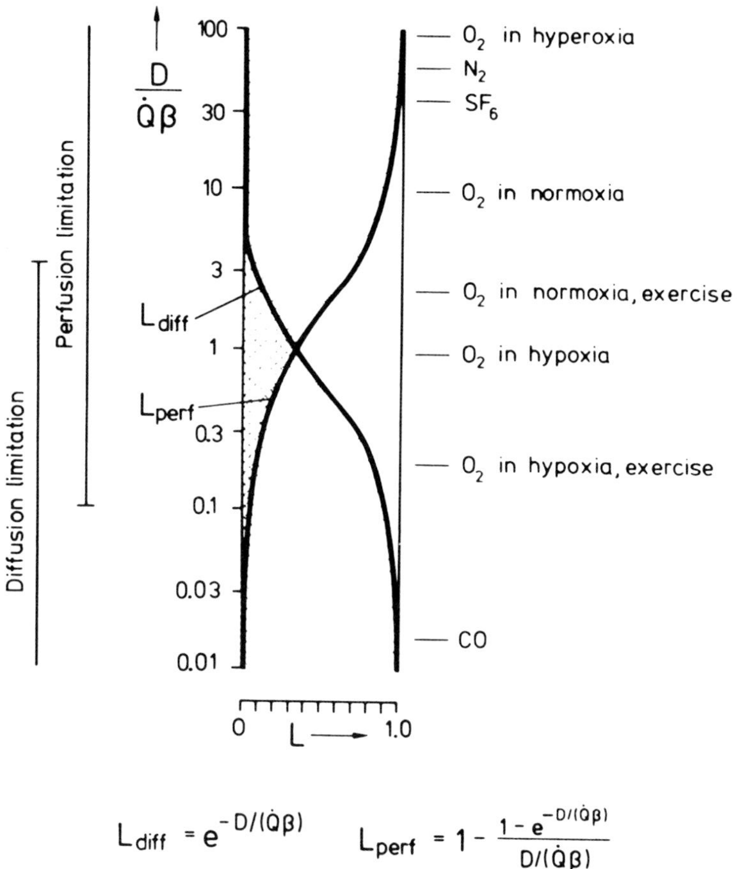

$$L_{diff} = e^{-D/(\dot{Q}\beta)} \qquad L_{perf} = 1 - \frac{1 - e^{-D/(\dot{Q}\beta)}}{D/(\dot{Q}\beta)}$$

Figure 5.5 Diagram to show the factors responsible for diffusion and perfusion limitation of gas transfer in the lung. L_{diff} and L_{perf} are measures of diffusion limitation and perfusion limitation respectively. Perfusion limitation is greatest at the top right of the diagram, and diffusion limitation is greatest at the bottom right. See text for details. (From Piiper and Scheid, 1980.)

P_{O_2}. Thirdly, the left shift of the curve caused by the respiratory alkalosis increases its slope. In fact, at extreme altitude, oxygen begins to resemble carbon monoxide to some extent.

For readers who prefer an intuitive explanation to the more formal analysis given above, the essential conclusion can be stated as follows. Diffusion limitation is likely when the 'effective solubility' of the gas in pulmonary capillary blood (that is, the slope of the dissociation curve) greatly exceeds the solubility of the gas in the tissues of the blood–gas barrier. This condition is met for carbon monoxide for which blood has an enormous avidity, and is approached for oxygen at high altitude because of the steepness of its dissociation curve at low P_{O_2} values, and the increased blood haemoglobin concentration.

5.3.7 Oxygen affinity of haemoglobin and diffusion limitation

It can be shown that increasing the affinity of haemoglobin for oxygen expedites the loading of oxygen in the pulmonary capillary under conditions of diffusion limitation at high altitude. The oxygen affinity of haemoglobin is conveniently expressed by the P_{50}, that is the P_{O_2} for 50% saturation of the haemoglobin. The normal value is about 27 mmHg.

Numerical analysis shows that increasing the affinity (leftward shift of the oxygen dissociation curve) results in more rapid equilibration between the P_{O_2} of alveolar gas and pulmonary capillary blood. A simplified way of looking at this is that the left-shifted curve keeps the blood P_{O_2} low in the initial stages of oxygen loading and thus maintains a large P_{O_2} difference between alveolar gas and capillary blood during much of the oxygenation time. This increased P_{O_2} difference therefore maintains the driving pressure and accelerates loading.

However a left-shifted oxygen dissociation curve interferes with the unloading of oxygen in peripheral capillaries because, for a given P_{O_2} in venous blood (required to maintain the diffusion head of pressure to the tissues), the blood unloads less oxygen. It is therefore not intuitively obvious whether the advantages of a left-shifted curve in assisting the loading of oxygen in the pulmonary capillaries outweigh the disadvantages of unloading the oxygen in the peripheral capillaries.

Several pieces of evidence suggest that a high oxygen affinity of haemoglobin is beneficial under hypoxic conditions. For example, the llama and vicuna, animals native to the Peruvian highlands, have left-shifted oxygen dissociation curves (Figure 5.6) as do some burrowing animals whose environment becomes oxygen depleted (Hall *et al.*, 1936). The human foetus, which is believed to have arterial P_{O_2} in the descending aorta of less than 25 mmHg, has a greatly increased oxygen affinity by virtue of its foetal haemoglobin which has a P_{50} at pH 7.4 of about 17 mmHg. Experimental studies have shown that rats with artificially left-shifted oxygen dissociation curves tolerate severe acute hypoxia better than rats with normal dissociation curves (Eaton *et al.*, 1974). Again, Hebbel and his colleagues (1978) described a family in which two of the four children had an abnormal haemoglobin (Andrew–Minneapolis) with a P_{50} of 17 mmHg. These two siblings had a higher $\dot{V}_{O_2}$ max at an altitude of 3100 m than the two with normal haemoglobin.

Numerical modelling gives some basis for these findings by showing

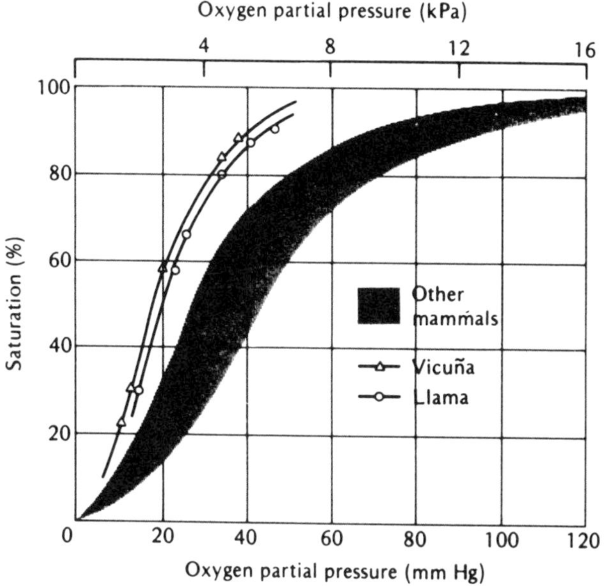

Figure 5.6 Oxygen dissociation curves of llama and vicuna blood compared with other mammals. The left-shifted curve for these high altitude natives indicates an increased affinity of the haemoglobin for oxygen which assists in oxygen loading along the pulmonary capillaries. (From Hall *et al.*, 1936.)

that the increased oxygen affinity of the haemoglobin improves oxygenation in the pulmonary capillaries under conditions of diffusion limitation more than it interferes with the release of oxygen by peripheral capillaries (Bencowitz *et al.*, 1982). Table 5.1 lists some of the strategies used by animals (including man) to increase the oxygen affinity of their haemoglobin under hypoxic conditions.

Climbers at high altitude tend to have an increased arterial blood pH which causes a leftward shift of the oxygen dissociation curve. This is caused by a partially compensated respiratory alkalosis and was the case for members of the American Medical Research Expedition to Everest who spent several weeks at an altitude of 6300 m. The mean arterial pH of three subjects was 7.47 (Winslow *et al.*, 1984) which is well above the normal range.

At extreme altitudes, there is evidence of extraordinary degrees of respiratory alkalosis. For example, when Pizzo took alveolar gas samples on the summit of Mt Everest, there is good evidence that his arterial pH exceeded 7.7. This value is based on a measured alveolar P_{CO_2} of 7.5 mmHg, and a base excess measured in venous blood taken on the following morning of $-5.9\,\text{mmol}\,\text{l}^{-1}$. This extreme respiratory

Table 5.1 Strategies for increasing oxygen affinity in chronic hypoxia

Strategy	*Subject*
Decrease in red cell 2,3-diphosphoglycerate	Foetus of dog, horse, pig
Decrease in ATP	Trout, eel (in hypoxic water)
Different type of haemoglobin	Human foetus, bar-headed goose, toadfish
Mutant haemoglobin (Andrew–Minneapolis)	Family in Minnesota (Hebbel *et al.*, 1978)
Different haemoglobin, small Bohr effect	Tadpole
Respiratory alkalosis	Climber at extreme altitude

alkalosis caused a marked leftward shift of the oxygen dissociation curve with a calculated *in vivo* P_{50} of about 19 mmHg. Thus a climber on the summit of Mt Everest develops conditions rather similar to those in the human foetus where the arterial P_{O_2} is less than 30 mmHg and the P_{50} is less than 20 mmHg.

5.4 PULMONARY DIFFUSING CAPACITY AT HIGH ALTITUDE

5.4.1 Acclimatized lowlanders

Barcroft and his colleagues measured the diffusing capacity for carbon monoxide in five members of the expedition to Cerro de Pasco in the Peruvian Andes in 1921–1922. They used the single breath method which had recently been described by Krogh (1915) and the measurements were made at rest. There was no consistent change from the sea-level values though the investigators believed that there was a slight tendency for the diffusing capacity to rise. They pointed out however that this small change would not be an important element in acclimatization (Barcroft *et al.*, 1923). Subsequent investigators have confirmed the absence of change or found only a very small (less than 10%) increase in diffusing capacity for carbon monoxide in resting subjects after periods of up to several months at altitudes of up to 4560 m (Kreuzer and van Lookeren Campagne, 1965; DeGraff *et al.*, 1970; Dempsey *et al.*, 1971; Guleria *et al.*, 1971).

Measurements on exercising subjects at altitudes up to 5800 m showed that, after seven to ten weeks of acclimatization, there was an increase in pulmonary diffusing capacity of 15–20% (Figure 5.7). However this small change could be wholly accounted for by the increased rate of

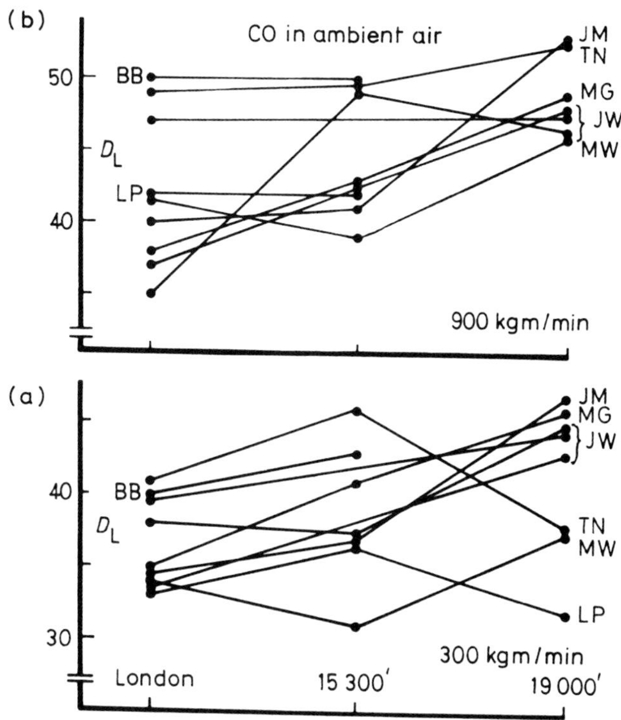

Figure 5.7 Diffusing capacities D_L in ml min^{-1} mmHg^{-1} measured at sea-level (London), 15 300 ft (4700 m) and 19 000 ft (5800 m) in acclimatized lowlanders exercising at: (a) 300 kg min^{-1} and (b) 900 kg min^{-1}. Note the moderate increase in diffusing capacity of carbon monoxide with altitude. (From West, 1962.)

reaction of carbon monoxide with haemoglobin due to hypoxia and by the increased blood haemoglobin concentration (West, 1962).

The mechanism of this increase can be explained by reference to Figure 5.2. The 'resistance' attributable to the rate of combination of oxygen with haemoglobin is given by $1/(\theta\ V_c)$. It has been found experimentally that the value of θ varies depending on the ambient P_{O_2}. At low P_{O_2} values, θ is increased and therefore the resistance to oxygen transfer is decreased. An additional factor is the increased blood haemoglobin concentration which, for a given value of V_c (capillary blood volume), increases the amount of haemoglobin present. Thus these factors completely accounted for the small observed increase in diffusing capacity for carbon monoxide at high altitude and indicated that there was no change in the diffusion properties of the lung itself after seven to ten weeks of acclimatization at an altitude of 5800 m.

5.4.2 High altitude natives

Several studies have shown that people who live permanently at high altitude (high altitude natives or highlanders) have pulmonary diffusing capacities that are about 20–50% higher than the predicted values, or than in lowlander controls (Figure 5.8). Remmers and Mithoefer (1969) showed that Andean Indians at an altitude of 3700 m had a diffusing capacity for carbon monoxide which was some 50% higher than predicted. High diffusing capacities have also been reported in Caucasians living at an altitude of 3100 m (DeGraff *et al.*, 1970; Dempsey *et al.*, 1971). The increased diffusing capacities were demonstrated both during rest and exercise.

A potential problem in such studies is the appropriateness of the predicted values for diffusing capacity. For example, in the study by

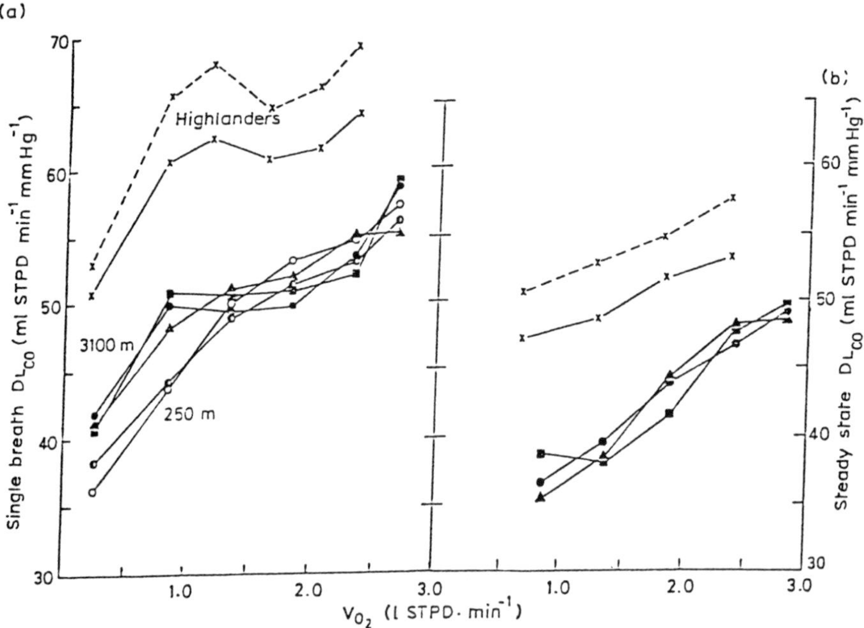

Figure 5.8 Diffusing capacities for carbon monoxide as obtained by the single breath method (a) and steady state method (b) in three groups of subjects; lowlanders at 250 m (○ and ◐), lowlanders sojourning at 3100 m (●, ▲ and ■ indicate different periods at this altitude), and native highlanders at 3100 m (×). The broken line indicates the measured data for highlanders while the continuous line shows the results after correction for 1/θ. All the measurements are on Caucasians, the 3100 m data being from Leadville, Colorado. Note the higher diffusing capacities of the highlanders both at rest and on exercise. (From Dempsey *et al.*, 1971.) (1 torr = 1 mmHg)

Remmers and Mithoefer (1969), predicted values were obtained from Caucasian North Americans and were applied to the South American high-altitude Indian population. This may introduce errors because of ethnic differences in body build. However in other studies such as that by Dempsey *et al.* (1971) diffusing capacities were compared between lowlanders and highlanders in similar ethnic groups (Figure 5.8).

The increased diffusing capacities can presumably be explained by the larger lungs which result in an increased alveolar surface area and capillary blood volume. Barcroft *et al.* (1923) commented on the remarkable chest development of the Peruvian natives in Cerro de Pasco and these early investigators made chest radiographs to confirm this. The radiographs showed that the ratio of chest width to height was greater in the high-altitude natives than in the Anglo–Saxon lowlanders. Subsequently it has been shown experimentally that animals exposed to low oxygen partial pressures during their active growth phase develop larger lungs and bigger diffusing capacities than animals reared in a normoxic environment (Figure 5.9) (Burri and Weibel, 1971; Bartlett and Remmers, 1971). This appears to be an adequate explanation for the observed high diffusing capacities, and would also account for the persistence of an increased diffusing capacity for carbon monoxide in highlanders after a prolonged period spent at sea-level as observed by Guleria and his co-workers (1971).

5.5 DIFFUSION LIMITATION OF OXYGEN TRANSFER AT HIGH ALTITUDE

The significance of pulmonary diffusion at high altitude is that it may be a limiting factor in oxygen uptake. A considerable amount of evidence now supports this.

One of the first groups to suggest diffusion limitation of oxygen uptake at altitude was Barcroft and his colleagues (1923). They concluded from their measurements of pulmonary diffusing capacity for carbon monoxide at an altitude of 4300 m that P_{O_2} equilibration between alveolar gas and the blood at the end of the capillary would not be achieved, especially on exercise. Subsequently Houston and Riley (1947) measured alveolar–arterial P_{O_2} differences in four subjects who spent 32 days in a low pressure chamber in which the pressure was gradually reduced from 760 to 320 mmHg (Operation Everest I). Measurements were made during rest and during relatively low levels of exercise (oxygen uptakes less than 1200 ml min^{-1} at simulated high altitude). During exercise, the alveolar–arterial P_{O_2} difference was increased to about 10 mmHg which they correctly ascribed to diffusion limitation.

During the Himalayan Scientific and Mountaineering Expedition of

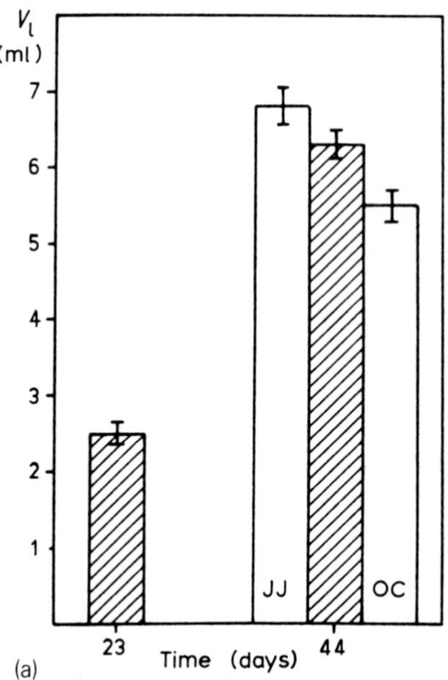

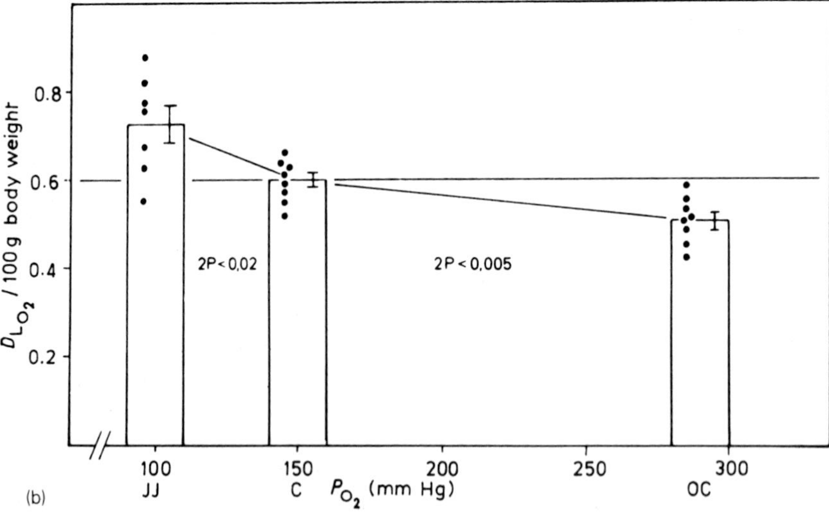

Figure 5.9 (a) shows the increase in lung volume V_1 from the 23rd to the 44th day of life in three groups of rats exposed to an altitude of 3450 m (JJ), sea-level (cross-hatched) and 40% oxygen at sea-level (OC). Note that lung volume increased most in the hypoxic animals and least in the hyperoxic. (b) shows the pulmonary diffusing capacity estimated morphometrically in the same three groups of animals at the 44th day. Note that the diffusing capacities reflected the changes in lung volume. C shows a control group. (From Burri and Weibel, 1971.)

1960–1961, measurements of arterial oxygen saturation by ear oximetry were made on five subjects who lived for four months at an altitude of 5800 m (P_B 380 mmHg) in a prefabricated hut. The average arterial oxygen saturation at rest was 67% and this fell at work levels of 300 and 900 kg min^{-1} to 63% and 56% respectively (West *et al.*, 1962). The progressive fall in arterial oxygen saturation as the work level was raised occurred in the face of an increasing alveolar P_{O_2} and was strong evidence for diffusion limitation of oxygen transfer. Alveolar–arterial differences were calculated and nine measurements at the maximal exercise level gave a mean P_{O_2} difference of 26 mmHg with a standard deviation of 4 mmHg. Calculations based on the Bohr integration procedure showed that the results were consistent with a maximum pulmonary diffusing capacity for oxygen of about 60 ml/min^{-1}/mmHg^{-1}.

Further evidence for diffusion limitation of oxygen transfer during exercise at very high altitudes was obtained on the American Medical Research Expedition to Everest in 1981. Fifteen subjects spent up to four weeks at an altitude of 6300 m (P_B 350 mmHg) and arterial oxygen saturation was measured by oximeter at rest and during increasing levels of work (Figure 5.10). Again there was a progressive fall in arterial oxygen saturation as the work level was increased from rest to 1200 kg min^{-1}, equivalent to an oxygen consumption of about 2.3 l min^{-1}. The calculated alveolar–arterial P_{O_2} difference at this highest work level was 21 mmHg (West *et al.*, 1983a).

Figure 5.10 also shows that additional measurements were made with subjects breathing 16% and 14% oxygen at this very high altitude. The latter gave an inspired P_{O_2} of 42 mmHg, equivalent to that encountered by a climber breathing air on the summit of Mt Everest. Note the very abrupt fall in arterial oxygen saturation as work rate was increased at this highest altitude on earth. Two subjects performed maximum exercise while breathing 14% oxygen and in one of them the oximeter reading fell to less than 10% oxygen saturation at one point during the experiment! Although the calibration of the oximeter at such values is unreliable, the actual saturation must have been extremely low.

A possible criticism of the measurements described so far is that no account was taken of ventilation–perfusion inequalities within the lung, and these may have contributed to the observed fall in arterial oxygen saturation and the increased alveolar–arterial P_{O_2} difference. Allowance for this possible factor can only be made if there is an independent measurement of ventilation–perfusion inequality. This was done by Wagner and his colleagues, both in an acute low pressure chamber study, and a 40-day simulated ascent of Mt Everest (Operation Everest II). These studies are important because they show that some increase in ventilation–perfusion inequality occurred at rest and on

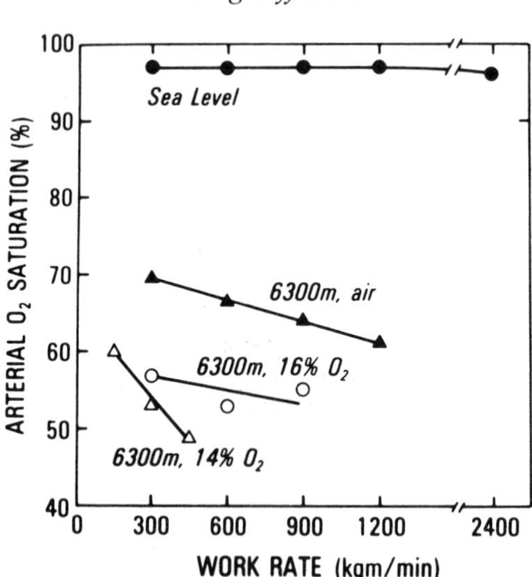

Figure 5.10 Arterial oxygen saturation as measured by ear oximetry plotted against work rate at sea-level and 6300 m altitude. The two lower lines were obtained with subjects breathing 16% and 14% oxygen at 6300 m. (From West *et al.*, 1983a.)

exercise both during acute exposure to low pressure and in subjects acclimatized to high altitude for periods up to 40 days. The measurements of ventilation–perfusion inequality were made using the multiple inert gas elimination technique (Wagner *et al.*, 1974). Inert gas exchange is not diffusion-limited, even during maximal exercise.

Figure 5.11 shows the increase in ventilation–perfusion inequality caused both by increasing altitude and increasing work level in the 40-day low pressure chamber experiment (Wagner *et al.*, 1987). The vertical scale shows the mean log standard deviation of the blood flow distribution which is one measure of ventilation–perfusion inequality. It can be seen that this index was about 0.5 during rest at sea-level but increased slightly when the oxygen consumption was raised to over $3 \, l \, min^{-1}$ during exercise at sea-level. At very high altitude, where the barometric pressure was 347 mmHg, the resting standard deviation rose to approximately 0.9 and it increased further to over 1.5 with exercise. The explanation of these intriguing data is uncertain but may be subclinical pulmonary oedema. There was evidence that rapid ascent was more likely to result in ventilation–perfusion inequality than slow ascent, suggesting that inadequate acclimatization may have been an important factor.

Using these independent measurements of the amount of ventilation–

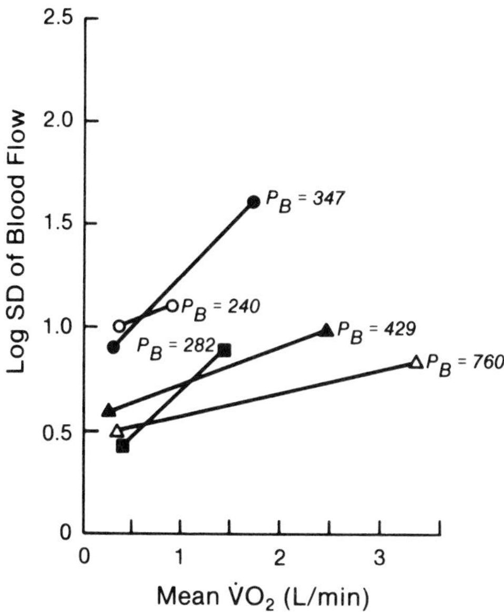

Figure 5.11 Relationship between the degree of ventilation–perfusion inequality in the lung and oxygen uptake in subjects during a simulated ascent of Mt Everest in a low pressure chamber (Operation Everest II). The ordinate shows the log SD of blood flow which is a measure of ventilation–perfusion inequality. Note that both a reduction of barometric pressure (P_B, measured in mmHg) and increase in work rate tended to increase the degree of ventilation–perfusion inequality. (From Wagner *et al.*, 1987.)

perfusion inequality present, it was possible to separate the contribution of diffusion limitation and ventilation–perfusion inequality on the observed increase of the alveolar–arterial P_{O_2} difference at high altitude. The results are shown in Figure 5.12. The arterial P_{O_2} was directly measured on arterial samples. It can be seen that the measured alveolar–arterial P_{O_2} difference increased to a mean of about 13 mmHg during maximal exercise at a barometric pressure of 347 mmHg where the oxygen consumption was a little over 2 l min^{-1}. At higher simulated altitudes, the maximum alveolar–arterial P_{O_2} differences were smaller. This can be explained by the smaller maximum oxygen uptakes, and the fact that the subjects were operating on the lower, steeper region of the oxygen dissociation curve.

Also shown in Figure 5.12 are the predicted alveolar–arterial P_{O_2} differences for the degree of ventilation–perfusion inequality measured at the same time by means of the multiple inert gas elimination technique. These predicted P_{O_2} differences decreased as the altitude

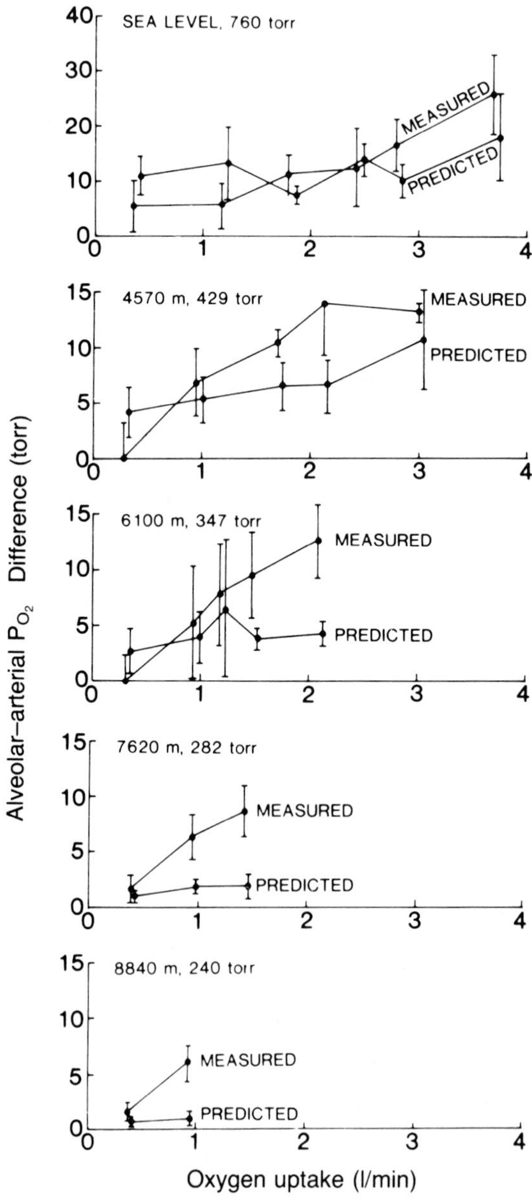

Figure 5.12 Relationship between the alveolar–arterial P_{O_2} difference and the oxygen uptake in Operation Everest II (compare Figure 5.11). The predicted difference refers to that calculated from the measured amount of ventilation–perfusion inequality. Note that, at the highest altitudes, the measured differences considerably exceeded the predicted values, indicating diffusion–limitation of oxygen uptake. For the measurements at 240 torr, the subjects breathed an oxygen mixture to give an inspired P_{O_2} of 43 torr. (From Wagner *et al.*, 1987.) (1 torr = 1 mmHg)

increased in spite of the broadening of the distributions of ventilation–perfusion ratios as shown in Figure 5.11. Again, the reason is that the P_{O_2} values are lower on the curvilinear oxygen dissociation curve. The data allow the total alveolar–arterial P_{O_2} difference to be divided into two components, one caused by ventilation–perfusion inequality, and the rest presumably attributable to diffusion limitation.

The results show that, at sea-level, essentially all of the alveolar–arterial P_{O_2} difference was attributable to ventilation–perfusion inequality up to an oxygen consumption of nearly $3\,l\,min^{-1}$. Above that high exercise level, some diffusion limitation apparently occurred. By contrast, at a barometric pressure of 429 mmHg, the measured alveolar–arterial P_{O_2} difference exceeded that predicted from the amount of ventilation–perfusion inequality when the oxygen uptake was above about $1\,l\,min^{-1}$. This was also true of a barometric pressure of 347 mmHg. At the higher simulated altitudes, with barometric pressures of 282 and 240 mmHg, almost all of the observed alveolar–arterial P_{O_2} difference during exercise could be ascribed to diffusion limitation. These elegant studies go a long way towards elucidating the role of diffusion in the hypoxaemia of high altitude during exercise.

REFERENCES

Barcroft, J., Cooke, A., Hartridge, H., *et al.* (1920) The flow of oxygen through the pulmonary epithelium. *J. Physiol. (London)*, **53**, 450–72.

Barcroft, J., Binger, C.A., Bock, A.V., *et al.* (1923) Observations upon the effect of high altitude on the physiological processes of the human body, carried out in the Peruvian Andes, chiefly at Cerro de Pasco. *Phil. Trans. Royal. Soc., Ser. B.*, **211**, 351–480.

Bartlett, D. and Remmers, J.E. (1971) Effects of high altitude exposure on the lungs of young rats. *Respir. Physiol.*, **13**, 116–25.

Bencowitz, H.Z., Wagner, P.D. and West, J.B. (1982) Effect of change in P_{50} on exercise tolerance at high altitude: a theoretical study. *J. Appl. Physiol.*, **53**, 1487–95.

Bohr, C. (1891) Uber die Lungenathmung. *Skand. Arch. Physiol.*, **32**, 236–69.

Bohr, C. (1909) Uber die spezifische Tatigkeit der Lungen bei der respiratorischen Gasaufnahmne und ihr verhalten zu der durch die Alveolarwand stattfindenden Gasdiffusion. *Skand. Arch. Physiol.*, **22**, 221–80. English translations of this and the previous paper are in *Translations in Respiratory Physiology*, (ed. J.B. West), 1981, Hutchinson Ross Publishing Company, Stroudsburg, Pennsylvania.

Burri, P.H. and Weibel, E.R. (1971) Morphometric estimation of pulmonary diffusion capacity. II. Effect of environmental P_{O_2} on the growing lung. *Respir. Physiol.*, **11**, 247–64.

DeGraff, A.C., Grover, R.F., Johnson, R.L., *et al.* (1970) Diffusing capacity of the lung in Caucasians native to 3100 m. *J. Appl. Physiol.*, **29**, 71–6.

Dempsey, J.A., Reddan, W.G., Birnbaum, M.L., *et al.* (1971) Effects of acute through life-long hypoxic exposure on exercise pulmonary gas exchange. *Respir. Physiol.*, **13**, 62–89.

Douglas, C.G., Haldane, J.S., Henderson, Y. and Schneider, E.C. (1913) Physiological observations made on Pike's Peak, Colorado, with special reference to adaptation to low barometric pressure. *Phil. Trans. R. Soc. London. Ser. B.*, **203**, 185–381.

Eaton, J.W., Skelton, T.D. and Berger, E. (1974) Survival at extreme altitude: protective effect of increased haemoglobin–oxygen affinity. *Science*, **183**, 743–4.

Filippi, F. de (1912) *Karakorum and Western Himalaya*. Constable, London.

Gehr, P., Bachofen, M. and Weibel, E.R. (1978) The normal human lung: ultrastructure and morphometric estimation of diffusing capacity. *Respir. Physiol.*, **32**, 121–40.

Gill, M.B., Milledge, J.S., Pugh, L.G.C.E. and West, J.B. (1962) Alveolar gas composition at 21 000 to 25 700 ft (6400–7830 m). *J. Physiol. (London)*, **163**, 373–7.

Guleria, J.S., Pande, J.N., Sethi, P.K. and Roy, S.B. (1971) Pulmonary diffusing capacity at high altitude. *J. Appl. Physiol.*, **31**, 536–43.

Haab, P., Perret, C. and Piiper, J. (1965) La capacite de diffusion pulmonaire pour l'oxygene chez l'homme normal jeune. *Helv. Physiol. Acta*, **23**, C23–5.

Haldane, J. and Smith, J.L. (1897) The absorption of oxygen by the lungs. *J. Physiol. (London)*, **22**, 231–58.

Haldane, J.S. and Priestley, J.G. (1935) Oxygen secretion in the lungs. In *Respiration*, 2nd edn, Yale University Press, New Haven, pp. 250–96.

Hall, F.G., Dill, D.B. and Barron, E.S.G. (1936) Comparative physiology in high altitudes. *J. Cell. Comp. Physiol.*, **8**, 301–13.

Hebbel, R.P., Eaton, J.W., Kronenberg, R.S., *et al.* (1978) Human llamas. Adaptation to altitude in subjects with high hemoglobin oxygen affinity. *J. Clin. Invest.*, **62**, 593–600.

Hinchliff, T.W. (1876) *Over the Sea and Far Away*, Longmans Green, London, p. 91.

Houston, C.S. and Riley, R.L. (1947) Respiratory and circulatory changes during acclimatization to high altitude. *Am. J. Physiol.*, **149**, 565–88.

Hyde, R.W., Forster, R.E., Power, G.G., *et al.* (1966) Measurement of O_2 diffusing capacity of the lungs with a stable O_2 isotope. *J. Clin. Invest.*, **45**, 1178–93.

Kreuzer, F. and van Lookeren Campagne, P. (1965) Resting pulmonary diffusing capacity for CO and O_2 at high altitude. *J. Appl. Physiol.*, **20**, 519–24.

Krogh, A. (1910) On the mechanism of the gas-exchange in the lungs. *Skand. Arch. Physiol.*, **23**, 248–78.

Krogh, A. and Krogh, M. (1910) On the tensions of gases in the arterial blood. *Skand. Archiv. Physiol.*, **23**, 179–92.

Krogh, M. (1915) The diffusion of gases through the lungs of man. *J. Physiol. (London)*, **49**, 271–96.

Piiper, J. and Scheid, P. (1980) Blood–gas equilibration in lungs. In *Pulmonary Gas Exchange, Volume 1, Ventilation, Blood Flow, and Diffusion*, (ed. J.B. West), Academic Press, New York, pp. 131–71.

Pugh, L.G.C.E. (1964) Cardiac output in muscular exercise at 5800 m (19 000 ft). *J. Appl. Physiol.*, **17**, 421–6.

Remmers, J.E. and Mithoefer, J.C. (1969) The carbon monoxide diffusing capacity in permanent residents at high altitudes. *Respir. Physiol.*, **6**, 233–44.

Riley, R.L., Shephard, R.H., Cohn, J.E., *et al.* (1954) Maximal diffusing capacity of the lungs. *J. Appl. Physiol.*, **43**, 357–64.

Roughton, F.J. (1945) Average time spent by blood in human lung capillary and its relation to the rates of CO uptake and elimination in man. *Am. J. Physiol.*, **143**, 621–33.

Roughton, F.J.W. and Forster, R.E. (1957) Relative importance of diffusion and chemical reaction rates in determining rate of exchange of gases in the human lung, with special reference to true diffusing capacity of pulmonary membrane and volume of blood in the lung capillaries. *J. Appl. Physiol.*, **11**, 291–302.

Schmidt-Nielsen, K. (1983) *Animal Physiology: Adaptation and Environment*, Cambridge University Press, Cambridge, p. 79.

Shepard, R.H., Varnauskas, E., Martin, H.B., *et al.* (1958) Relationship between cardiac output and apparent diffusing capacity of the lung in normal men during treadmill exercise. *J. Appl. Physiol.*, **13**, 205–10.

Turino, G.M., Bergofsky, E.H., Goldring, R.M. and Fishman, A.P. (1963) Effect of exercise on pulmonary diffusing capacity. *J. Appl. Physiol.*, **18**, 447–56.

Wagner, P.D. and West, J.B. (1972) Effects of diffusion impairment of O_2 and CO_2 time courses in pulmonary capillaries. *J. Appl. Physiol.*, **33**, 62–71.

Wagner, P.D., Saltzman, H.A. and West, J.B. (1974) Measurement of continuous distributions of ventilation–perfusion ratios: theory. *J. Appl. Physiol.*, **36**, 588–99.

Wagner, P.D., Sutton, J.R., Reeves, J.T., *et al.* (1987) Operation Everest II. Pulmonary gas exchange throughout a simulated ascent of Mt Everest. *J. Appl. Physiol.*, **63**, 2348–59.

Weibel, E.R. (1970) Morphometric estimation of pulmonary diffusion capacity. *Respir. Physiol.*, **11**, 54–75.

West, J.B. (1962) Diffusing capacity of the lung for carbon monoxide at high altitude. *J. Appl. Physiol.*, **17**, 421–6.

West, J.B. (1982) Diffusion at high altitude. *Fed. Proc.*, **41**, 2128–30.

West, J.B. and Wagner P.D. (1980) Predicted gas exchange on the summit of Mt Everest. *Respir. Physiol.*, **42**, 1–16.

West, J.B., Lahiri, S., Gill, M.B., *et al.* (1962) Arterial oxygen saturation during exercise at high altitude. *J. Appl. Physiol.*, **17**, 617–21.

West, J.B., Boyer, S.J., Graber, D.J., *et al.* (1983a) Maximal exercise at extreme altitudes on Mount Everest. *J. Appl. Physiol.*, **55**, 688–98.

West, J.B., Hackett, P.H., Maret, K.H., *et al.* (1983b) Pulmonary gas exchange on the summit of Mount Everest. *J. Appl. Physiol.*, **55**, 678–87.

Winslow, R.M., Samaja, M. and West, J.B. (1984) Red cell function at extreme altitude on Mount Everest. *J. Appl. Physiol.*, **56**, 109–16.

Zuntz, N., Loewy, A., Muller, F. and Caspari, W. (1906) Atmospheric pressure at high altitudes, in *Höhenklima und Bergwanderungen in ihrer Wirkung auf den Menschen*, Bong, Berlin, tables XI and XVIII in Appendix.

6

Cardiovascular system

6.1 INTRODUCTION

The cardiovascular system is an essential link in the process of transporting oxygen from the air to the mitochondria, and it therefore has an important role in acclimatization and adaptation to the oxygen depleted environment of high altitude. However aspects of the cardiovascular system at high altitude have not been as extensively studied as their importance may suggest. The chief reason for this is the difficulties of measurement, especially the invasive investigations necessary reliably to measure cardiac output and pulmonary artery pressure.

In this chapter we look at available data on many aspects of the cardiovascular system though, as will be seen, there are still many areas of ignorance. This chapter is closely related to some others. The cerebral circulation is discussed in Chapter 15, and changes in the capillary circulation in high altitude acclimatization and adaptation are considered in Chapter 9. High altitude pulmonary oedema and high-altitude cerebral oedema are discussed in Chapters 18 and 19.

6.2 HISTORICAL

Early travellers to high altitudes frequently complained of symptoms related to the cardiovascular system. Many of these accounts were collected by Paul Bert and set out in the first chapter of his classical book *La Pression Barométrique* (Bert, 1878, p. 29 in 1943 translation). For example, he quotes the great explorer Alexander von Humboldt at an altitude of 2773 'fathoms' on Chimborazo in the South American Andes complaining that 'blood issued from our lips and eyes'. Many other travellers gave accounts of bleeding from the mouth, eyes and nostrils, and they often attributed this to the low barometric pressure which they argued did not balance the pressures within the blood vessels. Of course this is fallacious reasoning because all vascular pressures fall along with the ambient atmospheric pressure (section 2.1). These early reports of bleeding are intriguing because this is not a typical feature of mountain sickness as we see it today.

Another common complaint of these early mountain travellers was cardiac palpitations especially on exercise. Typical is the passage quoted by Bert (1878, p. 37 in 1943 translation) from the explorer D'Orbigny who stated when he was on the crest of the Cordilleras that 'at the least movement, I felt violent palpitations'. The most observant travellers measured their pulse rate and noted that mild exercise such as riding caused it to increase dramatically while it was normal at rest. Cloves of garlic were frequently eaten to relieve these symptoms which often seem exaggerated to the modern reader.

An interesting historical vignette was the occurrence of oedema in cattle while grazing at high altitude in Utah and Colorado early in this century (Hecht *et al.*, 1962). The condition is known as Brisket Disease because the oedema is most prominent in that part of the animal between the forelegs and neck (brisket). The condition is apparently caused by right heart failure as a result of severe pulmonary hypertension caused, at least in part, by hypoxic pulmonary vasoconstriction.

Early climbers on Mt Everest who became fatigued were sometimes diagnosed as having 'dilatation' of the heart. This was thought to be one of the signs of failure to acclimatize. As late as 1934, Leonard Hill stated that 'degeneration of the heart and other organs due to low oxygen pressure in the tissues, is a chief danger which the Everest climbers have to face' (Hill, 1934).

6.3 CARDIAC FUNCTION

6.3.1 Cardiac output

It is generally accepted that acute hypoxia causes an increase in cardiac output both at rest and for a given level of exercise compared with normoxia. These responses are seen at sea-level following inhalation of low oxygen mixtures and upon acute exposure to high altitude (Asmussen and Consolazio, 1941; Honig and Tenney, 1957; Keys *et al.*, 1943; Kontos *et al.*, 1967; Vogel and Harris, 1967). There is also good evidence that in well acclimatized lowlanders at high altitude, the relationship between cardiac output and work rate returns to the sea-level value (Pugh, 1964; Reeves *et al.*, 1987). On the other hand there is some uncertainty about the changes following short periods of acclimatization.

Perhaps the first systematic studies of cardiac output at high altitude were made by Douglas, Haldane and their colleagues (1913) on the

Anglo–American Pike's Peak Expedition where they made measurements on themselves by means of ballistocardiography. No consistent changes in stroke volume of the heart were noted. They therefore concluded that cardiac output at rest was proportional to heart rate which they showed increased over the first 11 days at 4300 m and subsequently decreased. Barcroft and his colleagues (1923) used an indirect Fick technique to measure cardiac output in their study of themselves at Cerro de Pasco in the Peruvian Andes at an altitude of 4330 m. They reported a decreased cardiac output compared with sea-level but this has not been generally confirmed.

Grollman (1930) made an impressive series of measurements on Pike's Peak in 1929 using the acetylene rebreathing method. He reported that the cardiac output increased soon after reaching high altitude with a maximum value approximately five days later. However by the 12th day it had returned to its sea-level value. Similar changes were found by Christensen and Forbes (1937) during the International High Altitude Expedition to Chile.

Most recent investigators have reported similar findings. Figure 6.1 shows the increase in cardiac output during the first 40 h of acute exposure to simulated high altitude (Vogel and Harris, 1967). Klausen (1966) showed an increase in cardiac output following ascent to an altitude of 3800 m but after three to four weeks it had returned to its sea-level value. Similar findings were reported by Vogel and his colleagues (1967) on Pike's Peak at an altitude of 4300 m. However Alexander *et al.* (1967) reported a decrease in cardiac output during exercise after 10 days at 3100 m compared with sea-level. The decrease was caused by a fall in stroke volume.

In well acclimatized lowlanders at high altitude, and in high altitude natives, cardiac output in relation to work level is the same as at sea-level. This was shown by Pugh (1964) during the Silver Hut Expedition at an altitude of 5800 m where the measurements were made by acetylene rebreathing (Figure 6.2). Further measurements were made by Cerretelli (1976) at the Everest Base Camp where the subjects had acclimatized for two to three months. Reeves *et al.* (1987) reported the same finding on subjects during Operation Everest II where a remarkable series of measurements was made down to an inspired P_{O_2} of 43 mmHg, equivalent to that of the Everest summit (Figure 6.3).

High altitude natives also show the same relationship between cardiac output and oxygen consumption during exercise as at sea-level. Vogel *et al.* (1974) studied eight natives of Cerro de Pasco, Peru at an altitude of 4350 m and again after 8 to 13 days at Lima (sea-level) and showed that the results were almost superimposable (Figure 6.4).

It is perhaps surprising that cardiac output in well acclimatized lowlanders and high-altitude natives bears the same relationship to

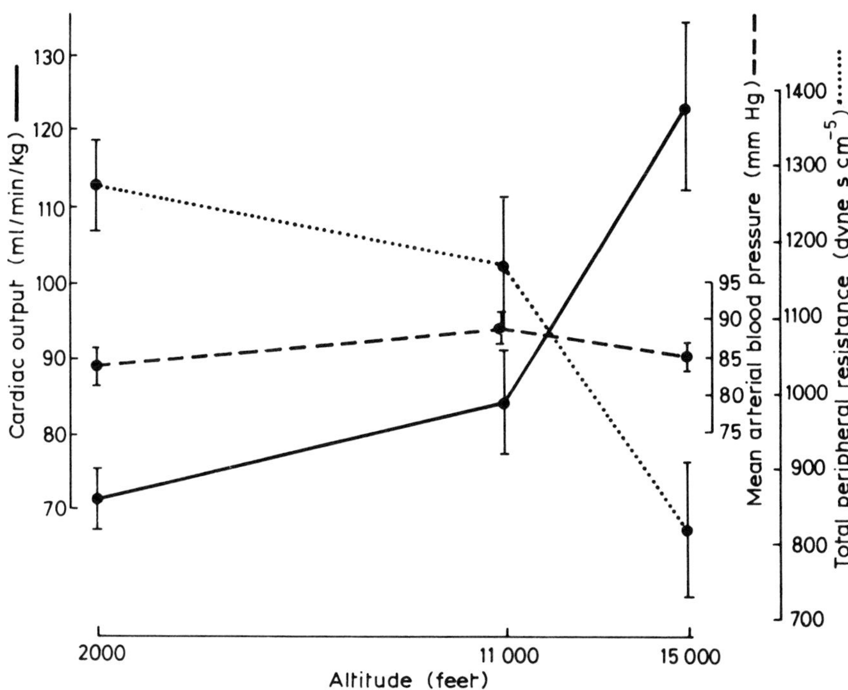

Figure 6.1 Cardiac output (solid line), mean systemic arterial pressure (dashed line), and calculated peripheral resistance (dotted line) during acute exposure to simulated altitudes of 2000 ft (610 m), 11 000 ft (3353 m) and 15 000 ft (4572 m). Measurements were made on 16 subjects after 10, 20, 30 and 40 h at each altitude. The results from the different altitude exposures were pooled. Mean ± SE indicated by vertical bars. (From Vogel and Harris, 1967.)

work rate (or power) as it does at sea-level. After all, there is plenty of evidence of severe tissue hypoxia during exercise at high altitude, and one way of increasing the tissue P_{O_2} would be to raise cardiac output and thus peripheral oxygen delivery. The fact that cardiac output returns to its sea-level value emphasizes how little we know about the control of cardiac output.

It should be remembered however that, in acclimatized subjects at high altitude, and in high altitude natives, the haemoglobin concentration is increased as a result of polycythaemia. Therefore although the cardiac output in relation to work level is unchanged, haemoglobin flow is appreciably increased. As long ago as 1929, Grollman suggested that the return of cardiac output to its sea-level value was related in some way to the increase in haemoglobin concentration of the blood.

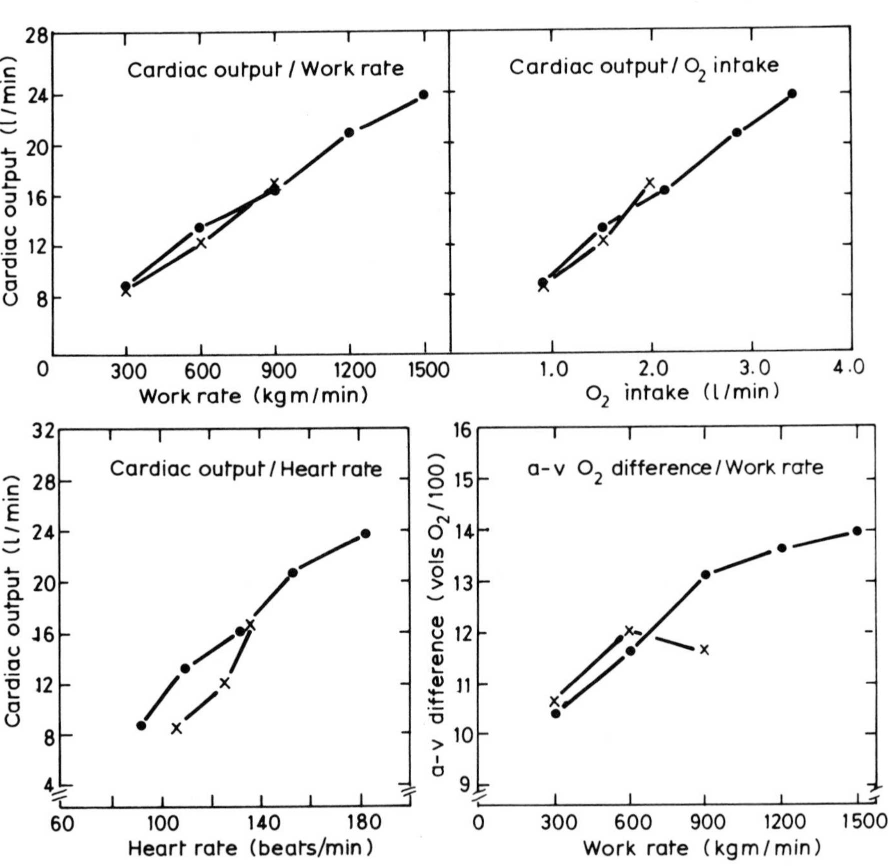

Figure 6.2 Cardiac output in relation to work rate and related variables as obtained from four well acclimatized subjects during the Himalayan Scientific and Mountaineering Expedition. Note that the cardiac output/work rate relationship is the same at an altitude of 5800 m (×, barometric pressure 380 mmHg) as at sea-level (●). (From Pugh, 1964.)

6.3.2 Heart rate

Acute hypoxia causes an increase in heart rate both at rest and for a given level of exercise just as is the case for cardiac output. The higher the altitude, the greater the increase in heart rate. At simulated altitudes of 4000–4600 m where acute exposure depresses the arterial P_{O_2} to 40–45 mmHg, resting heart rates increase by 40–50% of the sea-level values (Kontos *et al.*, 1967; Vogel and Harris, 1967).

In acclimatized subjects at high altitude, resting heart rates return to approximately the sea-level value up to an altitude of about 4500 m,

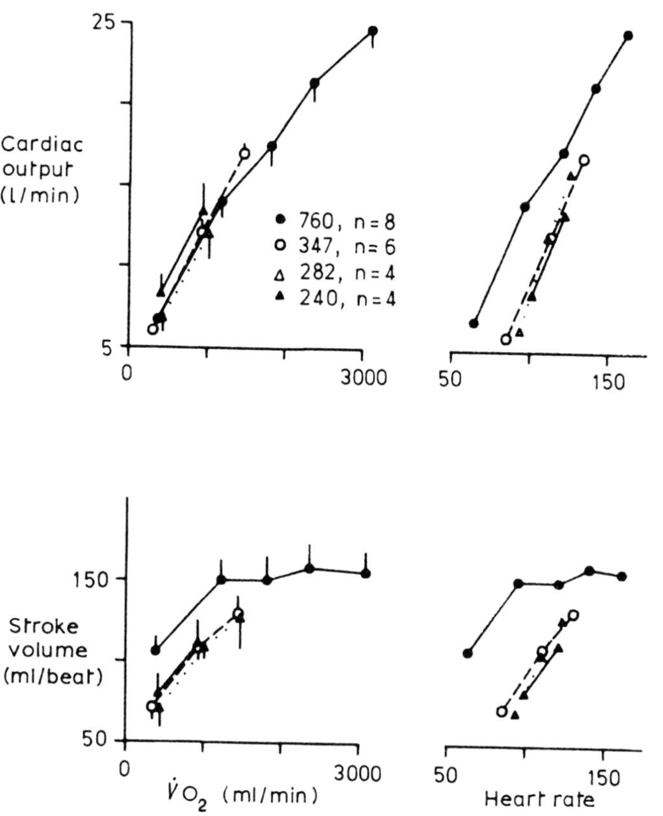

Figure 6.3 Cardiac output (by thermodilution) and stroke volume plotted against oxygen uptake and heart rate at barometric pressures of 760 (●), 347 (○), 282 (△) and 240 (▲) mmHg during Operation Everest II. For the measurements at 240 mmHg, the subjects breathed an oxygen mixture to give an inspired P_{O_2} of 43 mmHg. (From Reeves *et al.*, 1987.)

though there is some individual variation (Rotta *et al.*, 1956; Penaloza *et al.*, 1963). On exercise, heart rate for a given work rate or oxygen consumption exceeds the sea-level value. Figure 6.5 shows comparisons of heart rate at sea-level and at an altitude of 5800 m in four subjects from the Himalayan Scientific and Mountaineering Expedition who were well acclimatized to that altitude (Pugh, 1964). It can be seen that the sea-level values were generally lower than the high-altitude measurements. However in three of the four subjects the data points crossed at the highest work level that was tolerated at the high altitude. Note that, in every instance, this crossover was associated with a reduction in measured oxygen consumption suggesting that at the high

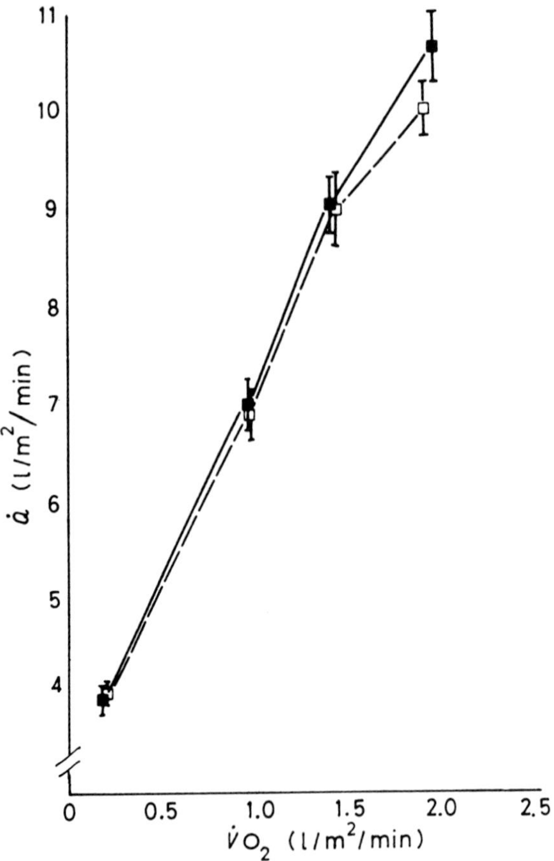

Figure 6.4 Cardiac index against oxygen uptake (both related to body surface area) in high altitude natives at 4350 m (□) and again after 8–13 days at sea-level (■). (From Vogel *et al.*, 1974.)

work rate, an increasing amount of work was being accomplished anaerobically.

Maximal heart rate, that is the heart rate at maximal exercise, is reduced in acclimatized subjects at high altitude. This is clearly seen from Figure 6.5. In Operation Everest II, maximal heart rates decreased from 160 ± 7 at sea-level to 137 ± 4 at a simulated altitude of 6100 m, 123 ± 6 at 7620 m, and 118 ± 3 at 8848 m (Reeves *et al.*, 1987). For a given work level, heart rates were greater at high altitude compared with sea-level though, interestingly, there seemed to be little difference between the measurements made at barometric pressures of 347, 282, and 240 mmHg as shown in Figure 6.6. This is possibly a reflection of

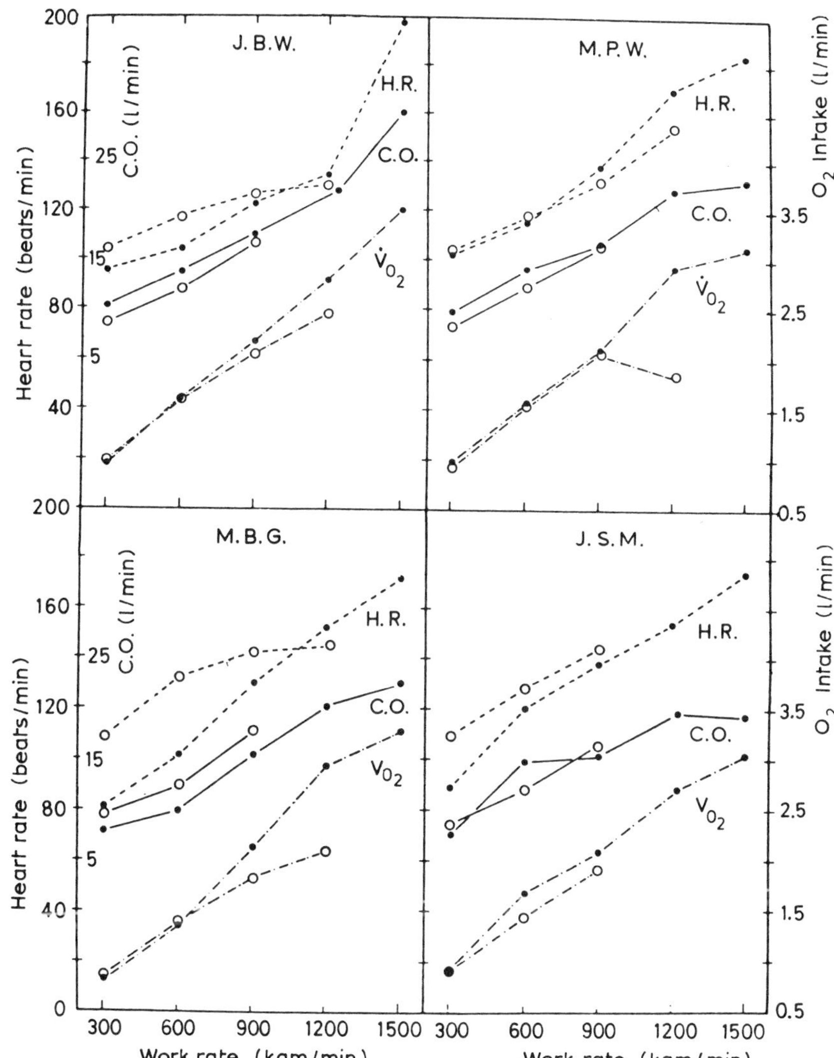

Figure 6.5 Heart rate (HR, ---) cardiac output (CO, —) and oxygen uptake ($\dot{V}_{O_2}$, –·– ·) against work rate in four well acclimatized subjects at an altitude of 5800 m. Measurements taken at sea level (●) and 5800 m (○, barometric pressure 380 mmHg). (From Pugh, 1964.)

the limited degree of acclimatization of the subjects at the higher altitudes (West, 1988).

Richalet (1990) has argued that the reduction of maximal heart rate in acclimatized subjects at high altitude represents a physiological

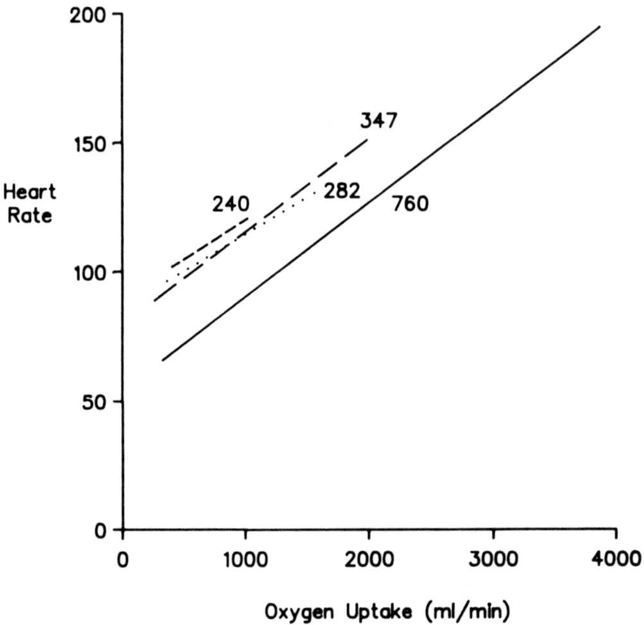

Figure 6.6 Regression lines for heart rate on oxygen uptake at barometric pressures of 760, 347, 282 and 240 mmHg during Operation Everest II. For the measurements at 240 mmHg, the subjects breathed an oxygen mixture to give an inspired P_{O_2} of 43 mmHg. (From Reeves *et al.*, 1987.)

adaptation which reduces cardiac work under conditions of limited oxygen availability. There is good evidence that hypoxia induces down regulation of β-adrenergic receptors in animal hearts (Voelkel *et al.*, 1981; Kacimi *et al.*, 1992). The role of the autonomic nervous system in controlling heart rate and cardiac output is well established. Short periods of exposure to hypoxia increase the plasma concentration of epinephrine and norepinephrine (Richalet, 1990) and the increase in heart rate caused by hypoxia is abolished by beta-blockers (Kontos and Lower, 1963).

However, the reduction of maximal heart rate in acclimatized subjects at high altitude can be interpreted differently. Since heart rate is actually increased both at rest and at a given work level compared with sea-level (except perhaps at the highest work level; Figure 6.5) it seems reasonable to regard the reduced maximal heart rate simply as a reflection of the reduced maximal work level. For example, it does not seem reasonable that a climber on the summit of Mt Everest where the $\dot{V}_{O_2max}$ is only $1\,l\,min^{-1}$ should have a maximal heart rate as high as the same person at sea level when the $\dot{V}_{O_2max}$ is $4–5\,l\,min^{-1}$.

Oxygen breathing in acclimatized subjects at high altitude reduces the heart rate for a given work level (Pugh *et al.*, 1964). This is shown in Figure 10.4 where it can be seen that the heart rate for a given work level was actually lower than the corresponding measurements at sea-level. Possible explanations include the fact that the arterial P_{O_2} at this altitude of 5800 m with 100% oxygen breathing is higher than at sea-level, and the fact that these subjects had much higher haemoglobin levels than at sea-level because of the high altitude polycythaemia. It is known that heart rate for a given work level is inversely related to haemoglobin concentration (Richardson and Guyton, 1959).

6.3.3 Stroke volume

Since stroke volume is determined by cardiac output divided by heart rate, its changes at high altitude can be deduced from those described in the last two sections.

Acute hypoxia causes approximately the same increase in cardiac output as heart rate. The result is no consistent change in stroke volume. This is true for both rest and exercise (Vogel and Harris, 1967).

After a few weeks' exposure to high altitude, the cardiac output response to work rate is the same as at sea-level (Figures 6.2 and 6.3) but heart rate remains high (Figures 6.5 and 6.6). This means that stroke volume is reduced. The fall in stroke volume has been attributed to depression of myocardial function as a result of myocardial hypoxia (Alexander *et al.*, 1967) but, as the next section shows, myocardial contractility is apparently well maintained up to extremely high altitudes. The reduction of stroke volume was also confirmed in Operation Everest II where it was shown that oxygen breathing did not increase stroke volume for a given pulmonary wedge or filling pressure. This suggested that the decline in stroke volume was not caused by severe hypoxic depression of contractility (Reeves *et al.*, 1987).

Studies of high-altitude natives at an altitude of 4350 m gave results similar to those found in acclimatized lowlanders. Cardiac output against oxygen consumption at high altitude was almost identical to the sea-level measurements (Figure 6.4), whereas heart rate was higher at high altitude and stroke volume was up to 13% less (Vogel *et al.*, 1974).

6.3.4 Myocardial contractility

As indicated above, stroke volume is reduced at high altitude both in acclimatized lowlanders and in high-altitude natives compared with sea-level. The reduced stroke volume could be caused either by reduced cardiac filling or impaired myocardial contractility. A fall in filling pressures could result either from an increased heart rate or a reduction of circulating blood volume or both.

During Operation Everest II, it was possible to measure both right atrial mean pressure (filling pressure for the right ventricle) and pulmonary wedge pressure (as an index of the filling pressure of the left ventricle). Both these measurements tended to fall as simulated altitude increased (Reeves *et al.*, 1987). It was interesting that the right atrial pressures tended to be low in spite of pulmonary hypertension (section 6.5). In general the relationship between stroke volume and right atrial pressure was maintained. This finding suggests maintenance of contractile function. In addition, as indicated above, oxygen breathing did not increase stroke volume for a given filling pressure, suggesting that the reduced stroke volume was not caused by hypoxic depression of contractility.

Additional evidence to support the finding of normal myocardial contractility came from a two-dimensional echocardiography study during Operation Everest II (Suarez *et al.*, 1987). It was found that the ventricular ejection fraction, the ratio of peak systolic pressure to end-systolic volume, and mean normalized systolic volume at rest were all sustained at a barometric presure of 282 mmHg corresponding to an altitude of about 8000 m. Indeed the surprising observation was made that during exercise at the level of 60 W, the ejection fraction was actually higher (79% ± 2 compared with 69% ± 8) at a barometric pressure of 282 mmHg compared with sea-level. The conclusion was that, despite the decreased cardiac volumes, the severe hypoxaemia and the pulmonary hypertension, cardiac contractile function appeared to be well maintained.

6.3.5 Abnormal rhythm

Abnormal rhythms (apart from sinus arrhythmia during periodic breathing) are uncommon at high altitude and perhaps this is surprising in view of the very severe arterial hypoxaemia. A resting climber on the summit of Mt Everest has an arterial P_{O_2} of less than 30 mmHg (West *et al.*, 1983; Sutton *et al.*, 1988). During exercise, the arterial P_{O_2} falls, principally because of diffusion limitation across the blood–gas barrier in the lung (West *et al.*, 1983). Thus the myocardium is exposed to extremely low oxygen levels and it is known that the hypoxic myocardium is prone to rhythm abnormalities (Josephson and Wellens, 1984).

In an electrocardiographic study of 19 subjects during the American Medical Research Expedition to Everest, only one subject had premature ventricular contractions and these were recorded at an altitude of 5300 m. Another climber showed premature atrial contractions at

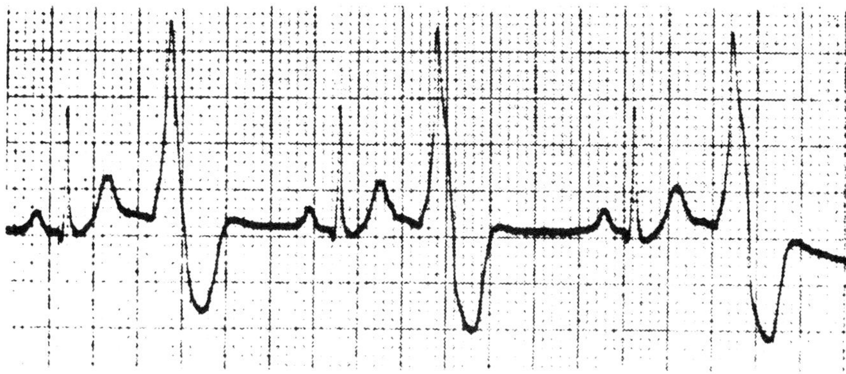

Figure 6.7 Electrocardiogram showing premature ventricular contractions occurring after exercise at 5800 m. (From Milledge, 1963.)

6300 m (Karliner *et al.*, 1985). One subject on the Himalayan Scientific and Mountaineering Expedition showed premature ventricular contractions after exercise at an altitude of 5800 m (Figure 6.7). However no other member of the expedition showed any dysrhythmia (Milledge, 1963). Occasional premature ventricular contractions and premature atrial contractions have been observed by others (Cummings and Lysgaard, 1981). Thus is appears that extreme hypoxia of the otherwise normal myocardium causes little abnormal rhythm even at the most extreme altitudes. This conclusion is consistent with the maintenance of normal myocardial contractility even during the extreme hypoxia of very great altitudes (Reeves *et al.*, 1987), as discussed in section 6.3.4.

Sinus arrythmia accompanying the periodic breathing of sleep is extremely common at high altitude (Chapter 12). Indeed the periodic slowing of the heart can be reliably used to identify the presence of periodic breathing at sea-level (Guilleminault *et al.*, 1984) and was used in this way with a Holter monitor to detect periodic breathing in climbers at an altitude of 8050 m during the American Medical Research Expedition to Everest (West *et al.*, 1986). It is likely that the most extreme arterial hypoxaemia for a given altitude occurs during the periodic breathing of sleep following the periods of apnoea. It is not surprising that occasional premature ventricular and premature atrial contractions are then sometimes seen. For example, during the four sleep studies at 8050 m, one individual had occasional premature ventricular contractions, another had atrial bigeminy and a third had occasional premature atrial beats (Karliner *et al.*, 1985).

6.3.6 Coronary circulation

The myocardium normally extracts a large proportion of the oxygen from the coronary arterial blood with the result that the venous P_{O_2} has one of the lowest values of all organs in the body. It is perhaps surprising therefore that coronary blood flow has been shown to be reduced in permanent residents of high altitude compared with people at sea-level. Moret (1971) measured coronary flow in two groups of people at La Paz (3700 m) and Cerro de Pasco (4375 m) and compared them with a group at sea-level. The flow per 100 g of left ventricle was some 30% less in the high-altitude natives. A reduction of blood flow in lowlanders following ascent to high altitude was found by Grover *et al.* (1970).

In spite of this, there appears to be little evidence of myocardial ischaemia in people living at high altitude (Arias-Stella and Topilsky, 1971). These authors showed that casts of the coronary vessels had a greater density of peripheral ramifications than sea-level controls. This might be part of the explanation for the apparent low incidence of angina and other features of myocardial ischaemia.

6.4 SYSTEMIC BLOOD PRESSURE

Acute hypoxia causes essentially no change in the mean systemic arterial blood pressure in humans, at least up to altitudes of 4600 m (Vogel *et al.*, 1967; Kontos *et al.*, 1967). This is in contrast to the dog, where acute hypoxia results in a rise of mean arterial pressure (Kontos *et al.*, 1967). Some measurements show that acclimatized lowlanders develop a rise in diastolic pressure with a corresponding decrease in pulse pressure (Brendel, 1956). However other studies suggest that the systemic blood pressure is lower in lowlanders living at high altitude than in sea-level residents, and a significantly lower prevalence of systemic hyertension has been reported at 4100 m and 4260 m in the Peruvian Andes compared with sea-level (Heath and Williams, 1977, p. 161). In another study, it was shown that a stay of one year at an altitude of 4500 m decreased systemic, systolic and diastolic pressures (Rotta *et al.*, 1956). It has been suggested that some patients with systemic hypertension who moved to an altitude of 3750 m showed a reduction in their level of systemic blood pressure (Penaloza, 1971). However no carefully controlled trials of the effect of high altitude on systemic blood pressure have been reported.

In high-altitude natives living at 4350 m, Vogel *et al.* (1974) found that the mean brachial arterial blood pressure was consistently higher during exercise than in the same subjects at sea-level. The increase in mean systemic arterial pressure which occurs during the course of heavy exercise is apparently the same in acclimatized lowlanders as it is in sea-level residents.

6.5 PULMONARY CIRCULATION

6.5.1 Pulmonary hypertension

One of the most striking cardiovascular changes at high altitude is the occurrence of pulmonary hypertension caused by an increase in pulmonary vascular resistance. This is seen in subjects exposed to acute hypoxia, in acclimatized lowlanders at high altitude, and in most high-altitude natives. The pulmonary hypertension of acute hypoxia is alleviated by oxygen breathing, but this is not the case in acclimatized lowlanders or high-altitude natives. In normal subjects at sea-level who are given low oxygen mixtures to breath, mean pulmonary artery pressure almost always increases. In early studies, Motley *et al.* (1947) reported an increase of 13–23 mmHg as a result of breathing 10% oxygen in nitrogen for 10 minutes. This study followed the initial demonstration by von Euler and Liljestrand (1946) that the pulmonary arterial pressure in the cat increased when the animals breathed 10% oxygen in nitrogen. The increase in pulmonary vascular resistance is caused by vasoconstriction, probably mainly as a result of contraction of smooth muscle in small pulmonary arteries.

Extensive studies of the effects of acute hypoxia on the pulmonary circulation have been made in humans and in a variety of animals. Figure 6.8 shows a typical study by Barer *et al.* (1970) in anaesthetized cats in which the left lower lobe of the lung was made hypoxic and its blood flow was plotted against the alveolar P_{O_2}. Note the typical non-linear stimulus–response curve. When the alveolar P_{O_2} was altered in the region above 100 mmHg, little change in blood flow and therefore vascular resistance was seen. However when the alveolar P_{O_2} was reduced to approximately 70 mmHg, obvious vasoconstriction occurred, and at very low P_{O_2} values approaching those of mixed venous blood, the local blood flow was almost abolished.

There are differences among species in the stimulus–response curves. In man, the vasoconstrictor response to acute hypoxia shows considerable variation between individuals leading Read and Fowler (1964) to refer to 'responders' and 'non-responders'. Indeed some people believe that the phenomenon of hypoxic pulmonary vasoconstriction is vestigial in the adult in that its most important function occurs in neonatal life. Here there is a release of pulmonary vasoconstriction when the newborn baby starts to breathe air, and the circulation transforms from the foetal placental to the adult lung mode.

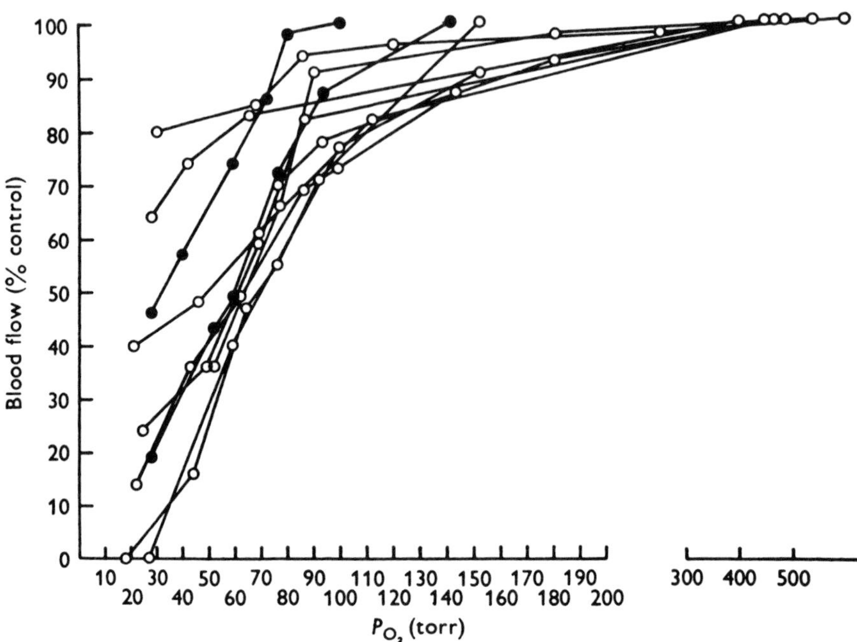

Figure 6.8 Blood flow from left lower lobe of open-chest anaesthetized cats against P_{O_2} of the pulmonary venous blood from the lobe. The lobe was ventilated with different inspired gas mixtures while the rest of the lung was breathing air (○) or 100% oxygen (●). (From Barer *et al.*, 1970.) (1 torr = 1 mmHg)

Presumably this is where the primary evolutionary pressure for the phenomenon is located.

Acclimatized lowlanders show pulmonary hypertension with a mean pulmonary arterial pressure increasing from its sea-level value of about 12 to a value of about 18 mmHg after one year at 4540 m (Rotta *et al.*, 1956; Sime *et al.*, 1974). This resting pulmonary arterial pressure increases considerably during exercise. Figure 6.9 shows the relationship between mean pulmonary vascular pressure gradient across the lung (mean pulmonary arterial pressure minus pulmonary wedge pressure) plotted against cardiac output in the subjects of Operation Everest II (Groves *et al.*, 1987). Note that the resting values of the gradient (determined primarily by the mean pulmonary artery pressure) increased, but the most dramatic change was in the slope of the pressure gradient with respect to cardiac output. This indicates the

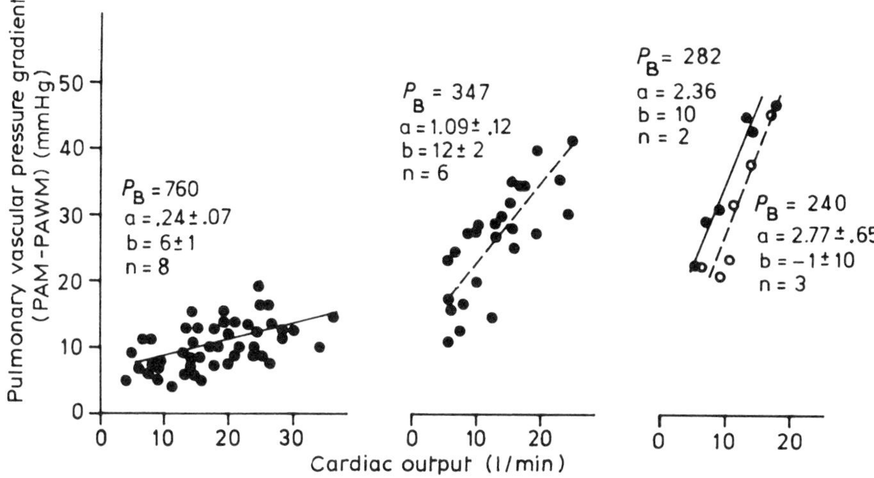

Figure 6.9 Mean pulmonary artery pressure minus mean pulmonary wedge pressure plotted against cardiac output (by thermodilution) at various barometric pressures (P_B) during Operation Everest II. For the measurements at 240 mmHg, the subjects breathed an oxygen mixture to give an inspired P_{O_2} of 43 mmHg, ● 282 mmHg, ○ 240 mmHg. (From Groves *et al.*, 1987.)

very striking increase in pulmonary vascular resistance at these great simulated altitudes.

High-altitude natives also show a substantial increase in mean pulmonary artery pressure during exercise. In one study, mean pulmonary artery pressure increased from 26 to 60 mmHg during exercise at an altitude of 4500 m (Sime *et al.*, 1974). This was a greater increase than that found in acclimatized lowlanders.

In contrast to the dramatic effect of oxygen breathing in acute hypoxia, which causes pulmonary vascular resistance to return to its prehypoxic level, oxygen breathing has relatively little effect in acclimatized lowlanders and high-altitude natives. For example, in Operation Everest II, 100% oxygen breathing was shown to lower cardiac output and pulmonary artery pressure but there was no significant fall in pulmonary vascular resistance (Groves *et al.*, 1987). In interpreting this result it should be recognized that a fall in cardiac output normally results in an *increase* in pulmonary vascular resistance because the reduction in capillary pressure causes derecruitment of capillaries and a reduction in calibre of those which remain open (Glazier *et al.*, 1969). Thus the fact that pulmonary vascular resistance did not change when it was expected to rise indicated that oxygen breathing probably reduced vascular resistance to some extent. Nevertheless it is remarkable that the subjects who were hypoxic for only two or three weeks when the measurements were made had a substantial degee of irreversibility of the increased pulmonary vascular resistance. This presumably implies that there were structural changes in the pulmonary blood vessels in addition to simple contraction of vascular smooth muscle.

High-altitude natives also show little response of their increased pulmonary vascular resistance to 100% breathing. In this case it is known that there are substantial structural changes in the lungs including a large increase in muscle in the small pulmonary arteries (section 6.5.2).

A study of a small sample of Tibetans suggested that they may have an unusually small degree of hypoxic pulmonary vasoconstriction compared with other high-altitude natives (Groves *et al.*, 1993). Five normal male residents of Lhasa (3658 m) were studied at rest and during near-maximal ergometer exercise. The resting mean pulmonary arterial pressure and pulmonary vascular resistance were within normal values for sea-level. Alveolar hypoxia resulted in a smaller rise of mean pulmonary artery pressure than in other high-altitude residents of North and South America (Reeves and Grover, 1975) (Figure 6.10). Exercise increased cardiac output more than three-fold but did not elevate pulmonary vascular resistance; 100% O_2 breathing during

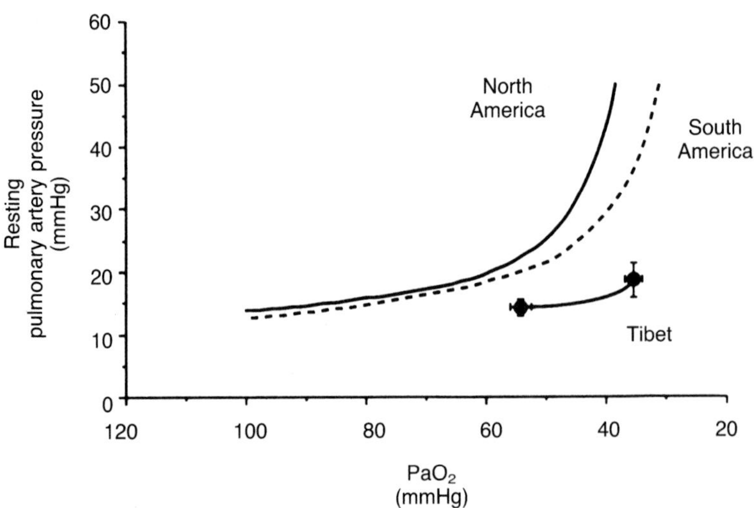

Figure 6.10 Change in mean pulmonary artery pressure during alveolar hypoxia in five Tibetans compared with high-altitude residents of North and South America. (From Groves *et al.*, 1993.)

exercise did not reduce pulmonary arterial pressure or vascular resistance. The authors argued that elevated pulmonary arterial pressure in high-altitude residents may be a maladaptive response to chronic hypoxia, and the findings indicated improved adaptation in a group that has been at high altitude for a very long period.

6.5.2 Mechanisms and structural changes

In acute hypoxia, the mechanism of hypoxic pulmonary vasoconstriction remains obscure in spite of a great deal of research. Since the phenomenon occurs in excised isolated lungs, it clearly does not depend on central nervous connections. Furthermore, excised segments of pulmonary artery can be shown to constrict if their environment is made hypoxic (Lloyd, 1965) so the response appears to be due to local action of the hypoxia on the artery itself. There is some evidence that the perivascular tissue of the artery plays a role because constriction does not occur in the absence of this (Lloyd, 1968). It is also known that it is the P_{O_2} of the alveolar gas, not the pulmonary arterial blood, which chiefly determines the response (Duke, 1954; Lloyd, 1965). This can be proved by perfusing a lung with blood of a high P_{O_2} while keeping the alveolar P_{O_2} low. Under these conditions the response is well seen.

The site of the vasoconstriction is still not certain but several pieces of evidence suggest that it is in the small pulmonary arteries (Kato and Staub, 1966; Glazier and Murray, 1971). Some studies indicate that the alveolar vessels may be partly responsible for the increased resistance, and contractile cells have been described in the interstitium of the alveolar wall, which could conceivably distort capillaries and increase their resistance (Kapanci *et al.*, 1974). However the fact that the pulmonary arterial pressure can increase to levels of 50 mmHg or more in subjects at high altitude without the occurrence of pulmonary edema suggests that the main site of constriction is upstream of the pulmonary capillaries from which the fluid leaks.

Having said this, it is also true that pulmonary edema does occur at high altitude from time to time (Chapter 18) and a likely mechanism is that the hypoxic pulmonary vasoconstriction is uneven (Hultgren, 1978) with the result that those capillaries which are not protected from the increased pulmonary arterial pressure develop ultrastructural damage to their walls. This results in a high-permeability type of edema. This topic is considered in more detail in section 18.5.2.

As indicated earlier, the mechanism of hypoxic pulmonary vasoconstriction is still unclear. Chemical mediators which have been studied in the past include catecholamines, histamine, angiotensin and prostaglandins (Fishman, 1985). Recently, a great deal of interest has been generated by the observation that inhaled nitric oxide (NO) reverses hypoxic pulmonary vasoconstriction.

NO has been shown to be an endothelium-derived relaxing factor for blood vessels (Ignarro *et al.*, 1987). NO is formed from L-arginine and is a final common pathway for a variety of biological processes (Moncada *et al.*, 1991). NO activates soluble guanylate cyclase which leads to smooth muscle relaxation through the synthesis of cyclic GMP. Nitro-vasodilators, such as nitroprusside and glycerol trinitrate, which have been used clinically for many years, are thought to act by these same mechanisms.

Inhibitors of NO synthesis have been shown to augment hypoxic pulmonary vasoconstriction in isolated pulmonary artery rings (Archer *et al.*, 1989), and attenuate pulmonary vasodilation in intact lambs (Fineman *et al.*, 1991). Inhaled NO reduces hypoxic pulmonary vasoconstriction in humans (Frostell *et al.*, 1993) and sheep (Pison *et al.*, 1993). The required inhaled concentration of NO is extremely low, being about 20 ppm, and the gas is highly toxic at high concentrations. The recognition of the role of NO has opened up a new era in understanding hypoxic pulmonary vasoconstriction.

Hypoxic pulmonary vasoconstriction has the effect of directing blood flow away from hypoxic regions of lung, caused, for example, by partial obstruction of an airway. Other things being equal, this will reduce the amount of ventilation–perfusion inequality in a lung and limit the depression of the arterial P_{O_2}. This is a useful response. However the pulmonary hypertension that is seen at high altitude appears to have no value except to cause a more uniform topographical distribution of blood flow (Dawson, 1972). In fact, the improvement in ventilation–perfusion relationships resulting from this more uniform distribution of blood flow is trivial in terms of overall gas exchange (West, 1962) and we must conclude that the pulmonary hypertension of high altitude has no useful function, and is responsible for the occurrence of high-altitude pulmonary edema. As stated earlier, the evolutionary pressure for the mechanism of hypoxic pulmonary vasoconstriction presumably comes from its value in the perinatal period.

The lungs of long term residents at high altitude show changes related to pulmonary hypertension (Heath and Williams, 1977, pp. 75–88). Bands of smooth muscle develop in the small pulmonary arteries (arterioles) of approximately 500 μm diameter which normally have a wall consisting only of a single elastic lamina. The result is that these small vessels develop a media of circularly-oriented smooth muscle bonded by internal and external elastic laminae (Figure 6.11). These changes are associated with narrowing of the lumen and an increase in pulmonary vascular resistance. Medial hypertrophy of the parent muscular pulmonary arteries is not a common feature (Arias-

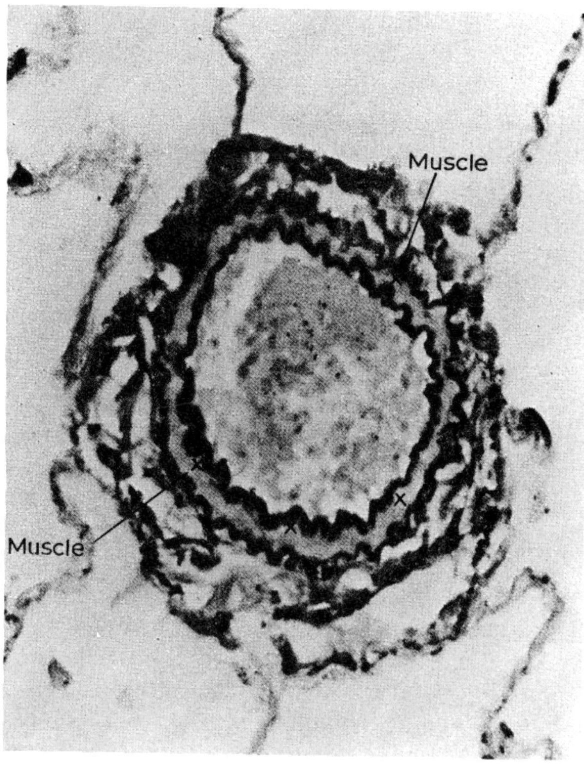

Figure 6.11 Histological section of a pulmonary arteriole from a Quechua Indian living at high altitude in the Peruvian Andes. Muscle tissue is seen between internal and external elastic laminae. Normally there is a single elastic lamina and no muscle tissue in a vessel of this size at sea-level. (Elastic van Gieson stain × 375.) (From Heath and Williams, 1977.)

Stella and Saldana, 1963) though it apparently occurs in some individuals (Wagenvoort and Wagenvoort, 1973). Occlusive intimal fibrosis apparently does not occur. However, longitudinal muscle fibres developing in the intima of pulmonary arterioles in highlanders have been described (Wagenvoort and Wagenvoort, 1973). Some authors have also described an increase in mast cell density in experimental animals exposed to long term hypoxia (Kay *et al.*, 1974). This is of interest because at one stage it was thought that mediators from mast cells, for example, histamine, might be involved in the vasoconstrictor response.

These structural changes are consistent with the fact that the pulmonary arterial pressure of high-altitude natives falls only slightly (by 15–20%) when oxygen is breathed (Penaloza *et al.*, 1962). These authors showed that inhabitants of Cerro de Pasco (4330 m) who moved to sea-level had their mean pulmonary arterial pressure halved from 24 to 12 mmHg after two years' residence at sea-level. The fact that lowlanders who are exposed to high altitude for two or three weeks develop pulmonary hypertension which is not completed reversed by 100% oxygen breathing (Groves *et al.*, 1987) suggests that their pulmonary blood vessels may also have developed some increased smooth muscle.

The structural changes that occur in pulmonary arteries when the pulmonary arterial pressure is raised as result of exposing the animal to hypoxia, are referred to as vascular remodelling (Riley, 1991). Meyrick and Reid (1978, 1980) exposed rats to half the normal barometric pressure for 1–52 days. The result was an increase in pulmonary artery pressure as a result of hypoxic pulmonary vasoconstriction. After two days they saw the appearance of new smooth muscle in small pulmonary arteries, and after ten days there was doubling of the thickness of the media and adventitia of the main pulmonary artery due to increased smooth muscle, collagen, elastin, and also oedema. There was some recovery after three days of normoxia, and after 14–28 days the thickness of the media was normal. However some increase in collagen persisted up to 70 days.

The molecular biology of the responses of the pulmonary blood vessels has been studied by several groups. Mecham *et al.* (1987) looked at the response of the pulmonary arteries of new-born calves to alveolar hypoxia. There was a 2–4-fold increase in elastin production in pulmonary arterial wall and medial smooth muscle cells. This was accompanied by a corresponding increase in elastin messenger RNA consistent with regulation at the transcriptional level. Poiani *et al.* (1990) exposed rats to 10% oxygen for 1–14 days. Within three days of exposure there was increased synthesis of collagen and elastin, and an increase in mRNA for pro α 1 (I) collagen.

Tozzi *et al.* (1989) placed rat main pulmonary artery rings in Krebs–Ringer bicarbonate. They applied mechanical tension equivalent to a transmural pressure of 50 mmHg for 4 h, and found increases in collagen synthesis (incorporation of ^{14}C proline), elastin synthesis (incorporation of ^{14}C valine), mRNA for pro α 1 (I) collagen, and mRNA for proto-oncogene v-*sis*. The last may implicate platelet-derived growth factor or transforming growth factor-β as a mediator. They were able to show that these changes were endothelium-dependent because they did not occur when the endothelium was removed from the arterial rings.

It is possible that this vascular remodelling is a general property of pulmonary vascular endothelium. It has been pointed out that the capillary wall has a dilemma in that it must be extremely thin for gas exchange but immensely strong to withstand the wall stresses when the capillary pressure rises during heavy exercise (West and Mathieu-

Costello, 1992). It appears that the extracellular matrix of the blood–gas barrier, at least on the thin side, is responsible for its strength, and it is known that in mitral stenosis, where the capillary pressure rises over long periods of time, there is an increase in thickness of the extracellular matrix (Kay and Edwards, 1973). Thus it may be that the capillary is continually regulating the structure of the wall in response to the capillary pressure which is sensed by the endothelium. The capillaries appear to be the most vulnerable vessels in the pulmonary circulation when the pressure rises. Thus vascular remodelling, which has been largely studied in larger blood vessels, may be a general property of the pulmonary vasculature, and its evolutionary advantage may be primarily the regulation of the strength of the walls of the capillaries.

The environment of the human foetus is similar in some respects to that of the high-altitude dweller in that the arterial P_{O_2} is apparently less than 30 mmHg, based on measurements on experimental animals (Itskovitz *et al.*, 1987). The foetus also has pulmonary hypertension because the pulmonary artery is connected to the systemic arterial system through the patent ductus arteriosus. In keeping with this, the foetal lung shows a high degree of muscularization of the pulmonary arteries. Babies born at a high altitude show persistence of this muscularization whereas the pulmonary arteries of those born at sea-level assume the adult appearance after only a few weeks.

6.5.3 Right ventricular hypertrophy

The pulmonary hypertension of high altitude causes right ventricular hypertrophy both in acclimatized lowlanders and in high-altitude natives. In one study it was shown in children of 2–10 years of age that, whereas at sea-level the ratio of left to right ventricular weights was about 1.8, it was less than 1.3 at high altitude (3700–4260 m) (Arias-Stella and Recavarren, 1962). Experimental studies on rats exposed to an altitude of 5500 m showed that they developed right ventricular hypertrophy within five weeks (Heath *et al.*, 1973).

Data on acclimatized lowlanders are not generally available though there is abundant indirect evidence of right ventricular hypertrophy from electrocardiographic changes (section 6.5.4). Occasionally, climbers returning from high altitude have shown evidence of right heart enlargement on the chest radiograph (Pugh, 1962).

6.5.4 Electrocardiographic changes

These are considered here because most of the changes are attributable to pulmonary hypertension. An extensive study was carried out during the American Medical Research Expedition to Everest (Karliner *et al.*,

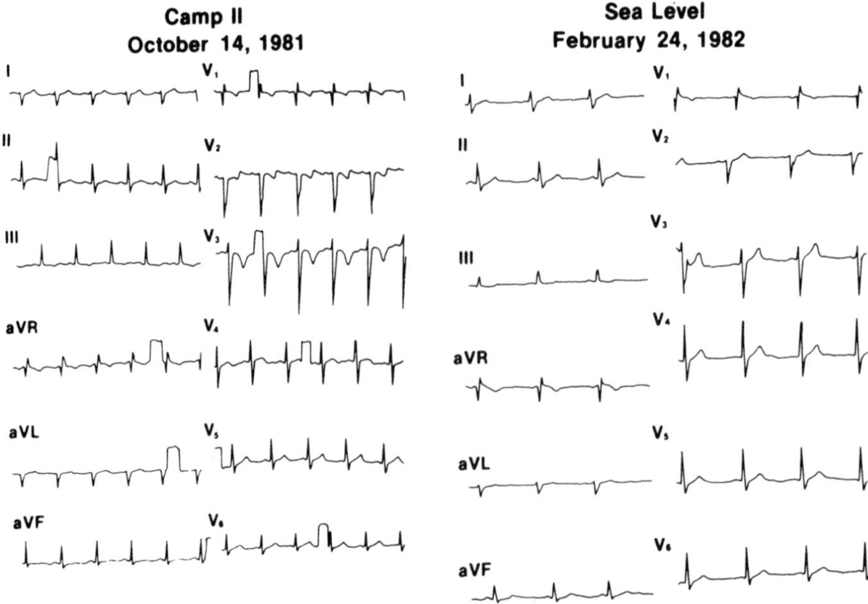

Figure 6.12 Twelve-lead electrocardiogram obtained at Camp 2 (6300 m) and about three months after return of the subject to sea-level. Sinus tachycardia and diffuse T-wave flattening present at altitude; the T waves in leads V_2 and V_3 exhibit terminal inversion. (From Karliner *et al.*, 1985.)

1985) when recordings were made at sea-level, 5400 m, 6300 m, and again at sea-level. A total of 19 subjects were studied though complete data were not obtained from all. Resting heart rate increased from a mean of 57 at sea-level to 70 at 5400 m and 80 to 6300 m (compare section 6.3.2). The amplitude of the P wave in standard lead 2 of the electrocardiogram increased by over 40% from sea-level to 6300 m, consistent with right atrial enlargement. Right axis deviation of the QRS axis was seen. The mean frontal plane QRS axis increased from +64° to +78° at 5400 m and +85° at 6300 m. Three subjects showed abnormalities of right bundle branch conduction at the highest altitude and three others showed changes consistent with right ventricular hypertrophy (posterior displacement of the QRS vector in the horizontal plane). Seven subjects developed flattened T waves and four showed T-wave inversions (Figure 6.12). All the changes returned to normal in tracings obtained at sea-level after the expedition.

Other investigators have reported similar findings in acclimatized lowlanders though generally on smaller numbers or at lower altitudes. Milledge (1963) made measurements during the Himalayan Scientific

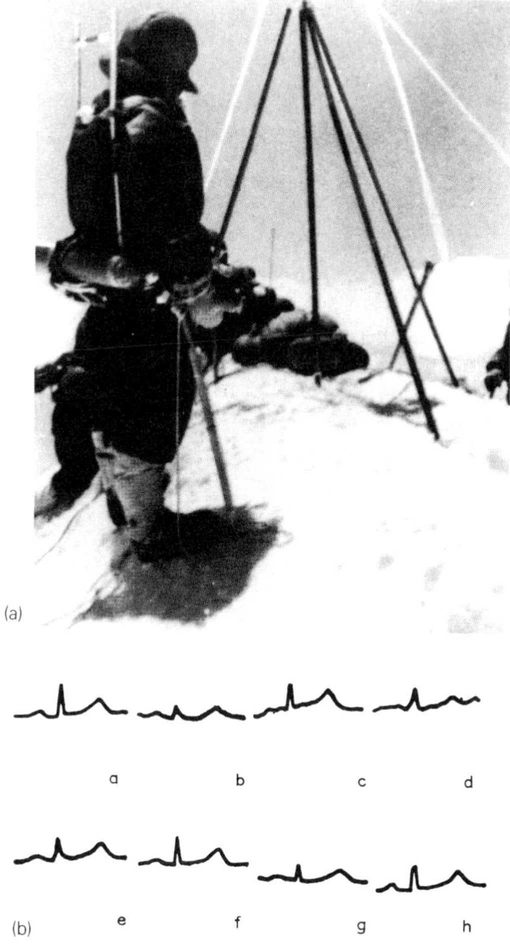

Figure 6.13 (a) Ms Phantog, Deputy Leader of the 1975 Chinese Expedition to Everest, lying under the tripod that was placed on the summit. Lead 1 of her electrocardiogram was telemetered to Base Camp (from *Another Ascent of the World's Highest Peak, Qomolangma* (no editor listed), Peking, Foreign Languages Press, 1975). (b) Standard lead 1 of the ECG of Ms Phantog from 50 m altitude to 8848 m (Everest summit) and back to 50 m. a, 50 m; b, 500 m; c, 6500 m; d, 8848 m (summit); e, back at 500 m; f, one month after returning to 50 m; g, two months after returning to 50 m; h, three months after returning to 50 m. No obvious changes are seen. (From Zhongyaun *et al.*, 1980.)

and Mountaineering Expedition and reported data on subjects who spent several months at an altitude of 5800 m. In addition some recordings were made as high as 7440 m in climbers who never used supplemental oxygen. He found T-wave inversions on the right precordial leads in six subjects, while two had left precordial T-wave inversion as well. Oxygen breathing had no effect on these changes. Das *et al.* (1983) reported on over 40 subjects who were rapidly transported to either 3200 or 3771 m. There was a tendency for a rightward axis shift which interestingly tended to resolve in most subjects after 10 days at high altitude.

A particularly remarkable measurement was made on Ms Phantog, deputy leader of the successful 1975 Chinese ascent of Mt Everest. She lay down on the summit under the newly erected tripod while her standard lead 1 was telemetered down to Base Camp (Figure 6.13(a) and (b)). Note that there were no changes from sea level to 8848 m and back again (Zhongyuan *et al.*, 1980). Other electrocardiographic studies at high altitude include those made by Aigner *et al.* (1980), Jackson and Davies (1960) Kapoor (1984), Malconian *et al.* (1990), and Penaloza and Echevarria (1957).

REFERENCES

Aigner, A., Berghold, F. and Muss, N. (1980) Investigations on the cardiovascular system at altitudes up to a height of 7800 meters. *Z. Kardiol.*, **69**, 604–10.

Alexander, J.K., Hartley, L.H., Modelski, M. and Grover, R.F. (1967) Reduction of stroke volume during exercise in man following ascent to 3100 m altitude. *J. Appl. Physiol.*, **23**, 849–57.

Archer, S.L., Tolins, J.P., Ralj, L. and Weir, E.K. (1989) Hypoxic pulmonary vasoconstriction is enhanced by inhibition of the synthesis of an endothelium derived relaxing factor. *Biochem. Biophys. Res. Commun.*, **164**, 1198–205.

Arias-Stella, J. and Recavarren, S. (1962) Right ventricular hypertrophy in native children living at high altitude. *Am. J. Pathol.*, **41**, 55–64.

Arias-Stella, J. and Saldana, M. (1963) The terminal portion of the pulmonary arterial tree in people native to high altitudes. *Circulation*, **28**, 915–25.

Arias-Stella, J. and Topilsky, M. (1971) Anatomy of the coronary circulation at high altitude, in *High Altitude Physiology: Cardiac and Respiratory Aspects*, (eds R. Porter and J. Knight), Churchill Livingstone, Edinburgh, p. 149.

Asmussen, E. and Consolazio, F.C. (1941) The circulation in rest and work on Mount Evans (4300 m). *Am. J. Physiol.*, **132**, 555–63.

Barcroft, J., Binger, C.A., Bock, A.V., *et al.* (1923) Observations upon the effect of high altitude on the physiological processes of the human body, carried out in the Peruvian Andes, chiefly at Cerro de Pasco. *Phil. Trans. R. Soc. London Ser. B.*, **211**, 351–480.

Barer, G.R., Howard, P. and Shaw, J.W. (1970) Stimulus–response curves for the pulmonary vascular bed to hypoxia and hypercapnia. *J. Physiol. (London)*, **211**, 139–55.

Bert, P. (1878) *La Pression Barométrique*, Masson, Paris. English translation (1943) by M.A. Hitchcock and F.A. Hitchcock, College Book Co., Columbus, Ohio, pp. 343–6.

Brendel, W. (1956) Anpassung von Atmung, Hamoglobin, Korpertemperatur und Kreislauf bei langfristigem Aufenthalten in grossen Hohen (Himalaya). *Pflugers Arch.*, **263**, 227–52.

Cerretelli, P. (1976) Limiting factors to oxygen transport on Mount Everest. *J. Appl. Physiol.*, **40**, 658–67.
Christensen, C.H. and Forbes, W.H. (1937) Der Kreislauf in grossen Hohen. *Skand. Arch. Physiol.*, **76**, 75–100.
Cummings, P. and Lysgaard, M. (1981) Cardiac arrhythmia at high altitude. *West. J. Med.*, **135**, 66–8.
Das, B.K., Tewari, S.C., Parashar, S.K., *et al.* (1983) Electrocardiographic changes at high altitude. *Indian Heart J.*, **35**, 30.
Dawson, A. (1972) Regional lung function during early acclimatization to 3100 m altitude. *J. Appl. Physiol.*, **33**, 218–23.
Douglas, C.G., Haldane, J.A., Henderson, Y. and Schneider, E.C. (1913) Physiological observations made on Pike's Peak, Colorado, with special reference to adaptation to low barometric pressures. *Phil. Trans. R. Soc. London Ser. B.*, **203**, 185–381.
Duke, H.N. (1954) Site of action of anoxia on the pulmonary blood vessels of the cat. *J. Physiol. (London)*, **125**, 373–82.
Fineman, J.R., Heymann, M.A. and Soifer, S.J. (1991) *N*-nitro-L-arginine attenuates endothelium-dependent pulmonary vasodilation in lambs. *Am. J. Physiol.*, **260**, (*Heart Circ. Physiol.*, **29**), H1299–306.
Fishman, A. (1985) Pulmonary circulation, in *Handbook of Physiology, Section 3: The respiratory system*, Vol. 1, (eds A.P. Fishman and A. Fisher), American Physiological Society, Bethesda, Maryland, pp. 93–165.
Frostell, C.G., Blomqvist, H., Hedenstierna, G., *et al.* (1993) Inhaled nitric oxide selectively reverses human hypoxic pulmonary vasoconstriction without causing systemic vasodilation. *Anesthesiology*, **78**, 427–35.
Glazier, J.B., Hughes, J.M.B., Maloney, J.E. and West, J.B. (1969) Measurements of capillary dimensions and blood volume in rapidly frozen lungs. *J. Appl. Physiol.*, **26**, 65–76.
Glazier, J.B. and Murray, J.F. (1971) Sites of pulmonary vasomotor reactivity in the dog during alveolar hypoxia and serotonin and histamine infusion. *J. Clin. Invest.*, **50**, 2550–8.
Grollman, A. (1930) Physiological variations of the cardiac output of man. VII. The effect of high altitude on the cardiac output and its related functions: an account of experiments conducted on the summit of Pike's Peak, Colorado. *Am. J. Physiol.*, **93**, 19–40.
Grover, R.F., Lufschanowski, R. and Alexander, J.A. (1970) Decreased coronary blood flow in man following ascent to high altitude. *Adv. Cardiol.*, **5**, 72–9.
Groves, B.M., Reeves, J.T., Sutton, J.R., *et al.* (1987) Operation Everest II: elevated high-altitude pulmonary resistance unresponsive to oxygen. *J. Appl. Physiol.*, **63**, 521–30.
Groves, B.M., Droma, T., Sutton, J.R., *et al.* (1993) Minimal hypoxic pulmonary hypertension in normal Tibetans at 3658 m. *J. Appl. Physiol.*, **74**, 312–8.
Guilleminault, C., Connolly, S., Winkle, R., *et al.* (1984) Cyclical variation of the heart rate in sleep apnoea syndrome. *Lancet*, **i**, 126–31.
Heath, D. and Williams, D.R. (1977) *Man at High Altitude*, Churchill Livingstone, London.
Heath, D., Edward, C., Winson, M. and Smith, P. (1973) Effects on the right ventricle, pulmonary vasculature, and carotid bodies of the rat exposure to, and recovery from, simulated high altitude. *Thorax*, **28**, 24–8.
Hecht, H.H., Kuida, H., Lange, R.L., *et al.* (1962) Brisket disease. II. Clinical features and hemodynamic observations in altitude-dependent right heart failure of cattle. *Am. J. Med.*, **32**, 171–83.

Hill, L. (1934) Foreword in *Oxygen and Carbon Dioxide Therapy*, (eds A. Campbell and E.P. Poulton), Oxford University Press, London.

Honig, C.R. and Tenney, S.M. (1957) Determinants of the circulatory response to hypoxia and hypercapnia. *Am. Heart J.*, **53**, 687–98.

Hultgren, H.N. (1978) High altitude pulmonary edema, in *Lung Water and Solute Exchange*, (ed. N.C. Staub), Dekker, New York, pp. 437–69.

Ignarro, L.J., Buga, G.M., Wood, K.S., *et al.* (1987) Endothelium-derived relaxing factor produced and released from artery and vein is nitric oxide. *Proc. Natl Acad. Sci. USA*, **84**, 9265–9.

Itskovitz, J., LaGamma, E.F. and Rudolph, A.M. (1987) Effects of cord compression on fetal blood flow distribution and O_2 delivery. *Am. J. Physiol. (Heart Circ. Physiol.)*, **21**, H100–9.

Jackson, F. and Davies, H. (1960) The electrocardiogram of the mountaineer at high altitude. *Br. Heart J.*, **22**, 671–85.

Josephson, M.E. and Wellens, H.J.J. (eds) (1984) *Tachycardia: mechanisms, diagnosis, treatment*, Lea and Febiger, Philadelphia.

Kacimi, R., Richalet, J.P., Corsin, A., *et al.* (1992) Hypoxia-induced downregulation of beta-adrenergic receptors in rat heart. *J. Appl. Physiol.*, **73**, 1377–82.

Kapanci, Y., Assimacopoulos, A., Irle, C., *et al.* (1974) 'Contractile interstitial cells' in pulmonary alveolar septa: a possible regulator of ventilation/perfusion ratio? *J. Cell. Biol.*, **60**, 375–92.

Kapoor, S.C. (1984) Changes in electrocardiogram among temporary residents at high altitude. *Defence Sci. J.*, **34**, 389–95.

Karliner, J., Sarnquist, F.H., Graber, D.J., *et al.* (1985) The electrocardiogram at extreme altitude: experience on Mt Everest. *Am. Heart J.*, **109**, 505–13.

Kato, M. and Staub, N.C. (1966) Response of small pulmonary arteries to unilobar hypoxia and hypercapnia. *Circ. Res.*, **19**, 426–40.

Kay, J.M. and Edwards, F.R. (1973) Ultrastructure of the alveolar-capillary wall in mitral stenosis. *J. Pathol.*, **111**, 239–45.

Kay, J.M., Waymire, J.C. and Grover, R.F. (1974) Lung mast cell hyperplasia and pulmonary histamine-forming capacity in hypoxic rats. *Am. J. Physiol.*, **226**, 178–84.

Keys, A., Stapp, J.P. and Violante, A. (1943) Responses in size, output and efficiency of the human heart to acute alteration in the composition of inspired air. *Am. J. Physiol.*, **138**, 763–71.

Klausen, K. (1966) Cardiac output in man in rest and work during and after acclimatization to 3800 m. *J. Appl. Physiol.*, **21**, 609–16.

Kontos, H.A., Levasseur, J.E., Richardson, D.W., *et al.* (1967) Comparative circulatory responses to systemic hypoxia in man and in unanesthetized dog. *J. Appl. Physiol.*, **23**, 381–6.

Kontos, H.A. and Lower, R.R. (1963) Rule of beta-adrenergic receptors in the circulatory response to high altitude hypexia. *Am. J. Physiol.*, **217**, 756–63.

Lloyd, T.C. (1965) Pulmonary vasoconstriction during histotoxic hypoxia. *J. Appl. Physiol.*, **20**, 488–90.

Lloyd, T.C. (1968) Hypoxic pulmonary vasoconstriction: role of perivascular tissue. *J. Appl. Physiol.*, **25**, 560–65.

Malconian, M.K., Rock, P.B., Hultgran, H.N., *et al.* (1990) The electrocardiogram at rest and exercise during a simulated ascent of Mt Everest (Operation Everest II). *Am. J. Cardiol.*, **65**, 1475–80.

Mecham, R.P., Whitehouse, L.A., Wrenn, D.S., *et al.* (1987) Smooth muscle-mediated connective tissue remodeling in pulmonary hypertension. *Science*, **237**, 423–6.

Meyrick, B. and Reid, L. (1978) The effect of continued hypoxia on rat pulmonary arterial circulation. An ultrastructural study. *Lab. Invest.*, **38**, 188.
Meyrick, B. and Reid, L. (1980) Hypoxia-induced structural changes in the media and adventitia of the rat hilar pulmonary artery and their regression. *Am. J. Pathol.*, **100**, 151–69.
Milledge, J.S. (1963) Electrocardiographic changes at high altitude. *Br. Heart J.*, **25**, 291–8.
Moncada, S.R., Palmer, M.J. and Higgs, E.A. (1991) Nitric oxide physiology, pathophysiology, and pharmacology. *Pharmacol. Rev.*, **43**, 109–42.
Moret, P.R. (1971) Coronary blood flow and myocardial metabolism in man at high altitude, in *High Altitude Physiology: Cardiac and Respiratory Aspects*, (eds R. Porter and J. Knight), Churchill Livingstone, Edinburgh, pp. 131–44.
Motley, H.L., Cournand, A., Werko, L., *et al.* (1947) Influence of short periods of induced acute anoxia upon pulmonary artery pressure in man. *Am. J. Physiol.*, **150**, 315–20.
Penaloza, D. (1971) Discussion, in *High Altitude Physiology: Cardiac and Respiratory Aspects*, (eds R. Porter and J. Knight), Churchill Livingstone, Edinburgh, p. 169.
Penaloza, D. and Echevarria, M. (1957) Electrocardiographic observations on ten subjects at sea level and during one year of residence at high altitudes. *Am. Heart J.*, **54**, 811–22.
Penaloza, D., Sime, F., Banchero, N. and Gamboa, R. (1962) Pulmonary hypertension in healthy man born and living at high altitudes. *Medicina Thoracalis*, **19**, 449–60.
Penaloza, D., Sime, F., Banchero, N., *et al.* (1963) Pulmonary hypertension in healthy men born and living at high altitudes. *Am. J. Cardiol.*, **11**, 150–7.
Pison, U., López, F.A., Heidelmeyer, C.F., *et al.* (1993) Inhaled nitric oxide reverses hypoxic pulmonary vasoconstriction without impairing gas exchange. *J. Appl. Physiol.*, **74**, 1287–92.
Poiani, G.J., Tozzi, C.A., Yohn, S.E., *et al.* (1990) Collagen and elastin metabolism in hypertensive pulmonary arteries of rats. *Circ. Res.*, **66**, 968–78.
Pugh, L.G.C.E. (1962) Physiological and medical aspects of the Himalayan Scientific and Mountaineering Expedition, 1960–61. *Br. Med. J.*, **2**, 621–7.
Pugh, L.G.C.E. (1964) Cardiac output in muscular exercise at 5800 m (19 000 ft). *J. Appl. Physiol.*, **19**, 441–7.
Pugh, L.G.C.E., Gill, M.B., Lahiri, S., *et al.* (1964) Muscular exercise at great altitudes. *J. Appl. Physiol.*, **19**, 431–40.
Read, J. and Fowler, K.T. (1964) Effect of exercise on zonal distribution of pulmonary blood flow. *J. Appl. Physiol.*, **19**, 672–8.
Reeves, J.T. and Grover, R.F. (1975) High-altitude pulmonary hypertension and pulmonary edema. *Prog. Cardiol.*, **4**, 99–118.
Reeves, J.T., Groves, B.M., Sutton, J.T., *et al.* (1987) Operation Everest II: preservation of cardiac function at extreme altitude. *J. Appl. Physiol.*, **63**, 531–9.
Richalet, J.-P. (1990) The heart and adrenergic system, in *Hypoxia: the Adaptations*, (eds J.R. Sutton, G. Coates and J.E. Remmers), Dekker, Philadelphia, pp. 231–40.
Richardson, T.Q. and Guyton, A.C. (1959) Effects of polycythemia and anemia on cardiac output and other circulatory factors. *Am. J. Physiol.*, **197**, 1167–79.
Riley, D.J. (1991) Vascular remodeling, in *The Lung: Scientific Foundations*, (eds R.G. Crystal and J.B. West), Raven Press, New York, pp. 1189–98.
Rotta, A., Canepa, A., Hurtado, A., *et al.* (1956) Pulmonary circulation at sea level and at high altitudes. *J. Appl. Physiol.*, **9**, 328–36.

Sime, F., Penaloza, D., Ruiz, L., *et al.* (1974) Hypoxemia, pulmonary hypertension, and low cardiac output in newcomers at low altitude. *J. Appl. Physiol.*, **36**, 561–5.

Suarez, J.M., Alexander, J.K. and Houston, C.S. (1987) Enhanced left ventricular systolic performance at high altitude during Operation Everest II. *Am. J. Cardiol.*, **60**, 137–42.

Sutton, J.R., Reeves, J.T., Wagner, P.D., *et al.* (1988) Operation Everest II. Oxygen transport during exercise at extreme simulated altitude. *J. Appl. Physiol.*, **64**, 1309–21.

Tozzi, C.A., Poiani, G.J., Harangozo, A.M., *et al.* (1989) Pressure-induced connective tissue synthesis in pulmonary artery segments is dependent on intact endothelium. *J. Clin. Invest.*, **84**, 1005–12.

Voelkel, N.F., Hegstrand, L., Reeves, J.T., *et al.* (1981) Effect of hypoxia on density of β-adrenergic receptors. *J. Appl. Physiol.*, **50**, 363–6.

Vogel, J.A. and Harris, C.W. (1967) Cardiopulmonary responses of resting man during early exposure to high altitude. *J. Appl. Physiol.*, **22**, 1124–8.

Vogel, J.A., Hansen, J.E. and Harris, C.W. (1967) Cardiovascular responses in man during exhaustive work at sea level and high altitude. *J. Appl. Physiol.*, **23**, 531–9.

Vogel, J.A., Hartley, L.H. and Cruz, J.C. (1974) Cardiac output during exercise in altitude natives at sea level and high altitude. *J. Appl. Physiol.*, **36**, 173–6.

Von Euler, U.S. and Liljestrand, G. (1946) Observations on the pulmonary arterial blood pressure in the cat. *Acta Physiol.*, **22**, 1115–23.

Wagenvoort, C.A. and Wagenvoort, N. (1973) Hypoxic pulmonary vascular lesions in man at high altitude and in patients with chronic respiratory disease. *Pathol. Microbiol.*, **39**, 276–82.

West, J.B. (1962) Regional differences in gas exchange in the lung of erect man. *J. Appl. Physiol.*, **17**, 893–8.

West, J.B. (1987) Tolerable limits to hypoxia – on high mountains, in *Hypoxia: The Tolerable Limits*, (eds J.R. Sutton, C.S. Houston and G. Coates), Benchmark Press, Indianapolis, pp. 353–62.

West, J.B. (1988) Rate of ventilatory acclimatization to extreme altitude. *Respir. Physiol.*, **74**, 323–33.

West, J.B. and Mathieu-Costello, O. (1992) Strength of the pulmonary blood–gas barrier. *Respir. Physiol.*, **88**, 141–8.

West, J.B., Hackett, P.H., Maret, K.H., *et al.* (1983) Pulmonary gas exchange on the summit of Mt Everest. *J. Appl. Physiol. Respir. Environ. Exercise Physiol.*, **55**, 678–87.

West, J.B., Peters, R.M., Aksnes, G., *et al.* (1986) Nocturnal periodic breathing at altitudes of 6300 and 8050 m. *J. Appl. Physiol.*, **61**, 280–7.

Zhongyuan, S., Xuehan, N., Shoucheng, Z., *et al.* (1980) Electrocardiogram made on ascending the Mount Qomolangma from 50 m A.S.L. *Sci. Sin.*, **23**, 1316–25.

7

Haematology

7.1 INTRODUCTION

Probably the best known adaptation to high altitude is the increase in the number of red blood cells per unit volume of blood. Paul Bert suggested in his book, *La Pression Barométrique* (published 1878), that adaptation to high altitude might include an increase in the number of red blood cells and the quantity of haemoglobin and thus the blood would be able to carry more oxygen. A few years later he was sent samples of blood from a number of domestic animals from La Paz, Bolivia (3500 m); he showed that these samples combined with 16.2–21.6 volumes of oxygen per 100 volumes of blood compared with 10–12 vols % in the blood of animals in France (West, 1981).

Viault, in 1890, made the first blood counts of men at high altitude. His own blood count at sea-level in Lima was $5 \times 10^6\,mm^{-3}$ and after three weeks at Morococha, a mining township at 4372 m in the Andes, the value had increased to $7.1 \times 10^6\,mm^{-3}$. We now know that most of this increase, early in altitude exposure, would be due to reduced plasma volume rather than an increase in red cell mass. He found these elevated counts present in a companion doctor from Lima and also in a number of the local Indian residents at altitude. He also noted that in a male llama the value was $16 \times 10^6\,mm^{-3}$. He called the llama, 'l'animal par excellence des grandes altitudes'. In 1891 Viault published further observations which confirmed Bert's work on the oxygen carrying capacity of high-altitude animals. He showed in two sheep and one dog that their oxygen carrying capacity was increased compared with similar animals in France.

Since then, almost all expeditions with any pretence at carrying out physiological research at high altitude have observed this increase in either red blood cell count, packed cell volume, or haemoglobin concentration [Hb].

The increase in red cell number and [Hb] increases the oxygen

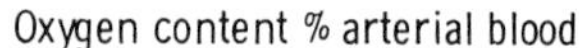

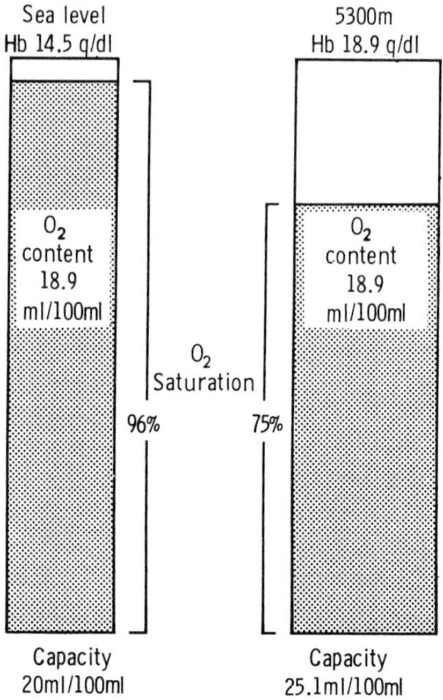

Figure 7.1 The oxygen content of arterial blood in an acclimatized subject at 5300 m and at sea-level.

carrying capacity in such a way that, up to at about 5300 m, fully acclimatized man has the same oxygen content in his blood as at sea-level (Figure 7.1).

The increased carrying capacity compensates for the reduced oxygen saturation. This affords physiology teachers a classical example of beneficial adaptation. However, it is unlikely that the mechanism of this adaptation evolved primarily to serve man at high altitude (section 7.2.1). The extent to which benefit can be gained by increasing [Hb] is fairly limited and indeed has been questioned as beneficial at all (Winslow and Monge, 1987a) (section 7.5.4).

7.2 REGULATION OF HAEMOGLOBIN CONCENTRATION

The [Hb] and packed cell volume (PCV) depend upon the ratio of the red cell mass (RCM) to plasma volume (PV). These two variables are regulated by different mechanisms. The RCM is determined by the rate of formation of red blood cells (erythropoiesis) and their rate of loss.

Red blood cells are lost by death (their natural length of survival is about 120 days), or by haemorrhage. Their death can be hastened by a variety of pathological states such as haemolytic anaemia. Erythropoiesis can be impaired by various deficiencies, such as iron or vitamin B_{12}, needed for haemoglobin synthesis or by disorders of the bone marrow. In the absence of these, erythropoiesis is thought to be controlled by the level of the hormone erythropoietin.

7.2.1 Erythropoietin and its regulation

Erythropoietin is produced mainly in the kidney though 10–15% of total production is in the liver (Erslev, 1987). The gene coding for the hormone has been cloned and expressed in cultured cells, allowing for sufficient material to be produced for clinical studies. It has been shown to stimulate erythropoiesis in patients anaemic with end-stage renal failure (Winearls *et al.*, 1986).

The two classical stimuli for erythropoietin secretion are hypoxia and blood loss, both of which result in tissue hypoxia. Of the two, blood loss is probably more important in evolutionary terms of survival of the organism since blood loss must be a far more common danger than is chronic hypoxia, and of course this system is no defence against acute hypoxia. The stimulus to erythropoietin secretion is hypoxia at some tissue site, probably in the kidney, possibly identical with the site of production of the hormone. It is instructive to compare this system with the other hypoxia sensitive system in the body, the hypoxic ventilatory response (HVR), mediated mainly via the carotid body:

- The HVR appears in seconds after a step change in arterial P_{O_2}, whereas there is no detectable rise in erythropoietin concentration for over an hour (114 min when exposed suddenly to 3000 m or 84 min at 4000 m) (Eckardt *et al.*, 1989).
- The carotid body is sensitive to reduction in P_{O_2} rather than oxygen content of the blood. Therefore it does not respond to anaemia, whereas anaemia stimulates erythropoietin secretion. From this observation it is assumed that, while the carotid body response is to arterial P_{O_2}, the sensing of P_{O_2} for erythropoietin secretion is at the venous or tissue level. In patients with a reversed flow through a patent ductus arteriosus, there is cyanosis (hypoxia) in the lower half of the body only. These patients have high [Hb] indicating that the P_{O_2} sensor is in the lower half of the body, presumably in the kidney. Fisher and Langston (1967) showed that erythropoietin was produced in the juxtaglomerular apparatus in the kidney and that hypoxia was sensed there, since the isolated dog kidney increased its output of erythropoietin when perfused with hypoxic blood.

7.2.2 Regulation of plasma volume

The central control of PV is probably by a feedback loop involving atrial natriuretic peptide (ANP) and the right atrium (Laragh, 1985). ANP is released in response to stretching of the right atrium. Physiologically, this is produced by increased right atrial pressure. This in turn may be due to shifts of blood volume from the periphery, mainly the lower body, or by increase in the total blood volume (i.e. PV). ANP causes the kidney to excrete sodium and with it water thus reducing the PV. This simple feedback loop is shown in Figure 7.2.

We can add on to this simple system a host of other factors which affect PV (Figure 7.3):

- Hydration and dehydration will obviously affect PV, along with all other body fluid compartments.
- The vascular capacity is determined by the tone of the vessels, especially the venous capacitance vessels and vessels in the skin. Vessel tone, in turn, depends upon a number of factors, such as temperature and catecholamine levels. Peripheral vasoconstriction shifts blood from the periphery to the centre, raising right atrial pressure and stimulating ANP release. Vasodilatation has the opposite effect. A change in vascular capacity also has a more direct effect on PV by shifting the balance of forces in the Starling equation. Vasodilatation will tend to reduce the intravascular pressure, favouring inward movement of fluid at the tissue level, vasoconstriction has the opposite effect. It is this direct effect that is depicted in Figure 7.3.
- Other factors which cause a shift of blood volume to the centre include posture: lying down, lower body immersion or G-suits. Zero

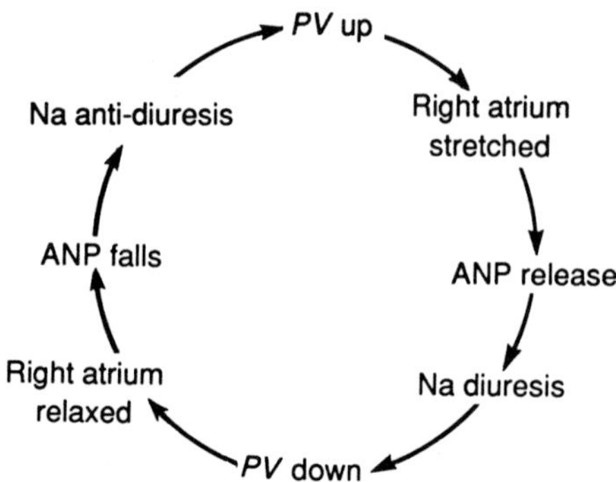

Figure 7.2 The regulation of plasma volume (PV) by atrial natriuretic peptide (ANP).

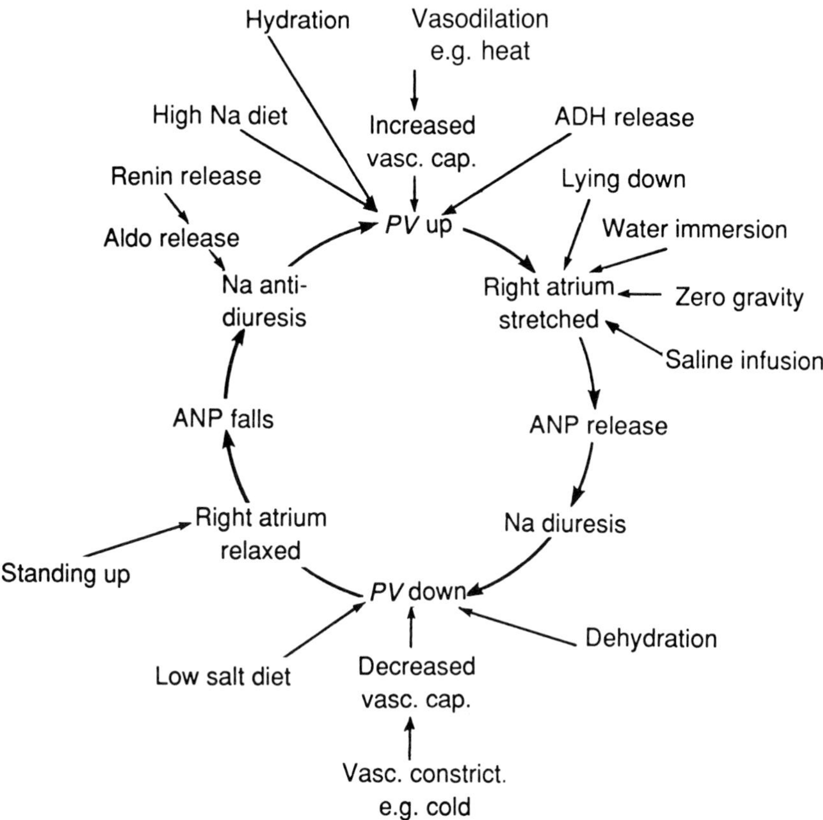

Figure 7.3 Some of the factors affecting plasma volume (PV) and its regulation by atrial natriuretic peptide (ANP), antidiuretic hormone (ADH), aldosterone (Aldo) and vascular capacity (vasc. cap.).

gravity experienced by astronauts has a similar effect. Right atrial pressure is raised and ANP excretion is increased. Conversely, the upright position tends to shift volume away from the centre to the lower body, reducing right atrial pressure and inhibiting ANP release.

- Antidiuretic hormone (ADH) secretion will result in increased PV by retaining water but there is another feedback loop involving plasma osmolality and ADH. If plasma volume increase is caused by hydration, osmolality falls and secretion of ADH is inhibited. A water diuresis then follows which restores the osmolality and ADH levels rise again. This loop is not shown in Figure 7.3, not to overload the diagram.
- The sodium status is important in determining the PV. A high sodium intake will tend to cause water retention and increase PV.

Then increase in ANP will compensate for this. Stimulation of the renin–angiotensin–aldosterone system causes sodium retention with the same result. Renin is stimulated by posture (the upright position) and by exercise, though posture and exercise have effects on PV via other mechanisms (section 7.2.3).

7.2.3 Posture and plasma volume

Seventy per cent of the blood volume is below the heart in the upright position and of this, 75% is in the distensible veins. On standing up, 500 ml of additional blood enters the legs so that reflex tachycardia and vasoconstriction is essential to prevent fainting. Vasoconstriction maintains the blood pressure and reduces flow, especially to the skin, muscles, kidneys and viscera. The capillaries are exposed to the hydrostatic pressure of the column of venous blood. This will tend to increase filtration of fluid out of the vascular compartment and haemoconcentration would be expected. These theoretical expectations have been confirmed by numerous investigators from Thompson *et al.* (1928) onwards. Thompson *et al.* found a reduction of plasma volume of 15% on assuming the upright position but the magnitude of this effect is variable and is influenced by many factors, including environmental and subject temperature, state of hydration etc.

Therefore the effect of posture is significant and needs to be taken into account when considering the effect of other variables such as hypoxia or exercise on plasma volume.

7.2.4 Exercise and plasma volume

Exercise can have an important effect on plasma volume and hence on [Hb] and PCV, but the effect varies according to the intensity, duration and type of exercise. The effect is modified by the temperature of the environment and the subject. It is also modified by posture (section 7.2.3). This is because temperature and posture affect the skin blood flow and hence the distribution of cardiac output to skin, working muscles, kidneys, splanchnic area etc. This, in turn, affects the capillary and venous pressures in these areas and hence the balance of forces in the Starling equation. Many studies on the effect of exercise have ignored the effect of posture and have taken control samples in a different posture from exercise samples.

Harrison (1985) has reviewed the literature and, with a number of reservations, comes to the conclusion that, for bicycle ergometer exercise, there is a reduction in the PV soon after starting exercise. This reduction is proportional to the intensity of exercise or, more precisely, to the rise in atrial pressure. Thereafter there is little change with continued exercise at normal room temperature but in high temperatures there is a further reduction in PV with time. However, these laboratory studies tend to look at fairly high intensity exercise (greater than 50% $\dot{V}_{O_2}$ max) for periods of up to an hour or two.

Exercise on mountains is taken over periods of many hours and may go on day after day. The availability of fluid for drinking will obviously make a difference. If this is not available, dehydration will certainly reduce PV, but usually fluid is available to climbers and exercise heat stress can usually be avoided. Under these circumstances exercise of 8 h or more at normal climbing rates (i.e. up to about 50% $\dot{V}_{O_2}$ max but averaging much less) an increase in PV is found. Pugh (1969) found an increase in blood volume of 7% after a 28-mile hill walk. Williams *et al.* (1979) found PV increased progressively for five days of strenuous daily hill walking to reach a 22% expansion. Both these studies were carried out under cold conditions and subjects avoided both overheating and cold stress. The changes in PV, interstitial and intracellular volumes are shown in Figure 7.4.

The mechanism is probably via activation of the renin–angiotensin–aldosterone system, which results in sodium retention and thus a

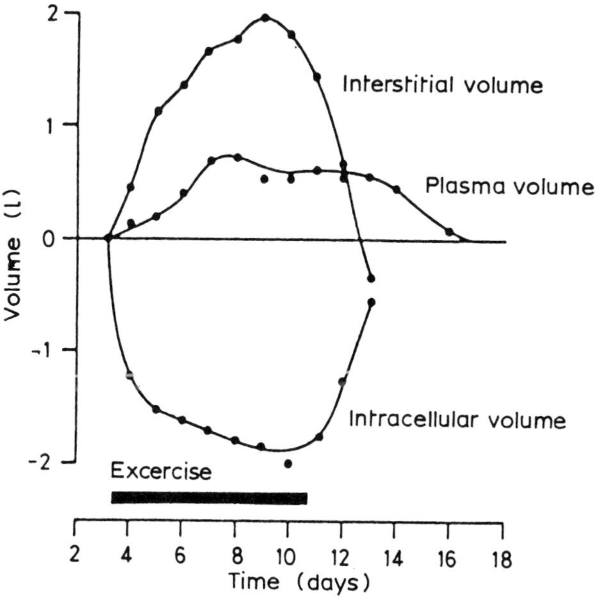

Figure 7.4 The effect of five consecutive days strenuous hill walking on body fluid compartments. The changes are calculated from changes in packed cell volume, and sodium and water balances. (Reproduced with permission from Williams *et al.* (1979).)

general expansion of the extracellular fluid volume including the PV (Milledge *et al.*, 1982). Under these circumstances the PCV decreased from a mean of 43.5% to 37.9% after five days of exercise.

7.3 EFFECT OF ALTITUDE ON PLASMA VOLUME

During the first few hours of altitude exposure the effect on PV is variable and data are scanty. In the field, the effect of hypoxia may be overshadowed by that of cold, dehydration and exercise but it seems that those subjects free from acute mountain sickness (AMS) have a diuresis and contract their PV. Singh *et al.* (1990) found a reduction in PV from 40.4 ml kg^{-1} at sea-level, to 37.7 ml kg^{-1} on the second day at 3500 m, and 37.0 ml kg^{-1} on the twelfth day. Wolfel *et al.* (1991) reported similar changes in PV on ascent to 4300 m; PV fell from 48.8 ml kg^{-1} to 42.5 ml kg^{-1} on arrival at altitude and to 40.2 ml kg^{-1} by day 21. However, subjects with AMS have an antidiuresis and probably expand their PV. Vigorous exercise taken on getting up to altitude or on arrival will also result in expansion of the PV, via the renin–aldosterone system (Milledge *et al.*, 1983).

The effect of acute hypoxia on body fluid volumes, especially in animal experiments, has been reviewed by Honig (1983). With exposure to moderate hypoxia equivalent to altitudes of 3000–6000 m there is a diuresis and natriuresis. After reviewing possible mechanisms via effects on the cardiovascular system, Honig presents evidence, from his own work, that the carotid body, stimulated by hypoxia, reduces the reabsorption of sodium by the kidney via neural pathways. This mechanism has not been demonstrated in man. (This comprehensive review ante-dates the recognition of the importance of atrial natriuretic peptide.)

After this early phase of altitude exposure, there is a definite reduction in PV over the next few weeks. Pugh (1964a) found a 21% reduction in PV after 18 weeks at altitudes above 4000 m in four members of the 1960–1961 Himalayan Scientific Expedition (Figure 7.5). During the following 7–14 weeks the PV returned towards control levels, values being on average 10% less than control when corrected for changes in body weight.

Sanchez *et al.* (1970) found altitude residents at Cerro de Pasco (4370 m) to have a mean PV two-thirds that of a group of students at Lima (sea-level). When allowance was made for the weight difference of the groups they still had a PV 27% less in a blood volume that was 14% greater.

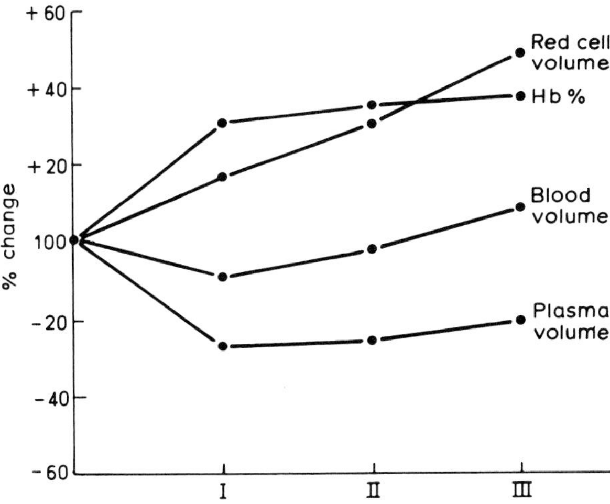

Figure 7.5 Changes in haemoglobin concentration (Hb%), red cell volume, blood volume and plasma volume in four subjects during the Silver Hut Expedition. I. after 18 weeks at between 4000 and 5800 m; II. after a further three to six weeks at 5800 m; III. after a further 9–14 weeks at or above 5800 m. (After Pugh (1964a).)

7.4 ALTITUDE AND ERYTHROPOIESIS

7.4.1 Altitude and serum erythropoietin concentration

Until about 1980, measurements of erythropoietin in blood were by bioassays which could not detect the hormone until its concentration was above normal sea-level values. Therefore, earlier work often relied on more indirect indices of erythropoietic activity such as intestinal iron absorption or reticulocyte counts. The latter is a rather late effect. Intestinal iron absorption has been shown to be independent of erythropoietin and to be promoted as a direct effect of hypoxia rather than secondary to plasma iron turnover or erythropoietic activity (Raja *et al.*, 1986). On going to altitude there is an elevation of erythropoietin concentration in the first 24–48 h (Albrecht and Little, 1972; Siri *et al.*, 1966). Newer methods of erythropoietin estimation using radioimmunoassays are sensitive to levels of erythropoietin well below the normal range (13–37 miu ml^{-1}). Using this type of assay it has been found that serum immunoreactive erythropoietin concentration (SiEp) begins to rise within 2 h of hypoxic exposure depending on the altitude (Eckardt *et al.*, 1989) and reaches a maximum at about 24–48 h. Thereafter, after three weeks, it declines to reach values not measurably

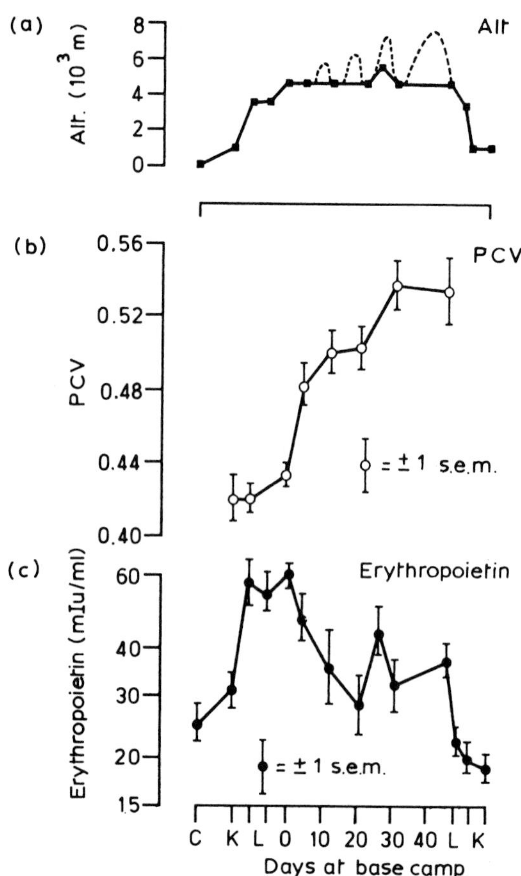

Figure 7.6 The effect of going to altitude on the serum erythropoietin concentration. The top panel shows the altitude/time profile for the eight subjects. The dotted line indicates ascent above base camp between blood samples. Note, the samples at 30 days were taken at 5500 m after four sample times at base camp (4500 m). Mean packed cell volume (PCV) is shown in the centre panel and mean erythropoietin concentration in the lower panel. (C), control, sea-level; (K), Kashgar (1200 m); (L), Karakol lakes (3500 m). (Reproduced with permission from Milledge and Cotes (1985).)

different from controls (Milledge and Cotes, 1985). This is shown in Figure 7.6, which also shows the rise in PCV on going to altitude.

The rise in SiEp with altitude shows great individual variability. In a recent study in the Andes, Richalet *et al.* (1993) found the increase to range from 3–134-fold in their group of subjects one week after arrival at 6540 m.

Figure 7.6 also shows that, even after three weeks above 4500 m, a rise in altitude to 5500 m caused another rise in SiEp. Quite a short pulse of hypoxia initiates a rise in SiEp which continues after normoxia is restored. For instance, 120 min breathing 10% oxygen caused SiEp to rise just after normoxia was restored and the rise continued for a further 120 min (Knaupp *et al.*, 1992).

It will be seen from Figure 7.6 that PCV continues to rise after SiEp falls to near control values. The rise in RCM continues even longer (section 7.4.2). In patients with polycythaemia secondary to hypoxic lung disease the SiEp was found to be within the normal range in over 50% (Wedzicha *et al.*, 1986). A continued erythropoiesis when levels of SiEp have fallen to near control values is unexplained.

7.4.2 Altitude and red cell mass

The result of increased erythropoiesis at altitude is an increase in RCM since the life span of the red blood cell is unchanged (Berlin *et al..*, 1954). Figure 7.5 shows the rise in RCM, which is quite slow at first but continues for a long time. After about six months at altitudes above 4000 m it had increased by a mean of 50% in absolute terms or 67.5% when corrected for loss of body weight. By this time the blood volume had increased over control by 7.3% or 22.8% corrected for body weight (Pugh, 1964a) (Figure 7.5). Sanchez *et al.* (1970) found altitude residents in the Andes to have a RCM 83% greater than sea-level residents when corrected for weight difference.

7.5 ALTITUDE AND HAEMOGLOBIN CONCENTRATION

7.5.1 Lowlanders going from sea-level to altitude

The combined effect of changes in PV and RCM result in an increase in haemoglobin concentration ([Hb]). This increase allows more oxygen to be carried per litre of blood at any given oxygen saturation. The price paid for this gain in oxygen capacity, however, is an increase in viscosity of the blood with the attendant increased risk of thrombosis (Chapter 21).

As discussed in section 7.3, the initial rise in [Hb] during the first few days and weeks at altitude is largely a result of reduction in PV. The [Hb] rise is roughly exponential, plateauing out at about six weeks at a given altitude. However, after that, the RCM continues to rise but so does the PV so that [Hb] remains approximately constant (Figure 7.5).

Pugh (1964b) reviewed results from five expeditions (51 observations in 40 subjects) and concluded that the [Hb] after about six weeks at altitude averaged 20.5 g dl^{-1} and was independent of altitude above

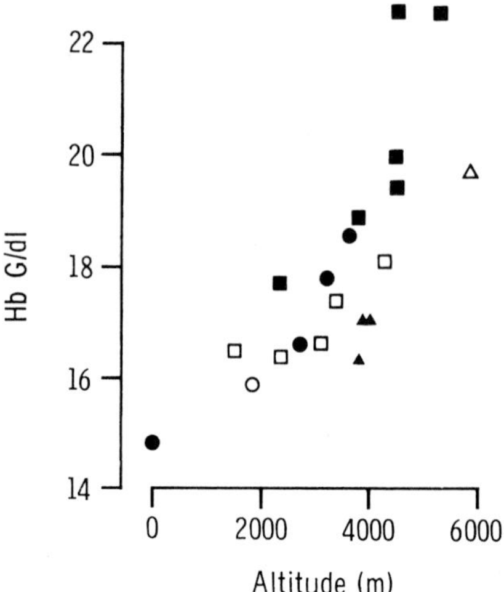

Figure 7.7 The effect of altitude on haemoglobin concentration in male residents at altitude. ●, from the Tien Shan; □ from Colorado mining camps; ○ from South Indian hill towns; ■ from the Andes; ▲ from Nepal (Sherpas); △ climbers after three months or more at altitude.

5500 m. Winslow *et al.* (1984), reviewing [Hb] values from the 1981 American Everest expeditions and two previous Everest expeditions, found the range of mean values was 17.8–20.6 $g\,dl^{-1}$ at altitudes of 5350–6300 m, with no correlation between altitude and [Hb] within this altitude range.

7.5.2 Residents at altitude

Figure 7.7 shows the rise in [Hb] with altitude in residents of high altitude from North and South America and Asia.

Andean subjects have been reported to have values in the region of 22 $g\,dl^{-1}$ at altitudes of 4300 m to 4500 m (Dill *et al.*, 1937; Talbot and Dill, 1938; Merino, 1950). However, these studies may include subjects who would now be considered to have chronic mountain sickness. More recent publications from South America give mean values nearer 20 $g\,dl^{-1}$ (Penaloza *et al.*, 1971).

In Sherpa subjects [Hb] is lower, a mean of 17 $g\,dl^{-1}$ at 4000 m is given by Adams and Strang (1975) and of 16.2 $g\,dl^{-1}$ by Morpurgo *et al.*, (1976). In this case the possibility that some subjects may be iron deficient cannot be ruled out. Morpurgo *et al.* argue that it represents greater adaptation over perhaps 100 000 years compared with about 20 000 years for Andean residents. However, results in residents of the Tien Shan, and Pamirs by Son (1979) give values closer to those from South America (Figure 7.7) and would seem not to support this hypothesis. A more likely explanation for the difference between Andean and Himalayan residents is that Sherpas move up and down in altitude more frequently than do Andean altitude dwellers on the altiplano.

A study from Tibet (Beall *et al.*, 1987) demonstrated a [Hb] of 18.2 g dl^{-1} in male subjects resident at an altitude of 4850–5450 m, a value higher than most results from the Andes at comparable altitude. However, even in populations of similar ethnic origin and at the same altitude in the Andes, quite different mean [Hb] values have been reported. Cassio (quoted by Winslow and Monge, 1987b) found residents at San Antonio (4600 m) to have almost 3 g dl^{-1} higher [Hb] than men at Tichlio (4600 m). The former are in line with most Andean results, the latter with results in Sherpa subjects and Beall *et al.*'s results in Tibetans. There is also the problem that, in comparing results from individual workers in the two continents, variation in methods may account for some of the reported differences. Winslow *et al.* (1989) used identical methods to compare Himalayan natives (Sherpas) to high-altitude Andean natives at similar altitudes in Khundi, Nepal and Ollague (Chile) at 3700 m. Mean haematocrit values in Nepal were significantly lower than in Chile (48.4 compared with 52.2). They also found SiEp concentrations to be higher in the Andean population, indicating that they were functionally anaemic even with the higher haematocrit!

Caucasian subjects resident in high-altitude towns in Colorado and acclimatized climbers tend to have lower [Hb] than Andean and Central Asian residents (Figure 7.7).

7.5.3 Polycythaemia of high altitude

Excessive rise of [Hb] (i.e. above 22 g dl^{-1} is generally considered to be pathological and diagnostic of chronic mountain sickness (Chapter 20). Both people native to high altitude and lowlanders resident at high altitude for some years are at risk of developing this condition. Huang *et al.* (1984) report that Han (Chinese) lowlanders resident on the Tibetan plateau have a higher incidence of this polycythaemia than Tibetans.

7.5.4 Optimum haemoglobin concentration

An increase in [Hb] increases the oxygen carrying capacity of blood since each gram of haemoglobin can carry 1.31 ml of oxygen (Gregory, 1974). The oxygen content of the blood is the product of capacity and saturation (Sa_{O_2}) plus the dissolved oxygen. Thus the increase in [Hb] with altitude compensates for a reduction in arterial Sa_{O_2}. At altitudes up to about 5300 m this compensation results in an arterial oxygen content approximately equal to that at sea-level in those who are acclimatized (Figure 7.1). However, increasing [Hb] results in increasing viscosity (Guyton *et al.*, 1973). This increase in viscosity is curvilinear so that, with [Hb] above about 18 g dl^{-1} viscosity increases rapidly. Eventually, this increased viscosity increases resistance in both systemic and pulmonary circulation so impeding blood flow and cardiac output falls. Oxygen supply to the tissues depends upon oxygen delivery which is the product of arterial oxygen content and cardiac output.

These considerations result in the concept of an optimum [Hb] below which oxygen delivery is reduced because of reduction in oxygen content, and above which it is reduced because the great increase in viscosity causes a reduction in cardiac output which more than offsets the increase in content. The major problem in calculating what should be the value of this optimum [Hb] is the viscosity of blood and its effect on cardiac output. Since blood is a non-Newtonian fluid a single value for viscosity cannot be assigned to it at any given [Hb]. The value will vary according to the way it is measured *in vitro*. *In vivo* the effect on resistance will vary according to the diameter of the vessel under consideration as well as to whether flow is streamlined or turbulent. Apparent resistance will also vary with flow. If we ignore the physics and just look at the effect of changing [Hb] on cardiac output in acute animal experiments, these may not reflect the human situation at altitude where the vascular system has time to adapt to the polycythaemia. The situation is so complex that it is clearly impossible, on theoretical grounds, to predict an optimum [Hb]. Another factor affecting the apparent viscosity is the deformability, or filterability, of the red cells. A recent study addressed this and concluded that altitude exposure resulted in an impaired filterability of red cells which was prevented by the administration of vitamin E (Simon-Schnass and Korniszewski, 1990).

From clinical experience, it would seem that the extremely high [Hb] concentration found in chronic mountain sickness (Chapter 20) and in some patients with chronic hypoxic lung disease is deleterious. Haemodilution by venesection alone or with intravenous fluid replacement results in clinical improvement. In such patients reduction of PCV from 61% to 50% resulted in a decrease in pulmonary artery pressure and resistance (Weisse *et al.*, 1975). Similarly Winslow *et al.* (1985) found in Andean high altitude residents that reduction of PCV from 62% to 42% resulted in increased cardiac output and mixed venous P_{O_2}. Willison *et al.* (1980) found that reducing the PCV from 54% to 48% in patients resulted in an increase of cerebral blood flow from 44 to 57 ml^{-1} min^{-1} per 100 g brain tissue. This would increase oxygen delivery to the brain by 15% and was accompanied by an increase in alertness.

In a study of climbers at altitude by Sarnquist *et al.* (1986) it was found that haemodilution produced no improvement or deterioration in measured physical performance though there was a small, significant improvement in psychomotor tests. However, the subjects studied, though having the highest PCV in the expedition, were not very polycythaemic. Their PCV ranged from 57% to 60% before heamodilution.

There is no obvious correlation between climbing performance and [Hb] within the range of values common on an expedition, at about 17–22 g dl^{-1} (Pugh, 1964b). Indeed it is usual to find that climbers who perform best are at the lower end of this range, suggesting that the optimum [Hb] at altitudes above about 5000 m is in the region of 18 g dl^{-1}. Winslow and Monge (1987a) conclude that, 'Excessive polycythemia serves no useful purpose. Indeed, it is doubtful whether there is any physiologic value in "normal" polycythemia.'

7.5.5 Haemoglobin concentration on descent from altitude

On descent from altitude arterial oxygen saturation will return to the normal 96–98% and this, together with the now raised [Hb], might be expected to inhibit erythropoietin secretion. However Milledge and Cotes (1985) reported that levels were 66% of control values eight and 20 hours after decent following two months at or above 4500 m. This reduced erythropoietin level presumably is sufficient to reduce erythropoiesis since [Hb] declines after descent and reaches normal sea-level values after about six weeks (Heath and Williams, 1981).

7.6 PLATELETS AND CLOTTING AT ALTITUDE

These topics are discussed more fully in Chapter 21.

In summary, it seems that the physiological response to hypoxia does not involve any important changes in platelet count or adhesiveness, or in clotting factors. However, there may be changes associated with AMS. If there are changes in clotting factors they may represent an effect or a complication of AMS rather than being essential in its genesis.

7.7 WHITE BLOOD CELLS

There seem to be variable changes in total white cell and differential count on going to altitude. One study reported a rise in granulocyte count on ascent to 4300 m (Simon-Schnass and Korniszewski, 1990) and another an increase in certain lymphocyte subsets. CD16+ or natural killer cells were particularly increased in seven subjects in a decompression chamber at 380 mmHg (Klokker *et al.*, 1993). There is anecdotal evidence that infections in the skin and subcutaneous tissues are slow to clear at altitude. One could speculate that the above finding might have a bearing on on this.

REFERENCES

Adams, W.H. and Strang, L.J. (1975) Haemoglobin levels in persons of Tibetan ancestry living at high altitude. *Proc. Soc. Exp. Biol. Med.*, **149**, 1036–9.

Albrecht, P.H. and Little, J.K. (1972) Plasma erythropoietin in men and mice during acclimatization to different altitudes. *J. Appl. Physiol.*, **32**, 54–8.

Beall, C.M., Goldstein, M.C. and the Tibetan Academy of Sciences (1987) Haemoglobin concentration of pastoral nomads permanently resident at 4850–5450 meters in Tibet. *Am. J. Phys. Anthropol.*, **73**, 433–8.

Berlin, N.I., Reynafarje, C. and Lawrence, J.H. (1954) Red cell life span in the polycythaemia of high altitude. *J. Appl. Physiol.*, **7**, 271–2.

Dill, D.B., Talbot, J.H. and Consolazio, W.V. (1937) Blood as a physiochemical system: XII. Man at high altitudes. *J. Biol. Chem.*, **118**, 649–66.

Eckardt, K., Boutellier, U., Kurtz, A., *et al.* (1989) Rate of erythropoietin formation in humans in response to acute hypobaric hypoxia. *J. Appl. Physiol.*, **66**, 1785–8.

Erslev, A. (1987) Erythropoietin coming of age. *N. Engl. J. Med.*, **316**, 101–3.

Fisher, J.W. and Langston, J.W. (1967) The influence of hypoxia and cobalt on erythropoietin production in the isolated perfused dog kidney. *Blood*, **29**, 114–25.

Gregory, I.C (1974) The oxygen and carbon monoxide capacities of foetal and adult blood. *J. Physiol.*, **236**, 625–34.

Guyton, A.C., Jones, C.E. and Coleman, T.G. (1973) *Cardiac Output and its Regulation*, 2nd edn, Saunders, Philadelphia, p. 396.

Harrison, M.H. (1985) Effects of thermal stress and exercise on blood volume in humans. *Physiol. Rev.*, **65**, 149–208.

Heath, D. and Williams, D.R. (1981) *Man at High* Altitude, 2nd edn. Churchill Livingstone, Edinburgh, p. 56.

Honig, A. (1983) Role of arterial chemoreceptors in the reflex control of renal function and body fluid volumes in acute arterial hypoxia, in *Physiology of the Peripheral Arterial Chemoreceptors*, (eds H. Acher and R.G. O'Regan), Elsevier, Amsterdam, pp. 395–429.

Huang, S.Y., Ning, X.H., Zhou, Z.N., *et al.* (1984) Ventilatory function in adaptation to high altitude: studies in Tibet, in *High Altitude and Man*, (eds J.B. West and S. Lahiri), American Physiological Society Bethesda, MA, pp. 173–7.

Klokker, M., Kharazmi, A., Galbo, H., *et al.* (1993) Influence of *in vivo* hypobaric hypoxia on function of lymphocytes, natural killer cells, and cytokines. *J. Appl. Physiol.*, **74**, 1100–6.

Knaupp, W., Khilnani, S., Sherwood, J., *et al.* (1992) Erythropoietin response to acute normobaric hypoxia in humans. *J. Appl. Physiol.*, **73**, 837–40.

Laragh, J.H. (1985) Atrial natriuretic hormone, the renin–aldosterone axis, and blood pressure–electrolyte homeostasis. *N. Engl. J. Med.*, **313**, 1330–40.

Merino, C.F. (1950) Studies on blood formation and destruction in the polycythaemia of high altitude. *Blood*, **5**, 1–31.

Milledge, J.S. and Cotes, P.M. (1985) Serum erythropoietin in humans at high altitude and its relation to plasma renin. *J. Appl. Physiol.*, **59**, 360–4.

Milledge, J.S., Bryson, E.I., Catley, D.M., *et al.* (1982) Sodium balance, fluid homeostasis and the renin–aldosterone system during the prolonged exercise of hill walking. *Clin. Sci.*, **62**, 595–604.

Milledge, J.S., Catley, D.M., Williams, E.S., *et al.* (1983) Effect of prolonged exercise at altitude on the renin–aldosterone system. *J. Appl. Physiol.*, **55**, 413–18.

Morpurgo, G., Arese, P., Bosia, A., *et al.* (1976) Sherpas living permanently at high altitude: A new pattern of adaptation. *Proc. Natl Acad. Sci. USA*, **73**, 747–51.

Penaloza, D., Sime, F. and Ruiz, L. (1971) Cor pulmonale in chronic mountain sickness: present concept of Monge's disease, in *High Altitude Physiology*, (eds. R. Porter and J. Knight), Churchill Livingstone, London, pp. 41–60.

Pugh, L.G.C.E. (1964a) Blood volume and haemoglobin concentration at altitudes above 18 000 ft (5500 m). *J. Physiol.*, **170**, 344–54.

Pugh, L.G.C.E. (1964b) Animals in high altitudes: man above 5000 m mountain exploration, in *Handbook of Physiology*, section 4, (eds D.B. Dill, E.F. Adolph and C.G. Wilber), Washington DC, pp. 861–8.

Pugh, L.G.C.E. (1969) Blood volume changes in outdoor exercise of 8–10 h duration. *J. Physiol. (London)*, **200**, 345–51.

Raja, K.B., Pippard, M.J., Simpson, R.J. and Peters, T.J. (1986) Relationship between erythropoiesis and the enhanced intestinal uptake of ferric iron in hypoxia in the mouse. *Br. J. Haematol.*, **64**, 587–93.

Richalet, J.-P., Souberbielle, J.-C., Antezana, A.-M., *et al.* (1993) Control of erythropoiesis in humans during prolonged exposure to the altitude of 6542 m. *Am. J. Physiol.*, **266**, R756–44.

Sanchez, C., Merino, C. and Figallo, M. (1970) Simultaneous measurement of plasma volume and cell mass in polycythemia of high altitude. *J. Appl. Physiol.*, **28**, 775–8.

Sarnquist, F.H., Schoene, R.B., Hackett, P.H. and Townes, B.D. (1986) Hemodilution of polycythemic mountaineers: Effects on exercise and mental function. *Aviat. Space Environ. Med.*, **57**, 313–7.

Simon-Schnass, I. and Korniszewski, L. (1990) The influence of vitamin E on rheological parameters in high altitude mountaineers. *Int. J. Vit. Nutr. Res.*, **60**, 26–34.

Singh, M.V., Rawal, S.B. and Tyagi, A.K. (1990) Body fluid status on induction, reinduction and prolonged stay at high altitude on human volunteers. *Int. J. Biometeorol.*, **34**, 93–7.

Siri, W.E., Van Dyke, D.C., Winchell, H.S., *et al.* (1966) Early erythropoietin, blood, and physiological responses to severe hypoxia in man. *J. Appl. Physiol.*, **21**, 73–80.

Son, Y.A. (1979) Quantitative estimation of haemoglobin and its fractions in permanent mountain dwellers in the Tyan'-Shan' and Pamir. *Hum. Physiol.*, **5**, 208–10.

Talbot, J.H. and Dill, D.B. (1938) Clinical observations at high altitude. *Am. J. Med. Sci.*, **192**, 626–37.

Thompson, W.O., Thompson, P.K. and Dailey, M.M. (1928) The effect of posture on the composition and volume of the blood in man. *J. Clin. Invest.*, **5**, 573–604.

Viault, F. (1890) Sur l'augmentation considérable du nombre des globules rouges dans le sang chez les habitants des hauts plateaux de l'Amérique du Sud. *Comptes Rendus* **111**, 917–8.

Viault, M. (1891) Sur la quantité d'oxygène contenue dans le sang des animaux des hauts plateaux de l'Amérique du Sud. *Comptes Rendus*, **112**, 295–8.

Wedzicha, J.A., Cotes, P.M., Empey, D.W., *et al.* (1985) Serum immunoreactive erythropoietin in hypoxic lung disease with and without polycythaemia. *Clin. Sci.*, **69**, 413–22.

Weisse, A.B., Moschos, C.B., Frank, M.J., *et al.* (1975) Haemodynamic effects of staged haematocrit reduction in patients with stable cor pulmonale and severely elevated haematocrit. *Am. J. Med.*, **58**, 92–8.

West, J.B. (1981) *High Altitude Physiology: Benchmark papers in physiology*, Vol. 15, Hutchinson Ross, Stroudsburg, PA.

Williams, E.S., Ward, M.P., Milledge, J.S., *et al.* (1979) Effect of the exercise of seven consecutive days hill-walking on fluid homeostasis. *Clin. Sci.*, **56**, 305–16.

Willison, J.R., Thomas, D.J., DuBoulay, G.H., *et al.* (1980) Effects of high haematocrit on alertness. *Lancet*, **1**, 846–8.

Winearls, C.G., Oliver, D.O., Pippard, M.J., *et al.* (1986) Effect of human erythropoietin derived from recombinant DNA on the anaemia of patients maintained by chronic haemodialysis. *Lancet*, **2**, 1175–7.

Winslow, R.M., Samaja, M. and West, J.B. (1984) Red cell function at extreme altitude on Mount Everest. *J. Appl. Physiol.*, **56**, 109–16.

Winslow, R.M., Monge, C.C., Brown E.G., *et al.* (1985) Effects of hemodilution on O_2 transport in high-altitude polycythemia. *J. Appl. Physiol.*, **59**, 1495–502.

Winslow, R.M. and Monge, C.C. (1987a) *Hypoxia, Polycythemia, and Chronic Mountain Sickness*, Johns Hopkins University Press, Baltimore, p. 203.

Winslow, R.M. and Monge, C.C. (1987b) *Hypoxia, Polycythemia, and Chronic Mountain Sickness*, Johns Hopkins University Press, Baltimore, p. 37.

Winslow, R.M., Chapman, K.W., Gibson, C.C., *et al.* (1989) Different haematologic response to hypoxia in Sherpas and Quechua Indians. *J. Appl. Physiol.*, **66**, 1561–9.

Wolfel, E.E., Groves, B.M., Brooks, G.A., *et al.* (1991) Oxygen transport during steady state submaximal exercise in chronic hypoxia. *J. Appl. Physiol.*, **70**, 1129–36.

8

Blood gas transport and acid–base balance

8.1 INTRODUCTION

Physiological changes in the blood play an important role in acclimatization and adaptation to high altitude. In this chapter, the main topics considered are the changes in oxygen affinity of haemoglobin, and the alterations of the acid–base status of the blood. The increase in red cell concentration of the blood was discussed in Chapter 7 where the regulation of erythropoiesis was described. Some of the consequences of an altered oxygen affinity of haemoglobin are alluded to in other chapters, especially Chapter 5 on diffusion of oxygen across the blood–gas barrier, and Chapter 11 on limiting factors at extreme altitude.

8.2 HISTORICAL

The honour of first plotting the oxygen and carbon dioxide dissociation curves apparently belongs to Paul Bert. In his monumental book *La Pression Barométrique* he showed the relationships between partial pressure and blood gas concentration for both oxygen and carbon dioxide as experimental animals were exposed to lower and lower barometric pressures, or as they were gradually asphyxiated by rebreathing in a closed space (Bert, 1878; pp. 135–8 in 1943 translation). However he did not discover the S-shaped curve for oxygen because he did not reduce the P_{O_2} far enough.

The first oxygen dissociation curve over its whole range was published by Christian Bohr in 1885. The measurements were made on dilute solutions of haemoglobin (Bohr, 1885) and were obviously not compatible with the data obtained by Bert in experimental animals. Hüfner (1890) published a similar curve for haemoglobin solutions and argued that a hyperbolic shape would be expected from the simple equation:

$$Hb + O_2 \rightleftharpoons HbO_2$$

An important advance was made by Bohr when he used whole blood rather than haemoglobin solutions and he thereby discovered the now familiar S-shaped curve. In the following year, in collaboration with Hasselbalch and Krogh, he showed that the dissociation curve was shifted to the right when the P_{CO_2} of the blood was increased, a phenomenon which came to be known as the Bohr effect (Bohr *et al.*, 1904). A few years later, Barcroft showed that the addition of acid displaced the dissociation curve to the right (Barcroft and Orbeli, 1910), and also that an increase in temperature had the same effect (Barcroft and King, 1909). Astrup and Severinghaus (1986) have written a useful historical review of blood gases and acid–base balance.

It was not long after these important modulators of oxygen affinity for haemoglobin were discovered that physiologists wondered about their importance at high altitude. For example, when Barcroft accompanied the first international high altitude expedition to Mt Tenerife in 1910, he made a special study of the position of the oxygen dissociation curve, expecting it to be displaced to the left by the low arterial P_{CO_2}. In the event, he found that the oxygen dissociation curves of some members of the expedition at 2130 and 3000 m were shifted to the right when measured at the normal sea-level P_{CO_2} of 40 mmHg. However when he repeated the equilibrations at the subject's actual P_{CO_2} at altitude, the positions of the curves were essentially the same as at sea level (Barcroft, 1911). He concluded that the decrease in carbonic acid in the blood was compensated for by an increase in some other acid, possibly lactic acid. One year later Barcroft went to Mosso's laboratory, the Capanna Regina Margherita on Monte Rosa (nearly 4600 m), and reported a slight excess acidity at that altitude (Barcroft *et al.*, 1914).

Some ten years later during the 1921–1922 Anglo–American Expedition to Cerro de Pasco in Peru, Barcroft and his colleagues found an increased oxygen affinity in acclimatized lowlanders as a result of the increased alkalinity of the blood. It also appeared that the increase in affinity was greater than could be explained by the change in acid–base status (Barcroft *et al.*, 1923).

The question of haemoglobin–oxygen affinity was examined again on the International High Altitude Expedition to Chile in 1935. It was found that the 'physiological' dissociation curves (that is, measured at a subject's own P_{CO_2}) were displaced slightly to the left of the sea-level values up to about 4270 m, but that above that altitude, the curves were displaced increasingly to the right of the sea-level positions (Keys *et al.*, 1936). Measurements of oxygen affinity of the haemoglobin were also made at constant pH and these showed a uniform tendency to a decreased affinity. The investigators argued that this rightward shift of the curve might be advantageous at high altitude because it would facilitate oxygen unloading to the tissues.

An important discovery was made in 1967 by two groups working independently (Benesch and Benesch, 1967; Chanutin and Curnish, 1967) that a fourth factor (in addition to P_{CO_2}, pH and temperature) had an important effect on the oxygen affinity of haemoglobin. This was the concentration of 2,3-diphosphoglycerate (2,3-DPG) within the red cells. This unexpected development raised doubts about much earlier work where this important factor had not been controlled. It was subsequently shown that 2,3-DPG increased at high altitude (Lenfant *et al.*, 1968) and it was argued that the resulting decrease in oxygen affinity, which facilitated unloading of oxygen in the tissues, was an important part of the adaptation process (Lenfant and Sullivan, 1971).

Until recently very little information was available on the oxygen affinity of haemoglobin at extreme altitude. A few measurements from the Himalayan Scientific and Mountaineering Expedition for 1960–1961 showed that lowlanders who were well acclimatized to 5800 m had an almost fully compensated respiratory alkalosis (West *et al.*, 1962). Data above this altitude did not exist.

It was therefore astonishing to find on the 1981 American Medical Research Expedition to Everest that climbers near the summit apparently had an extreme degree of respiratory alkalosis which greatly increased the oxygen affinity of their haemoglobin. The arterial pH of Pizzo on the Everest summit was calculated to exceed 7.7 (section 8.3.5).

Turning now to the early history of acid–base balance at high altitude, it is clear from the above that it overlaps considerably with a discussion of oxygen affinity of haemoglobin. However the reaction of the blood (as it was called) at high altitude created a great deal of interest in its own right. Indeed the acid–base status of the blood played an important role in early theories of the control of breathing at high altitude (Kellogg, 1980). As long ago as 1903, Galeotti found that, in various experimental animals taken to Mosso's Capanna Regina Margherita laboratory on Monte Rosa, the amount of acid needed to bring their haemolysed blood to a standard pH (determined from litmus paper) was decreased compared with sea-level (Galeotti, 1904). He interpreted this decrease in titratable alkalinity to mean that there was an increase in some acid substance in the blood. It was known that hypoxia caused lactic acid production (Araki, 1891) and that acid blood stimulated breathing (Zuntz *et al.*, 1906). It was therefore natural to conclude that this explained the hyperventilation of high altitude, and that the P_{CO_2} fell as a consequence (Boycott and Haldane, 1908). Winterstein (1911) formulated what became known as the 'reaction theory' of breathing which stated that the effects of both hypoxia and carbon dioxide as stimulants of ventilation could be explained by the fact that they both acidified the blood.

The correct explanation of how hypoxia stimulates ventilation at high altitude had to wait for discovery of the peripheral chemoreceptors by Heymans and Heymans (1925). Meanwhile Winterstein (1915) provided evidence against his own theory when he showed that in acute hypoxia, the blood becomes alkaline rather than acid. A few years later, Henderson (1919) and Haldane *et al.* (1919) correctly explained the alkalinity as being secondary to the lowered P_{CO_2} caused by hyperventilation. Nevertheless it is true that even today the control of ventilation during chronic hypoxia is not fully understood (Chapter 4) and a good deal of interest still remains in the acid–base status of the extracellular fluid which forms the environment of the central chemoreceptors.

8.3 OXYGEN AFFINITY OF HAEMOGLOBIN

8.3.1 Basic physiology

Figure 8.1 shows the oxygen dissociation curve of human whole blood and the four factors that shift the curve to the right, that is decrease the affinity of haemoglobin for oxygen. These four factors are increases in: P_{CO_2}, hydrogen ion concentration, temperature, and the concentration of 2,3-diphosphoglycerate in the red cells. Increasing the ionic concentration of the plasma also reduces oxygen affinity.

Almost all of the change in oxygen affinity caused by P_{CO_2} can be ascribed to its effect on hydrogen ion concentration, although a change in P_{CO_2} has a small effect in its own right (Margaria, 1957). The mechanism of the alteration of oxygen affinity through hydrogen ion concentration (Bohr effect) is through a change in configuration of the haemoglobin molecule which makes the binding site less accessible to molecular oxygen as the hydrogen ion concentration is raised. The molecule exists in two forms: one in which the chemical subunits are maximally chemically bonded (T form) and another where some bonds are ruptured and the structure is relaxed (R form). The R form has a higher affinity for oxygen because the molecule can more easily enter the region of the haem. The approximate magnitudes of the effects of change in P_{CO_2} and pH on the oxygen dissociation curve are shown in the right insets of Figure 8.1.

Increase in temperature has a large effect on the oxygen affinity of haemoglobin as shown in the top inset of Figure 8.1. The temperature

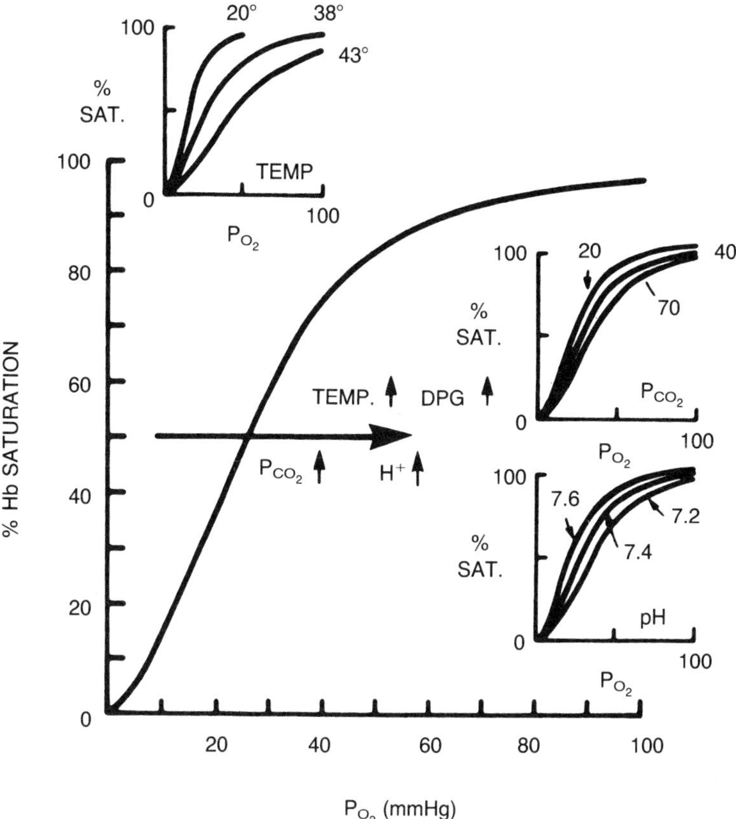

Figure 8.1 Normal oxygen dissociation curve and its displacement by increases in H^+, P_{CO_2}, temperature and 2,3-diphosphoglycerate (DPG). (Reproduced from West, 1994.)

effect follows from thermodynamic consideration: the combination of oxygen with haemoglobin is exothermic so that an increase in temperature favours the reverse reaction, that is dissociation of the oxyhaemoglobin.

The compound 2,3-diphosphoglycerate is a product of red cell metabolism as shown in Figure 8.2. An increased concentration of this material within the red cell reduces the oxygen affinity of the haemoglobin by increasing the chemical binding of the subunits and converting more haemoglobin to the low affinity T form.

A useful number to describe the oxygen affinity of haemoglobin is the P_{50}, that is the P_{O_2} for 50% saturation of the haemoglobin with oxygen. The normal value for adult whole blood at a P_{CO_2} of 40 mmHg,

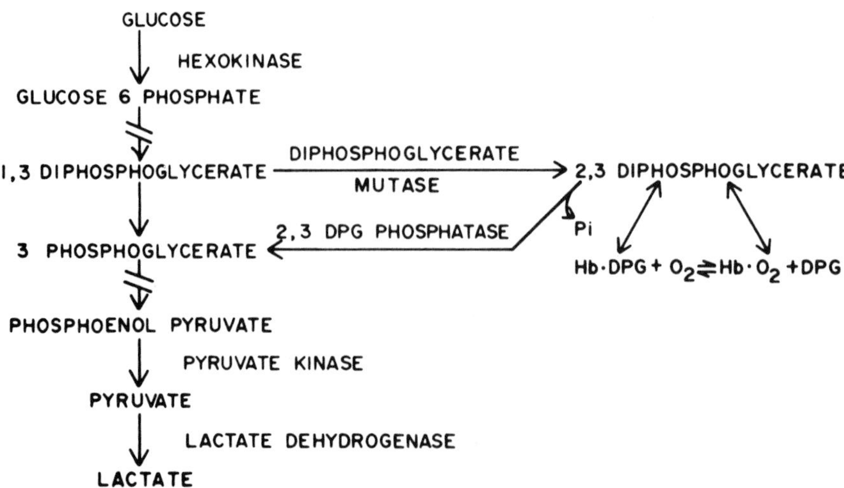

Figure 8.2 Formation of 2,3-diphosphoglycerate in erythrocytes. The vertical chain at the left shows the glycolytic pathway in cells other than erythrocytes. In red blood cells, the enzyme DPG mutase catalyses the conversion of much of the 1,3-DPG to 2,3-DPG. (From Mines, 1981.)

pH 7.4, temperature 37°C, and normal 2,3-DPG concentration is 26–27 mmHg. Human foetal blood has a P_{50} of about 19 mmHg because of the different chemical structure of foetal haemoglobin. An increase of 2,3-DPG within the red cell increases the P_{50} by about 0.5 mmHg mole^{-1} of 2,3-DPG. The magnitude of the Bohr effect is usually given in terms of the increase in $\log P_{50}$ per pH unit. The normal value for human blood is 0.4 at constant P_{CO_2}. Note that although historically the 'Bohr effect' referred to the change in affinity caused by P_{CO_2}, in modern usage the term is restricted to the effect of pH. The temperature effect is 0.024 for the change in $\log P_{50}$ (mmHg °C^{-1}).

Much can be learned about the effect of changes in the oxygen affinity of haemoglobin on the physiology of high altitude by modelling the oxygen transport system using computer subroutines for the oxygen and carbon dioxide dissociation curves (Bencowitz *et al.*, 1982). Kelman described useful subroutines for the oxygen dissociation curve (Kelman, 1966a,b) and the carbon dioxide dissociation curve (Kelman, 1967). The practical use of these procedures has been described (West and Wagner, 1977). These procedures are able to accommodate changes in P_{CO_2}, pH, temperature and 2,3-DPG concentration, and allow the investigator to answer questions about the interactions of these variables which would otherwise be impossibly complicated.

8.3.2 Animals native to high altitude

It has been known for many years that animals who live at high altitude tend to have increased oxygen affinity of their haemoglobin. Figure 5.6 shows part of the oxygen dissociation curves of the vicuna and llama which are native to high altitude in the South American Andes (Hall *et al.*, 1936). The diagram also shows the range of dissociation curves for eight lowland animals including man, horse, dog, rabbit, pig, peccary, ox and sheep. It can be seen that the high-altitude native animals have a substantially increased oxygen affinity of their haemoglobin. This adaptation to high altitude is of genetic origin as is shown by the fact that a llama brought up in a zoo at sea-level has the same high oxygen affinity.

High-altitude birds also show these phenomena. Hall and his colleagues (1936), during the 1935 International High Altitude Expedition to Chile, reported that the high-altitude ostrich and huallata have higher oxygen affinities than a group of six lowland birds including the pigeon, muscovy duck, domestic goose, domestic duck, Chinese pheasant and domestic fowl. A particularly interesting example is the bar-headed goose which is known to fly over the Himalayan ranges as it migrates between its breeding grounds in Siberia and its wintering grounds in India. This remarkable animal has a blood P_{50} about 10 mmHg lower than its close relatives from moderate altitudes (Black and Tenney, 1980).

Deer mice, *Peromyscus maniculatus*, show the same relationships. A study was carried out on ten subspecies who live from below sea-level in Death Valley in California to the high mountains of the nearby Sierra Nevada (4350 m) and it was found that there was a strong correlation between the habitat altitude and the oxygen affinity of the blood. The genetic source of this relationship was proved by moving one subspecies to another location and showing that the oxygen affinity was unchanged. Moreover the relationship persisted in second generation animals (Snyder *et al.*, 1982).

8.3.3 Animals in oxygen-deprived environments

High altitude is just one of the oxygen-deprived environments in which animals are found, and it is interesting to consider the variety of strategies that have been adopted to mitigate the problems posed by oxygen deficiency. Table 8.1 shows examples of some of the strategies that have been adopted through genetic adaptation. The first two groups increase the oxygen affinity of their haemoglobin by decreasing the concentration of organic phosphates. This is done with 2,3-DPG in the foetus of the dog, horse and pig, and by decreasing the concentration of ATP in the trout and eel.

Table 8.1 Strategies for increasing oxygen affinity of haemoglobin in hypoxia

Strategy	*Subject*
Decrease in 2,3-DPG	Foetus of dog, horse, pig
Decrease in ATP	Trout, eel
Different type of Hb	Bar-headed goose, toad-fish
Mutant Hb (Andrew–Minneapolis)	Family in Minnesota
Different Hb, small Bohr effect	Tadpole
Respiratory alkalosis	Climber at extreme altitude

Several animals have evolved special types of haemoglobin with high oxygen affinities. These include the bar-headed goose referred to above, and the toad-fish. Some species of tadpoles which frequently live in stagnant pools have a high oxygen affinity haemoglobin whereas the adult frogs produce a different type of haemoglobin with a lower affinity which fits their higher oxygen environment. Note also that the tadpole blood shows a smaller Bohr effect. This is useful because low oxygen and high carbon dioxide pressures are likely to occur together in stagnant water, and a large Bohr effect would be disadvantageous because it would decrease the oxygen affinity of the blood when a high affinity was most needed.

As indicated earlier, the human foetus also has a high oxygen affinity by virtue of its foetal haemoglobin. This is essential because the arterial P_{O_2} of the fetus is less than 30 mmHg. Indeed the human foetus and the adult climber on the summit of Mt Everest have some similar features in that in both cases the arterial P_{O_2} is extremely low, and the P_{50} of the arterial blood (at the prevailing pH) is also very low (Section 8.4.4).

A particularly interesting example of a human 'animal' with an unusual haemoglobin was described by Hebbel *et al.* (1978). The authors studied a family in which two of the siblings had a mutant haemoglobin (Andrew–Minneapolis) with a P_{50} of 17.1 mmHg. They showed that the siblings with the abnormal haemoglobin tolerated exercise at an altitude of 3100 m better than the normal siblings.

The last row in Table 8.1 refers to the climber at extreme altitude who has a marked respiratory alkalosis which greatly increases the oxygen affinity of the haemoglobin. This is discussed in detail below.

8.3.4 High-altitude natives

Barcroft *et al.* (1923) measured the oxygen dissociation curves of three natives of Cerro de Pasco (4330 m) at the prevailing P_{CO_2} (between 25 and 30 mmHg) and showed that the curves were displaced to the left, that is there was an increased oxygen affinity. A similar result was found in acclimatized members of the expedition. Barcroft (1925) believed that part of the leftward shift was caused by increased alkalinity of the blood but part was also due to a real change in the affinity of haemoglobin.

During the International High Altitude Expedition to Chile in 1935, a number of measurements were made on high-altitude natives who were living at 5340 m (P_B 401 mmHg). Some of the men were accustomed to work each day at 5700 m. The dissociation curves were found to be within normal limits for men at sea-level, or perhaps shifted slightly to the right (Keys *et al.*, 1936). Measurements were also made on dilute solutions of haemoglobin taken both from high-altitude residents and from acclimatized lowlanders (Hall, 1936). The results were very similar to those obtained at sea-level but the high-altitude residents seemed to have a slightly reduced oxygen affinity.

Aste-Salazar and Hurtado (1944) measured the oxgyen dissociation curves of 17 healthy Pervuians in Lima at sea-level and 12 other permanent residents of Morococha (4540 m). These studies were subsequently extended to a total of 40 subjects in Lima and 30 in Morococha (Hurtado, 1964). The mean value of the P_{50} at pH 7.4 was 24.7 mmHg at sea-level and 26.9 mmHg at high altitude (Figure 8.3). It was argued that the rightward displacement of the curve would enhance the unloading of oxygen from the peripheral capillaries.

Recently Winslow and his colleagues (1981) reported oxygen dissociation curves on 46 native Peruvians in Morococha (4540 m, P_B 432 mmHg) and confirmed that at pH 7.4 the P_{50} was significantly higher in the high-altitude population than in the sea-level controls (31.2 mmHg as opposed to 29.2 mmHg, $P < 0.001$). However these investigators also found that the acid–base status of the high-altitude subjects was that of partially compensated respiratory alkalosis with a mean plasma pH of 7.44. When the P_{50} values were corrected to the subjects' actual plasma pH, the mean value of 30.1 mmHg could no longer be distinguished from that of the sea-level controls (Figure 8.4). The conclusion was that the small increase in P_{50} resulting from the increased concentration of 2,3-diphosphoglycerate in the red cells was offset by the mild degree of respiratory alkalosis, with the net result that the position of the oxygen dissociation curve was essentially the same as that in sea-level controls.

In a controversial study Morpurgo *et al.* (1976) reported that Sherpas living permanently at an altitude of 4000 m in the Nepalese Himalayas had a substantially increased oxygen affinity at standard pH. The P_{50} value of the high-altitude Sherpas was 22.6 mmHg compared with 27.1 mmHg in low-altitude Caucasians. The Sherpa blood was also

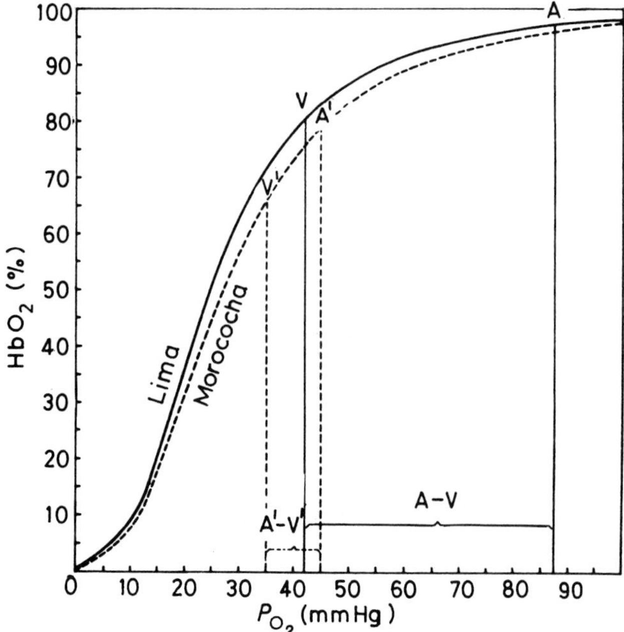

Figure 8.3 Mean positions of the oxygen dissociation curves of Peruvians in Lima (sea-level) and Morococha (4540 m). Note that the high-altitude natives have a slightly reduced oxygen affinity. Mean values of the P_{O_2} in arterial (A) and mixed venous (V) blood for the two groups are also shown. (From Hurtado, 1964.)

reported to have an unusually large Bohr effect. Interestingly, Sherpas living at low altitude appeared to have an increased P_{50} value of 36.7 mmHg. A weakness of this study was that the oxygen dissociation curves were determined five to six days after the blood was taken. A subsequent study by Samaja *et al.* (1979) failed to confirm these provocative findings. Samaja *et al.* also showed that the oxygen affinity could be completely accounted for by the known effectors of haemoglobin function: pH, P_{CO_2}, 2,3-DPG and temperature.

8.3.5 Acclimatized lowlanders

As discussed in section 8.2, Barcroft (1911) was perhaps the first person to measure the position of the oxygen dissociation curve in acclimatized lowlanders. This was done at altitudes of 2130 and 3000 m on Tenerife, and he reported that the curve was shifted to the right if measured at the normal P_{CO_2} of 40 mmHg, but if the P_{CO_2} for those altitudes was

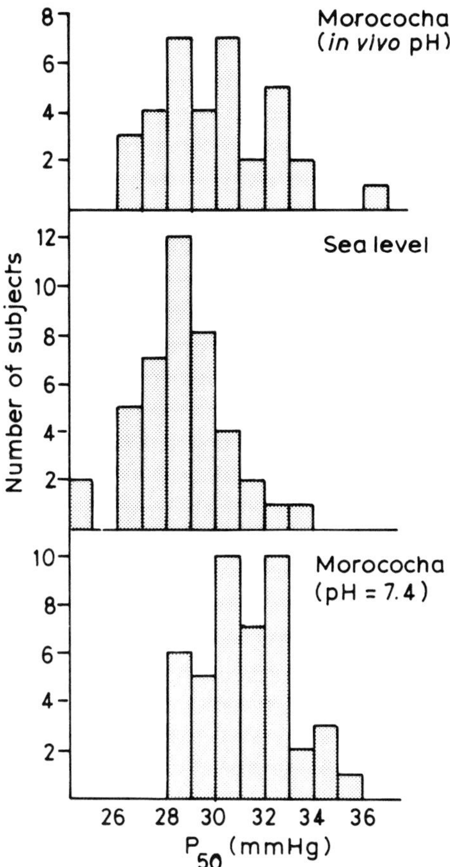

Figure 8.4 Distribution of P_{50} values at sea-level and high altitude. In the top panel, values are expressed at the *in vivo* pH; in the bottom at pH 7.4. When corrected for the subjects' plasma pH, the *in vivo* P_{50} at high altitude falls in the sea-level range in all but one subject. (From Winslow *et al.*, 1981.)

used, the curves had the same position at sea-level. Barcroft made additional measurements on Monte Rosa in 1911 (Barcroft *et al.*, 1914) and reported a slight rightward shift of the curves at the prevailing P_{CO_2}. However during the expedition to Cerro de Pasco in 1922, a leftward shift was observed at the prevailing arterial P_{CO_2} of between 25 and 30 mmHg (Barcroft *et al.*, 1923). He made the point that this might be beneficial because of enhanced oxygen uptake in the lung owing to the increased oxygen affinity of the haemoglobin.

During the International High Altitude Expedition to Chile 1935, three ways of measuring the oxygen affinity of the haemoglobin were employed, namely whole blood at normal pH, whole blood at the prevailing pH, and dilute solutions of haemoglobin. At constant pH, Keys *et al.* (1936) reported that the oxygen affinity of the haemoglobin was apparently slightly reduced with a change in P_{50} of approximately 3.5 mmHg. However the 'physiological' dissociation curves were displaced to the left from sea-level up to an altitude of approximately 4270 m, though above that they were displaced increasingly to the right of the sea-level positions. On dilute haemoglobin solutions, Hall (1936) showed that the oxygen affinity of the haemoglobin was essentially unchanged compared with sea-level.

These somewhat confusing results were substantially clarified when the role of 2,3-diphosphoglycerate in the red cell was appreciated (Chanutin and Curnish, 1967; Benesch and Benesch, 1967). They showed that this normal product of red cell metabolism reduced the oxygen affinity of haemoglobin, and it was clear that many previous measurements were unreliable because of ignorance of this factor. Lenfant and his colleagues (Lenfant *et al.*, 1968, 1969, 1971) showed that the concentration of 2,3-DPG was increased in lowlanders when they became acclimatized to high altitude. The primary cause of the increase in 2,3-DPG was the increase in plasma pH above the normal sea-level value as a result of the respiratory alkalosis. When subjects were made acidotic with acetazolamide there was no increase in plasma pH or red cell 2,3-DPG concentration at high altitude, and the oxygen dissociation curve did not shift to the right. It was argued that the increase in 2,3-DPG was an important feature of the acclimatization process of lowlanders, and the adaptation to high altitude of highlanders (Lenfant and Sullivan, 1971).

Subsequent measurements on lowlanders at high altitude have confirmed these changes although there is still some uncertainty about whether acclimatized lowlanders develop complete metabolic compensation for their respiratory alkalosis (that is, whether the pH returns to 7.4). Certainly this does not happen at extremely high altitudes. During the American Medical Research Expedition to Everest in 1981, Winslow *et al.* (1984) made an extensive series of measurements on acclimatized lowlanders at an altitude of 6300 m. They also obtained data on two subjects who reached the summit (8848 m). These measurements were made on venous blood samples taken at an altitude of 8050 m the morning after the summit climb. Winslow and his colleagues found that the red cell concentration of 2,3-DPG increased with altitude (Figure 8.5) and that this was associated with a slightly increased P_{50} value when expressed at pH 7.4. However because the respiratory alkalosis was not fully compensated, the subjects' *in vivo* P_{50} at 6300 m (27.6 mmHg) was slightly less than at-sea level (28.1 mmHg). The esti-

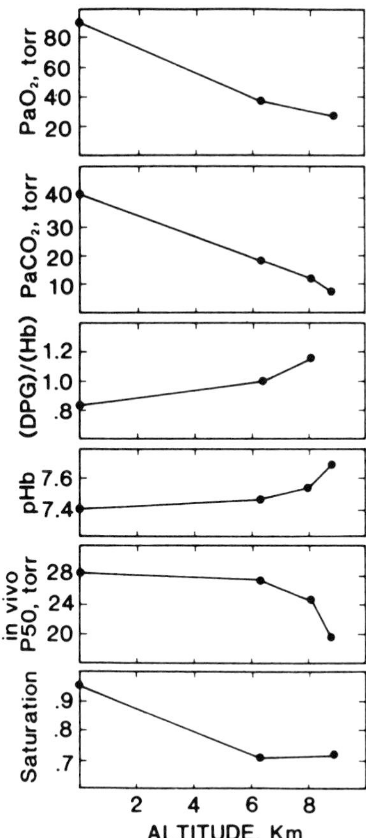

Figure 8.5 Blood variables measured on the 1981 American Medical Research Expedition to Everest at sea-level, 6300 m, 8050 m and 8848 m (summit). (From Winslow *et al.*, 1984.) (1 torr = 1 mmHg)

mated *in vivo* P_{50} was found to become progressively lower at 8050 m (24.9 mmHg), and on the summit at 8848 m it was as low as 19.4 mmHg in one subject. Thus these data show that, at extreme altitudes, the blood oxygen dissociation curve shifts progressively leftward (increased oxygen affinity of haemoglobin) primarily because of the respiratory alkalosis. Indeed this effect completely overwhelms the relatively small tendency for the curve to shift to the right because of the increase in red cell 2,3-DPG.

The results obtained on Operation Everest II were generally in agreement with these (Sutton *et al.*, 1988) except that the P_{CO_2} values at extreme altitude were higher, and the blood pH values therefore lower. These differences can probably be explained by the inadequate acclimatization because of the limited time available in the low-pressure chamber.

8.3.6 Physiological effects of changes in oxygen affinity

As indicated above, there have been differences of opinion on whether a decreased or an increased oxygen affinity is beneficial at high altitude. Barcroft *et al.* (1923) found a slightly increased affinity and argued that this would enhance oxygen loading in the lung. However Aste-Salazar and Hurtado (1944) reported a slight decrease in oxygen affinity in high-altitude natives at Morococha and reasoned that this would enhance oxygen unloading in peripheral capillaries. The same argument was used by Lenfant and Sullivan (1971) when the influence of the increased red cell concentration of 2,3-DPG on the oxygen dissociation curve was appreciated. They stated that the decreased oxygen affinity would help the peripheral unloading of oxygen, and that this was one of the many features both of acclimatization of lowlanders to high altitude and of the genetic adaptation of highlanders.

However there is now strong evidence that an increased oxygen affinity (left-shifted oxygen dissociation curve) is beneficial, especially at higher altitudes, and particularly on exercise (Bencowitz *et al.*, 1982). Indeed this should not come as a surprise when it is appreciated that many animals increase the oxygen affinity of their blood in oxygen-deprived environments by a variety of strategies (section 8.3.3; Table 8.1). In addition, Eaton *et al.* (1974) reported that rats whose oxygen dissociation curve had been left-shifted by cyanate administration showed an increased survival when they were decompressed to a barometric pressure of 233 mmHg. The controls were rats with a normal oxygen affinity. Turek *et al.* (1978) also studied cyanate-treated rats and found that they maintained better oxygen transfer to tissues during severe hypoxia than normal animals. In addition, we have already referred to the studies of Hebbel *et al.* (1978) who found a family with two members who had a haemoglobin with a very high affinity (Hb Andrew–Minneapolis, P_{50} 17.1 mmHg). These two members performed better during exercise at an altitude of 3100 m than two siblings with normal blood.

Theoretical studies show that a high oxygen affinity is beneficial at high altitude, especially on exercise (Bencowitz *et al.*, 1982; Turek *et al.*, 1973). In one study, oxygen transfer from air to tissues was modelled for a variety of altitudes and a range of oxygen uptakes (Bencowitz *et al.*, 1982). The oxygen dissociation curve was shifted both to the left and right with P_{50} of 16.8 mmHg (left-shifted), 26.8 mmHg (normal), and 36.8 mmHg (right-shifted). The pulmonary diffusing capacity for oxygen was varied over a wide range and all the determinants of oxygen transport, including temperature, base excess, haemoglobin concentration and haematocrit, were taken into account.

The results showed that in the presence of diffusion-limitation of oxygen transfer across the blood–gas barrier in the lung, a left-shifted curve resulted in the highest P_{O_2} of mixed venous blood (which was taken as an index of tissue P_{O_2}) (Figure 8.6). In other words, in the presence of diffusion-limitation, an increased oxygen affinity of haemoglobin results in a higher tissue P_{O_2}. The explanation is that the increased affinity enhances the loading of oxygen in the lung more than it interferes with unloading in peripheral capillaries. This appears to be the physiological justification for the increased oxygen affinity so frequently seen among animals who live in low oxygen environments (Table 8.1).

The role of an increased oxygen affinity is seen dramatically in a climber on the summit of Mt Everest. In spite of some increase of 2,3-DPG concentration within the red cell, the extremely low P_{CO_2} of 7.5 mmHg as a result of the enormous increase in ventilation causes a dramatic degree of respiratory alkalosis with an arterial pH calculated to exceed 7.7 (West *et al.*, 1983). As a result, the *in vivo* P_{50} is about 19 mmHg which is very similar to the value of the human foetus *in utero*. The resulting striking increase in oxygen affinity of haemoglobin plays a major role in allowing the climber to survive this extremely hypoxic environment (Chapter 11).

8.4 ACID–BASE BALANCE

8.4.1 Introduction

This topic overlaps with that of the previous section, oxygen affinity of haemoglobin, because the affinity at high altitude is primarily determined by the pH of the blood together with the concentration of 2,3-diphosphoglycerate in the red cells. However, for convenience, available information on acid–base status is set out here.

8.4.2 During acclimatization

When a lowlander goes to high altitude, hyperventilation occurs as a result of stimulation of the peripheral chemoreceptors by the hypoxaemia (Chapter 4), the arterial P_{CO_2} falls, and the arterial pH rises in accordance with the Henderson–Hasselbalch equation:

$$\mathrm{pH} = \mathrm{p}K + \log\frac{[\mathrm{HCO_3}^-]}{0.03\ P_{CO_2}}$$

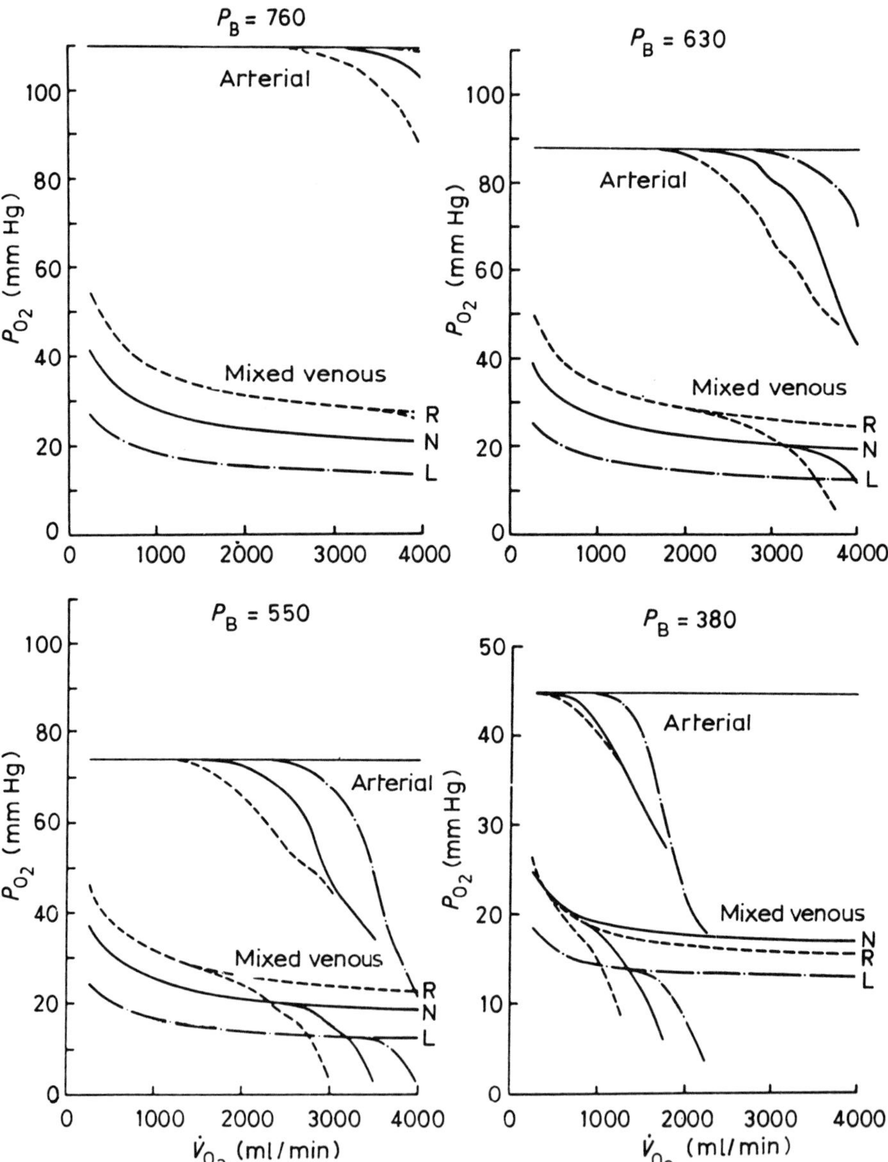

Figure 8.6 Results of a theoretical study showing changes in calculated arterial and mixed venous P_{O_2} with increasing oxygen uptake at four altitudes for three values of P_{50}. The P_{50} values are normal (N, 26.8 mmHg) right-shifted (R, 36.8 mmHg) and left-shifted (L, 16.8 mmHg). The nearly horizontal lines labelled 'mixed venous' show the P_{O_2} values for an infinitely high pulmonary oxygen diffusing capacity. The curved lines peeling away from these lines show the results of diffusion-limitation. In this example, the diffusing capacity of the membrane for oxygen (DMO_2) is 80 ml min^{-1} mmHg^{-1}. Note that at the highest levels of exercise, and especially at high altitude, the left-shifted curved gives the highest values of P_{O_2} in mixed venous blood and therefore the tissues. (From Bencowitz *et al.*, 1982.) (1 torr = 1 mmHg)

where the bicarbonate comcentration [HCO_3^-] is in millimoles per litre and the P_{CO_2} is in mmHg. However the kidney responds by eliminating bicarbonate ion, being prompted to do this by the decreased P_{O_2} in the renal tubular cells. The result is a more alkaline urine because of decreased reabsorption of bicarbonate ions. The resulting decrease in plasma bicarbonate then moves the bicarbonate/P_{CO_2} ratio back towards its normal level. This is known as metabolic compensation for the respiratory alkalosis. The compensation may be complete, in which case the arterial pH returns to 7.4 or, more usually, incomplete with a steady-state pH that exceeds 7.4.

The time course of the changes in arterial pH when normal subjects are taken abruptly to high altitude has been studied by several investigators (Severinghaus *et al.*, 1963; Dempsey *et al.*, 1978; Lenfant *et al.*, 1971). In one study, lowlanders were taken from sea-level to an altitude 4509 m (P_B 446 mmHg) in less than five hours, where they remained for four days. The arterial pH rose to a mean of about 7.47 within 24 h and then apparently slowly declined but was still about 7.45 at the end of the four-day period. On return to sea-level the pH fell steadily to reach the normal value of 7.4 after about 48 h (Lenfant *et al.*, 1971).

In another study, four normal subjects were taken abruptly to 3800 m for eight days. The arterial pH rapidly rose from a mean of 7.424 at sea-level to 7.485 after two days, and remainded essentially constant being 7.484 at the end of eight days (Severinghaus *et al.*, 1963). In a further study, 11 lowlanders moved to 3200 m altitude where they remained for 10 days (Dempsey *et al.*, 1978). The arterial pH rose by 0.03 to 0.04 units within two days and then remained essentially unchanged. In all instances, the arterial P_{CO_2} continued to fall as did the plasma bicarbonate concentration. However it appears that the return of the arterial pH to (or near to) its sea-level value is very slow.

8.4.3 High-altitude natives

Most authors have reported a fully compensated respiratory alkalosis in high-altitude natives with arterial pH values close to 7.4. Table 8.2 shows a summary of a number of published papers prepared by Winslow and Monge (1987). This is perhaps the expected finding. The body generally maintains the arterial pH within very narrow limits in health, and it seems reasonable that people who are born and bred at high altitude would fully compensate for their reduced P_{CO_2} by eliminating bicarbonate and restoring the pH to the normal sea-level value.

However Winslow *et al.* (1981) measured the arterial pH in 46 high-altitude natives of Morococha (4540 m, P_B 432 mmHg) and reported that the mean plasma pH was 7.439 ± 0.065. In other words these

Table 8.2 Blood-gas and pH values in high-altitude natives (From Winslow and Monge, 1987)

Altitude (m)	*N*	*Hct (Hb)**	*Pa_{O_2} (torr)*	*Sa_{O_2} (%)*	*Pa_{CO_2} (torr)*	*pH*	*Source*
4300	3	—	46.7	84.6	—	—	(1)
4300	12	—	—	—	—	7.360	(2)
4500	40	(20.6)	45.1	80.1	33.3	7.370	(3)
4515	22	(19.5)	—	82.8	33.8	7.400	(4)
4300	6	56.0	—	—	32.5	7.431†	(5)
4300	5	73.8	—	—	39.0	7.429†	(5)
3700	—	—	—	—	3.0	7.431†	(6)
4545	—	—	—	—	—	7.424†	(6)
4820	—	—	—	—	—	7.426†	(6)
3960	3	—	—	—	—	—	(7)‡
4880	4	—	—	—	—	7.399	(7)‡
4500	6	73.4	—	—	—	—	(8)
4500	10	65.5	—	—	—	—	(8)
4300	6	54.4	45.2	74.7	31.6	7.414	(9)
4500	4	63.3	44.1	73.3	32.2	7.405	(9)
4300	4	—	50.8	—	32.9	7.405	(10)
4500	35	61.0	51.7	85.7	34.0	7.395	(11)

Sources: (1) Barcroft et al., 1923; (2) Aste-Salazar and Hurtado, 1944; (3) Hurtado, Velásquez, Reynafarje *et al.*, 1956; (4) Chiodi, 1957; (5) Monge, Lozano and Carcelén, 1964; (6) Severinghaus and Carclén, 1964; (7) Lahiri *et al.*, 1967; (8) Lenfant *et al.*, 1969; (9) Torrance, 1970; (10) Rennie, 1971; and (11) Winslow *et al.*, 1981. Please refer to Winslow and Monge (1987) for details

* Numbers in parentheses are haemoglobin concentration ($g\,dl^{-1}$)

† Plasma pH

‡ Himalayan subjects

1 torr = 1 mmHg

highlanders did not have a fully compensated respiratory alkalosis but their blood lay slightly on the alkaline side of normal. As pointed out in section 8.3.4, the result of this mild respiratory alkalosis was to restore the oxygen dissociation curve to the normal sea-level position because there was an increase in red cell 2,3-DPG concentration which tended to move the curve to the right.

The interpretation of these results is complicated by the fact that Winslow *et al.* (1981) believed that the increased red cell concentration that is seen at high altitude had an effect on the glass electrode for measuring pH (Whittembury *et al.*, 1968). If the observed pH is corrected for this effect of increased red cell concentration, the calculated plasma pH becomes 7.395 as shown in the bottom row of Table 8.2. However no other investigators have corrected the pH in this way and the conclusion from the work of Winslow and his colleagues is that high-altitude natives have a mildly uncompensated respiratory alkalosis with an arterial pH that exceeds 7.4.

8.4.4 Acclimatized lowlanders

When sufficient time is allowed for extended acclimatization to high altitude, the arterial pH returns close to the normal value of 7.4, at least up to altitudes of 3000 m. For example, during the 1935 International High Altitude Expedition to Chile, Dill and his colleagues (1937) found that the arterial pH increased little if at all up to this altitude, but above 3000 m, higher values of pH were found with a mean of about 7.45 at an altitude of 5340 m. A few measurements on acclimatized subjects at an altitude of 5800 m during the Himalayan Scientific and Mountaineering Expedition indicated values of between 7.41 and 7.46 (West *et al.*, 1962).

Extensive measurements were made by Winslow *et al.* (1984) during the 1981 American Medical Research Expedition to Everest. The mean arterial pH of acclimatized lowlanders living at an altitude 6300 m was 7.47 (Figure 8.7). It was also possible to calculate the arterial pH at altitudes of 8050 m (Camp 5) and the Everest summit (8848 m). The

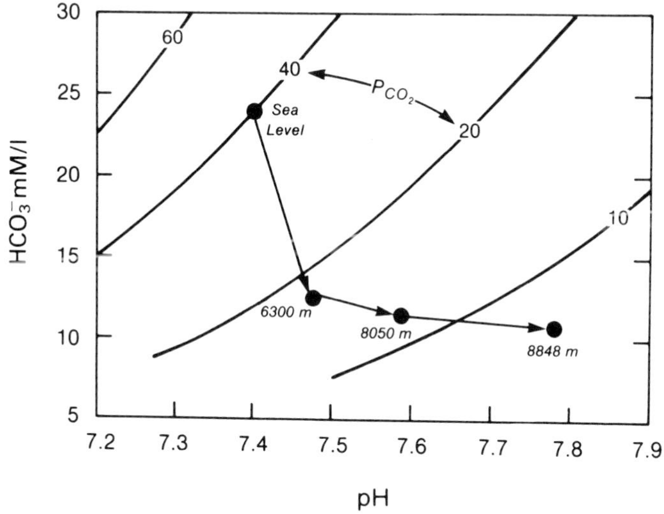

Figure 8.7 Davenport diagram showing the pH, P_{CO_2} and plasma bicarbonate concentration of arterial blood during the 1981 American Medical Expedition to Everest at altitudes of 6300 m, 8050 m and 8848 m (summit). Note the increasingly severe respiratory alkalosis at the extreme altitudes. The points for 8050 and 8848 m are from Pizzo. (Data from Winslow *et al.*, 1984.)

calculations were made from the base excess measured on venous blood samples taken at 8050 m, and measurements of alveolar P_{CO_2} on sealed samples of alveolar gas brought back to the USA. It was assumed that the arterial and alveolar P_{CO_2} values were the same, and also that base excess did not change over the 24 h between the summit and Camp 5. As discussed in section 8.4.5, there is evidence that base excess was changing very slowly at this great altitude. The mean arterial pH of two climbers at 8050 m was 7.55, and the one subject, whose alveolar P_{CO_2} was measured as 7.5 mmHg on the summit gave a calculated arterial pH of over 7.7.

These climbers were not 'acclimatized' to 8050 or 8848 m in the sense that they had spent long periods at these great altitudes. However it is not possible to spend an extended time at an altitude such as 8000 m because high-altitude deterioration occurs so rapidly. Thus the values probably represent the inevitable respiratory alkalosis which occurs in climbers who go so high.

8.4.5 Metabolic compensation for respiratory alkalosis

An interesting feature of the studies at extreme altitude referred to above is that metabolic compensation for the respiratory alkalosis appears to be extremely slow. The mean base excess measured on three subjects who were living at an altitude of 6300 m was $-7.9\,\text{mmol}\,\text{l}^{-1}$. The measurements made on venous blood taken from two climbers at 8050 m gave a mean value of $-7.2\,\text{mmol}\,\text{l}^{-1}$, essentially the same. The 8050 m measurements were taken several days after the climbers had left Camp 2 at 6300 m, and the data therefore suggest that metabolic compensation was proceeding extremely slowly in spite of the fact that the P_{CO_2} had fallen considerably. For example, the mean P_{CO_2} at 6300 m was 18.4 mmHg, at 8050 m 11.0 mmHg, and at 8848 m (summit) 7.5 mmHg. The last value was obtained from only one subject.

The reason for the very slow change in bicarbonate at these great altitudes in unclear. One possible factor is chronic dehydration. Blume *et al.* (1984) measured serum osmolality at sea level, 5400 m and 6300 m in 13 subjects of the expedition and showed that the mean value rose from $290 \pm 1\,\text{mmol}\,\text{kg}^{-1}$ at sea-level to 295 ± 2 at 5400 m, and to 302 ± 4 at 6300 m. This volume depletion occurred in spite of adequate fluids to drink and a reasonably normal life-style. An interesting feature of the fluid balance studies was that plasma arginine–vasopressin concentrations remained unchanged from sea-level to 6300 m in spite of the hyperosmolality. A possible factor in the volume depletion was the large insensible loss of fluid at these great altitudes as a result of hyperventilation. However the failure of the vasopressin levels to change suggests that there is some abnormality of body fluid regulation.

It is known that the kidney is slow to correct an alkalosis in the presence of volume depletion. It appears that of the two options, correcting fluid balance and correcting acid–base balance, the kidney gives a higher priority to fluid balance. In order to correct the respiratory alkalosis, bicarbonate ion excretion must be increased (or reabsorption decreased) and this entails the loss of a cation which inevitably aggravates the hyperosmolality. This would explain the reluctance of the kidney to correct a respiratory alkalosis in the presence of volume depletion.

A different explanation was offered by Gonzalez *et al.* (1990), when they studied the slow metabolic compensation of respiratory alkalosis in a chronically hypoxic rat model. They found that the rate of metabolic compensation was indeed slower than in acute hypoxia, and they attributed this to the lower plasma bicarbonate concentration resulting from chronic hypoxia. They argued that, because proton secretion and reabsorption of bicarbonate are functions of the bicarbonate load offered to the renal proximal tubule, it is probable that the slower increase in bicarbonate excretion of the chronically hypoxic animals was ultimately the result of the lower plasma bicarbonate concentration.

REFERENCES

Araki, T. (1891) Ueber die Bildung von Milchsaure und Glycose im Organisms bei Sauerstoffmangel. *Z. Physiol. Chem.*, **15**, 335–70.

Aste-Salazar, H. and Hurtado, A. (1944) The affinity of haemoglobin for oxygen at sea level and at high altitudes. *Am. J. Physiol.*, **142**, 733–43.

Astrup, P. and Severinghaus, J.W. (1986) *The History of Blood Gases, Acids and Bases*, Munksgaard, Copenhagen.

Barcroft, J. (1911) The effect of altitude on the dissociation curve of blood. *J. Physiol. (London)*, **42**, 44–63.

Barcroft, J. (1925) *The Respiratory Function of the Blood. Part I. Lessons from High Altitudes*. Cambridge University Press, Cambridge.

Barcroft, J. and King, W.O.R. (1909) The effect of temperature on the dissociation curve of blood. *J. Physiol. (London)*, **39**, 374–84.

Barcroft, J. and Orbeli, L. (1910) The influence of lactate acid upon the dissociation curve of blood. *J. Physiol. (London)*, **41**, 355–67.

Barcroft, J., Camis, M., Mathison, C.G., *et al.* (1914) Report of the Monte Rosa Expedition of 1911. *Phil. Trans. R. Soc. London Ser. B.*, **206**, 49–102.

Barcroft, J., Biner, C.A., Bock, A.V., *et al.* (1923) Observations upon the effect of high altitude on the physiological processes of the human body, carried out in the Peruvian Andes, chiefly at Cerro de Pasco. *Phil. Trans. R. Soc. London Ser. B.*, **211**, 351–480.

Bencowitz, H.Z., Wagner, P.D. and West, J.B. (1982) Effect of change in P_{50} on exercise tolerance at high altitude: a theoretical study. *J. Appl. Physiol. Respir. Environ. Exercise Physiol.*, **53**, 1487–95.

Benesch, R. and Benesch, R.E. (1967) The effect of organic pyrophosphates from human erythrocyte on the allosteric properties of haemoglobin. *Biochem. Biophys. Res. Commun.*, **26**, 162–7.

Bert, P. (1878) *La Pression Barométrique*, Masson, Paris. English translation by M.A. Hitchcock and F.A. Hitchcock. College Book Co, Columbus, Ohio, 1943.

Black, C.P. and Tenney, S.M. (1980) Oxygen transport during progressive hypoxia in high-altitude and sea-level waterfowl. *Respir. Physiol.*, **39**, 217–39.

Blume, F.D., Boyer, S.J., Braverman, L.E., *et al.* (1984) Impaired osmoregulation at high altitude. *J. Am. Med. Assoc.*, **252**, 524–6.

Bohr, C. (1885) *Experimentale Untersuchungen über die Sauerstoffaufnahme des Blutfarbstoffes*, O.C. Olsen & Co.'s Buchdruckerei, Copenhagen.

Bohr, C. Hasselbalch, K. and Krogh, A. (1904) Ueber einen biologischer Beziehung wichtigen Einfluss, den die Kohlensaurespanning des Blutes auf dessen Sauerstoff-binding übt. *Skand. Arch. Physiol.*, **16**, 402–12.

Boycott, A.E. and Haldane, J.S. (1908) The effects of low atmospheric pressures on respiration. *J. Physiol. (London)*, **37**, 355–77.

Chanutin, A. and Curnish, R.R. (1967) Effect of organic and inorganic phosphatases on the oxygen equilibrium of human erythrocyte. *Arch. Biochem. Biophys.*, **121**, 96–102.

Dempsey, J.A., Forster, H.V., Chosy, L.W., *et al.* (1978) Regulation of CSF [HCO_3] during long-term hypoxic hypocapnia in man. *J. Appl. Physiol.*, **44**, 175–82.

Dill, D.B., Talbott, J.H. and Consolazio, W.V. (1937) Blood as a physiochemical system. *J. Biol. Chem.*, **118**, 649–66.

Eaton, J.W., Skelton, T.D. and Berger, E. (1974) Survival at extreme altitude: protective effect of increased hemoglobin-oxygen affinity. *Science*, **183**, 743–4.

Galeotti, G. (1904) Les variations de l'alcalinite du sang sur le sommet du Mont Rosa. *Arch. Ital. Biol.*, **41**, 80–92.

Gonzalez, N.C., Albrecht, T., Sullivan, L.P. and Clancy, R.L. (1990) Compensation of respiratory alkalosis induced after acclimatization to simulated altitude. *J. Appl. Physiol.*, **69**, 1380–6.

Haldane, J.S., Kellas, A.M., and Kennaway, E.L. (1919) Experiments on acclimatization to reduced atmospheric pressure. *J. Physiol. (London)*, **53**, 181–206.

Hall, F.G. (1936) The effect of altitude on the affinity of haemoglobin for oxygen. *J. Cell. Comp. Physiol.*, **115**, 484–90.

Hall, F.G., Dill, D.B. and Guzman-Barron, E.S. (1936) Comparative physiology at high altitudes. *J. Cell. Comp. Physiol.*, **8**, 301–13.

Hebbel, R.P., Eaton, J. W., Kronenberg, R.S., *et al.* (1978) Human llamas: adaptation to altitude in subjects with high haemoglobin oxygen affinity. *J. Clin. Invest.*, **62**, 593–600.

Henderson, Y. (1919) The physiology of the aviator. *Science*, **49**, 431–41.

Heymans, J.F. and Heymans, C. (1925) Sur le mécanisme de l'apnée réflexe ou pneumogastrique. *Comptes Rendus Soc. Biol.*, **92**, 1335–8.

Hüfner, C.G. (1890) Uber das Gesetz der Dissociation des Oxyhamoglobins und über einige daran sich knupfende wichtige Fragen aus der Biologie. *Arch. Pathol. Anat. Physiol.*, 1–27.

Hurtado, A. (1964) Animals in high altitudes: resident man, in *Handbook of Physiology, section IV, Adaptation to the Environment*, (ed. D.B. Dill), American Physiological Society, Washington DC, pp. 843–60.

Kellogg, R.H. (1980) Acid–base balance in high altitude: historical perspective, in *Environmental Physiology: Aging, Heat and Altitude*, (eds S.M. Horvarth and M.K. Yousef), Elsevier, New York, pp. 295–308.

Kelman, G.R. (1966a) Digital computer subroutine for the conversion of oxygen tension into saturation. *J. Appl. Physiol.*, **21**, 1375–6.

Kelman, G.R. (1966b) Calculation of certain indices of cardio-pulmonary function using a digital computer. *Respir. Physiol.*, **1**, 335–43.

Kelman, G.R. (1967) Digital computer procedure for the conversion of PCO_2 into blood CO_2 content. *Respir. Physiol.*, **3**, 335–43.

Keys, A., Hall, F.G. and Guzman-Barron, E.S. (1936) The position of the oxygen dissociation curve of human blood at high altitude. *Am. J. Physiol.*, **115**, 292–307.

Lenfant, C. and Sullivan, K. (1971) Adaptation to high altitude. *N. Engl. J. Med.*, **284**, 1298–309.

Lenfant, C., Torrance, J., English, E., *et al.* (1968) Effect of altitude on oxygen binding by hemoglobin and on organic phosphate levels. *J. Clin. Invest.*, **47**, 2652–6.

Lenfant, C., Ways, P., Aucutt, C. and Cruz, J. (1969) Effect of chronic hypoxic hypoxia on the O_2-Hb dissociation curve and respiratory gas transport in man. *Respir. Physiol.*, **7**, 7–29.

Lenfant, C. Torrance, J.D. and Reynafarje, C. (1971) Shift of the O_2–Hb dissociation curve at altitude: mechanism and effect. *J. Appl. Physiol.*, **30**, 625–31.

Margaria, R. (1957) The contribution of hemoglobin to acid-base equilibrium of the blood in health and disease. *Clin. Chem.*, **3**, 306–18.

Mines, A.H. (1981) *Respiratory Physiology*, Raven Press, New York.

Morpurgo, G., Arese, P., Bosia, A., *et al.* (1976) Sherpas living permanently at high altitude: a new pattern of adaptation. *Proc. Natl Acad. Science, USA*, **73**, 747–51.

Samaja, M., Veicsteinas, A. and Cerretelli, P. (1979) Oxygen affinity of blood in altitude Sherpas. *J. Appl. Physiol.*, **47**, 337–41.

Severinghaus, J.W., Mitchell, R.A., Richardson, B.W. and Singer, M.M. (1963) Respiratory control at high altitude suggesting active transport regulation of CSF pH. *J. Appl. Physiol.*, **18**, 1155–66.

Snyder, L.R.G., Born, S. and Lechner, A.L. (1982) Blood oxygen affinity in high- and low-altitude populations of the deer mouse. *Respir. Physiol.*, **48**, 89–105.

Sutton, J.R., Reeves, J.T., Wagner, P.D., *et al.* (1988) Operation Evesest II: oxygen transport during exercise at extreme simulated altitude. *J. Appl. Physiol.*, **64**, 1309–21.

Turek, Z., Kreuzer, F. and Hoofd, L.J.C. (1973) Advantage or disadvantage of a decrease of blood oxygen affinity for tissue oxygen supply at hypoxia; a theoretical study comparing man and rat. *Pflugers Arch.*, **342**, 185–97.

Turek, Z., Kreuzer, F. and Ringnalda, B.E.M. (1978) Blood gases at several levels of oxygenation in rats with a left shifted blood oxygen dissociation curve. *Pflugers Arch.*, **376**, 7–13.

West, J.B. (1994) *Respiratory Physiology – The Essentials*, 5th edn, Williams & Wilkins, Baltimore.

West, J.B. and Wagner, P.D. (1977) Pulmonary gas exchange, in *Bioengineering Aspects of the Lung*, (ed. J.B. West), Decker, New York, pp. 361–457.

West, J.B., Lahiri, S., Gill, M.B., *et al.* (1962) Arterial oxygen saturation during exercise at high altitude. *J. Appl. Physiol.*, **17**, 617–21.

West, J.B., Hackett, P.H., Maret, K.H., *et al.* (1983) Pulmonary gas exchange on the summit of Mt Everest. *J. Appl. Physiol. Respir. Environ. Exercise Physiol.*, **55**, 678–87.

Whittembury, J., Lozano, R. and Monge, C.C. (1968) Influence of cell concentration in the electrometric determination of blood pH. *Acta Physiol. Lat. Am.*, **18**, 263–5.

Winslow, R.M. and Monge, C. (1987) *Hypoxia, Polycythemia and Chronic Mountain Sickness*, Johns Hopkins University Press, Baltimore.

Winslow, R. M., Monge, C.C., Statham, N.J., *et al.* (1981) Variability of oxygen affinity of blood: human subjects native to high altitude. *J. Appl. Physiol.*, **51**, 1411–16.

Winslow, R.M., Samaja, M. and West, J.B. (1984) Red cell function at extreme altitude on Mount Everest. *J. Appl. Physiol. Respir. Environ. Exercise Physiol.*, **56**, 109–16.

Winterstein, H. (1911) Die Regulierung der Atmung durch das Blut. *Pflugers Arch. Ges. Physiol.*, **138**, 167–84.

Winterstein, H. (1915) Neue Untersuchungen über die physikalisch-chemische Regulierung der Atmung. *Biochem. Z.*, **70**, 45–73.

Zuntz, N., Loewy, A., Müller, A.F. and Caspari, W. (1906) *Höhenklima und Bergwanderungen in ihrer Wirkung auf den Menschen*, Bong, Berlin.

9

Peripheral tissues

9.1 INTRODUCTION

The diffusion of oxygen from the peripheral capillaries to the mitochondria, and its consequent utilization by these organelles, constitutes the final link of the oxygen cascade which begins with the inspiration of air. In spite of its critical importance, many uncertainties remain concerning the changes that occur in peripheral tissues both in acclimatized lowlanders, and in the adaptation of high-altitude natives. An obvious reason for this paucity of knowledge is the difficulty of studying peripheral tissues in intact man. Much of our information necessarily comes from measurements on experimental animals exposed to low barometric pressures, though additional studies have been made on tissue biopsies in humans.

It is probable that tissue factors play a very important role in the remarkable tolerance of high-altitude natives to exercise at high altitude. As was pointed out in Chapter 4, people born at high altitude have a reduced ('blunted') ventilatory response to hypoxia. At first sight this is counterproductive because it will result in a lower alveolar P_{O_2}, and therefore a lower arterial P_{O_2}, other things being equal. There is no reason to think that oxygen transfer from the lungs to the peripheral capillaries is very different in high-altitude natives compared with acclimatized lowlanders although there is some evidence that they may have a higher pulmonary diffusing capacity. However their better exercise performance at high altitude in the face of a blunted ventilatory response to hypoxia certainly suggests that there are important adaptations within the tissues of which we are so far ignorant.

The present chapter overlaps with others to some extent. The principles of diffusion of gases through tissues were dealt with in Chapter 5, and there is a discussion in Chapter 10 of how diffusion-limitation in peripheral tissues may limit oxygen delivery during exercise. This topic is also alluded to in Chapter 11 in the discussion of limiting factors at extreme altitudes.

9.2 HISTORICAL

Early physiologists interested in high altitude did not attach much importance to tissue changes. For example, Paul Bert in *La Pression Barométrique* hardly refers to the possibility of tissue acclimatization although he deals at some length with changes in respiration and circulation. At one point he wonders whether the metabolism of high-altitude natives is different from that of lowlanders:

> . . . just as a Basque mountaineer furnished with a piece of bread and a few onions makes expeditions which require of the member of the *Alpine Club* who accompanys him the absorption of a pound of meat, so it may be that the dwellers in high places finally lessen the consumption of oxygen in their organism, while keeping at their disposal the same quantity of vital force, either for the equilibrium of temperature, or the production of work. Thus we could explain the acclimatization of individuals, of generations, of races.
>
> *(Paul Bert, 1878; p. 1004 in 1943 translation)*

Incidentally we now know that the oxygen requirements of a given amount of work are no different at high altitude compared with sea-level, or in high-altitude natives compared with lowlanders. Bert goes on, 'But we should consider not only the acts of nutrition, but also the stimulation, perhaps less, which an insufficiently oxygenated blood causes in the muscles, the nerves, and the nervous centers . . .' However he does not carry his speculations any further.

There is a delightful section where Bert suggests that there may be changes in the blood at high altitude:

> We might ask first whether, by a harmonious compensation of which general natural history gives us many examples, either by a modification in the nature or the quantity of haemoglobin or by an increase in the number of red corpuscles, his blood has become qualified to absorb more oxygen under the same volume, and thus to return to the usual standard of the seashore.
>
> *(Paul Bert, 1878, p. 1000 in 1943 translation)*

He goes on to say that this hypothesis would be very easy to test. Since it had recently been shown:

> that the capacity of the blood to absorb oxygen does not change after putrefaction, nothing would be easier than to collect the venous blood of a healthy vigorous man (an acclimated European or an Indian) or of an animal, defibrinate it, and send it in a well-corked flask; it would then be sufficient to shake it vigorously in the air to judge its capacity of absorption during life.
>
> *(Paul Bert, 1878, p. 1008 in 1943 translation)*

This beautiful research project handed to the research community on a silver plate was taken up by Viault (1890) with exactly the results predicted by Bert. However this was a change in the blood compartment of the body rather than the peripheral tissues with which this chapter is chiefly concerned.

Following the work of Krogh (1919, 1929) on the increase in the number of open capillaries in muscle when the oxygen demands were raised by exercise, it was natural to wonder whether increased capillarization was a feature of tissue acclimatization in response to chronic hypoxia. It was subsequently reported that capillaries in the brain, heart and liver were significantly dilated and that their number was apparently increased after hypoxic exposure (Mercker and Schneider, 1949; Optiz, 1951; Valdivia, 1958). As we shall see later, more recent measurements suggest that the number of capillaries in muscle tissue does not increase as a result of chronic hypoxia, but the intercapillary diffusion distance lessens because the muscle fibres become smaller.

Hurtado and his co-workers (1937) reported an increase in the intracellular concentration of the oxygen-carrying pigment, myoglobin, in high-altitude animals. The measurements were made on dogs born and raised in Morococha (4540 m) and the increased concentrations were found in the diaphragm, myocardium and muscles of the chest wall and leg. The controls were dogs from Lima at sea-level. Since then a number of other investigators have reported increased tissue myoglobin levels at high altitude.

An increase in mitochondrial density was shown in the myocardium of cattle born and raised at high altitude by Ou and Tenney (1970). Changes in mitochondrial enzymes in muscle of high-altitude natives were reported by Reynafarje (1962). He found alterations in the enzyme systems NADH-oxidase, NADPH-cytochrome c-reductase, $NAD[P]^+$ transhydrogenase and others. These measurements were made on muscle biopsies taken from permanent residents of Cerro de Pasco at an altitude of 4400 m. The sea-level controls were residents of Lima.

9.3 DIFFUSION IN PERIPHERAL TISSUES

9.3.1 Principles

Oxygen moves from the peripheral capillaries to the mitochondria, and carbon dioxide moves in the opposite direction by the process of diffusion. Fick's law of diffusion was discussed in section 5.3.2. It states that the rate of transfer of a gas through a sheet of tissue is proportional to the area of the tissue, and to the difference in gas partial pressure between the two sides, and inversely proportional to the tissue thickness.

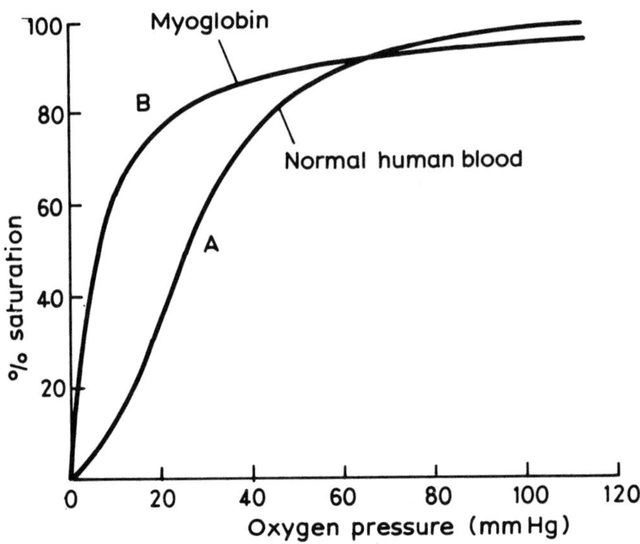

Figure 9.1 Comparison of the oxygen dissociation curves for normal human blood (curve A) and myoglobin (curve B). The P_{50} values are approximately 27 and 5 mmHg respectively. (From Roughton, 1964.)

In discussing the lung, it was pointed out that the blood–gas barrier of the human lung is extremely thin, being only 0.3 μm in many places. By contrast, the diffusion distances in peripheral tissues are typically much greater. For example, the distance between open capillaries in resting muscle is of the order of 50 μm. However, during exercise, when the oxygen consumption of the muscle increases, additional capillaries open up thus reducing the diffusion distance and increasing the capillary surface area available for diffusion. As discussed in section 5.3.2, carbon dioxide diffuses about 20 times faster than oxygen through tissues because of its much higher solubility, and therefore the elimination of carbon dioxide poses less of a problem then oxygen delivery.

Early workers believed that the movement of oxygen through tissues was by simple passive diffusion. However it is now believed that facilitated diffusion of oxygen probably occurs in muscle cells as a result of the presence of myoglobin. This haem–protein has a structure which resembles haemoglobin but the dissociation curve is a hyperbola, as opposed to the S-shape of the oxygen dissociation curve of whole blood (Figure 9.1). Another major difference is that myoglobin takes up oxygen at a much lower P_{O_2} than haemoglobin, that is it has a very low P_{50} of about 5 mmHg. This is a necessary property if the myoglobin is to be of any use in muscle cells where the tissue P_{O_2} is very low.

Scholander (1960) and Wittenberg (1959) have shown experimentally that myoglobin can facilitate oxygen diffusion.

Other modes of oxygen transport are possible within cells. Streaming movements of cytoplasm have been observed and it is conceivable that such movements, known as 'stirring', enhance the transport of oxygen by convection. Another hypothesis is that oxygen moves into some cells along invaginations of the lipid cell membrane in which it has a high solubility (Longmuir and Betts, 1987).

There is good evidence that the P_{O_2} in the immediate vicinity of the mitochondria is very low, of the order 1 mmHg. In fact many models of oxygen transfer in tissues assume that the mitochondrial P_{O_2} is so low that it can be neglected in the context of the P_{O_2} of the capillary blood which is of the order of 30–50 mmHg. In measurements of suspensions of liver mitochondria *in vitro*, oxygen consumption has been shown to continue at the same rate until the P_{O_2} of the surrounding fluid falls to the region of 3 mmHg. Measurements of P_{O_2} at the sites of oxygen utilization based on the spectral characteristics of cytochromes also indicate that the P_{O_2} is probably less than 1 mmHg (Chance, 1957; Chance *et al.*, 1962). Thus it appears that the purpose of the much higher P_{O_2} of capillary blood is to ensure an adequate pressure for diffusion of oxygen to the mitochondria and that, at the actual sites of oxygen utilization, the P_{O_2} is extremely low.

9.3.2 Tissue partial pressures

A classical model to analyse the distribution of P_{O_2} values in tissue was described by August Krogh (1919). He considered a hypothetical cylinder of tissue around a straight thin capillary into which blood entered with a known P_{O_2}. As oxygen diffuses away from the capillary, oxygen is consumed by the tissue and the P_{O_2} falls. If simplifying assumptions are made, such as uniform consumption rate of oxygen in every part of the tissue, an equation can be written to describe the P_{O_2} profile (Krogh, 1919; Piiper and Scheid, 1986).

Another model is shown in Figure 9.2 (Hill, 1928). In (a) we see a cylinder of tissue which is supplied with oxygen by capillaries at its periphery: in (1) the balance between oxygen consumption and delivery (determined by the capillary P_{O_2}, the intercapillary distance R_c, and the oxygen consumption rate of the tissue) results in an adequate P_{O_2} throughout the cyclinder; in (2) the intercapillary distance or the oxygen consumption has been increased until the P_{O_2} at one point in the tissue falls to zero. This is referred to as a *critical* situation; in (3) there is an anoxic region where aerobic (that is, oxygen-utilizing) metabolism is impossible. Under anoxic conditions the tissue energy requirements

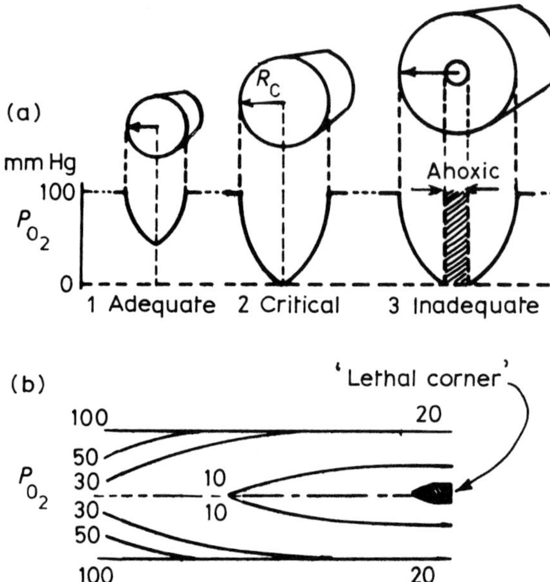

Figure 9.2 Scheme showing the fall in P_{O_2} between adjacent capillaries. In (a) three hypothetical cylinders of tissue are shown and oxygen is diffusing into these cylinders from capillaries at the periphery. In (2) the cylinder had a critical radius R_c while in (3) the radius of the cylinder is so large that there is an anoxic zone in the middle of the cylinder. (b) shows a section along the hypothetical cylinder of tissue. The P_{O_2} in the blood adjacent to the tissue is assumed to fall from 100 to 20 mmHg along the capillary. Lines of equal P_{O_2} are shown. Note the possibility of a 'lethal corner' in the middle of the cylinder at the venous end. (From West, 1985.)

must be met by obligatory anaerobic glycolysis with the consequent formation of lactic acid.

The situation *along* the tissue cylinder is shown in (b). It is assumed that the P_{O_2} in the capillaries at the periphery of the tissue cylinder falls from 100 to 20 mmHg as shown from left to right. As a consequence the P_{O_2} in the centre of the tissue cylinder falls towards the venous end of the capillary. It is clear that, on the basis of this model, the most vulnerable tissue is that furthest from the capillary at its downstream end. This was referred to as the 'lethal corner' by Krogh. It is possible that this pattern of focal anoxia is responsible for some tissue damage at high altitude. For example it may explain how some nerve cells of the brain are damaged at great altitudes causing the residual impairment of central nervous system function. This is discussed in Chapter 15.

The concept of a cylinder of tissue surrounded by a network of capillaries is supported by recent studies emphasizing the tortuosity of capillaries around skeletal muscle cells (Potter and Groom, 1983; Mathieu-Costello, 1987). Although at first sight the capillaries of skeletal muscle chiefly appear to run parallel to the muscle fibres, this is an oversimplification because of the connections between adjacent capillaries, and also the tortuosity which increases considerably as a result of muscle shortening (Mathieu-Costello, 1987). Thus a reasonable model of oxygen delivery to muscle is a syncytium of capillaries surrounding a tubular muscle cell.

Recent studies by Honig and his associates (1991) have indicated that the P_{O_2} profiles shown in Figure 9.2 may be misleading in skeletal muscle. These investigators rapidly froze working muscles of experimental animals and then measured the degree of oxygen saturation of the intracellular myoglobin using a spectrometer with a narrow light beam. The intracellular P_{O_2} was inferred from the myoglobin oxygen saturation. These data and theoretical work by the same group suggest that the major resistance to oxygen diffusion from capillary to muscle fibre mitochondria is at the capillary–fibre interface. That is the thin carrier-free region including plasma, endothelium and interstitium. This in turn necessitates a large driving force (P_{O_2} difference) at that site to deliver oxygen to the muscle fibres. Theoretical results are shown in Figure 9.3 where it can be seen that most of the fall of P_{O_2} apparently occurs in the immediate vicinity of the peripheral capillary and that, throughout the muscle cell, the P_{O_2} is remarkably uniform and very low (of the order of 1–3 mmHg). This pattern results chiefly from the presence of myoglobin which facilitates the diffusion of oxygen within the muscle fibres.

9.4 CAPILLARY DENSITY

One way to improve tissue diffusion under conditions of oxygen deprivation such as high altitude is to reduce the intercapillary distance. The technical name for the number of capillaries per unit area of tissue is capillary density. It has been known since the time of Krogh (1919) that the number of open capillaries in a muscle depends on the degree of metabolic activity. During exercise additional capillaries open up thus reducing the diffusing distance and increasing the diffusing surface area. Exercise training is known to increase the number of capillaries in skeletal muscle (Saltin and Gollnick, 1983).

Early studies apparently showed increased vascularization of the brain, retina, skeletal muscle and liver of experimental animals exposed to low barometric pressures over several weeks (Mercker and Schneider, 1949; Optiz, 1951; Valdivia, 1958; Cassin *et al.*, 1971). Tenney and Ou

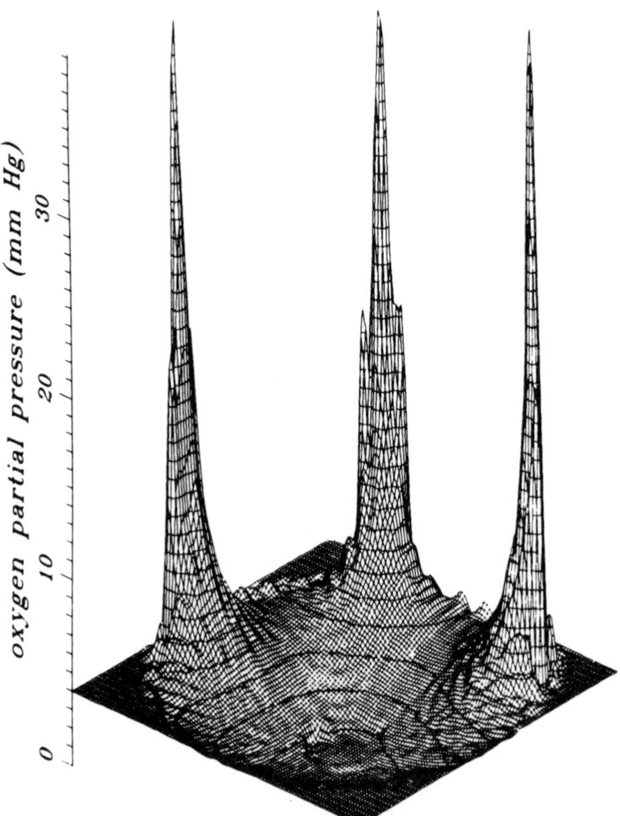

Figure 9.3 Calculated distribution of P_{O_2} around three capillaries in a heavily working red fibre of skeletal muscle. P_{O_2} contours are at intervals of 1 mmHg. There is a rapid fall of P_{O_2} in the immediate vicinity of the capillary, and within the muscle cell the P_{O_2} is relatively uniform and very low. (From Honig *et al.*, 1991.)

(1970) measured the rate of loss of carbon monoxide from subcutaneous gas pockets in rats after three weeks of simulated exposure to 5600 m and concluded that there was a 50% increase in capillary number.

However some of these studies were questioned by Banchero (1982) who argued that the results obtained by Valdivia (1958) and Cassin *et al.* (1971) might be influenced by technical errors. The consensus now seems to be that, although capillary density increases in skeletal muscles with exposure to high altitude, this is not caused by the formation of new capillaries, but by a reduction in size of the muscle fibres. This result has been found in guinea pigs (Figure 9.4) which were studied at

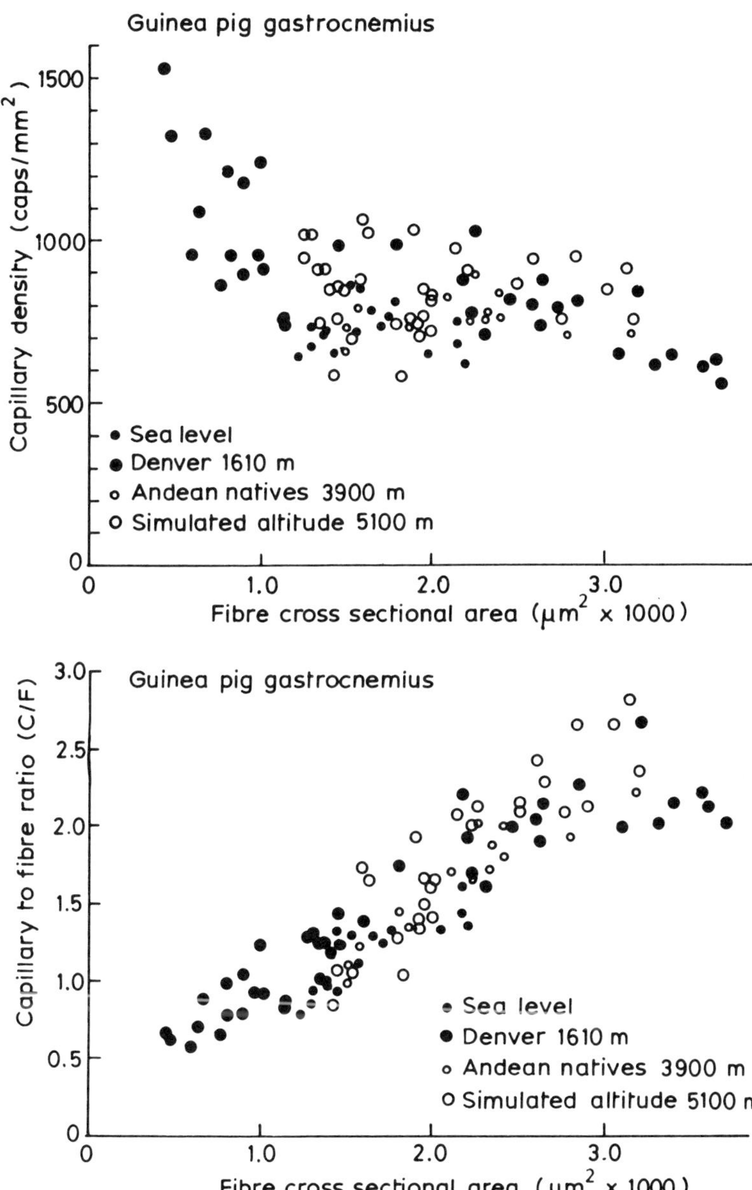

Figure 9.4 Data showing capillary density (number of capillaries per mm^2 of cross section) and capillary/fibre ratio (number of capillaries per muscle fibre) in gastrocnemius muscle of four groups of guinea pigs. These were studied at sea-level, in Denver at 1610 m, at 3900 m (Andean natives) and at simulated altitude of 5100 m. The data are consistent with the increase in capillary to fibre ratio being explained by a decrease in cross-sectional area of the muscle fibres. (From Banchero, 1982.)

sea-level, in Denver at 1610 m, at 3900 m (in a species native to the Andes), and at a simulated altitude of 5100 m (Banchero, 1982).

The same pattern has been described in acclimatized man where muscle samples were obtained by biopsy. For example, Cerretelli and his co-workers obtained muscle biopsies on climbers immediately after they had spent several weeks attempting to climb Lhotse Shar (8398 m) and showed that, although the capillary density was somewhat raised, the increase could be wholly accounted for by a reduction of muscle fibre size (Cerretelli *et al.*, 1984; Boutellier *et al.*, 1983). A similar result was found in Operation Everest II in six volunteers who were gradually decompressed to the simulated altitude of Mt Everest over a period of 40 days. Needle biopsies from the vastus lateralis showed a significant (25%) decrease in cross sectional area of Type I fibres, and a 26% decrease (non-significant) for Type II fibres. Capillary to fibre ratios were unchanged and there was a trend (non-significant) towards an increase in capillary density (MacDougall *et al.*, 1991).

Although these studies show that the number of new capillaries in skeletal muscle does not increase as a result of exposure to prolonged hypoxia, it has been suggested that there are changes in the configuration of the capillaries with increased tortuosity which would effectively increase capillary surface area and enhance gas diffusion (Appell, 1978). However this result has not been confirmed by Mathieu-Costello and Poole (Mathieu-Costello, 1989; Poole and Mathieu-Costello, 1990) who showed that muscle capillary tortuosity does not increase with chronic exposure to hypoxia when account is taken of sarcomere length. These investigators believe that Appell's results may be explained by failure to control the state of contraction of the muscle. It is known that the degree of capillary tortuosity increases during muscle shortening (Mathieu-Costello, 1987).

This lack of increase in the number of capillaries per muscle fibre at high altitude should be contrasted with the increase in muscle capillarity which occurs with training. Longitudinal studies in humans have shown that exercise training increases muscle capillarity including both the capillary/fibre ratio and number of capillaries per mm^2 within several weeks (Andersen and Henriksson, 1977; Brodal *et al.*, 1977; Ingjer and Brodal, 1978). Furthermore it has been demonstrated that the increased capillary supply is proportional to the increased maximum oxygen uptake (Andersen and Henriksson, 1977). The increase in capillaries is found in all fibre types provided that they are recruited during training (Andersen and Henriksson, 1977; Nygaard and Nielsen, 1978). If studies of acclimatization to high altitude involve increased levels of exercise, it is important to take account of this effect. Table 9.1 compares some of the tissue changes caused by training with those resulting from exposure to high altitude.

Table 9.1 Comparison of tissue changes caused by training, and associated with exposure to high altitude

Tissue changes	*Endurance training*	*High altitude*
Capillary density in skeletal muscle	Increased due to new capillaries	Increased due to reduction in diameter of muscle fibres
Fibre diameter of skeletal muscle	May be increased	Decreased
Myoglobin concentration	No change in humans	Increased in skeletal, heart muscle
Muscle enzymes	No change in glycolytic, increase in oxidative	Similar changes at moderate altitudes; at extreme altitudes, increase in glycolytic and decrease in oxidative

9.5 MUSCLE FIBRE SIZE

As indicated above, one way to increase capillary density and thus reduce diffusion distance within skeletal muscle is to reduce the size of the muscle fibres. There is now good evidence that this occurs during high-altitude acclimatization (Boutellier *et al.*, 1983; Cerretelli *et al.*, 1984; MacDougall *et al.*, 1991). This topic is discussed further in Chapter 13.

The mechanism of muscle atrophy at high altitude is not well understood. It has been suggested that one contributing factor is lack of muscular activity. Certainly lowlanders who go to very high altitudes easily become fatigued and often spend much of their time at a reduced level of physical activity. Indeed Tilman (1952) once remarked that a hazard of Himalayan expeditions was bedsores!

However, reduced physical activity is unlikely to be the whole story as evidenced by the experience obtained on the 1960–1961 Himalayan Scientific and Mountaineering Expedition. During several months at 5800 m, the level of physical activity was well maintained with opportunities for daily skiing and yet the expedition members suffered a relentless and progressive loss of weight which averaged 0.5 to 1.5 kg per week (Pugh, 1964). Moreover, reasonable estimates of calorie intake were made and it was shown that these were more than adequate for the level of activity. It is true that gastrointestinal absorption is apparently impaired at high altitude (Chapter 13) but it seems very likely that there is some change in protein metabolism which results in extensive breakdown of muscle protein.

9.6 VOLUME OF MITOCHONDRIA

The muscle mitochondria are the primary sites of oxygen utilization by the body and thus constitute the final link of the oxygen cascade. In general, mitochondrial volume density (volume of mitochondria per unit volume of tissue) in skeletal muscle is related to maximal oxygen uptake and, for example, is greater in highly aerobic animals such as the horse compared with less active animals such as the cow (Hoppeler *et al.*, 1987). It is also known that physical training increases mitochondrial volume density (Holloszy and Coyle, 1984).

We might therefore expect that at high altitude where maximal oxygen uptake is reduced (Chapter 10) mitochondrial density would decrease. However Ou and Tenney (1970) showed that the number of mitochondria in samples of myocardium was 40% greater in cattle born and raised at 4250 m compared with cattle at sea-level (Figure 9.5). The size of individual mitochondria was found to be the same and it was argued that the increase in mitochondrial number was advantageous because it reduced the diffusion distance of the intracellular oxygen.

These interesting results may not apply to all species. Another investigation of the mitochondrial density of the myocardium of rabbits

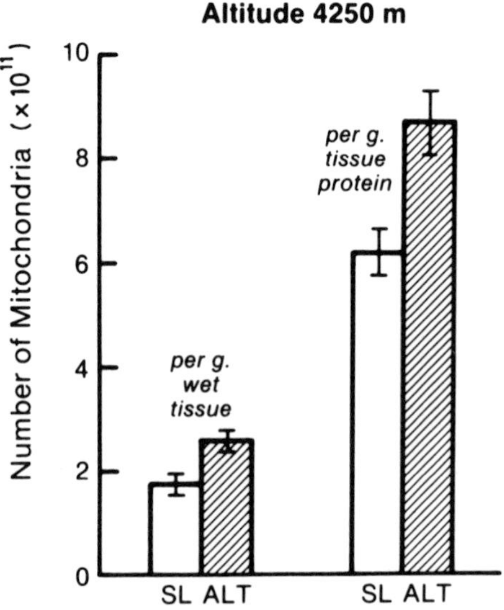

Figure 9.5 Increase in number of mitochondria in myocardium of cattle born and raised at 4250 m (ALT) compared with another group born and raised at sea-level (SL). The left-hand columns show the number of mitochondria ($\times 10^{11}$) per gram of wet tissue, while the right hand columns show the number per ($\times 10^{11}$) gram of tissue protein. (Data from Ou and Tenney, 1970.)

and guinea pigs from Cerro de Pasco (4330 m) compared with those at sea-level showed no increase in density (Kearney, 1973).

Recent work indicates that the mitochondrial volume in human skeletal muscle decreases with high-altitude acclimatization. In a study on muscle biopsies of climbers returning from two Swiss Himalayan expeditions, mitochondrial volume decreased by 20%. This was associated with a decrease of 10% in muscle mass. The net result was a decrease in absolute mitochondrial volume of nearly 30% (Hoppeler *et al.*, 1990). There was no significant increase in mitochondrial volume density in biopsies of vastus lateralis in subjects of Operation Everest II (MacDougall *et al.*, 1991).

9.7 MYOGLOBIN CONCENTRATION

As stated above, early studies by Hurtado and his colleagues (1937) showed increased concentrations of myoglobin in several muscles of dogs born and raised in Morococha (4540 m). The controls were dogs in Lima at sea-level. Increased myoglobin concentrations were found in the diaphragm, adductor muscles of the leg, pectoral muscles of the chest, and the myocardium (Figure 9.6).

Reynafarje (1962) measured myoglobin concentrations in the sartorius muscle of healthy humans native to Cerro de Pasco (4400 m) and in

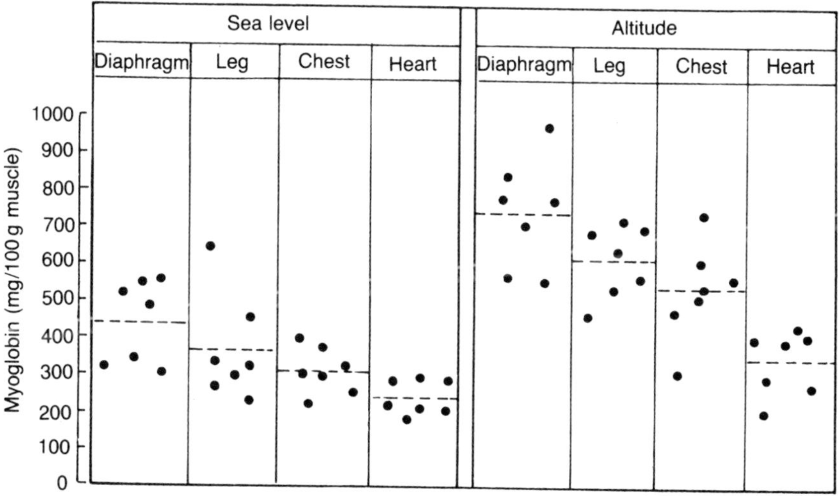

Figure 9.6 Myoglobin concentration (mg per 100 g of muscle) from seven sea-level dogs compared with seven born and raised at 4540 m. (From Hurtado *et al.*, 1937.)

other Peruvians native to sea-level. Higher concentrations of myglobin were found in the high-altitude natives ($7.03\,\mathrm{mg\,g^{-1}}$ tissue) than in the sea-level controls ($6.07\,\mathrm{mg\,g^{-1}}$). The result was interpreted as a true high-altitude effect because it was accompanied by an increased nitrogen content of the muscle, while the lean body mass and body water content were the same as at sea-level. This point was important because in another study (Anthony *et al.*, 1959) a reported increase in myoglobin content of skeletal muscle in rats could possibly have been caused by a decrease in body weight as a result of dehydration. Other studies which have shown an increase in myoglobin as a result of acclimatization to hypoxia include those of hamster heart muscle (Clark *et al.*, 1952), rat heart and diaphragm (Vaughan and Pace, 1956) and various guinea pig tissues (Tappan and Reynafarje, 1957).

As discussed above, the chief value of myoglobin may be that it facilitates oxygen diffusion through muscle cells. However it may also serve to buffer regional differences of P_{O_2} (Figure 9.3) and act as an oxygen store for short periods of very severe oxygen deprivation. It has been shown that increased levels of exercise raise the myoglobin content of muscles in experimental animals (Lawrie, 1953; Pattengale and Holloszy, 1967). Animals which exhibit large oxygen uptakes in conditions of reduced oxygen availability, such as seals, typically have very large amounts of myoglobin (Castellini and Somero, 1981). However, a study comparing trained and untrained human subjects (Jansson *et al.*, 1982), and another study of short term training in man (Svedenhag *et al.*, 1983) both failed to show any effect of training on muscle myoglobin concentration.

9.8 INTRACELLULAR ENZYMES

Enzymes are essential to all aspects of the metabolic pathways involved in energy production. Figure 9.7 summarizes the three main stages in energy metabolism: (a) conversion of glucose units (from either glucose or glycogen, known as glycolysis), amino acids and fatty acids to acetyl CoA, (b) citric acid or Krebs cycle, and (c) electron transport chain. Because oxygen is not required for the glycolytic breakdown of glucose or glycogen, glycolysis represents an important though temporary source of energy under conditions of oxygen shortage or absence. By contrast neither the Krebs cycle not the electron transport chain can produce energy in the absence of oxygen.

There is evidence that chronic hypoxia caused by moderate or high altitude increases the concentration or activities of certain important enzymes involved in oxidative metabolism but hypoxia does not appear to affect enzymes in the glycolytic pathway. However, it must be stressed that endurance exercise training also causes profound changes

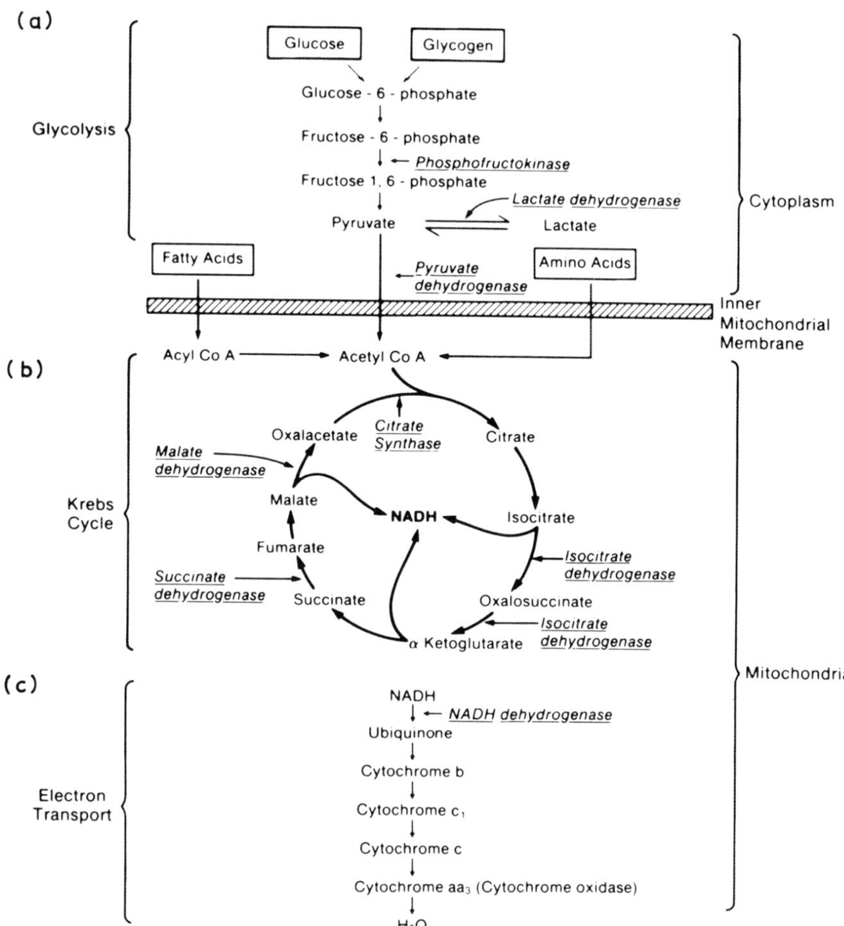

Figure 9.7 Major energy-yielding pathways in muscle. Principal controlling enzymes are indicated. Altitude or hypoxic exposure and exercise training do not affect glycolytic capacity appreciably but cause substantial increases in oxidative capacity as demonstrated by augmented mitochondrial volume in some species and activity of major enzymes of the citric acid cycle and the electron transport chain.

in the oxidative enzyme systems and it is difficult to maintain a given level of physical activity during exposure to chronic hypoxia. Similarly, it is also difficult to match sea-level residents with residents at altitude with respect to physical activity.

Perhaps the first study of the enzymatic activity of human muscle at high altitude was that by Reynafarje (1962). The measurements were made on biopsies taken from the sartorius muscles of natives of Cerro de Pasco (4400 m) and these were compared with biopsies from residents of Lima at sea-level. Reynafarje measured the activities of enzymes of glycolysis (lactate dehydrogenase), Krebs cycle (isocitrate dehydrogenase) and the electron transport chain (NADH and NADPH-cytochrome c-reductase and $NAD[P]^+$ transhydrogenase). In this study Reynafarje found that the activity of NADH-oxidase, NADPH-cytochrome c-reductase and $NAD[P]^+$ transhydrogenase were significantly increased in the altitude residents.

Harris *et al.* (1970) reported on the levels of succinate dehydrogenase (Krebs cycle) and lactate dehydrogenase (glycolysis) activity in myocardial homogenates from guinea pigs, rabbits and dogs indigenous to high altitude (4380 m) and compared the measurements with those made on the same species at sea-level. They found a consistent increase in the activity of succinate dehydrogenase in the high-altitude animals but no significant difference in lactate dehydrogenase. Ou and Tenney (1970) also found increased levels of succinate dehydrogenase and several enzymes of the electron transport chain including cytochrome oxidase, NADH-oxidase and NADH-cytochrome c-reductase in high-altitude cattle.

In contrast to the effects of moderately high altitude (4000–5000 m), it appears that extreme altitude (above 6000 m) may cause a reduction in the activity of certain enzymes. The effect of exposure to extreme altitude on muscle enzyme systems has recently been studied by taking muscle biopsies from climbers before and after the Swiss expeditions to Lhotse Shar in 1981 (Cerretelli, 1987) and Mt Everest in 1986 (Howald *et al.*, 1990) and also from experimental subjects before and after prolonged decompression during Operation Everest II (Green *et al.*, 1989). All of these studies have reported decreased activities of oxidative enzymes. Results on three subjects from the Lhotse Shar expedition suggest that extreme altitude reduces the activity of both Krebs cycle (succinate dehydrogenase) and glycolytic (phosphofructokinase, lactate dehydrogenase) enzymes (Cerretelli, 1987). In a more comprehensive study of seven climbers from the Swiss 1986 expedition, reduced activity of enzymes of the Krebs cycle (citrate synthase, malate dehydrogenase) and electron transport chain (cytochrome oxidase) were reported (Howald *et al.*, 1990). In contrast to the Lhotse Shar study this latter study found increases in enzyme activities of glycolysis. In Operation Everest II, significant reductions were found in succinate dehydrogenase (21%), citrate synthase (37%) and hexokinase (53%) at extreme altitudes (Green *et al.*, 1989).

Interestingly, the enhanced capacity for oxidative metabolism found in the face of an unchanged glycolytic potential after high-altitude (below 5000 m) exposure is qualitatively similar to the changes found in skeletal muscle after endurance exercise training (Holloszy and Coyle, 1984). This observation supports the contention that tissue hypoxia may be responsible for the changes in mitochondrial density and oxidative enzyme capacity under both conditions.

It has been argued that the primary importance of an augmented oxidative capacity of skeletal muscle lies not in the ability to achieve a higher maximum oxygen uptake but, rather, to sustain a given submaximal oxygen uptake with less intracellular metabolic disturbance (i.e. change of ADP and P_i, both potent stimulators of glycolysis) (Gollnick and Saltin, 1982; Holloszy and Coyle, 1984; Dudley *et al.*, 1987). Thus, for strenuous exercise where fatigue is associated with depletion of muscle glycogen stores, an augmented muscle oxidative capacity enables a given oxygen uptake to be sustained at lower intracellular ADP and P_i concentrations. Consequently, muscle glycogen stores would be conserved and fat oxidation would contribute proportionally more to the energetic output of the muscle, resulting in an enhanced endurance capacity (Holloszy and Coyle, 1984; Dudley *et al.*, 1987).

In conclusion, these changes in tissue enzymes (with the exception of those at extreme altitudes) are consistent with the assumption that the muscles are improving their ability for oxidative metabolism in the face of oxygen deprivation or deficiency. This is an area of research that has received relatively little attention up till now and one in which we can expect rapid progress in the future.

REFERENCES

Andersen, P. and Henriksson, J. (1977) Capillary supply of the quadriceps femoris muscle of man: adaptive response to exercise. *J. Physiol. (London)*, **270**, 677–90.

Anthony, A., Ackerman, E. and Strother, G.K. (1959) Effects of altitude acclimatization on rat myoglobin. Changes in myoglobin content of skeletal and cardiac muscle. *Am. J. Physiol.*, **196**, 512–16.

Appell, H.J. (1978) Capillary density and patterns in skeletal muscles. III. Changes of the capillary pattern after hypoxia. *Pflügers Arch.*, **377**, R-53 (abstract).

Banchero, N. (1982) Long-term adaptation of skeletal muscle capillarity. *Physiologist*, **25**, 385–9.

Bert, P. (1878) *La Pression Barométrique*. Masson, Paris. English translation by M.A. Hitchcock and F.A. Hitchcock. College Book Co., Columbus, Ohio, 1943.

Boutellier, U., Howald H., di Prampero, P.E., *et al.* (1983) Human muscle adaptations to chronic hypoxia. *Prog. Clin. Biol. Res.*, **136**, 273–81.

Brodal, P., Ingjer, F. and Hermansen, L. (1977) Capillary supply of skeletal muscle fibers in untrained and endurance-trained men. *Am. J. Physiol.*, **232**, H705–12.

Cassin, S.R., Gilbert, D., Bunnell, C.F. and Johnson, E.M. (1971) Capillary development during exposure to chronic hypoxia. *Am. J. Physiol.*, **220**, 448–51.

Castellini, M.A. and Somero, G.N. (1981) Buffering capacity of vertebrate muscle: correlations with potentials for anaerobic function. *J. Comp. Physiol.*, **143**, 191–8.

Cerretelli, P. (1987) Éxtreme hypoxia in air breathers, in *Comparative Physiology of Environmental Adaptations*, (ed. P. Dejours), Karger, Basel.

Cerretelli, P., Marconi, C., Deriaz, O. and Giezendanner, D. (1984) After effects of chronic hypoxia on cardiac output and muscle blood flow at rest and exercise. *Eur. J. Appl. Physiol.*, **53**, 92–6.

Chance, B. (1957) Cellular oxygen requirements. *Fed. Proc.*, **16**, 671–80.

Chance, B., Cohen, P., Jobsis, F. and Schoener, B. (1962) Intracellular oxidation reduction states *in vivo*. *Science*, **137**, 499–508.

Clark, R.T., Criscuolo, D. and Coulson, D.K. (1952) Effects of 20 000 feet simulated altitude on myoglobin content of animals with and without exercise. *Fed. Proc.*, **11**, 25.

Dudley, G.A., Tullson, P.C. and Tyerjung, R.L. (1987) Influence of mitochondrial content on the sensitivity of respiratory control. *J. Biol. Chem.*, **262**, 9109–14.

Gollnick, P.D. and Saltin, B. (1982) Significance of muscle oxidative enzyme enhancement with endurance training. *Clin. Physiol.*, **2**, 1–12.

Green, H.J., Sutton, J.R., Cymerman, A. and Houston, C.S. (1989) Operation Everest II: Adaptations in human skeletal muscle. *J. Appl. Physiol.*, **66**, 2454–61.

Harris, P., Castillo, Y., Gibson, K., *et al.* (1970) Succinic and lactic dehydrogenase activity in myocardial homogenates from animals at high and low altitude. *J. Mol. Cell. Cardiol.*, **1**, 189–93.

Hill, A.V. (1928) The diffusion of oxygen and lactic acid through tissues. *Proc. R. Soc. London Ser. B.*, **104**, 39–96.

Holloszy, J.O. and Coyle, E.F. (1984) Adaptations of skeletal muscle to endurance exercise and their metabolic consequences. *J. Appl. Physiol.*, **56**, 831–8.

Hoppeler, H., Kayar, S.R., Claassen, H., *et al.* (1987) Adaptive variation in the mammalian respiratory system in relation to energetic demand: III. Skeletal muscles: setting the demand for oxygen. *Respir. Physiol.*, **69**, 27–46.

Hoppeler, H., Howald, H. and Cerretelli, P. (1990) Human muscle structure after exposure to extreme altitude. *Experientia*, **46**, 1185–7.

Honig, C.R., Gayeski, T.E.J. and Goebe, K. (1991) Myoglobin and oxygen gradients, in *The Lung: Scientific Foundations*, (eds R.G. Crystal and J.B. West), Raven Press, New York, pp. 1489–96.

Howald, H., Pette, D. and Simoneau, J.A., *et al.* (1990) Effect of chronic hypoxia on muscle enzyme activities. *Int. J. Sports Med.*, 11 (**suppl 1**), S10–14.

Hurtado, A., Rotta, A., Merino, C. and Pons, J. (1937) Studies of myohemoglobin at high altitude. *Am. J. Med. Sci.*, **194**, 708–13.

Ingjer, F. and Brodal, P. (1978) Capillary supply of skeletal muscle fibers in untrained and endurance-trained women. *Eur. J. Appl. Physiol.*, **38**, 291–9.

Jansson, E., Sylven, C. and Nordevang, E. (1982) Myoglobin in the quadriceps femoris muscle of competitive cyclists and untrained men. *Acta Physiol. Scand.*, **114**, 627–9.

Kearney, M.S. (1973) Ultrastructural changes in the heart at high altitude. *Pathol. Microbiol.*, **39**, 258–65.

Krogh, A. (1919) Number and distribution of capillaries in muscles with calculations of the oxygen pressure head necessary to supplying the tissue. *J. Physiol.* (*London*), **52**, 409–15.

Krogh, A. (1929) *The Anatomy and Physiology of Capillaries*, Yale University Press, New York.

Lawrie, R.A. (1953) Effect of enforced exercise on myoglobin concentration in muscle. *Nature*, **171**, 1069–70.

Longmuir, I.S. and Betts, W. (1987) Tissue acclimation to altitude. *Fed. Proc.*, **46**, 794.

MacDougall, J.D., Green, H.J., Sutton, J.S., *et al.* (1991) Operation Everest II: Structural adaptations in skeletal muscle in response to extreme simulated altitude. *Acta Physiol. Scand.*, **142**, 421–7.

Mathieu-Costello, O. (1987) Capillary tortuosity and degree of contraction or extension of skeletal muscle. *Microvasc. Res.*, **33**, 98–117.

Mathieu-Costello, O. (1989) Muscle capillary tortuosity in high altitude mice depends on sarcomere length. *Respir. Physiol.*, **76**, 289–302.

Mercker, H. and Schneider, M. (1949) Uber capillarveranderungen des gehirns bei hohenanpassung. *Pflugers Arch.*, **251**, 49–55.

Nygaard, E. and Nielsen, E. (1978) Skeletal muscle fibre capillarization with extreme endurance training in man, in *Swimming Medicine IV*, (eds B. Eriksson and B. Furberg), University Park, Baltimore.

Optiz, E. (1951) Increased vascularization of the tissue due to acclimatization to high altitude and its significance of oxygen transport. *Exp. Med. Surg.*, **9**, 389–403.

Ou, L.C. and Tenney, S.M. (1970) Properties of mitochondria from hearts of cattle acclimatized to high altitude. *Respir. Physiol.*, **8**, 151–9.

Pattengale, P.K. and Holloszy, J.O. (1967) Augmentation of skeletal muscle myoglobin by a program of treadmill running. *Am. J. Physiol.*, **213**, 783–5.

Piiper, J. and Scheid, P. (1986) Cross-sectional P_{O_2} distributions in Krogh cylinder and solid cylinder models. *Respir. Physiol.*, **64**, 241–51.

Poole, D.C. and Mathieu-Costello, O. (1990) Effects of hypoxia on capillary orientation in anterior tibialis muscle of highly active mice. *Respir. Physiol.*, **82**, 1–10.

Potter, R.F. and Groom, A.C. (1983) Capillary diameter and geometry in cardiac and skeletal muscle studied by means of corresion casts. *Microvasc. Res.*, **25**, 68–84.

Pugh, L.G.C.E. (1964) Animals in high altitudes: man above 5000 meters – mountain exploration, in *Handbook of Physiology, Adaptation to the Environment*, (ed. D.B. Dill), American Physiological Society, Washington DC, pp. 861–8.

Reynafarje, B. (1962) Myoglobin content and enzymatic activity of muscle and altitude adaptation. *J. Appl. Physiol.*, **17**, 301–5.

Roughton, F.J.W. (1964) Transport of oxygen and carbon dioxide, in *Handbook of Physiology, Section 3, Respiration*, Vol 1, (eds. W.O. Fenn and H. Rahn), American Physiological Society, Washington DC, pp. 767–825.

Saltin, B. and Gollnick, P.D. (1983) Skeletal muscle adaptability: significance for metabolism and performance, in *Handbook of Physiology, Section 10*, (ed. L.D. Penchy), American Physiological Society, Washington DC, pp. 555–631.

Scholander, P. (1960) Oxygen transport through hemoglobin solution. *Science*, **131**, 585–90.

Svedenhag, J., Henriksson, J. and Sylven, C. (1983) Dissociation of training effects on skeletal muscle mitochondrial enzymes and myoglobin in man. *Acta Physiol. Scand.*, **117**, 213–18.

Tappan, D.V. and Reynafarje, B.D. (1957) Tissue pigment manifestation of adaptation to high altitude. *Am. J. Physiol.*, **190**, 99–103.

Tenney, S.M. and Ou, L.C. (1970) Physiological evidence for increased tissue capillarity in rats acclimatized to high altitude. *Respir. Physiol.*, **8**, 137–50.

Tilman, H.W. (1952) *Nepal Himalaya*, Cambridge University Press, Cambridge, p. 79.

Valdivia, E. (1958) Total capillary bed in striated muscle of guinea pigs native to the Peruvian mountains. *Am. J. Physiol.*, **194**, 585–9.

Vaughan, B.E. and Pace, N. (1956) Changes in myoglobin content of the high altitude acclimatized rat. *Am. J. Physiol.*, **185**, 549–56.

Viault, F. (1890) Sur l'augmentation considerable du nombre des globule rouges dans le sang chez les habitants des haut plateaux de l'Amerique du Sud. *Comptes Rendus, Hebdomaire Des Seances de l'Academie Des Sciences, Paris*, **111**, 917–8. English translation (1981) in *High Altitude Physiology*, (ed. J.B. West), Hutchinson Ross Publishing Company, Strandsburg PA, pp. 333–4.

West, J.B. (ed.) (1985) *Best and Taylor's Physiological Basis of Medical practice*, 11th edn, Williams and Wilkins, Baltimore.

Wittenberg, J.B. (1959) Oxygen transport: a new function proposed for myoglobin. *Biol. Bull.*, **117**, 402–3.

10

Exercise

10.1 INTRODUCTION

The hypoxia of high altitude puts stress on the oxygen transfer system of the body even at rest. If the oxygen requirements are further increased by exercise, the problems of oxygen delivery to the mitochondria of the working muscles are correspondingly exaggerated. Indeed one of the most obvious consequences of going to high altitude is a reduced exercise tolerance.

In this chapter we examine the physiology of oxygen transfer from the air to the mitochondria in the face of the reduced inspired P_{O_2}. The steps in the oxygen cascade include getting the oxygen to the alveoli via pulmonary ventilation, diffusion of oxygen across the blood–gas barrier, uptake by the pulmonary capillary blood, removal from the lung by the cardiac output, transport to the tissues via the arterial blood, diffusion of oxygen to the mitochondria, and utilization of oxygen by the cellular biochemical reactions. The present chapter synthesizes information, some of which occurs in other chapters. The subject of limitation of oxygen uptake under the conditions of extreme altitude is dealt with in Chapter 11. The literature on exercise at altitude is very extensive and the present chapter is necessarily selective. Many monographs and reviews have been published including Cerretelli, 1992; Cerretelli and Whipp, 1980; Jokl, 1968; Margaria, 1967; Sutton *et al.*, 1983; and Sutton, Houston, and Coates, 1987.

10.2 HISTORICAL

A reduced exercise tolerance at high altitude has been recognized since man began to climb high mountains. For example, extreme fatigue was often reported in the early climbs of the European Alps and in fact this led to one of the popular theories of mountain sickness. The argument ran that the normal barometric pressure was necessary to maintain the proper articulation of the head of the femur in the acetabulum of the pelvis, and that at high altitude, when the reduced barometric pressure did not assist this as it should, the muscles became fatigued as a result (Bert, 1878).

Some of the earliest measurements of exercise at high altitude were made by Zuntz, Durig and their colleagues in the first few years of this century (Zuntz *et al.*, 1906; Durig, 1911). For example, Zuntz showed that there was a decline in oxygen consumption but increase in ventilation at high altitude when trekkers walked at the speed that they normally adopted in an Alpine setting.

Douglas, Haldane and their colleagues (Douglas *et al.*, 1913) studied muscular exercise during walking uphill on Pike's Peak during the Anglo–American Expedition of 1911. They made the important observation that a given amount of work required the same amount of oxygen at 4300 m altitude as at sea level.

Colourful descriptions of the great difficulties of exercise at very high altitudes were common in the early Everest expeditions. Indeed the accounts of the 1921 reconnaissance expedition (Howard-Bury, 1922), and the expeditions of 1922 (Bruce, 1923) and 1924 (Norton, 1925) make graphic reading even today. Typical is E.F. Norton's account of his climb to nearly 8600 m without supplementary oxygen in 1924 (Norton, 1925). He wrote 'our pace was wretched. My ambition was to do 20 consecutive paces uphill without a pause to rest and pant elbow on bent knee, yet I never remember achieving it – 13 was nearer the mark'. Norton was accompanied to just below that altitude by the surgeon T.H. Somervell who subsequently wrote 'for every step forward and upward, 7 to 10 complete respirations were required' (Somervell, 1925).

Of course these were observations by lowlanders who were at extreme altitudes after relatively short periods of time for acclimatization. It is interesting to compare the observations of Barcroft who led an expedition at about the same time (winter of 1921–1922) to Cerro de Pasco at an altitude of 4330 m (14 200 ft) in the Peruvian Andes (Barcroft *et al.*, 1923). Naturally this was at a considerably lower altitude than the summit of Mt Everest. Nevertheless the lowlanders were amazed at the capacity of the high-altitude residents for physical work, and they were astonished at the popularity of energetic sports such as soccer football. The contrast between poorly acclimatized lowlanders and native high-altitude dwellers, who had been at the same altitude for perhaps generations, was very clear.

Valuable findings on exercise at high altitude were made during the 1935 International High Altitude Expedition to Chile (Keys, 1936). The expedition members studied their own maximal working capacity and showed how this fell as the altitude increased in spite of acclimatization.

Christensen (1937) made measurements up to an altitude of 5340 m using a bicycle ergometer and confirmed the findings of Douglas *et al.* (1913) that the efficiency of muscle exercise was independent of altitude, that is that the oxygen consumption for a given work level was the same. In addition he showed that although exercise ventilation measured at BTPS (body temperature, ambient pressure, saturated with water vapour) was greatly increased at high altitudes, ventilation expressed at STPD (standard temperature and pressure, dry gas) was independent of altitude over a wide range of altitudes and work rates.

An interesting observation was made by Edwards who discovered a curious paradox about lactate levels in the blood on exercise. Generally, exhaustive exercise is accompanied by relatively high blood lactate levels, especially in unfit subjects, as the muscles outstrip their capacity for aerobic work and resort to anaerobic glycolysis. It would be natural to expect this to occur to an extreme extent at high altitude, but Edwards found the opposite. Exhaustive work at very high altitude was associated with very low levels of blood lactate (Edwards, 1936).

The expedition members were also surprised by the tolerance of the miners for energetic physical activity at the Aucanquilcha mine which they believed was at an altitude of 5800 m (19 000 ft). We now know that the mine is actually higher, the altitude being 5950 m (19 500 ft). The exercise level of the miners is indeed astonishing as they break large pieces of sulphur ore (caliche) with sledge hammers (McIntyre, 1987). The miners are predominantly Bolivians who were born at moderately high altitudes and since most of them live at Amincha (altitude 4200 m) they have a considerable degree of high-altitude acclimatization.

In preparation for the British expedition of 1953 to Mt Everest, Pugh measured oxygen uptake on climbers in the field near Cho Oyu in the Nepal Himalayas in 1952. These data were then used to determine the amount of oxygen to be carried by the 1953 expedition during which Pugh made further measurements of exercise physiology (Pugh, 1958). He subsequently greatly extended this programme in the ambitious Himalayan Scientific and Mountaineering Expedition of 1960–1961 in which several physiologists spent the winter in a prefabricated hut at an altitude of 5800 m (Pugh, 1962). Further measurements of maximal oxygen consumption were carried out in the spring when the expedition moved to Mt Makalu (8481 m) and a bicycle ergometer was erected on the Makalu Col (altitude 7440 m) (Figure 1.6). Those measurements of maximal work remain the highest ever made (Pugh *et al.*, 1964). The data assembled by Pugh and his co-workers (Figure 10.1) were of great interest because they predicted that, near the summit of Mt Everest, the maximal oxygen uptake would be very close to the basal oxygen requirements, and therefore it seemed problematical whether man

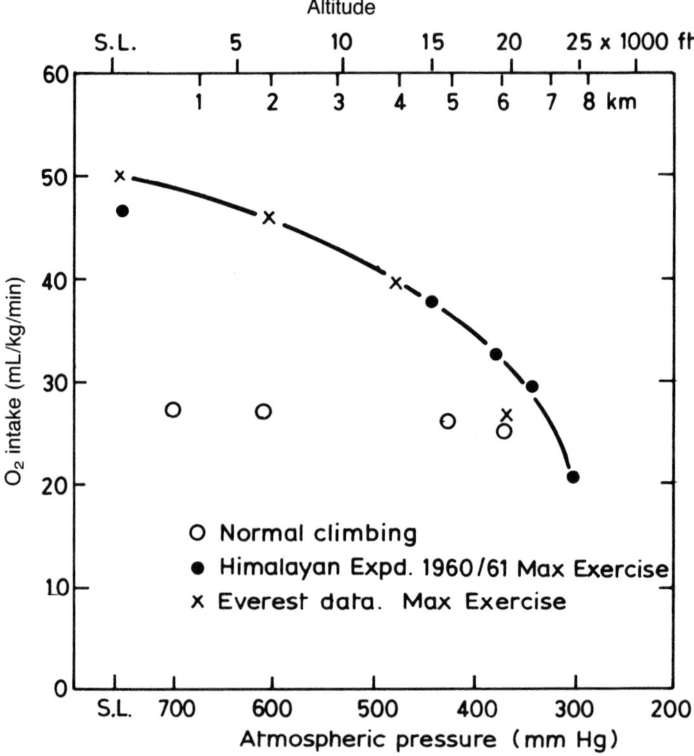

Figure 10.1 $\dot{V}_{O_2}$ max against barometric pressure in acclimatized subjects (●, ×) as reported by Pugh *et al.* (1964). Data from normal climbing rates are also shown (○).

could ever reach the summit without supplementary oxygen (West and Wagner, 1980).

Additional measurements of maximal oxygen consumption were made by Cerretelli during an Italian expedition to Mt Everest in 1973 (Cerretelli, 1976a). All the data were obtained at Base Camp (altitude 5350 m) but they included meaurements on climbers who had been above 8000 m. One of the many interesting observations was the failure of the maximal oxygen uptake of acclimatized subjects at 5350 m to return to the sea-level value when pure oxygen was breathed. The explanation of this finding, also made by Pugh and others, is still unclear.

The issue of whether the partial pressure of oxygen at the summit of Mt Everest was sufficient for man to reach it without supplementary oxygen was finally answered in 1978 by Reinhold Messner and Peter Habeler. However their accounts make it clear that neither had much in reserve (Messner, 1979; Habeler, 1979). The intriguing question of how the body is just able to transport sufficient oxygen to the exercising muscles under these conditions of profound hypoxia is considered in detail in Chapter 11.

During the American Medical Research Expedition to Everest of 1981 (AMREE), extensive measurements of maximal oxygen uptake were made in the main laboratory camp, altitude 6300 m. However data were also obtained for exercise at higher altitudes by giving the well-acclimatized subjects inspired mixtures containing low concentrations of oxygen. For example, when the inspired P_{O_2} was only 42.5 mmHg, corresponding to that on the summit of Mt Everest, the measured maximal oxygen consumption was just over $1 l min^{-1}$ (West *et al.*, 1983a). Although this is very low, being equivalent to that of someone walking slowly on the level, it is apparently just sufficient to explain how a climber can reach the summit without supplementary oxygen (Chapter 11).

A further extensive series of exercise measurements were made during Operation Everest II in the autumn of 1985 (Houston *et al.*, 1987). The eight subjects spent 40 days in a large low-pressure chamber being gradually decompressed to the barometric pressure existing at the summit of Mt Everest, and a series of measurements of maximal exercise were made using a bicycle ergometer. The measured oxygen consumptions agreed well with those found in the field by the 1981 expedition (Sutton *et al.*, 1988) but Operation Everest II had the great additional advantage that many invasive measurements could be made which were impracticable in the field. These included extensive measurements of pulmonary vascular pressures, muscle volume, and muscle biopsies (Sutton *et al.*, 1987).

10.3 VENTILATION

Exercise at high altitude is accompanied by very high levels of ventilation. Indeed this was one of the most obvious features of climbing at extreme altitudes in the early Everest expeditions as evidenced by the quotations from Norton and Somervell in the preceding section.

Ventilation is normally expressed at body temperature, ambient pressure, and with the gas saturated with water vapour (BTPS). This is because the volumes of gas moved then correspond to the volume excursions of the chest and lungs. Ventilation can also be expressed at standard temperature and pressure for dry gas (STPD). These volumes are very much smaller at high altitude and bear no obvious relationship to the actual chest movements. However the oxygen consumption and carbon dioxide output are traditionally expressed in these units so that the values are independent of altitude.

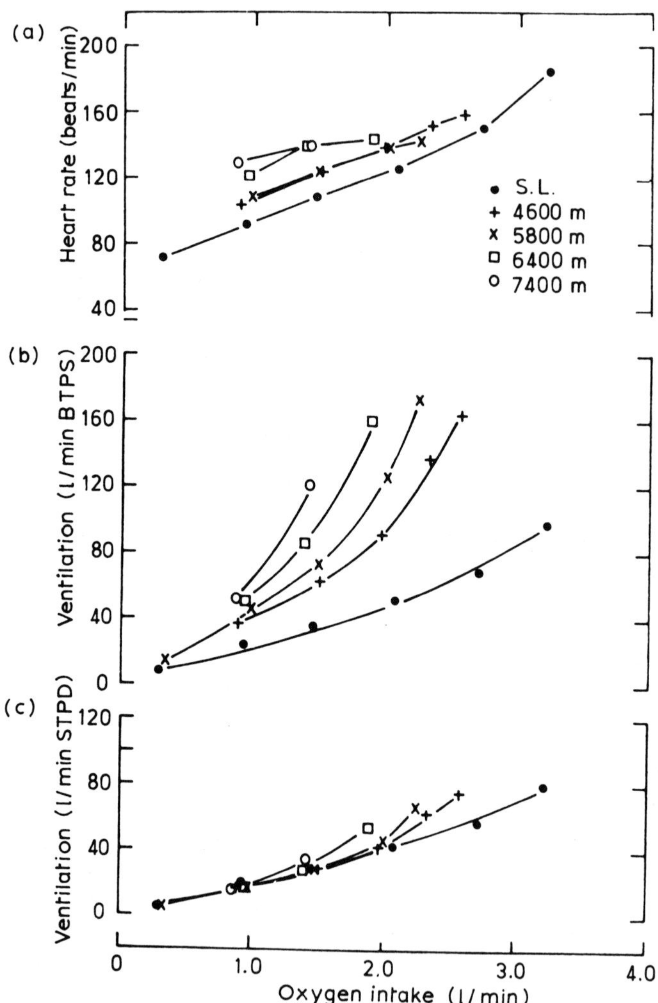

Figure 10.2 Relationship between ventilation, both BTPS and STPD, and oxygen uptake at various altitudes. Heart rate is also shown. (From Pugh *et al.*, 1964.)

For a given work level, the ventilation expressed as BTPS increases at high altitude. Typical results are shown in Figure 10.2(b) which shows data obtained during the 1960–1961 expedition (Pugh *et al.*, 1964). Figure 10.2(c) shows ventilations expressed as STPD. Here the values also tend to be somewhat higher than those measured at sea-level, especially at work levels approaching the maximum for the altitude, but the differences are clearly much less than for BTPS ventilation.

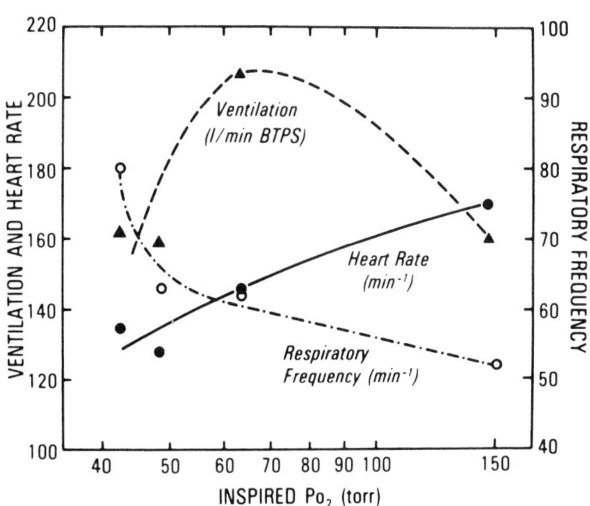

Figure 10.3 Maximal ventilation (BTPS), maximal respiratory frequency, and maximal heart rate plotted against inspired P_{O_2} on a log scale. This scale was chosen only because otherwise the high-altitude points fall very close together. Note that both maximal ventilation and heart rate fall at extreme altitudes because work levels become so low. However respiratory frequency continues to increase. (From West *et al.*, 1983a.) (1 torr = 1 mmHg)

Ventilation (BTPS) can reach extremely high levels as evidenced by data obtained during the 1981 AMREE expedition at an altitude of 6300 m (P_B 351 mmHg). In eight subjects who exercised at a work rate of 1200 kg min^{-1} the mean ventilation (BTPS) was 207.2 l min^{-1} with a mean respiratory frequency of 62 breaths per minute. These values were for a mean oxygen consumption of 2.31 l min^{-1}. These levels of ventilation far exceed anything ever seen at sea level and are approaching the maximal voluntary ventilation (MVV), that is the maximal amount of air that can be moved per minute by breathing in and out as rapidly and deeply as possible, usually measured over 15 s.

It is interesting that these extremely high levels of ventilation are not seen at the highest altitudes. For example, when two subjects on the 1981 expedition were given a 14% oxygen mixture to breath at an altitude of 6300 m (inspired P_{O_2} 42.5 mmHg), the maximal exercise ventilation was only 161.9 l min^{-1}. This inspired P_{O_2} corresponded to that at the Everest summit. A reasonable explanation for the lower exercise ventilation is that the work rate was very much lower, being only 450 kg min^{-1} as opposed to 1200 at the altitude of 6300 m while breathing air. Figure 10.3 shows maximal exercise ventilation plotted against inspired P_{O_2} (dashed line) and the fact that there is a maximal value is clearly seen although there are only four points on the curve. A similar pattern was found during the 1960–1961 expedition. For example, the maximal exercise ventilation at 5800 m had a mean value of 173.1 l min^{-1}. At the higher altitude of 6400 m this had fallen to 160.9, while at the highest altitude of 7440 m, the value was only 121.5 l min^{-1}. Corresponding to the fall in maximal exercise ventilation, the $\dot{V}_{O_2}$ max decreased from 1200 kg min^{-1} at 5800 m, to 900 kg min^{-1} at 6400 m, to 600 kg min^{-1} at 7400 m.

These extremely high exercise ventilations are facilitated by the reduced work of breathing as a result of the lowered density of the air at high altitude. The reduced density also results in an increased maximal voluntary ventilation (or maximum breathing capacity) as altitude is increased (Cotes, 1954). For example, Cotes showed that the maximal voluntary ventilation increased from 158 at sea-level to 197 l min^{-1} (BTPS) at a simulated altitude of 5180 m in a low-pressure chamber. In a further study, a mean value of 203 l min^{-1} was observed at a simulated altitude of 8250 m (Cotes, 1954). The increase in MVV was compatible with the hypothesis that the work of maximum breathing remains constant at high altitude. The reduction in the work of breathing at high altitude caused by the change in gas density was also analysed by Petit *et al.* (1963).

Oxygen breathing reduces exercise ventilation for a given work rate at high altitude. However, as Figure 10.4 shows, the ventilations do not return to the sea-level values but are intermediate between the high-altitude and sea-level values for ambient air.

The pattern of breathing during exercise at high altitude is characterized by very high frequencies and relatively small tidal volumes. Somervell's observation referred to in section 10.2 of '7 to 10 complete respirations' per step is evidence for that. The highest measurements of respiratory frequency and tidal volume yet made were those on Pizzo during the 1981 Everest expedition (West *et al.*, 1983a). He climbed for about seven minutes at an altitude of 8300 m (P_B 271 mmHg) while measuring his ventilation with a turbine flow meter, the output of which was registered on a slow-running tape recorder. During the middle four minutes of this period, his mean respiratory frequency was 86 ± 2.8 (SD) breaths per minute, mean tidal volume was 1.26 l, and mean ventilation was 107 l min^{-1} at BTPS. Thus his breathing was shallow and extremely rapid. Reference has already been made to the measurements of maximal exercise at an inspired P_{O_2} of 42.5 mmHg corresponding to that on the Everest summit which was obtained by making the subjects inspire 14% oxygen at an altitude of 6300 m. For two subjects, the mean respiratory frequency was 80 breaths per minute.

This pattern of breathing is consistent with the very powerful hypoxic

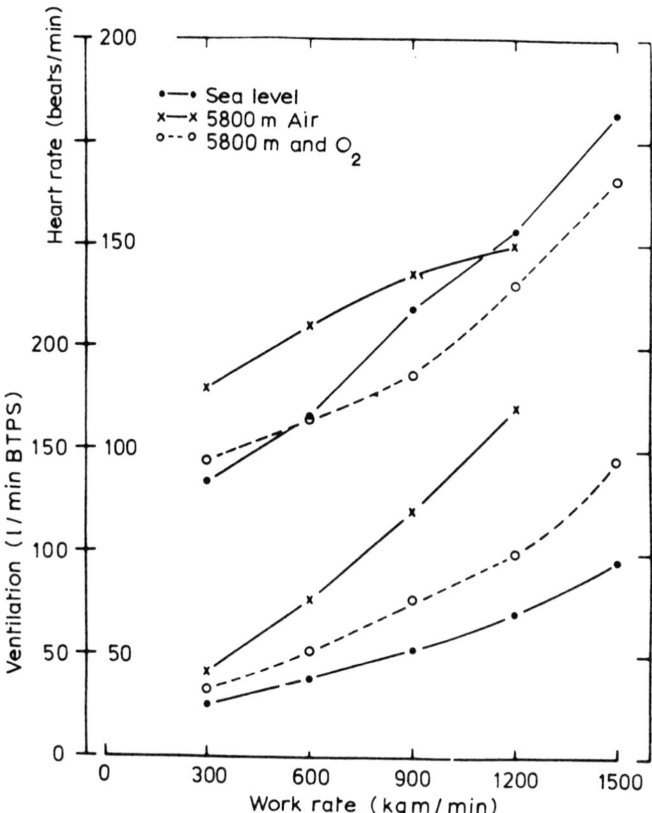

Figure 10.4 Effect of breathing oxygen at sea-level pressure on ventilation and heart rate in acclimatized subjects at 5800 m. The points are mean values from two subjects. (From Pugh *et al.*, 1964.)

drive via the peripheral chemoreceptors. As pointed out in Chapter 4, it is remarkable that the hypoxic drive is so strong under these conditions because the arterial P_{CO_2} is less than 10 mmHg and the arterial pH is over 7.7. A very low P_{CO_2} and high pH normally inhibit ventilation.

10.4 DIFFUSION

As discussed in Chapter 5, there is strong evidence that diffusion-limitation of oxygen transfer in the lung occurs during exercise at high altitude. This is the primary reason for the fall in arterial P_{O_2} and arterial oxygen saturation which has been consistently observed. Analysis of the situation at extreme altitude indicates that the diffusing capacity of the blood–gas barrier is one of the chief limiting factors for maximal exercise (Chapter 11).

There is no evidence that the diffusing capacity of the blood–gas barrier increases during acclimatization to high altitude in normal subjects. Measurements from the 1960–1961 Himalayan Scientific and Mountaineering Expedition showed that the diffusing capacity of the blood–gas barrier for a given level of exercise was the same as at sea-level (West, 1962). Overall pulmonary diffusing capacity for carbon monoxide increased by 19% at an altitude of 5800 m, but this could be attributed to the more rapid rate of combination of carbon monoxide with oxygen because of the low prevailing P_{O_2}. The volume of blood in the pulmonary capillaries as determined by measuring the diffusing capacity at two values of alveolar P_{O_2} showed no change or possibly a slight fall. This may have been due to hypoxic pulmonary vasconstriction.

These results also infer that, in acclimatized subjects, the transit time for red cells in the pulmonary capillaries at a given work level is approximately the same as at sea-level. The transit time of the pulmonary capillary blood is given by the pulmonary capillary blood volume divided by the cardiac output (Roughton, 1945). As discussed in Chapter 6, there is good evidence that, in acclimatized lowlanders at high altitude, the cardiac output for a given work level is the same as at sea-level (Pugh, 1964; Reeves *et al.*, 1987). Thus since both the pulmonary capillary blood volume and the cardiac output are essentially unchanged, this indicates that the transit time through the pulmonary capillaries will also be the same as at sea-level.

10.5 VENTILATION–PERFUSION RELATIONSHIPS

Until recently it was believed that the only change in ventilation–perfusion relationships at high altitude was a more uniform topographical distribution of blood flow. This is caused by the increased pulmonary arterial pressure as a result of hypoxic pulmonary vasoconstriction (Chapter 6). For example, measurements with radioactive xenon have shown that the topographical differences of blood flow between apex and base of the upright lung are reduced at an altitude of 3100 m (Dawson, 1972). As discussed in Chapter 11, measurements by Wagner and his co-workers show a broadening of the distribution of ventilation–perfusion ratios during severe exercise at high altitude, the cause of which is unclear. The change in the distribution takes the form of a shoulder on the left of the blood flow distribution (plotted against ventilation–perfusion ratio), that is, an increase in blood flow to poorly-ventilated lung units.

These changes have now been seen in normal subjects who are

exercising while acutely exposed to hypoxia in a low pressure chamber (Gale *et al.*, 1985), exercising normal subjects who are inhaling low oxygen mixtures (Hammond *et al.*, 1986), and normal subjects during a 40-day exposure to low pressure in a chamber during Operation Everest II (Wagner *et al.*, 1988b). Evidence from this last study suggests that the ventilation–perfusion abnormalities are most likely to be seen in poorly-acclimatized subjects after a rapid ascent. In general, the abnormalities were most marked at the most severe levels of hypoxia, and at the heaviest exercise levels.

A reasonable hypothesis is that these changes are caused in some way by subclinical pulmonary oedema which results in inequality of ventilation. As discussed in Chapter 18, high-altitude pulmonary oedema is a well-known complication of going to high altitude. The likely mechanism is uneven hypoxic pulmonary vasoconstriction, which allows some capillaries to be exposed to high pressure with subsequent damage to their walls (West and Mathieu-Costello, 1992). The increase in pulmonary artery pressure is exaggerated during heavy exercise (Groves *et al.*, 1987).

10.6 CARDIOVASCULAR RESPONSES

These are discussed in Chapter 6. In non-acclimatized and poorly acclimatized lowlanders who go to high altitude, cardiac output at rest and during exercise for a given work level is increased compared with sea-level values. The same is true of heart rate.

In acclimatized lowlanders, cardiac output for a given work level returns to its sea-level value as shown by Pugh (1964) during the Himalayan Scientific and Mountaineering Expedition, and more recently during Operation Everest II (Reeves *et al.*, 1987). However, heart rate for a given level of exercise remains higher at altitude and therefore stroke volume is less. Measurements of contractile function of the heart during Operation Everest II in exercising subjects at all altitudes showed remarkable preservation in spite of the very severe hypoxaemia (Reeves *et al.*, 1987).

Pulmonary artery pressures are increased during exercise at altitude compared with sea-level values at the same work level. The elevated pressures are seen in both unacclimatized (Kronenberg *et al.*, 1971) and acclimatized (Groves *et al.*, 1987) lowlanders and in native highlanders (Penaloza *et al.*, 1963; Lockhart *et al.*, 1976). The basic cause of the pulmonary hypertension is presumably hypoxic pulmonary vasoconstriction. However it is of considerable interest that in the subjects of Operation Everest II, the pulmonary vascular pressures did not return to normal when 100% oxygen was breathed even though the subjects had been at high altitude only two or three weeks (Groves *et al.*, 1987).

This presumably indicates some structural changes in the pulmonary arteries in addition to hypoxic vasoconstriction.

10.7 ARTERIAL BLOOD GASES

At high altitude, the resting pattern of a low arterial P_{O_2} and P_{CO_2} is also seen during exercise. Arterial P_{O_2} typically falls further on exercise because of diffusion-limitation. In addition, at high work levels, the arterial P_{CO_2} often falls below the resting value, indicating that alveolar ventilation increases more than CO_2 production. The falling P_{CO_2} is associated with an increased respiratory exchange ratio which may rise to values over 1.2 at the highest work loads at very high altitudes (West *et al.*, 1983a). This represents an unsteady state since the respiratory quotient of the metabolizing tissues cannot exceed 1.0. At sea-level, such an increase in respiratory exchange ratio is often associated with lactate production from exercising muscles as a result of anaerobic glycolysis. However, at very high altitude, blood lactate levels remain surprisingly low even following exhausting exercise (Edwards, 1936; Cerretelli, 1980; West, 1986).

Arterial pH is near normal in well-acclimatized subjects up to altitudes of about 5400 m though Winslow believes there is often a small degree of uncompensated respiratory alkalosis, even in native highlanders (Winslow *et al.*, 1981; Winslow and Monge, 1987). At higher altitudes the arterial pH at rest tends to increase and there is evidence that it exceeds 7.7 on the Everest summit (West *et al.*, 1983b). Presumably the respiratory alkalosis is exaggerated on exercise because the arterial P_{CO_2} tends to fall and levels of blood lactate are low.

As stated in section 10.2, the observation that blood lactate is low in acclimatized subjects at high altitude, even during maximal work, was first made by Edwards (1936) during the 1935 International High Altitude Expedition to Chile. Figure 10.5 is redrawn from Edward's paper and shows that the levels of blood lactate during exercise at high altitude (up to 5340 m) were essentially the same as at sea-level. This means that the blood lactate levels for a given work level were apparently independent of tissue P_{O_2}. The only clear exceptions to this were the points shown by the open circles which were obtained at the lowest altitude of 2810 m. The small numbers over these points indicate the number of days that the subject had spent at this lowest altitude when the measurement was made, and it is clear that in most instances these data were obtained before the subject had had time to become fully acclimatized. Since maximal work capacity declines markedly with increasing altitude, the data of Figure 10.6 imply that maximal blood lactate falls in acclimatized subjects as altitude increases.

These results have been extended by Cerretelli (1976a, 1976b, 1980)

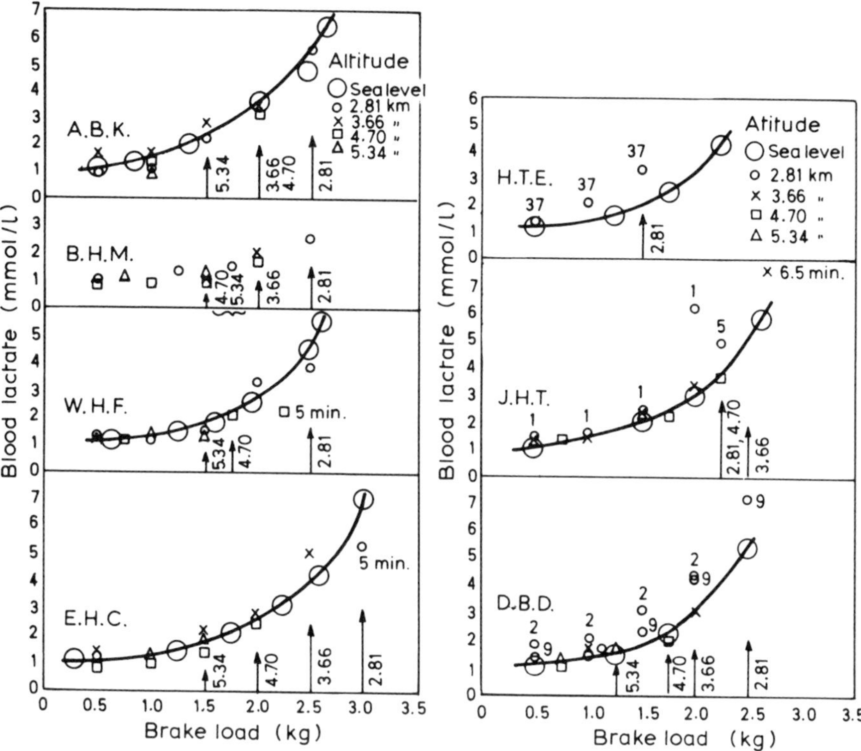

Figure 10.5 Venous blood lactate after exercise as reported by Edwards from the 1935 International High Altitude Expedition to Chile. The lines are drawn through the sea-level values. In general, lactate levels at high altitude lie on the same line, the only obvious exceptions being measurements made at the lowest altitude of 2.81 km. The small figures above these points indicate the number of days spent at that altitude and in most instances this was insufficient for acclimatization. (From Edwards, 1936.)

with additional measurements made at an altitude of 6300 m on the 1981 AMREE expedition (West *et al.*, 1983a). Figure 11.5 summarizes the data on resting and maximal blood lactate (West, 1986) and suggests the surprising conclusion that, after maximal exercise at altitudes exceeding 7500 m, there will be no increase in lactate in the blood at all in spite of the extreme oxygen deprivation. Possible reasons for this are discussed in more detail in Chapter 11.

10.8 PERIPHERAL TISSUES

The changes which occur in peripheral tissues at high altitude were discussed in Chapter 9. Animal studies indicate an increase in capillary

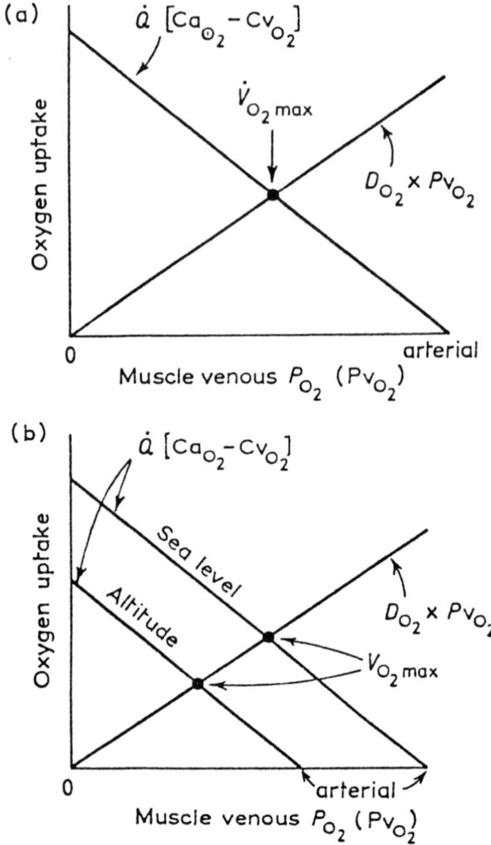

Figure 10.6 (a) Diagram to show how $\dot{V}_{O_2}$ max is determined assuming that oxygen diffusion from the peripheral capillary to the mitochondria is the limiting factor. The two lines show the oxygen uptake available from the Fick principle on the one hand, and Fick's law of diffusion on the other. The $\dot{V}_{O_2}$ max is given by the intersection of the two lines. See text for more details. (From Wagner, 1988a.) (b) As (a) except an additional line has been added to represent the Fick equation at high altitude. This reduces the $\dot{V}_{O_2}$ max as shown. See text for further details. (From Wagner, 1988a.)

density in some tissues as a result of chronic hypoxia. However data available from human muscle biopsies indicate that the number of capillaries remains constant in acclimatized lowlanders, but the average distance over which oxygen diffuses is reduced because the muscle fibres become smaller. There are changes in intracellular enzymes, and some studies show an increase in muscle myoglobin which may enhance oxygen diffusion. All these factors will play an important role in oxygen delivery and utilization during exercise.

Recently there has been considerable interest in the possible role of oxygen diffusion from capillaries to mitochondria as a factor limiting exercise at high altitude. Traditionally, many physiologists have argued that the power of working muscles at high altitude is determined by the amount of oxygen reaching them via the arterial blood. Oxygen delivery defined as the arterial oxygen concentration multiplied by the blood flow to the muscle has often been regarded as the critical variable.

Wagner and his co-workers have analysed the relationship between oxygen uptake and the P_{O_2} of muscle capillary blood on the assumption that the uptake is limited by oxygen diffusion from the capillaries to the mitochondria (Hogan *et al.*, 1988a). Figure 10.6(a) shows a diagram relating oxygen uptake to the P_{O_2} of muscle venous blood, taken as an index of muscle capillary P_{O_2}. The line sloping from top left to bottom right shows the amount of oxygen being delivered to the muscle by the capillaries (Fick principle). The line from bottom left to top right shows the pressure gradient available to cause oxygen diffusion from the red cells to the mitochondria (Fick's law) assuming that the mitochondrial P_{O_2} is nearly zero. The slope of this line is the lumped 'diffusing capacity of oxygen' of the tissues. The point where the two diagonal lines cross represents the $\dot{V}_{O_2}$ max. Regions to the left of this indicate situations where ample oxygen is available in the blood but the diffusing head of pressure is inadequate. Regions to the right indicate a more than adequate diffusing head of pressure but inadequate amounts of oxygen in the blood.

Figure 10.6(b) shows the same diagram with another line added indicating the presumed situation at high altitude. Because the oxygen concentration of the arterial blood is low, the line representing the Fick principle is displaced downwards and to the left. The $\dot{V}_{O_2}$ max is therefore lower. The diagram assumes that the 'diffusing capacity for oxygen' of the tissue is the same at sea-level and at altitude, which may not be the case if the diffusing distance is reduced by the appearance of more capillaries, or the size of muscle fibres is reduced. In these cases, the lump 'tissue diffusing capacity' would be increased.

Several pieces of evidence now support this concept. For example, a retrospective analysis of data from Operation Everest II showed that the points relating the P_{O_2} of mixed venous blood to oxygen uptake tend to lie on a straight line passing through the origin. On the assumption that the P_{O_2} of mixed venous blood reflects the P_{O_2} of the blood in the capillaries of the exercising muscles, this relationship supports the notion. Indeed, it was this observation that prompted the hypothesis.

More direct evidence comes from a prospective study in which normal subjects exercised at high work loads breathing hypoxic mixtures, and samples of femoral venous blood were taken via an indwelling catheter (Roca *et al.*, 1989). Again a plot of the P_{O_2} of femoral venous blood against oxygen uptake for different inspired oxygen concentrations showed the points lying close to a straight line passing near to the origin. A similar plot was found when the calculated mean capillary P_{O_2} was substituted for femoral venous P_{O_2}.

Additional studies have been carried out on an isolated dog gastrocnemius preparation where the muscle was supplied with hypoxic blood and stimulated maximally. Again a good relationship was found between the P_{O_2} of the effluent blood and the maximal oxygen uptake at different levels of hypoxia (Hogan *et al.*, 1988a). This preparation allowed a test of two competing hypotheses, that referred to above, and an alternative hypothesis that $\dot{V}_{O_2}$ max is determined by the amount of oxygen delivered to the muscle via the blood. The test was made by supplying the isolated muscle with the same amounts of oxygen (arterial oxygen concentration × blood flow) but using different blood flows (and therefore oxygen concentrations). The results showed that $\dot{V}_{O_2}$ max was more closely related to the P_{O_2} of muscle venous blood than to the oxygen delivered via the arterial blood, and therefore the results support the hypothesis of diffusion limitation (Hogan *et al.*, 1988b).

10.9 MAXIMAL OXYGEN UPTAKE AT HIGH ALTITUDE

Many investigators have documented the fall in maximal oxygen uptake at high altitude since the early studies of Zuntz *et al.* (1906), and the results of Pugh and his co-workers are shown in Figure 10.1. Figure 10.7(a) shows data from a number of studies collated by Cerretelli (1980). Note that, even at the very modest altitude of 2500 m, there is already an average decrease of $\dot{V}_{O_2}$ max of 5–10% as compared to sea-level. Cerretelli pointed out that these data do not show any consistent differences between subjects exposed to acute hypoxia and those who have had the advantage of acclimatization to high altitude. This conclusion goes against the experience of many climbers who feel that they can work harder at high altitude after acclimatization, and the conclusion cannot presumably be true at the most extreme altitudes where acute exposure to the prevailing barometric pressure (for example, on the summit of Mt Everest) results in loss of consciousness within a few minutes in most unacclimatized individuals who are acutely exposed. It is of interest that elite high altitude climbers have only moderately high levels of maximal oxygen consumption at sea-level (Oelz *et al.*, 1986).

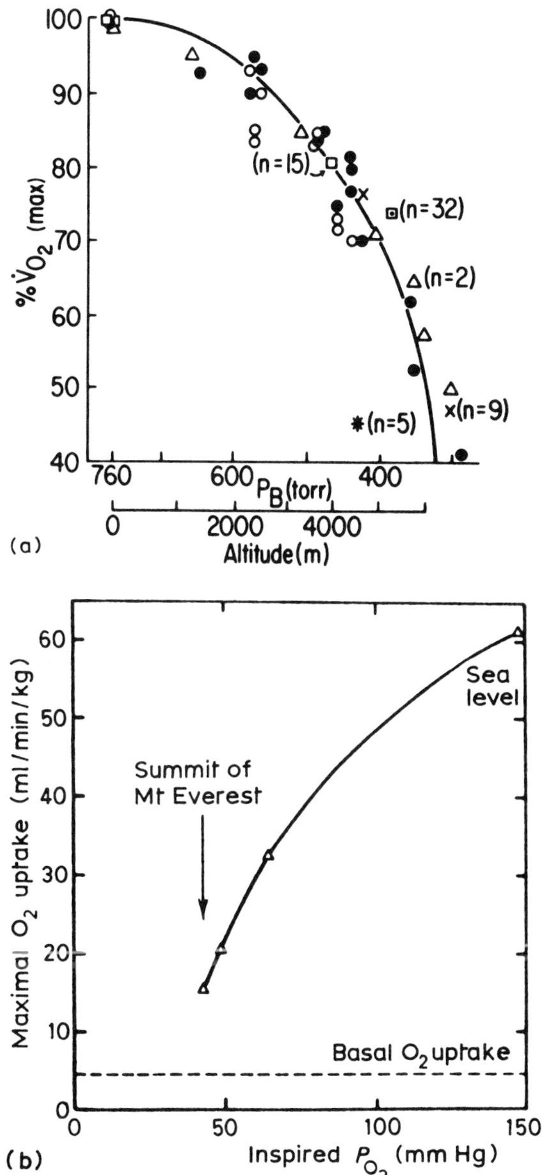

Figure 10.7 (a) $\dot{V}_{O_2}$ max as a percentage of the sea-level value plotted against barometric pressure and altitude. (○, △), acute hypoxia; (●), chronic hypoxia; (×), high-altitude natives. See original text for complete explanation of symbols. (From Cerretelli, 1980.) (b) Maximal oxygen uptake against inspired P_{O_2} as measured on the 1981 American Medical Research Expedition to Everest. The lowest point was obtained by giving well-acclimatized subjects at an altitude of 6300 m an inspired gas mixture containing 14% oxygen. The inspired P_{O_2} was 42.5 mmHg which is equivalent to that on the Everest summit. Compare Figure 10.2. (Modified from West *et al.*, 1983a.) (1 torr = 1 mmHg)

These data on maximal oxygen uptake were extended by the 1981 AMREE, where measurements were made at an altitude of 6300 m on subjects breathing ambient air, but also breathing 16 and 14% oxygen (West *et al.*, 1983a). The last gave an inspired P_{O_2} of 42.5 mmHg equivalent to that on the Everest summit. The results are shown in Figure 10.8(b) where it can be seen that in these subjects who were well acclimatized to very high altitude, the $\dot{V}_{O_2}$ max fell to 15.3 ml min^{-1} kg^{-1} which was equivalent to 1.07 l min^{-1}. Thus at the highest point on earth, the maximal oxygen uptake is reduced to between 20% and 25% of the sea-level value. As pointed out in Chapter 11, this oxygen uptake is equivalent to that seen when a subject walks slowly on the level but nevertheless is apparently sufficient to explain how Messner and Habeler were able to reach the Everest summit without supplementary oxygen in 1978. Indeed Messner's statement that the last 100 m took more than an hour to climb fits with this measured oxygen uptake (Messner, 1979).

Measurements of $\dot{V}_{O_2}$ max at various altitudes were also made during Operation Everest II and the data are almost superimposable on those shown in Figure 10.7(b) at the highest altitudes (Sutton *et al.*, 1987). This is interesting because the subjects of Operation Everest II were not as well acclimatized to the extreme altitudes as the members of the 1981 expedition as judged from their alveolar gas composition (West, 1987). The values for $\dot{V}_{O_2}$ max at any given altitude as determined by the 1981 Everest expedition (Figure 10.7(b)) are higher than those earlier reported by Pugh *et al.* (1964) based on measurements made during the Himalayan Scientific and Mountaineering Expedition and previous measurements on Mt Everest. This can be explained by the higher level of fitness of subjects on the 1981 expedition. For example, several of the expedition members were competitive marathon runners.

Several studies since the early measurements of Douglas *et al.* (1913) have shown that the relationship between oxygen uptake and work rate (or power) is independent of altitude. Figure 10.8(a) shows a comparison of data from the 1960–1961 Himalayan Scientific and Mountaineering Expedition, and Figure 10.8(b) from the 1981 Everest expedition. The message of the two plots is the same but note the much higher work rates at sea-level recorded prior to the 1981 expedition which is further evidence of the high level of athletic ability of these subjects.

As indicated earlier, breathing pure oxygen at high altitude does not return the $\dot{V}_{O_2}$ max to the sea-level value as shown by Cerretelli (1976a) and others. The reason is unclear; the opposite might be expected since the subjects acclimatized to high altitude have higher blood haemoglobin levels. It has been suggested that the reduced $\dot{V}_{O_2}$ max is caused by the loss of muscle mass at high altitude, and that if $\dot{V}_{O_2}$ max were

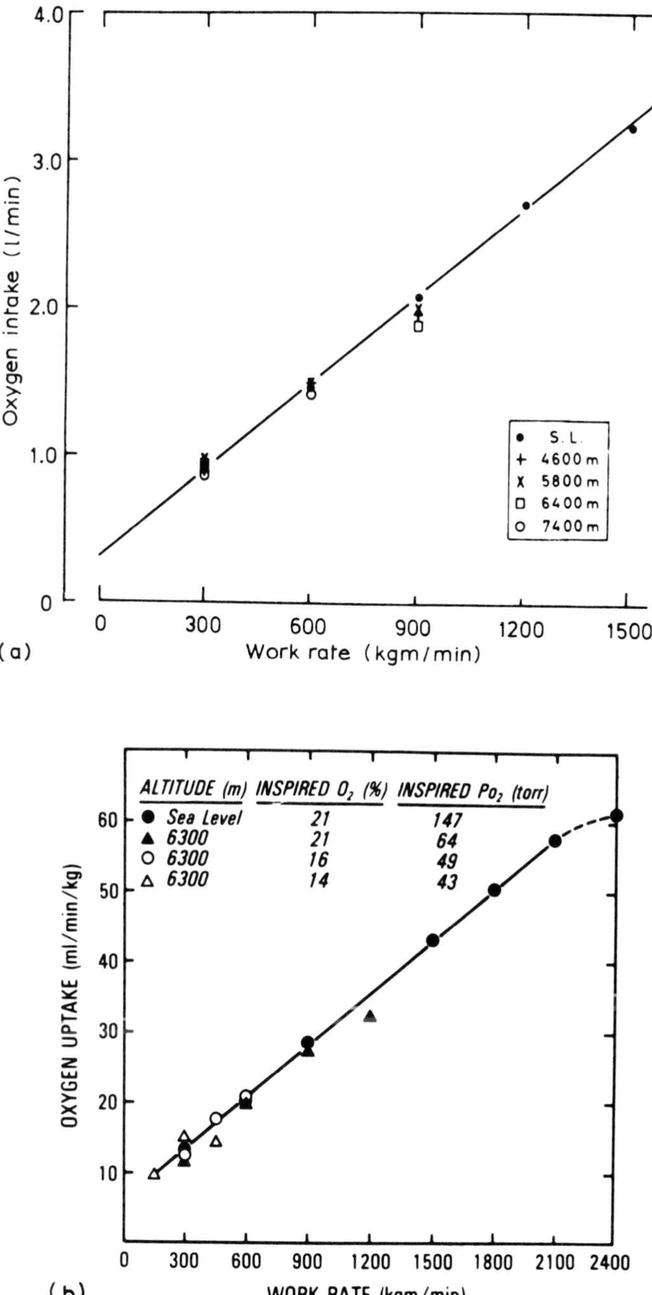

Figure 10.8 (a) Oxygen uptake plotted against work rate at various altitudes during HSME showing that the relationship remains essentially the same as at sea level. (From Pugh *et al.*, 1964). (b) Similar plot as in (a) but showing the much higher work rates at sea-level obtained during the 1981 AMREE expedition. (From West *et al.*, 1983a.) (1 torr = 1 mmHg)

related to lean body mass, the reduction would not be found. As discussed in Chapter 9, the diameter of muscle fibres decreases during acclimatization. Another possibility is that the increased red blood cell concentration causes uneven blood flow and sludging in peripheral capillaries and this interferes with oxygen unloading.

Does a period of acclimatization at high altitude improve $\dot{V}_{O_2}$ max at sea-level? Again the answer is not clear. Cerretelli (1976a) measured $\dot{V}_{O_2}$ max in a group of subjects at sea-level shortly before they were exposed to an altitude of 5350 m for 10–12 weeks, and again at sea-level about four weeks after return from altitude. Although there was an approximately 11% increase in haemoglobin concentration, this was not accompanied by a statistically significant rise in $\dot{V}_{O_2}$ max. On the other hand, more recent studies involving the reinjection of a subject's own red cells in order to raise the haematocrit have shown a small but significant increase in $\dot{V}_{O_2}$ max at sea-level (Spriet *et al.*, 1986). This result would suggest that a period at medium altitude (certainly lower than 5350 m) may improve exercise tolerance at sea-level. Perhaps the reduction of muscle fibre size at very high altitudes is the explanation for the failure to see an increase in $\dot{V}_{O_2}$ max after acclimatization at very high altitude.

It should be pointed out that the $\dot{V}_{O_2}$ max determined at any particular altitude is something of an artificial measurement because climbers, for example, do not ordinarily exercise at that intensity. Pugh (1958) showed that climbers typically select an oxygen uptake of one-half to three-quarters of their maximum for normal climbing at altitudes up to 6000 m. Actual values of oxygen uptake measured by Pugh during normal climbing are included in Figure 10.1.

10.10 ANAEROBIC PERFORMANCE AT HIGH ALTITUDE

Reference has already been made to the paradoxically low levels of blood lactate following exhaustive exercise at extreme altitude (section 10.7, Figure 10.5). This phenomenon may be related to the reduced plasma bicarbonate concentration which interferes with buffering of hydrogen ion as discussed in Chapter 11. Cerretelli (1992) has recently shown that the rate of increase of $\dot{V}_{O_2}$ when exercise is suddenly begun was slower in subjects after return from the 1981 Swiss Lhotse Expedition compared with before departure. This finding may be related to changes in anaerobic performance. However it was also shown that maximal anaerobic (alactic) 'peak' power as measured by a standing jump was not affected by exposure of up to three weeks at 5200 m. Thereafter it tended to fall along with the reduction of muscle mass.

REFERENCES

Barcroft, J., Binger, C.A., Bock, A.V., *et al.* (1923) Observations upon the effect of high altitude on the physiological processes of the human body, carried out in the Peruvian Andes, chiefly at Cerro de Pasco. *Phil. Trans. R. Soc. London Ser. B.*, **211**, 351–480.

Bert, P. *La Pression Barométrique*. Masson, Paris. (1878) English translation by M.A. Hitchcock and F.A. Hitchcock. College Book Co., Columbus, Ohio, 1943, pp. 343–6.

Bruce, C.G. (1923) *The Assault on Mt Everest 1922*, Arnold, London.

Cerretelli, P. (1976a) Limiting factors to oxygen transport on Mount Everest. *J. Appl. Physiol.*, **40**, 658–67.

Cerretelli, P. (1976b) Metabolismo ossidativo ed anaerobico nel soggetto acclimatato alla altitudine. *Minerva Aerosp.*, **67**, 11–26.

Cerretelli, P. (1980) Gas exchange at high altitude, in *Pulmonary Gas Exchange*, Vol. II, (ed. J.B. West), Academic Press, New York, pp. 97–147.

Cerretelli, P. (1992) Energy sources for muscular exercise. *Int. J. Sports Med*, **13(Suppl 1)**, S106–10.

Cerretelli, P. and Whipp, B.J. (1980) *Exercise, Bioenergetics and Gas Exchange*. Elsevier/North Holland Biomedical Press, Amsterdam.

Christensen, E.H. (1937) Sauerstoffaufnahme und respiratorische Funktionen in grossen Hohen. *Scand. Arch. Physiol.*, **76**, 88–100.

Cotes, J.E. (1954) Ventilatory capacity at altitude and its relation to mask design. *Proc. R. Soc. London Ser. B.*, **143**, 32–9.

Dawson, A. (1972) Regional lung function during early acclimatization to 3100 m altitude. *J. Appl. Physiol.*, **33**, 218–23.

Douglas, C.G., Haldane, J.A., Henderson, Y. and Schneider, E.C. (1913) Physiological observations made on Pike's Peak, Colorado, with special reference to adaptation to low barometric pressures. *Phil. Trans. R. Soc. London Ser. B.*, **203**, 185–381.

Durig, A. (1911) Ergebnisse der Monte Rosa Expedition vom Jahre 1906. Uber den Gaswechsel beim Geben. *Denkschr. Akad. Wiss. Wien*, **86**, 293–347.

Edwards, H.T. (1936) Lactic acid in rest and work at high altitude. *Am. J. Physiol.*, **116**, 367–75.

Gale, G.E., Torre-Bueno, J.R., Moon, R.E., *et al.* (1985) Ventilation–perfusion inequality in normal humans during exercise at sea-level and simulated altitude. *J. Appl. Physiol.*, **58**, 978–88.

Groves, B.M., Reeves, J.T., Sutton, J.R., *et al.* (1987) Operation Everest II: elevated high-altitude pulmonary resistance unresponsive to oxygen. *J. Appl. Physiol.*, **63**, 521–30.

Habeler, P. (1979) *Everest: Impossible Victory*, Arlington, London.

Hammond, M.D., Gale, G.E., Kapitan, K.S., *et al.* (1986) Pulmonary gas exchange in humans during normobaric hypoxic exercise. *J. Appl. Physiol.*, **61**, 1749–57.

Hogan, M.C., Roca, J., Wagner, P.D. and West, J.B. (1988a) Limitation of maximal O_2 uptake and performance by acute hypoxia in dog muscle *in situ*. *J. Appl. Physiol.*, **65**, 815–21.

Hogan, M.C., Roca, J., West, J.B., and Wagner, P.D. (1988b) Dissociation of maximal O_2 uptake from O_2 delivery in canine gastrocnemius *in situ*. *J. Appl. Physiol.*, **66**, 1219–26.

Houston, C.S., Sutton, J.R., Cymerman, A. and Reeves, J.T. (1987) Operation Everest II: man at extreme altitude. *J. Appl. Physiol.*, **63**, 877–82.

Howard-Bury, C.K. (1922) *Mt Everest: The Reconnaissance 1921*, Arnold, London.

Jokl, E. (1968) *Exercise and Altitude*, Karger, Basel.

Keys, A. (1936) The physiology of life at high altitude: the International High Altitude Expedition to Chile 1935. *Sci. Mon.*, **43**, 289–312.

Kronenberg, R.S., Safar, P., Lee, J., *et al.* (1971) Pulmonary artery pressure and alveolar gas exchange in man during acclimatization to 12470 ft. *J. Clin. Invest.*, **50**, 827–37.

Lockhart, A., Zelter, M., Mensch-Dechene, M., *et al.* (1976) Pressure–flow–volume relationships in pulmonary circulation of normal highlanders. *J. Appl. Physiol.*, **41**, 449–56.

McIntyre, L. (1987) The high Andes. *Nat. Geogr.*, **171**, 422–59.

Margaria, R. (ed.) (1967) *Exercise at Altitude*, Excerpta Medica Foundation, Amsterdam.

Messner, R. (1979) The mountain, in *Everest: Expedition to the Ultimate*. Kaye & Ward, London, pp. 47–217.

Norton, E.G. (1925) Norton and Somervell's attempt, in *The Fight for Everest*, (ed. E.G. Norton), Arnold, London, pp. 99–119.

Oelz O., Howald, H., dePrampero, P.E., *et al.* (1986) Physiological profile of world-class high-altitude climbers. *J. Appl. Physiol.*, **60**, 1734–42.

Penaloza, D., Sime, F., Banchero, N., *et al.* (1963) Pulmonary hypertension in healthy men born and living at high altitudes. *Am. J. Cardiol.*, **11**, 150–7.

Petit, J.M., Milic-Emili, J. and Troquet, J. (1963) Travail dynamique pulmonaire et altitude. *Rev. Med. Aerosp.*, **2**, 276–9.

Pugh, L.G.C.E. (1958) Muscular exercise on Mt Everest. *J. Physiol. (London)*, **141**, 233–61.

Pugh, L.G.C.E. (1962) Physiological and medical aspects of the Himalayan Scientific and Mountaineering Expedition, 1960–1961. *Br. Med. J.*, **2**, 621–7.

Pugh, L.G.C.E. (1964) Cardiac output in musclar exercise at 5800 m (19 000 ft). *J. Appl. Physiol.*, **19**, 431–40.

Pugh, L.G.C.E., Gill, M.B., Lahiri, S., *et al.* (1964) Muscular exercise at great altitude. *J. Appl. Physiol.*, **19**, 431–40.

Reeves, J.T., Groves, B.M., Sutton, M.P., *et al.* (1987) Operation Everest II: preservation of cardiac function at extreme altitude. *J. Appl. Physiol.*, **63**, 531–9.

Roca, J.M., Hogan, M.C., Storey, D., *et al.* (1989) Evidence for tissue limitation of $\dot{V}_{O_2}$ max in normal man. *J. Appl. Physiol.*, **67**, 291–9.

Roughton, F.J. (1945) Average time spent by blood in human lung capillary and its relation to the rates of CO uptake and elimination in man. *Am. J. Physiol.*, **143**, 621–33.

Somervell, T.H. (1925) Note on the composition of alveolar air at extreme height. *J. Physiol. (London)*, **60**, 282–85.

Spriet, L.L., Gledhill, N., Froese, A.B. and Wilkes, D.L. (1986) Effect of graded erythrocythemia on cardiovascular and metabolic responses to exercise. *J. Appl. Physiol.*, **61**, 1942–8.

Sutton, J.R., Houston, C.S. and Jones, N.L. (1983) *Hypoxia, Exercise and Altitude*, Liss, New York.

Sutton, J.R., Houston, C.R. and Coates, G. (1987) *Hypoxia: The Tolerable Limits*. Benchmark Press, Indianapolis.

Sutton, J.R., Reeves, J.T., Wagner, P.D., *et al.* (1988) Operation Everest II: Oxygen transport during exercise at extreme simulated altitude. *J. Appl. Physiol.*, **64**, 1309–21.

Wagner, P.D. (1988a) An integrated view of the determinants of maximum oxygen uptake, in *Oxygen Transfer from Atmosphere to Tissues*, Vol. 227, (eds N.C. Gonzalez and M.R. Fedde), Plenum, New York, pp. 246–56.

Wagner, P.D., Sutton, J.R., Reeves, J.T., *et al.* (1988b) Operation Everest II. Pulmonary gas exchange during a simulated ascent of Mt Everest. *J. Appl. Physiol.*, **63**, 2348–59.

West, J.B. (1962) Diffusing capacity of the lung for carbon monoxide at high altitude. *J. Appl. Physiol.*, **17**, 421–6.

West, J.B. (1986) Lactate during exercise at extreme altitude. *Fed. Proc.*, **45**, 2953–7.

West, J.B. (1987) Tolerable limits to hypoxia – on high mountains, in *Hypoxia: The Tolerable Limits*, (eds J. Sutton, C. Houston and G. Coates), Benchmark Press, Indianapolis, pp. 353–62.

West, J.B. and Mathieu-Costello, O. (1992) High altitude pulmonary edema is caused by stress failure of pulmonary capillaries. *Int. J. Sports Med.*, **13(suppl 1)**, S54–S58.

West, J.B. and Wagner, P.D. (1980) Predicted gas exchange on the summit of Mt Everest. *Respir. Physiol.*, **42**, 1–16.

West, J.B., Boyer, S.J., Graber, D.J., *et al.* (1983a) Maximal exercise at extreme altitudes on Mount Everest. *J. Appl. Physiol. Respir. Environ. Exercise Physiol.*, **55**, 688–98.

West, J.B., Hackett, P.H., Maret, K.H., *et al.* (1983b) Pulmonary gas exchange on the summit of Mt Everest. *J. Appl. Physiol. Respir. Environ. Exercise Physiol.*, **55**, 678–87.

Winslow, R.M. and Monge, C.C. (1987) *Hypoxia, Polycythemia and Chronic Mountain Sickness*, Johns Hopkins University Press, Baltimore.

Winslow, R.M., Monge, C.C., Statham, N.J., *et al.* (1981) Variability of oxygen affinity of blood: human subjects native to high altitude. *J. Appl. Physiol.*, **51**, 1411–16.

Zuntz, N., Loewy, A., Muller, F. and Caspari, W. (1906) *Höhenklima und Bergwanderungen in ihrer Wirkung auf den Menschen*, Bong, Berlin.

11

Limiting factors at extreme altitude

11.1 INTRODUCTION

It is a remarkable coincidence that when man is well-acclimatized to high altitude, he can just reach the highest point on earth without breathing supplementary oxygen. This feat was only realized in 1978 and many physiologists and physicians interested in high altitude had previously predicted that it would not be possible. It was truly the end of an era when Messner and Habeler stood on the summit of Mt Everest on 8 May, 1978.

This chapter examines the profound physiological changes which are necessary for man to survive and do small amounts of work at extreme altitudes like the summit of Mt Everest. It includes an analysis of the factors which limit performance at these great altitudes and shows that such ascents are only possible if both the physiological make-up of the climber and physical factors such as barometric pressure are right.

11.2 HISTORICAL

11.2.1 Sixteenth to nineteenth centuries

It has been known for many centuries that very high altitude has a deleterious effect on the human body and that the amount of work that a man can do becomes more and more limited. One of the first descriptions of the disabling effects of high altitude was given by the Jesuit missionary Joseph de Acosta who accompanied the early Spanish conquistadores to Peru in the sixteenth century. He described how as he travelled over a high mountain, he 'was suddenly surprised with so mortall and strange a pang, that I was ready to fall from the top to the ground.' His dramatic description was first published in 1590 (Acosta, 1590).

In the eighteenth century, climbers in the European Alps reported a variety of disagreeable sensations which now seem to us greatly exaggerated. For example, the physicist De Saussure, who was the third person to reach the summit of Mont Blanc, reported during the climb: 'When I began this ascent, I was quite out of breath from the rarity of the air . . . The kind of fatigue which results from the rarity of the air is absolutely unconquerable; when it is at its height, the most terrible danger would not make you take a single step further.' When he was near the summit he complained of extreme exhaustion 'This need of rest was absolutely unconquerable; if I tried to overcome it, my legs refused to move, I felt the beginning of a faint, and was seized by dizziness . . .'. On the summit itself he reported 'When I had to get to work to set out the instruments and observe them, I was constantly forced to interrupt my work and devote myself to breathing' (De Saussure, 1786–1798). All these complaints at an altitude of 4807 m (15 782 ft) or less reflect a combination of an almost complete lack of acclimatization and the fear of the unknown.

In the nineteenth century numerous ascents were made of higher mountains including those in the Andes and there were abundant accounts of the disabling effects of extreme altitude. In 1879, Whymper made the first ascent of Chimborazo and described how, at an altitude of 16 664 ft (5079 m), he was incapacitated by the thin air:

> . . . in about an hour I found myself lying on my back, along with both the Carrels [guides], placed *hors de combat*, and incapable of making the least exertion . . . We were unable to satisfy our desire for air, except by breathing with open mouths . . . Besides having our normal rate of breathing largely accelerated, we found it impossible to sustain life without every now and then giving spasmodic gulps, just like fishes when taken out of water.
>
> *(Whymper, 1891)*

However, Whymper and his two guides gradually recovered their strength and in fact his lively account shows that he was aware of the beneficial effects of high-altitude acclimatization.

In the latter part of the nineteenth century, there was considerable interest in the highest altitude that could be tolerated by climbers. Thomas W. Hinchliff, President of the (British) Alpine Club (1875–1877), wrote an account of his travels around the world and described his feelings as he looked at the view from Santiago in Chile.

> Lover of mountains as I am, and familiar with such summits as those of Mont Blanc, Monte Rosa, and other Alpine heights, I could not repress a strange feeling as I looked at Tupungato and Aconcagua, and reflected that endless successions of men must in

all probability be forever debarred from their lofty crests . . . Those who, like Major Godwin Austen, have had all the advantages of experience and acclimatization to aid them in attacks upon the higher Himalayas, agree that 21 500 ft [6553 m] is near the limit at which man ceases to be capable of the slightest further exertion.

(Hinchliff, 1876)

11.2.2 Twentieth century

In 1909, the aristocratic Italian climber, the Duke of the Abruzzi attempted an ascent of K2 in the Karakorum Mountains, and though his party was unsuccessful in reaching the summit, they reached the remarkable altitude of 7500 m (24 600 ft) without supplementary oxygen. According to the Duke's biographer, one of the reasons given for this expedition was 'to see how high man can go' (Filippi, 1912), and certainly the climb had a dramatic effect on both the mountaineering and the medical communities interested in high-altitude tolerance. In contrast to the florid accounts of paralysing fatigue and breathlessness given by De Saussure, Whymper and others at much lower altitudes, the Duke made light of the physiological problems associated with this great altitude. However, as we saw earlier (Chapter 5), his feat prompted heated arguments among physiologists about whether the lungs actively secreted oxygen at this previously unheard of altitude.

Ten years later, a milestone in the history of the physiology of extreme altitude was provided by the British physiologist, Alexander M. Kellas, whose contributions have been almost completely overlooked. Kellas was lecturer in chemistry at the Middlesex Hospital Medical School in London during the first two decades of the century, but, in spite of this full time faculty position, managed to make eight expeditions to the Himalayas, and probably spent more time above 20 000 ft (6100 m) than anyone else. In 1919 he wrote an extensive paper entitled *A consideration of the possibility of ascending Mt Everest*, which unfortunately was only published in French in a very obscure place (Kellas, 1921). In this he analysed the physiology of a climber near the Everest summit including a discussion of the summit altitude, barometic pressure, alveolar P_{O_2}, arterial oxygen saturation, maximal oxygen consumption, and maximal ascent rate. On the basis of his study he concluded that, 'Mt Everest could be ascended by a man of excellent physical and mental constitution in first-rate training, without adventitious aids [supplementary oxygen] if the physical difficulties of the mountain are not too great.' The importance of this study was not so much that he reached the correct conclusion. He had so few data that many of his calculations were incorrect. However Kellas asked all the right questions and he can claim the distinction of being the first physiologist seriously to analyse the limiting factors at the highest point on earth. It was not until almost 60 years later that his prediction was fulfilled.

Kellas was a member of the first official reconnaissance expedition to Everest in 1921, but tragically he died during the approach march just as the expedition had its first view of the mountain they came to climb. Three years later, E.F. Norton, who was a member of the third Everest expedition reached a height of about 8589 m (28 150 ft) on the north side of Everest without supplementary oxygen. He was accompanied to just below that altitude by Dr T.H. Somervell, who collected alveolar gas samples at an altitude of 7010 m (23 000 ft) though unfortunately these were stored in rubber bladders through which the carbon dioxide rapidly diffused (Somervell, 1925). Somervell also referred to the extreme breathlessness at that altitude stating that 'for every step forward and upward, 7 to 10 complete respirations were required.'

The summit of Everest was finally attained in 1953 by Hillary and Tensing (Hunt, 1953). Naturally this was a landmark event in the physiology of extreme altitude but the fact that the two climbers used supplementary oxygen still did not answer the question of whether it was possible to reach the summit breathing air. Hillary did remove his oxygen mask on the summit for about ten minutes and at the end of the time reported, 'I realized that I was becoming rather clumsy-fingered and slow-moving, so I quickly replaced my oxygen set and experienced once more the stimulating effect of even a few litres of oxygen.' Nevertheless the fact that he could survive for a few minutes without additional oxygen came as a surprise to some physicians who had predicted that he would lose consciousness.

However, there was a precedent for surviving for this period on the summit in the experiment Operation Everest I, carried out by Houston and Riley in 1945. As briefly described in Chapter 1, four volunteers spent 34 days in a low-pressure chamber and two were able to tolerate 20 minutes without supplementary oxygen on the 'summit'. In fact, the equivalent altitude was even higher because the standard atmosphere pressure was inadvertently used (section 11.3.2).

Additional information on whether there was enough oxygen in the air to allow a climber to reach the Everest summit while breathing air was obtained by Pugh and his colleagues during the Himalayan Scientific and Mountaineering Expedition of 1960–1961 (Pugh *et al.*, 1964). Measurements of maximal oxygen consumption were made using a bicycle ergometer on a group of physiologists who wintered at an altitude of 5800 m (19 000 ft) and who were therefore extremely well-acclimatized to this altitude. Figure 11.1 (lower curve) shows the results of measurements made up to an altitude of 7440 m (24 400 ft). Note that extrapolation of the line to a barometric pressure of 250 mmHg on the

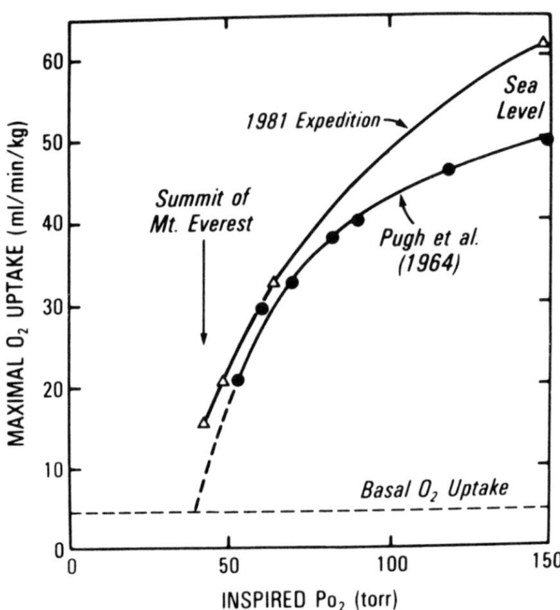

Figure 11.1 Maximal O_2 uptake against inspired P_{O_2}. The lower line shows data from Pugh *et al.* (1964) suggesting that all the oxygen available at the Everest summit would be required for basal O_2 uptake. However as the upper line shows, the 1981 AMREE measured an O_2 uptake of just over $1\,l\,min^{-1}$ for an inspired P_{O_2} of 43 mmHg. (From West *et al.*, 1983a.) (1 torr = 1 mmHg)

Everest summit suggested that almost all the oxygen available would be required for the basal oxygen uptake. (For details of the extrapolation procedure refer to West and Wagner (1980).) Thus these results strongly suggested that, if man could reach the Everest summit without supplementary oxygen, he would be very near the limit of human tolerance.

The ultimate climbing achievement occurred when Reinhold Messner and Peter Habeler reached the summit of Everest without supplementary oxygen in May 1978. Messner's account (Messner, 1979) makes it clear that he had very little in reserve: 'After every few steps, we huddle over our ice axes, mouths agape, struggling for sufficient breath . . . As we get higher it becomes necessary to lie down to recover our breath . . . Breathing becomes such a strenous business that we scarcely have strength to go on.' And when he eventually reaches the summit, 'in my state of spiritual abstraction, I no longer belong to myself and to my eyesight. I am nothing more than a single, narrow gasping lung, floating over the mists and the summits.'

The long period of 25 years between the first ascent of Everest in

1953 and this first 'oxygenless' ascent also suggests that we are near the limit of man's tolerance. Again, as indicated earlier, Norton and Somervell ascended to within 300 m of the Everest summit as early as 1924, but it was not until 1978 that climbers reached the top without supplementary oxygen. Thus the last 300 m took 54 years!

Since that historic climb, Messner has further confirmed his outstanding tolerance to the extreme hypoxia of great altitudes. In 1980, he became the first man to ascend Everest alone without supplementary oxygen (Messner, 1981), and in 1986 he became the first man to climb all fourteen of the 8000 m peaks without supplementary oxygen. These accomplishments assure him a place not only in the history of mountaineering but in the history of the physiology of extreme altitude.

11.3 PHYSIOLOGY OF EXTREME ALTITUDE

11.3.1 Introduction

This section is devoted to human performance at altitudes over 8000 m (26 250 ft). There has been a renewed interest in this topic since Messner and Habeler climbed Everest without supplementary oxygen in 1978 but, as indicated above, the issue of whether man would be able to tolerate the highest altitude on earth was raised early in this century, notably by Kellas in 1919.

The following analysis is based primarily on data from three studies. The first was the Himalayan Scientific and Mountaineering Expedition of 1960–1961 during which data were obtained on maximal oxygen consumptions as high as 7440 m (P_B 300 mmHg) and alveolar gas samples were taken as high as 7830 m (P_B 288 mmHg). These measurements were extended to the Everest summit by the American Medical Research Expedition to Everest (AMREE) in 1981 where measurements on the summit included barometric pressure, alveolar gas samples and electrocardiograms, with additional measurements made between the summit and the highest camp situated at 8050 m (P_B 284 mmHg). The third study was Operation Everest II in the autumn of 1985 when eight volunteers were gradually decompressed to a barometric pressure of 240 mmHg over a period of 40 days in a low pressure chamber. Although the rate of simulated ascent was too fast for optimal acclimatization, much valuable data were obtained particularly in the areas of cardiopulmonary and muscle physiology.

11.3.2 Barometric pressure

Barometric pressure is a critical variable in physiological performance at extreme altitude because it determines the inspired P_{O_2}. This is the first link in the chain of the oxygen cascade from the atmosphere to the mitochondria. As pointed out in Chapter 2, there has been considerable confusion in the past about the relationships between barometric pressure and altitude on high mountains such as the Himalayan chain. The resulting errors are particularly important at extreme altitude because it can be shown that maximal oxygen consumption is exquisitely sensitive to barometric pressure. It is remarkable that Paul Bert gave essentially the correct value of barometric pressure for the Everest summit in Appendix I of his classical book *La Pression Barométrique* (Bert, 1878). His figure of 248 mmHg was based on an extrapolation of measurements made by Jourdanet at various locations including the Andes (Jourdanet, 1875).

However, when the standard atmosphere was introduced and used extensively by aviation physiologists in the 1930s and 1940s, it was erroneously applied to Mt Everest, giving the value of 236 mmHg which was much too low. Nevertheless this number was used by several high-altitude physiologists. For example, during Operation Everest I when four naval recruits were gradually decompressed to what was thought to be the simulated altitude of Mt Everest, they were exposed to a pressure of 236 mmHg and their alveolar P_{O_2} fell to as low as 21 mmHg (Riley and Houston, 1951)! As the next section shows, this is about 14 mmHg less than that of a well-acclimatized climber on the summit of Mt Everest.

As described in Chapter 2, Dr Christopher Pizzo measured a barometric pressure of 253 mmHg on the Everest summit on 24 October, 1981. This was about 2 mmHg higher than that expected from the mean barometric pressure for that month based on extensive weather balloon data (Figure 2.4). The discrepancy can be accounted for by normal variation and the high pressure system which made the weather ideal for climbing. The reading of 253 mmHg was within 1 mmHg of the pressure predicted for an altitude of 8848 m from radio-sonde balloons released in New Delhi, India on the same day (West *et al.*, 1983c).

As section 11.4 shows, exercise performance at these extreme altitudes is exquisitely sensitive to barometric pressure. This is chiefly because the lung is working very low on the oxygen dissociation curve where the slope is steep. As a consequence, a fall of barometric pressure of as little as 3 mmHg (less than twice the daily standard deviation) will apparently cause a reduction of maximal oxygen uptake of over 5%. This means that even the daily variations of barometric pressure caused by weather can affect physical performance.

Seasonal variations of barometric pressure can be expected to have a marked effect on maximal oxygen uptake. As Figure 2.4 shows, mean barometric pressure falls from nearly 255 mmHg in the summer months to only 243 mmHg in mid-winter. This decrease is predicted to reduce maximal oxygen uptake by some 25%. It is noteworthy that Mt Everest has only once been climbed during winter without supplementary oxygen (December 1987) in spite of several attempts, and although the very cold temperatures and high winds are naturally a factor, the reduced barometric pressure must certainly contribute (section 2.2.8).

As pointed out in Chapter 2, the location of Mt Everest at 28°N latitude is fortunate because the barometric pressure at its summit is considerably higher than would be the case if it were at a higher latitude. As an example, if Mt McKinley were 8848 m high, its barometric pressure for May and October (preferred climbing months for Everest) would be only 223 mmHg. It would be impossible to reach the summit without supplementary oxygen under these conditions.

A similar argument would apply if the barometric pressure on the Everest summit were only 236 mmHg, as predicted from the standard atmosphere model. The reduction of pressure by 17 mmHg below that measured by Pizzo would reduce the maximal oxygen consumption by over 30% according to the analysis presented in the present chapter. It seems certain that climbing Everest without supplementary oxygen under these conditions would be impossible. Thus the higher pressure that Everest enjoys because of its near equatorial latitude makes it just possible for man to reach the highest point on earth.

11.3.3 Alveolar gas composition

On ascent to high altitude, the alveolar P_{O_2} falls because of the reduction in the inspired P_{O_2}. At the same time, alveolar P_{CO_2} falls because of increasing hyperventilation. As described in Chapter 4, Rahn and Otis (1949) clarified the differences between unacclimatized and fully-acclimatized subjects at high altitude by plotting their alveolar gas P_{O_2} and P_{CO_2} values on an oxygen–carbon dioxide diagram (Figure 4.6).

Figure 11.2 shows alveolar P_{CO_2} plotted against barometric pressure at extreme altitude. The closed circles show data reported by Greene (1934), Warren (1939), Pugh (1957) and Gill *et al.* (1962). The triangles show data obtained on the AMREE (West *et al.*, 1983b). It can be seen that alveolar P_{CO_2} declines approximately linearly as barometric pressure falls and that the pressure on the summit of Mt Everest is about 7.5 mmHg. The measurements made on the summit itself were marred by high respiratory exchange ratio (R) values for reasons which are not clear. However the data obtained at the slightly lower altitude of 8400 m (P_B 267 mmHg) had a mean R value of 0.82 with a P_{CO_2} of 8.0 mmHg which means we can be confident of the very low values at this great altitude.

Figure 11.3 shows the line drawn by Rahn and Otis (1949) for fully-acclimatized subjects (lower line on Figure 4.6) together with additional

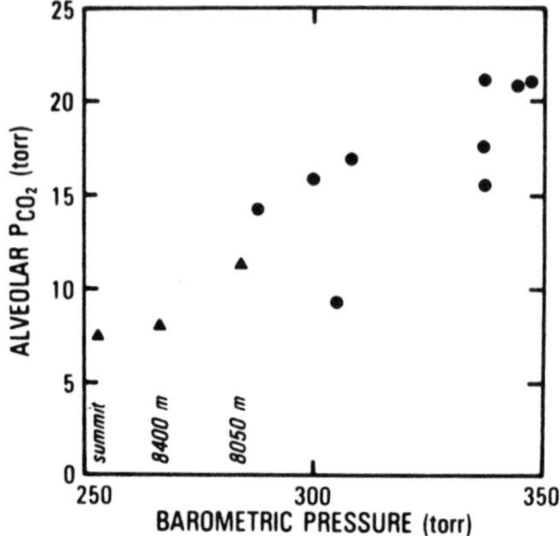

Figure 11.2 Alveolar P_{CO_2} against barometric pressure at extreme altitudes. Triangles (▲) show the means of measurements on the AMREE. Circles (●) are results from previous investigators at barometric pressures below 350 mmHg (Table 11.1). (From West *et al.*, 1983b.) (1 torr = 1 mmHg)

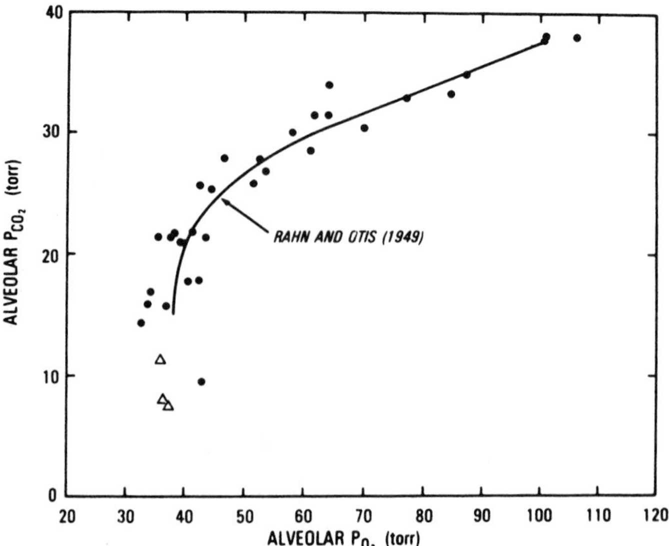

Figure 11.3 O_2–CO_2 diagram showing alveolar gas values collated by Rahn and Otis (1949) (●) together with values obtained at extreme altitudes by the AMREE (△). (From West *et al.*, 1983b.) (1 torr = 1 mmHg)

Table 11.1 Alveolar P_{O_2} and P_{CO_2} in acclimatized subjects at barometric pressures below 350 mmHg

Source	*Barometric pressure*	*Partial pressure* O_2 (P_{O_2})	*Partial pressure* CO_2 (P_{CO_2})	*Respiratory exchange ratio* R
Greene, 1934	337	40.7	17.7	0.87
	305	43.0	9.2	0.79
Warren, 1939	337*	37.0	15.6	0.60
Pugh, 1957	347	39.3	21.0	0.87
	337	35.5	21.3	0.87
	308	34.1	16.9	0.77
Gill *et al.*, 1962	344	38.1	20.7	0.82
	300	33.7	15.8	0.78
	288	32.8	14.3	0.77
West *et al.*, 1983b	284	36.1	11.0	0.78
	267	36.7	8.0	0.82
	253	37.6	7.5	1.49

All pressure values are given in mmHg
*Barometric pressure estimated from curve of Zuntz *et al.* (1906)

data obtained at barometric pressures below 350 mmHg (Table 11.1). Note that the AMREE data (triangles) fit well with the extrapolation of the line. This method of plotting the data shows that, as well-acclimatized man goes to higher and higher altitudes, the P_{O_2} falls because of the decreasing inspired P_{O_2}, and the P_{CO_2} falls because of the increasing hyperventilation. However above an altitude of about 7000 m (23 000 ft; P_B 325 mmHg) the alveolar P_{O_2} becomes essentially constant at a value of about 35 mmHg. This means that successful climbers are able to defend their alveolar P_{O_2} by the process of extreme hyperventilation. In other words, they insulate the P_{O_2} of their alveolar gas from the falling value in the atmosphere around them. This appears to be one of the most important features of acclimatization at extreme altitude.

Not everyone can generate the enormous increase in ventilation required for the very low P_{CO_2} values shown in Figures 11.2 and 11.3. This explains why climbers with a large hypoxic ventilatory response tolerate extreme altitude better than those with a more modest response (Schoene *et al.*, 1984). Indeed, experience on the AMREE expedition showed that individuals who had an unusually low hypoxic ventilatory response were not able to remain at the higher camps (West, 1985).

The pattern of alveolar gas values shown in Figure 11.3 is only

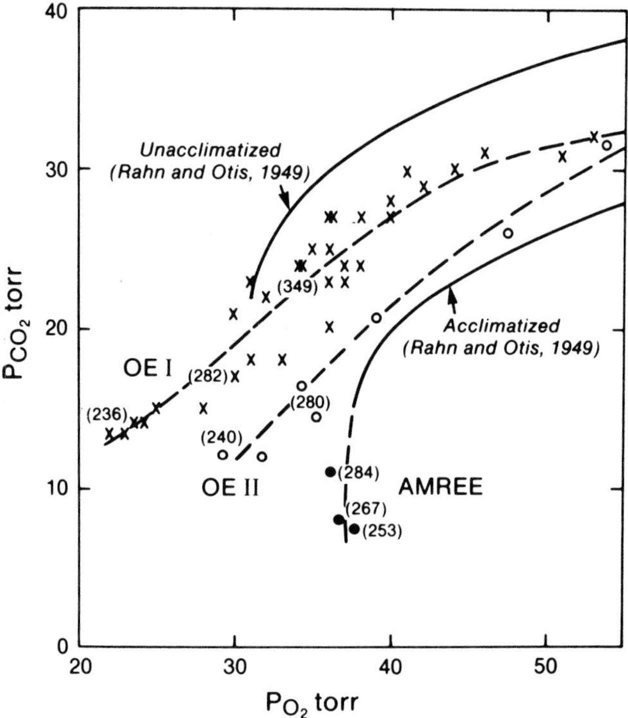

Figure 11.4 O_2–CO_2 diagram showing the two lines described by Rahn and Otis (1949) for unacclimatized and acclimatized subjects at high altitude (compare Figure 4.6). In addition data from Operation Everest I (OE I) and Operation Everest II (OE II) are included. The numbers in brackets show barometric pressure. Note that the OE I subjects were poorly acclimatized at extreme altitudes while the OE II had intermediate values. (From West, 1988.) (1 torr = 1 mmHg)

obtained if sufficient time is allowed for full respiratory acclimatization. Figure 11.4 compares the results found in unacclimatized and fully-acclimatized subjects at high altitude (Figures 4.6, 11.3) with alveolar gas data reported from two low-pressure chamber experiments in which the simulated rate of ascent was much faster. It can be seen that in Operation Everest I (Riley and Houston, 1951) the subjects reached the simulated summit after only 31 days and at the extreme altitudes the data fell close to the region predicted by the line for unacclimatized man. In Operation Everest II (Malconian *et al.*, 1993) the ascent was a little slower with the first simulated summit excursion occurring after 36 days. However the alveolar gas values at extreme altitudes still deviated considerably from those found in fully-acclimatized subjects. Little information is available about the time required for full respiratory acclimatization at extreme altitudes, say over 8000 m, but Figure 11.4 suggests that 36 days are inadequate whereas 77 days are sufficient.

11.3.4 Acid–base status

Relatively little is known about acid–base changes at extreme altitude in spite of the importance of this topic. Some data are available from two well acclimatized subjects of the AMREE, based on blood samples removed during the morning after they had reached the summit. Venous blood samples taken at the highest camp (8050 m; P_B 267 mmHg) showed a mean base excess of $-7.2\,\text{mmol}\,\text{l}^{-1}$. This was a considerably higher base excess than expected (in other words the base deficit was less than predicted) and the result was an extremely high arterial pH of over 7.7 calculated for the Everest summit (West *et al.*, 1983b). This calculation assumes that there was no change in base excess in the previous 24 h and that a climber resting on the summit had a negligible blood lactate concentration (see below). In addition, the measured alveolar P_{CO_2} of 7.5 mmHg is assumed to apply to the arterial blood.

A remarkable feature of these base excess values is that they were essentially unchanged from those measured in 14 subjects living for several weeks at Camp 2 (6300 m, P_B 351 mmHg) where the mean value was $-8.7 \pm 1.7\,\text{mmol}\,\text{l}^{-1}$. This suggests that base excess was changing extremely slowly above an altitude of 6300 m. The reason for this is not known but may be related to the chronic volume depletion which was observed in climbers living at 6300 m. At this altitude the serum osmolality was $302 \pm 4\,\text{mmol}\,\text{kg}^{-1}$ which was significantly higher ($P <$ 0.01) than in the same subjects at sea-level where the value was $290 \pm 1\,\text{mmol}\,\text{kg}^{-1}$ (Blume *et al.*, 1984). It is known that the kidney gives a higher priority to correcting dehydration than acid–base disturbances, and in order to excrete more bicarbonate to reduce the base excess, it would be necessary to lose corresponding cations which would aggravate the volume depletion. This may be the basis for the slow renal bicarbonate excretion.

These acid–base changes may be part of the explanation of why climbers can spend only a relatively short time at extreme altitudes, say above 8000 m. It was pointed out in Chapter 5 that the marked respiratory alkalosis which increases the oxygen affinity of the haemoglobin at extreme altitude is beneficial because it accelerates the loading of oxygen by the pulmonary capillaries. If a climber remains at extreme altitude for several days, presumably there is some renal excretion of bicarbonate (though this appears to be slow) and the resulting metabolic

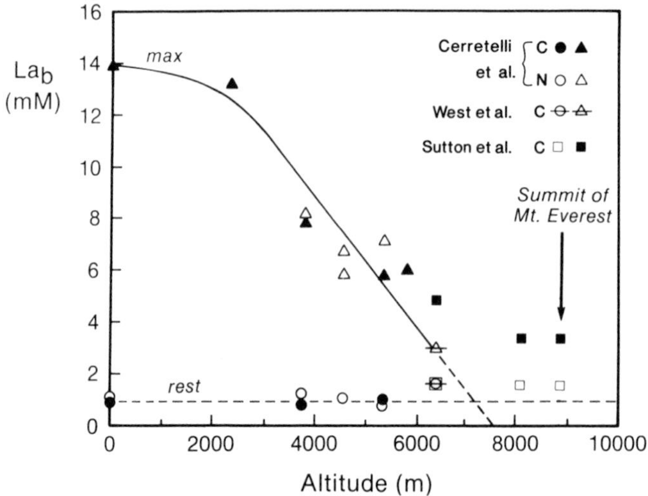

Figure 11.5 Maximal blood lactate La_b as a function of altitude. Most of the data are redrawn from Cerretelli (1980). The filled circles and triangles show data for acclimatized Caucasians (C); the open circles and triangles are for high-altitude natives (N). The data for 6300 m are from the AMREE for acclimatized lowlanders. (From West, 1986). The points marked Sutton *et al.* are from Operation Everest II (Sutton *et al.*, 1988).

compensation would move the pH back towards 7.4. Thus the advantage of a left-shifted dissociation curve would tend to be lost.

One way to counter this disadvantage during a climb of Mt Everest would be to set up the high camps and then return to base camp at a lower altitude for several days. This period at medium altitude would then allow the body to adjust again to this more moderate oxygen deprivation and enable the blood pH to stabilize nearer its normal value. The final summit assault would then be as rapid as possible to take advantage of the nearly uncompensated respiratory alkalosis. In fact this was the pattern adopted by Messner and Habeler in their first ascent of Mt Everest without supplementary oxygen in 1978.

Blood lactate is known to be very low in acclimatized subjects at high altitude even during maximal work, an observation first made by Edwards (1936) during the International High Altitude Expedition to Chile in 1935. Figure 11.5 shows data on resting and maximal blood lactate obtained by Cerretelli (1980). Also shown are measurements made at 6300 m after maximal exercise at the rate of 900 kg min^{-1}, that is, an oxygen uptake of 1.75 l min^{-1} (West, 1986). The mean value after exercise at 6300 m was only 3.0 mmol l^{-1} in spite of arterial P_{O_2} of less than 35 mmHg and, presumably, extreme tissue hypoxia. Note that extrapolation of the line relating maximal blood lactate concentration to altitude suggests that, after maximal exercise at altitudes exceeding 7500 m, there will be no increase in lactate in the blood at all in spite of the extreme oxygen deprivation. This is indeed a paradox.

It is worth noting that the blood lactate concentrations after maximal exercise were appreciably higher on Operation Everest II (Sutton *et al.*, 1988). For example, at an inspired P_{O_2} of 63 mmHg, the mean lactate concentration following maximal exercise was 4.7 mmol l^{-1}, that is about 56% higher than on the AMREE for the same inspired P_{O_2}. Moreover the 'summit' measurements on Operation Everest II gave a blood lactate concentration of 3.4 mmol l^{-1}, a higher value than that found at only 6300 m on the AMREE (Figure 11.5). It is known that the low lactate concentrations following maximal exercise at high altitude come about as a result of high-altitude acclimatization, because acute hypoxia causes very high lactate levels. Presumably therefore the higher values seen on Operation Everest II compared with the AMREE and other field studies can be explained by the limited degree of acclimatization.

The reasons for the low blood lactate levels following maximal exercise in well-acclimatized subjects at high altitude are unknown. One hypothesis is that the bicarbonate depletion which occurs as a result of acclimatization interferes with the buffering of released lactate and hydrogen ions, and the consequent fall in local pH inhibits the enzyme phosphofructokinase in the glycolytic cycle and thus puts a break on glycolysis (Figure 9.7). It is known that the activity of phosphofructokinase is reduced as the pH is lowered. Certainly Cerretelli has shown that the changes in blood H^+ concentration as a result of increases in blood lactate are higher in acclimatized than unacclimatized subjects (Cerretelli, 1980). However many other factors affect blood lactate and the issue is far from settled.

11.3.5 Cardiac output

Intuitively it would be reasonable to expect an increased cardiac output for a given work level at extreme altitude compared with sea-level. It is known that cardiac output increases as a result of acute hypoxia (Chapter 6). Furthermore, the oxygen concentration of the arterial blood is extremely low at very high altitude, and an increase in cardiac output would help to compensate for the reduced oxygen delivery. Paradoxically however, the relationship between cardiac output and oxygen uptake in acclimatized subjects at an altitude of 5800 m is essentially the same as at sea-level (Figure 6.2) and this apparently holds true even at extreme altitudes, although data are sparse. Reeves *et al.* (1987) showed that the sea-level relationship was maintained down to a barometric pressure of 282 mmHg, and almost maintained at an inspired P_{O_2} equivalent to the summit of Mt Everest, though at that extreme altitude the cardiac output appeared to be slightly higher (Figure 6.3). The explanation for the deviation at extreme altitude may be that the subjects were not fully acclimatized.

11.3.6 Pulmonary diffusing capacity

As discussed in Chapter 5, oxygen transfer during exercise at high altitude is, in part, diffusion-limited, and all calculations suggest that this limitation will be exaggerated at the extreme altitudes near the summit of Mt Everest. However very few data on diffusing capacity at high altitude are available. Available measurements at an altitude of 5800 m (P_B 380 mmHg) indicate that the diffusing capacity for carbon monoxide during exercise is essentially unchanged from the sea-level value except for the expected increase caused by the faster rate of combination of carbon monoxide with haemoglobin under the prevailing hypoxic conditions (West, 1962). These data suggest that the diffusing capacity of the pulmonary membrane itself is unaltered by acclimatization.

Measurements of the diffusing capacity for carbon monoxide at different alveolar P_{O_2} values allow calculation of the pulmonary capillary blood volume. Again, in measurements made at 5800 m altitude, there appeared to be little change in capillary blood volume although there was a suggestion that it was slightly lower, possibly as a result of hypoxic pulmonary vasoconstriction (West, 1962). If we accept the conclusion that capillary blood volume is unchanged, and that the cardiac output/oxygen consumption relationship is the same as at sea-level (section 11.3.5) this implies that capillary transit time in the lung is normal since this is given by capillary blood volume divided by cardiac output (Roughton, 1945).

Using these data it is possible to calculate the changes in P_{O_2} along the pulmonary capillary for a climber at rest on the summit of Mt Everest (Figure 5.4). This show that the rate of oxygenation is extremely slow and that the end-capillary P_{O_2} is much lower than the alveolar value, indicating severe diffusion limitation of oxygen transfer.

11.3.7 P_{O_2} of venous blood

During maximal exercise at extreme altitude, the extraction of oxygen by the peripheral tissues results in very low values of venous P_{O_2} in the exercising muscles. This in turn reduces the P_{O_2} of mixed venous blood. In order to analyse the relationships between the many variables and determine what limits exercise performance at extreme altitude, a reasonable assumption is that the body will not tolerate a P_{O_2} of mixed venous blood below a certain value, for example 15 mmHg (2.0 kPa) (West and Wagner, 1980; West, 1983). This assumption received strong support from Operation Everest II where direct measurements of the P_{O_2} in mixed venous blood gave very similar values (Sutton *et al.*, 1988). For example, on the 'summit' during 60 watts of exercise, the P_{O_2} of mixed venous blood had a mean value of 14.8 mmHg, and at 120 watts, which was the highest work level, the mean P_{O_2} was 13.8 mmHg.

11.3.8 Heat loss by hyperventilation

Mathews (1954) argued that tolerance to extreme altitude might be limited by the high rate of heat loss from the lungs as a result of the extreme hyperventilation. However, subsequent experience has not borne this out. Calculations of net heat loss are complex because the upper respiratory tract acts as a heat exchanger. During expiration, expired gas warms the respiratory tract, and this heat is then available to warm the cold inspired gas. Climbers who have reached the summit of Mt Everest without supplementary oxygen have not been affected by cold beyond the extent expected from the very low temperatures of the environment. When Pizzo reached the summit to take his alveolar gas samples during the course of the AMREE, he became overheated during the climb and photographs taken on the summit when he was breathing air show that he was not even wearing his down jacket which he carried with him stored in his backpack (West, 1985, facing p. 51).

11.3.9 Oxygen cost of ventilation

A climber at extreme altitude has considerable hyperventilation at rest, and even more during moderate exercise. An alveolar P_{CO_2} of 7.5 mmHg was measured on the Everest summit and, since it is known that the CO_2 production both at rest and for a given work level is independent of altitude, we can conclude that the alveolar ventilation on the summit was at least five times the resting value. Even small amounts of physical activity will greatly increase this. If we take the normal resting ventilation to be 7–8 l min^{-1}, this means that the resting ventilation on the summit is at least 40 l min^{-1}.

It is likely that the oxygen cost of this hyperventilation is a significant proportion of the resting oxygen consumption. Measurements at sea-level suggest that increasing the ventilation from 8 to 40 l min^{-1} increases the oxygen consumption by about 20–40 ml min^{-1} (Otis, 1964). However there is considerable variability in measurements of the oxygen cost of hyperventilation. In addition, at great altitudes where the density of the air is much less, the work of breathing is reduced (Petit *et al.*, 1963). Nevertheless it appears that the oxygen cost of ventilation may be 10% of the total oxygen uptake at rest, and that it contributes a higher proportion of the total oxygen uptake during moderate exercise. It is possible that the situation arises where an attempt at additional physical activity requires such an increase in ventilation that the resulting oxygen cost negates any additional external work.

11.4 WHAT LIMITS EXERCISE PERFORMANCE AT EXTREME ALTITUDE?

11.4.1 Concept of limitation

The oxygen cascade from the atmosphere to the mitochondria includes the processes of convective ventilation of oxygen to the alveoli, diffusion of oxygen across the blood–gas barrier, uptake of oxygen by the haemoglobin in the pulmonary capillaries, convective flow of the blood to the peripheral capillaries, unloading of the oxygen from the haemoglobin, diffusion to the mitochondria, and utilization of oxygen by the electron transport system. How can we determine which of these factors is (or are) limiting exercise at extreme altitude?

One approach is to use the analogy of a turbine which is fed by water flowing through a pipe which has a series of constrictions in it (Figure 11.6). Clearly all sections of the pipe limit the flow of water to some extent. However, a useful description of the extent to which flow is limited by any particular section of the pipe can be found by calculating the percentage change in total flow for a given (say 5%) change in diameter at that point. In carrying out this calculation, we assume that all other factors remain unchanged. Clearly such an analysis can only be carried out if the whole system is modelled using a computer.

11.4.2 Limitations to oxygen uptake on the summit of Mt Everest

The model analysis described above has been carried out for a hypothetical subject exercising on the summit of Mt Everest (West, 1983). A number of assumptions and extrapolations are necessary because so few data have yet been obtained at these great altitudes. In general, the physiological variables were those set out in section 11.3. Table 11.2 summarizes some of the key variables. The whole oxygen transport system was modelled using numerical procedures previously described (West and Wagner, 1977; West and Wagner, 1980).

Figure 11.7 shows the calculated changes in the P_{O_2} of alveolar gas,

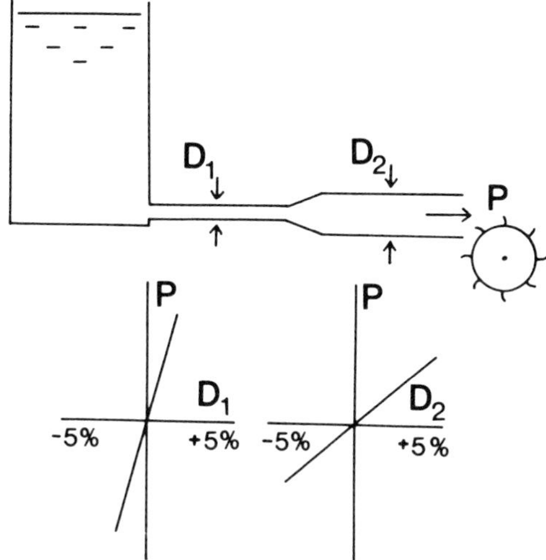

Figure 11.6 Hydraulic analogy to clarify the concept of limitation of oxygen transfer. Each part of the pipe limits the flow of water to some extent. However the extent of the limitation can be determined by noting the change in flow for a given (say 5%) change in diameter (D) at a particular point. P is pressure at turbine.

arterial blood, and mixed venous blood as the oxygen uptake is increased for a climber on the summit of Mt Everest. For clarity, a maximum membrane oxygen diffusing capacity of 100 ml min^{-1} mmHg^{-1} has been used for all values of oxygen uptake, though in practice the diffusing capacity would presumably be smaller at the lower work levels. Note the relentless fall in the P_{O_2} of the arterial and mixed venous bloods as the oxygen demand is increased. The decrease in arterial P_{O_2} in the face of a constant or rising alveolar P_{O_2} is the hallmark of diffusion-limited oxygen transfer. The slight rise in alveolar P_{O_2} at low work levels reflects the assumed increase in respiratory exchange ratio (R) from 0.8 at rest to 1.0 on moderate exercise.

To calculate maximal oxygen uptake ($\dot{V}_{O_2}$ max) it was assumed that the P_{O_2} of mixed venous blood could not fall below 15 mmHg. As discussed in section 11.3.7, direct measurements of the P_{O_2} of mixed venous blood during Operation Everest II support this assumption. The calculated $\dot{V}_{O_2}$ max shown in Figure 11.8 of just over 1 l min^{-1} agrees well with results obtained on the AMREE when well-acclimatized subjects performed maximal exercise with an inspired P_{O_2} of 42.5 mmHg, equivalent to that on the Everest summit (West *et al.*, 1983a). In addition, essentially the same value for $\dot{V}_{O_2}$ max was reported by Sutton *et*

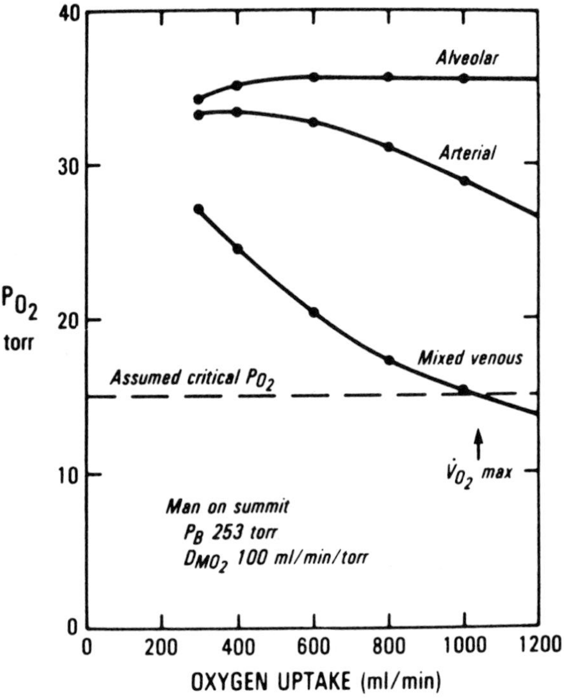

Figure 11.7 Predicted changes in the P_{O_2} of alveolar gas and arterial and mixed venous blood as oxygen uptake is increased for a climber on the summit of Mt Everest. It is assumed that $\dot{V}_{O_2}$ max will occur when P_{O_2} of venous blood falls to 15 torr. Lower values of venous P_{O_2} may allow higher values of $\dot{V}_{O_2}$. (From West, 1983.) (1 torr = 1 mmHg)

Table 11.2 Key variables for analysis factors limiting oxygen uptake on the summit of Mt Everest

Measured	
Barometric pressure	253 mmHg
Alveolar P_{CO_2}	7.5 mmHg
Haemoglobin concentration	$18.4\,g\,dl^{-1}$
P_{50} at pH 7.4	29.6 mmHg
Base excess	$-7.2\,mmol\,l^{-1}$
Assumed	
Respiratory exchange ratio	1.0
Cardiac output/O_2 uptake	Same as sea-level
Maximal DM_{O_2}*	$100\,ml\,min^{-1}\,mmHg^{-1}$
Capillary transit time	0.75 s

1 mmHg = 1 torr
* DM_{O_2} = diffusing capacity of the membrane for oxygen

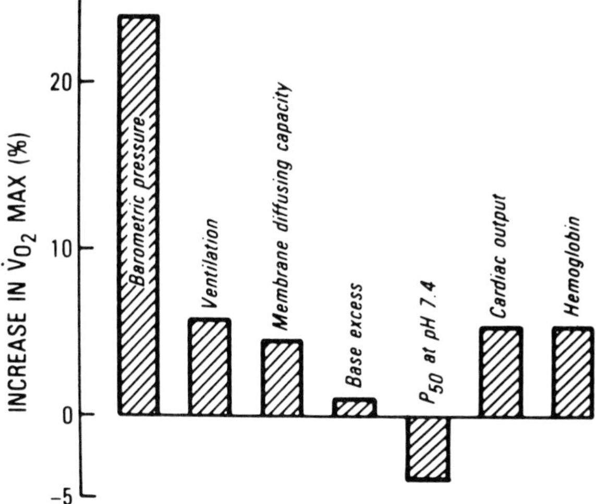

Figure 11.8 Sensitivity of calculated maximal oxygen consumption to changes in variables for a climber on the summit of Mt Everest. The initial conditions are those shown in Table 11.2, and each variable was increased by 5% leaving all the others constant. Refer to text for details. (From West, 1983.)

al. (1988) in their measurements during Operation Everest II when the subjects had an inspired P_{O_2} of 43 mmHg.

Figure 11.8 shows the sensitivity of $\dot{V}_{O_2}$ max to the variables in this theoretical study using the type of analysis shown in Figure 11.6. Note that the calculated $\dot{V}_{O_2}$ max is exquisitely sensitive to barometric pressure, a 5% increase in this variable resulting in a 25% increase in $\dot{V}_{O_2}$ max when all the other variables were held constant. This is the basis for the assertion made in section 11.3.2 that even day by day variations of barometric pressure at these extreme altitudes may measurably effect exercise performance.

Figure 11.8 also shows that $\dot{V}_{O_2}$ max is very sensitive to the level of alveolar ventilation and the magnitude of the membrane oxygen diffusing capacity. The ventilation is important because any increase raises the alveolar P_{O_2}. The diffusing capacity is important because oxygen transfer under these conditions is diffusion-limited (Chapter 5).

An increase in base excess results in a small rise in calculated $\dot{V}_{O_2}$ max. The reason is that for a given level of ventilation, and therefore arterial P_{CO_2}, a rise in base excess causes an increase in pH which moves the oxygen dissociation curve further to the left and increases the oxygen affinity of the haemoglobin. This assists in the loading of oxygen in the pulmonary capillaries (section 5.3.7).

By the same token, an increase in P_{50} of the oxygen dissociation curve reduces the calculated $\dot{V}_{O_2}$ max. The reason is the same: a reduced oxygen affinity of haemoglobin slows down the loading of oxygen in the pulmonary capillaries. This is an interesting point because it has often been claimed that the increase in 2,3-diphosphoglycerate which is seen in the red cells at high altitude is a useful feature of acclimatization (Lenfant *et al.*, 1971).

Increases of cardiac output and haemoglobin would also theoretically improve the $\dot{V}_{O_2}$ max. However there are reasons to believe that these apparent gains would not be realized in practice. As discussed in Chapter 6, the relationship between cardiac output and $\dot{V}_{O_2}$ max in acclimatized subjects at high altitude appears to be the same as at sea-level, in spite of the apparent advantage that an increased blood flow would have in delivering more oxygen to the tissues. Increases in polycythaemia may also be deleterious. High values of haematocrit cause flow abnormalities in small blood vessels including unevenness of blood flow and sludging of red cells, and it is possible that these untoward effects outweigh the possible advantages of an increased arterial oxygen concentration.

The chief conclusions from the analysis shown in Figure 11.8 are as follows:

- A climber attempting an ascent of Mt Everest without supplementary oxygen should ideally choose a day with a relatively high barometric pressure. Indeed this appears to be the most critical variable. Fortunately climbers generally try to make a summit assault when the weather is fine and usually this means a high pressure. Note however that this factor makes a winter ascent of Mt Everest without supplementary oxygen particularly difficult.
- The climber should have a high hypoxic ventilatory response because this is critical in maintaining an adequate alveolar P_{O_2}.
- It is advantageous to have a high oxygen diffusing capacity at a moderate work level.
- The climber should have as high a base excess as possible. Presumably one way to ensure this is to avoid prolonged stays at extreme altitudes.
- Any rise in the level of 2,3-diphosphoglycerate in the red cell is a liability because it increases the P_{50} and interferes with the loading of oxygen by the pulmonary capillaries.
- From a theoretical point of view, increases in cardiac output and haemoglobin concentration are advantageous to the oxygen transport system but in practice these advantages may not be realized.

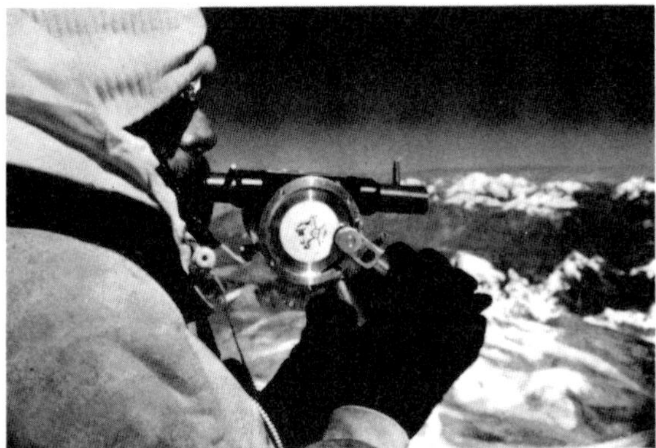

Figure 11.9 Dr Chris Pizzo taking alveolar gas samples on the summit of Everest (8848 m) (taken during the American Medical Research Expedition to Everest, October 1981).

11.4.3 How high can man climb without supplementary oxygen?

We have seen that the $\dot{V}_{O_2}$ max in acclimatized subjects with an inspired P_{O_2} of 43 mmHg equivalent to that on the Everest summit, is only a little over $1\,l\,min^{-1}$. This oxygen uptake is equivalent to walking slowly on level ground. Clearly man at the highest point on earth is very close to the limit of hypoxic tolerance.

Nevertheless, it is interesting to speculate on how much higher man could climb. The answer from Figure 11.8 seems to be very little. For example, only a 5% decrease in barometric pressure from 253 to 240 mmHg is calculated to reduce the $\dot{V}_{O_2}$ max by 25%, or to less than $800\,ml\,min^{-1}$. This would occur at an altitude of about 9250 m at the latitude of Everest, that is 400 m above the summit. Note also that the pressure of 240 mmHg is still above that predicted for the summit of Mt Everest by the standard atmosphere (Chapter 2), indicating again that it is only the equatorial bulge in barometric pressure (Figures 2.3 and 2.5) which allows man to reach the highest mountain top without supplementary oxygen.

REFERENCES

Acosta, J. de (1590) *Historia Natural y Moral de las Indias* . . . Iuan de Leon, Seville, Lib. 3, Cap. 9.

Bert, P. *La Pression Barométrique*. (1878) Masson, Paris, English translation by M.A. Hitchcock and F.A. Hitchcock. College Book Company, Columbus, Ohio, (1943).

Blume, F.D., Boyer, S.J., Braverman, L.E. and Cohen A. (1984) Impaired osmoregulation at high altitude. *J. Am. Med. Assoc.*, **252**, 1580–5.

Cerretelli, P. (1980) Gas exchange at high altitude, in *Pulmonary Gas Exchange*, Vol. 2, (ed. J.B. West), Academic Press, New York, pp. 97–147.

De Saussure, H.B. (1786–1798) *Voyages dans les alpes*, 4 Vol., Louis Fauche-Borel, Neuchatel.

Edwards, H.T. (1936) Lactic acid in rest and work at high altitude. *Am. J. Physiol.*, **116**, 367–75.

Filippi, F. de (1912) *Karakorum and Western Himalaya*, Constable, London.

Gill, M.G., Milledge, J.S., Pugh, L.G.C.E. and West J.B. (1962) Alveolar gas composition at 21 000 to 25 000 ft (6400–7830 m). *J. Physiol. (London)*, **163**, 373–7.

Greene, R. (1934) Observations on the composition of alveolar air on Everest. *J. Physiol. (London)*, **32**, 481–5.

Hinchliff, T.W. (1876) *Over the Sea and Far Away*, Longmans Green, London.

Hunt, J. (1953) *The Ascent of Everest*, Hodder and Stoughton, London.

Jourdanet, D. (1875) *Influence de la Pression de l'Air sur la Vie de l'Homme*, Masson, Paris.

Kellas, A.M. (1921) Sur les possibilites de faire l'ascension du Mount Everest. *Congres de l'Alpinisme, Monaco, 1920. Comptes Rendus des Seances*, Paris, **1**, 451–521.

Lenfant, C., Torrance, J.D. and Reynafarje, C. (1971) Shift of the O_2–Hb dissociation curve at altitude: mechanism and effect. *J. Appl. Physiol.*, **30**, 625–31.

Malconian, M.K., Rock, P.B., Reeves, J.T., Houston, C.S., *et al.* (1993) Operation Everest II: Gas tensious in expired air and arterial blood at extreme altitude. *Aviat. Space Environ. Med.*, **64**, 37–42.

Mathews, B. (1954) Limiting factors at high altitude. *Proc. R. Soc. London Ser. B.*, **143**, 1–4.

Messner, R. (1979) *Everest: Expedition to the Ultimate*, Kaye & Ward, London.

Messner, R. (1981) At my limit. *Natl Geogr.*, **160**, 553–66.

Otis, A.B. (1964) The work of breathing, in *Handbook of Physiology Respiration*, Vol. 1, American Physiological Society, Washington DC, pp. 463–76.

Petit, J.M., Milic-Emili, G. and Troquet, J. (1963) Travail dynamique pulmonaire et altitude. *Rev. Med. Aeronautique*, **2**, 276–9.

Pugh, L.G.C.E. (1957) Resting ventilation and alveolar air on Mount Everest: with remarks on the relation of barometric pressure to altitude in mountains. *J. Physiol. (London)*, **135**, 590–610.

Pugh, L.G.C.E., Gill, M.G., Lahiri, S., *et al.* (1964) Muscular exercise at great altitude. *J. Appl. Physiol.*, **19**, 431–40.

Rahn, H. and Otis, A.B. (1949) Man's respiratory response during and after acclimatization to high altitude. *Am. J. Physiol.*, **157**, 445–9.

Riley, R.L. and Houston, C.S. (1951) Composition of alveolar air and volume of pulmonary ventilation during long exposure to high altitude. *J. Appl. Physiol.*, **3**, 526–34.

Reeves, J.T., Groves, B.M., Sutton, J.R., *et al.* (1987) Operation Everest II: preservation of cardiac function at extreme altitude. *J. Appl. Physiol.*, **63**, 531–69.

Roughton, F.J. (1945) Average time spent by blood in human lung capillary and its relation to the rates of CO uptake and elimination in man. *Am. J. Physiol.*, **143**, 621–33.

Schoene, R.B., Lahiri, S., Hackett, P.H., *et al.* (1984) Relationship of hypoxic ventilatory response to exercise performance on Mount Everest. *J. Appl. Physiol.*, **56**, 1478–83.

Somervell, T.H. (1925) Note on the composition of alveolar air at extreme heights. *J. Physiol. (London)*, **60**, 282–5.

Sutton, J.R., Reeves, J.T., Wagner, P.D., *et al.* (1988) Operation Everest II: oxygen transport during exercise at extreme simulated altitude. *J. Appl. Physiol.*, **64**, 1309–21.

Warren, C.B.M. (1939) Alveolar air on Mount Everest. *J. Physiol. (London)*, **96**, 34–5.

West, J.B. (1962) Diffusing capacity of the lung for carbon monoxide at high altitude. *J. Appl. Physiol.*, **17**, 421–6.

West, J.B. (1983) Climbing Mt Everest without supplementary oxygen: an analysis of maximal exercise during extreme hypoxia. *Respir. Physiol.*, **52**, 265–79.

West, J.B. (1985) *Everest – The Testing Place*, McGraw-Hill, New York.

West, J.B. (1986) Lactate during exercise at extreme altitude. *Fed. Proc.*, **45**, 2953–7.

West, J.B. (1988) Rate of ventilatory acclimatization to extreme altitude. *Respir. Physiol.*, **74**, 323–33.

West, J.B. and Wagner, P.D. (1977) Pulmonary gas exchange, in *Bioengineering Aspects of the Lung*, (ed. J.B. West), Marcel Dekker, New York, pp. 361–457.

West, J.B. and Wagner, P.D. (1980) Predicted gas exchange on the summit of Mt Everest. *Respir. Physiol.*, **42**, 1–16.

West, J.B., Boyer, S.J., Graber, D.J., *et al.* (1983a) Maximal exercise at extreme altitudes on Mount Everest. *J. Appl. Physiol.*, **55**, 688–98.

West, J.B., Hackett, P.H., Maret, K.H., *et al.* (1983b) Pulmonary gas exchange on the summit of Mount Everest. *J. Appl. Physiol.*, **55**, 678–87.

West, J.B., Lahiri, S., Maret, K.H., *et al.* (1983c) Barometric pressures at extreme altitudes on Mt Everest: physiological significance. *J. Appl. Physiol.*, **54**, 1188–94.

Whymper, E. (1891) *Travels Amongst the Great Andes of the Equator*, Murray, London.

Zuntz, N., Lowey, A., Muller, F. and Caspari, W. (1906) Atmospheric pressure at high altitudes, in *Höhenklima und Bergwanderungen in ihrer Wirkung auf den Menschen*. Bong, Berlin. An English translation (1981) of the relevant pages can be found in *High Altitude Physiology*, (ed. J.B. West), Hutchinson Ross, Stroudsburg PA, pp. 78–80.

12

Sleep

12.1 INTRODUCTION

Everyone who has been to high altitude knows that sleeping is often impaired. This ubiquitous problem affects the skier or trekker who sleeps at altitudes of 2500–3000 m, as well as the well-acclimatized climber who spends a night as high as 8000 m. The altitude of many modern skiing resorts is over 2700 m (8900 ft) and many people who move rapidly from sea-level to that altitude have difficulties with sleep for the first two or three nights. Often they cannot get to sleep for a long period, or they wake frequently, and often they complain in the morning they do not awake refreshed. This last comment is also frequently heard from climbers at great altitudes on expeditions (Pugh and Ward, 1956). Some people trying to sleep at high altitude complain that the mind races with a kaleidoscope of thoughts tumbling through it; this is certainly the case with the writer who recognizes this as a very characteristic feature of the first night or two at high altitude.

Climbers at high altitude are often urged to climb high during the day but sleep low during the night. This advice acknowledges the increased incidence of difficulties during sleep. Many climbers over an altitude of about 7000 m find that a very low flow of supplementary oxygen of perhaps $1 \, l \, min^{-1}$ greatly improves the quality of sleep.

Periodic breathing during sleep at high altitude has been recognized since the last century. It is extremely common and may pose a hazard at extreme altitude because of the severe arterial hypoxaemia which follows the apnoeic periods (West *et al.*, 1986). Indeed this may be one of the factors that influences tolerance to very great altitudes. From a scientific point of view, periodic breathing during sleep at high altitude throws light on the control of breathing under these special conditions.

The present chapter overlaps the material of Chapter 4 on the control of ventilation, and also has some links with Chapter 6 on cardiovascular responses because of the alterations in heart rate that occur with periodic breathing.

12.2 HISTORICAL

12.2.1 Quality of sleep

There have been a number of anectodal references to the poor quality of sleep at high altitude. A particularly colourful description was given by Barcroft when he recounted his experiences during the glass chamber experiment carried out at Cambridge (Barcroft *et al.*, 1920). On this occasion he spent six days in a closed chamber in which the concentration of oxygen was regulated so that the initial equivalent altitude was 10 000 ft (3048 m) and the final altitude 16 000 ft (4877 m). He wrote:

> In the glass case experiment I had the opportunity of judging a little more exactly of anoxaemic sleeplessness than is usually the case. A committee of undergraduate pupils of mine made up their minds that I was never to be left alone, two of them therefore sat up each night outside the case lest help of any sort should be required. I used to ask them in the morning how I had slept, and each morning except perhaps the last they said I had slept well. My own view of the matter was quite otherwise. I thought I had been awake half the night and was unrefreshed in the morning. I was conscious of their moving about and looking in through the glass to see whether or not I was awake. I used to count my pulse at intervals. The two opinions can only be reconciled on the hypothesis that whilst I spent most of the night in sleep, the slumber was very light and fitful with incessant dreams. Even some low degree of consciousness which fell short of wakefulness. At Cerro it was the same: measured in hours we slept well, but the quality of the sleep in most cases was of an inferior order. The night seemed long and we woke unrefreshed. *(Barcroft, 1925)*

12.2.2 Periodic breathing

Various references to the uneven pattern of breathing during sleep at high altitude were made during the last century. One was by the eminent English physicist Tyndall who was one of the most ardent Alpine mountaineers in the middle of the century. Paul Bert commented that 'every year sees him planting his alpenstock on some new summit' (Bert, 1878). During Tyndall's first ascent of Mont Blanc in 1857, he became very fatigued. 'I stretched myself upon a composite couch of snow and granite, and immediately fell asleep. My friend, however, soon aroused me "You quite frighten me" he said, "I listened for some minutes and have not heard you breathe once."' On renewing the ascent, Tyndall complained of palpitations. 'At each pause my heart throbbed audibly, as I leaned upon my staff, and the subsidence of this action was always the signal for further advance' (Tyndall, 1860).

Another early comment on periodic breathing was made by Egli-Sinclair (1894) in an article on mountain sickness. He noted that at an altitude of 4400 m, respiration 'had the Stokes character, that is, it seemed regular during a certain time, after which a few rapid and profound breaths were drawn, a total suspension of a few seconds then following.' Here he was referring to the Irish physician, Dr William Stokes, who described the pattern of breathing which 'consists in the occurrence of a series of inspirations, increasing to a maximum and then declining in force and length until a state of apparent apnoea is established' (Stokes, 1854). Another Irish physician, John Cheyne had described the same pattern in 1818 (Cheyne, 1818) and so the breathing pattern is often known as Cheyne–Stokes breathing. However Ward (1973) pointed out that John Hunter had given a lucid and succinct description of the same condition in 1781 (Hunter, 1781).

The first extensive studies of periodic breathing at high altitude were made by Angelo Mosso, professor of physiology at the University of Turin, Italy. As mentioned earlier, he was responsible for the construction of the Capanna Regina Margherita on the Monte Rosa at an altitude of 4559 m. He measured the breathing movements by means of a pneumograph around the chest and abdomen. An example of one of his measurements on his brother, Ugolino Mosso, is shown in Figure 12.1(a). The periods of apnoea lasted about 12 s. Note that in this instance, the first breath after the apnoeic period was the largest. A more typical pattern is that shown in Figure 12.1(b) which was obtained on Francioli, keeper of the Regina Margherita hut. In this instance the waxing and waning of breathing movements is clearly seen and the periods of apnoea are shorter (Mosso, 1898).

A curious feature of Mosso's measurements was that he concluded that ventilation was actually decreased at high altitude, apparently because he converted his readings to standard conditions (0°C and 1000 mmHg in his case) rather than BTPS (body temperature and pressure saturated). Interestingly, Paul Bert also believed that hyperventilation did not occur at high altitude (Bert, 1878; p. 106 in the 1943 translation). He wrote, 'What is really certain is that . . . a dweller in lofty altitudes, does not even try to struggle against the decrease of oxygen is his arterial blood by speeding up his respirations excessively, as was first supposed. The observations of Dr Jourdanet are conclusive.' Bert probably reached this conclusion because he worked exclusively with low-pressure chambers that only allowed short term observations. It was not until Mosso built the Capanna Regina Margherita a few years later that measurements were easily made on subjects exposed to

(a)

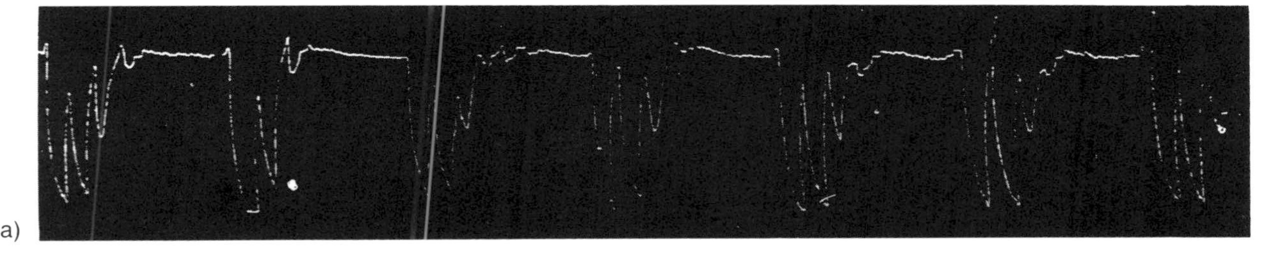

(b)

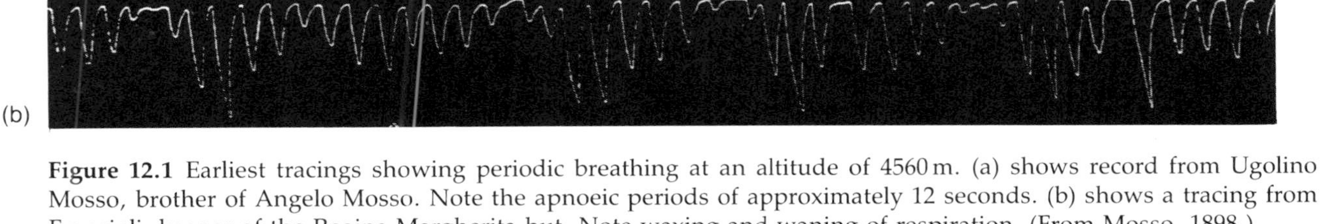

Figure 12.1 Earliest tracings showing periodic breathing at an altitude of 4560 m. (a) shows record from Ugolino Mosso, brother of Angelo Mosso. Note the apnoeic periods of approximately 12 seconds. (b) shows a tracing from Francioli, keeper of the Regina Margherita hut. Note waxing and waning of respiration. (From Mosso, 1898.)

high altitude for several days although, as indicated above, he thought that ventilation was decreased.

Mosso realized that the alveolar P_{CO_2} was reduced in people living in the Capanna Regina Margherita at 4559 m, but instead of attributing this to an increased ventilation, he argued that the low pressure at high altitude extracted carbon dioxide from the blood just as does a mercury pump in a blood–gas analysis apparatus. Barcroft (1925) could not follow Mosso's argument and remarked: 'I speak with all deference, but Mosso seems to me to have overlooked the fact that the body is exposed to what is practically a vacuum of CO_2, whether it be at the Capanna Margherita or in his own laboratory at Turin.' Mosso introduced the term 'acapnia' to refer to the reduction of P_{CO_2} and believed that this was an important factor in the development of acute mountain sickness. Indeed it may well be that the symptoms of this condition are related in part to the respiratory alkalosis. However Barcroft (1925) pointed out that Mosso's theory was not supported by their experience at the Alta Vista hut (3350 m) on Mt Tenerife during the First International High Altitude Expedition of 1910. Barcroft had an almost normal alveolar P_{CO_2} (38 mmHg) but was incapacitated by the altitude, whereas Douglas whose P_{CO_2} was only 32 mmHg was 'perfectly free from all symptoms'. Thus hypoxia (which was more severe in Barcroft because he did not increase his ventilation) rather than the low P_{CO_2} was implicated in the aetiology of mountain sickness.

12.3 PHYSIOLOGY OF SLEEP

In spite of the fact that we spend up to one-third of our lives in the sleeping state, the physiology is not completely understood. Sleep can be defined as a state of unconsciousness from which the subject can be aroused by sensory or other stimuli. As such it can be distinguished from deep anaesthesia and diseased states which cause coma, though these have some features in common with true sleep.

Two major types of sleep are recognized.

12.3.1 Slow wave sleep (SWS)

This is often called non-REM (rapid eye movement) or NREM sleep, or sometimes normal sleep. It is characterized by decreased activity of the reticular activating system, and is called slow wave sleep because of the predominance of slow delta waves in the EEG. These slow waves have a high voltage and occur at a rate of one or two per second. In the early stages of sleep, the alpha rhythm (8–13 Hz), which is always present during wakefulness, becomes more obvious. In addition, sleep spindles (14–16 Hz) may appear. These features are sometimes used to divide SWS into four stages (I–IV). The delta waves probably originate in the cortex of the brain when it is not driven from below because of the reduced level of activity of the reticular activating system. Slow wave sleep is dreamless, very restful, and associated with a decreased peripheral vascular tone, blood pressure, respiratory rate and basal metabolic rate.

12.3.2 Paradoxical or REM sleep

This is called REM (rapid eye movement) sleep because, although the eyes remain closed, there are rapid horizontal eye movements. In a normal night of sleep, bouts of REM sleep lasting 5–20 min usually appear on the average about every 90 min. Often the first such period occurs 80–100 min after the subject falls asleep. The EEG tracing resembles the waking state, but the person is actually more difficult to arouse than during NREM sleep. REM sleep is usually associated with active dreaming; the muscle tone throughout the body is greatly depressed, but there may be occasional muscular twitching and limb jerking. The heart rate and respiration usually become irregular. Thus in this type of sleep, the brain is quite active but the activity is not channelled in the proper direction for the person to be aware of his surroundings.

In experimental animals, sleep can be produced by electrically stimulating the raphe nuclei in the pons and medulla. There are extensive nerve fibre connections between these nuclei and the reticular formation. These nerve fibres secrete serotonin and some physiologists believe that this is a major transmitter substance associated with the production of sleep. However other possible transmitter substances may play a role in the onset of sleep.

Sleep deprivation impairs mental function, the higher brain functions being the most susceptible. There are similarities between the behaviour of sleep-deprived subjects and people at high altitude whose brains are affected by the hypoxia. In both instances, mental activities which are 'mechanical' in nature, such as tabulating a set of data, can be accurately accomplished, whereas activities that require problem solving and initiative are seriously affected (Chapter 15). It may be that some of the impairment of CNS function in individuals living at high altitude can be ascribed to the poor quality of sleep, but the direct effects of hypoxia on the brain also clearly play a role.

12.4 CHARACTERISTICS OF SLEEP AT HIGH ALTITUDE

12.4.1 Increased frequency of arousals

Persons at high altitude often report that they wake more frequently during the night than at sea-level, and this is confirmed by careful studies (Reite *et al.*, 1975; Weil *et al.*, 1978). The subjects had continuous recordings of the EEG, electromyogram (EMG) and eye movements, and an arousal was recognized by the occurrence of EMG activation, eye movements and alpha wave activity on the EEG. In one study an average of 36 arousals per night occurred at an altitude of 4300 m compared with 20 at sea-level (Weil *et al.*, 1978). Administration of the drug acetazolamide, which is known to stimulate ventilation at high altitude, reduced the frequency of arousals.

Some investigators believe that the arousals are caused in some way by periodic breathing. There is some evidence that arousals are more frequent when the strength of periodic breathing is high. It is easy to imagine that the strenuous muscular activity required to generate large breaths after a prolonged period of apnoea could contribute to an arousal. A common nightmare at high altitude is that the tent has been covered with snow by an avalanche and the subject wakes violently feeling suffocated and very short of breath. This may be associated with the air hunger caused by a long apnoeic period as part of periodic breathing. However arousals are more frequent at high altitude even in individuals who do not have periodic breathing (Reite *et al.*, 1975).

12.4.2 Changes of sleep state

EEG studies confirm that there is a deterioration in the quality of sleep at high altitude. Light sleep (stages I and II of NREM) is increased whereas there are decreases both in deep sleep (stages III and IV of NREM) and in REM sleep. In some studies, REM sleep is virtually abolished (Megirian *et al.*, 1980; Pappenheimer, 1977). These studies of the electrical activity of the brain support the subjective conclusions of climbers that sleep at high altitude is often of poor quality, and not as refreshing as sleep at sea-level.

Studies on rats by Pappenheimer (1977, 1984) have clarified the alterations in sleep at high altitude. In one study rats were exposed to 10% oxygen, equivalent to an altitude of approximately 5490 m. The proportion of time spent in slow wave (NREM) sleep was measured from EEG recordings via chronically implanted cortical electrodes. Rats typically sleep on and off during the day, and during this period the proportion of time spent in slow wave sleep was 45% when the rats breathed air, but only 27% when they breathed the low oxygen mixture. Adding carbon dioxide to the inspired gas failed to prevent the reduction of slow wave sleep during hypoxia. This indicated that the effects of hypoxia on sleep depended on the changes in P_{O_2} rather than the changes in P_{CO_2}.

The effect of sleep and hypoxia on the pattern of breathing was also studied. Slow wave sleep decreased breathing frequency and minute volume by 10–20%. However when the animals inhaled the hypoxic mixture, the frequency increased markedly when the animals entered slow wave sleep though the minute volume was not significantly changed. It was concluded that stimulation of breathing by hypoxia was greater during slow wave sleep than during wakefulness.

In a subsequent study (Pappenheimer, 1984) the amplitudes of the cortical slow waves were measured during NREM sleep, and the relative amounts of REM and NREM sleep were also assessed. It was found that acute exposure of rats to 10.5% O_2 (5030 m altitude equivalent) during daylight hours virtually abolished REM sleep. In addition, the distribution of amplitudes of the EEG of slow wave sleep shifted towards the values seen in awake animals. Adding carbon monoxide to the inspired gas sufficient to increase the concentration of carboxyhaemoglobin to 35% did not alter respiration rate and alveolar ventilation. It was therefore inferred that hypoxic stimulation of sleep was not mediated by peripheral chemoreceptors regulating breathing.

Pappenheimer also measured the amplitude of the cortical slow waves during sleep and showed that this was greatly reduced at the simulated high altitude (Figure 12.2). In fact the primary effects of hypoxia were to reduce the amplitude of the EEG slow waves, and to shift the distribution of amplitudes towards the awake values as shown in Figure 12.2. He suggested that this reduction in amplitude reflected the poor quality of the NREM sleep. In other words, even if the duration of NREM sleep as determined by conventional EEG recordings is not greatly reduced at high altitude, the quality of the NREM sleep may be greatly impaired. This conclusion fits with the assessments of the poor quality of sleep at high altitude given by many climbers, and Barcroft's colourful description quoted in section 12.2.1.

12.5 PERIODIC BREATHING

12.5.1 Characteristics

Early records of chest movements during periodic breathing are shown in Figure 12.1. This pattern has now been confirmed in many studies carried out at various altitudes from sea-level up to an altitude of 8050 m (Douglas and Haldane, 1909; Douglas *et al.*, 1913; Weil *et al.*, 1978; Sutton *et al.*, 1979; Berssenbrugge *et al.*, 1983; Lahiri *et al.*, 1983; West *et al.*, 1986).

A typical pattern recorded at an altitude of 6300 m (P_B 351 mmHg in a well-acclimatized lowlander using modern equipment is shown in Figure 12.3 (West *et al.*, 1986). Note that the tidal volume waxed and waned during each burst of breathing with apnoeic periods of about 8 s. Arterial oxygen saturation as measured by ear oximeter fluctuated

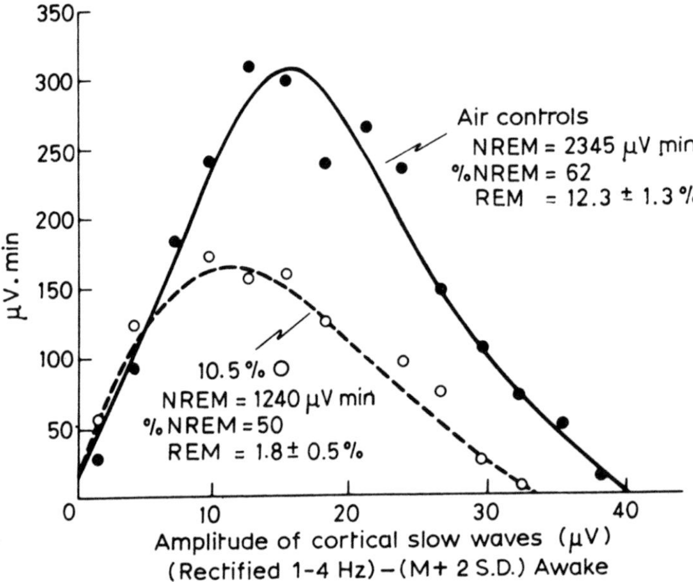

Figure 12.2 Effects of acute hypoxia on EEG pattern of sleeping rats. The ordinate shows the product of EEG amplitude and time. Hypoxia shifts the distribution of slow waves to lower amplitudes (light sleep), and reduces the amount of both NREM and REM sleep. (From Pappenheimer, 1984.)

with the same frequency as the periodic breathing. Note the phase difference; the highest arterial oxygen saturation (inverted scale) occurred at approximately the end of the apnoeic period. This can be accounted for by the circulation time from the lung capillaries to the ear where the oxygen saturation was measured. Heart rate was measured from the ECG and showed marked fluctuations with the same frequency as the periodic breathing. Note that the highest heart rate appeared at the end of the burst of ventilation.

Nocturnal periodic breathing is extremely common in lowlanders who ascend to high altitude. In the study from which Figure 12.3 is taken, all eight subjects who were living at an altitude of 6300 m showed obvious periodic breathing during the several weeks over which the measurements were made.

Table 12.1 shows some of the features of periodic breathing during this study. Measurements were made over a period of about 1–3.5 h late at night and the proportion of the study period during which periodic breathing was seen varied between 57% and 90%. In general the percentage of time occupied by periodic breathing increases with altitude. For example Waggener *et al.* (1984) reported that periodic

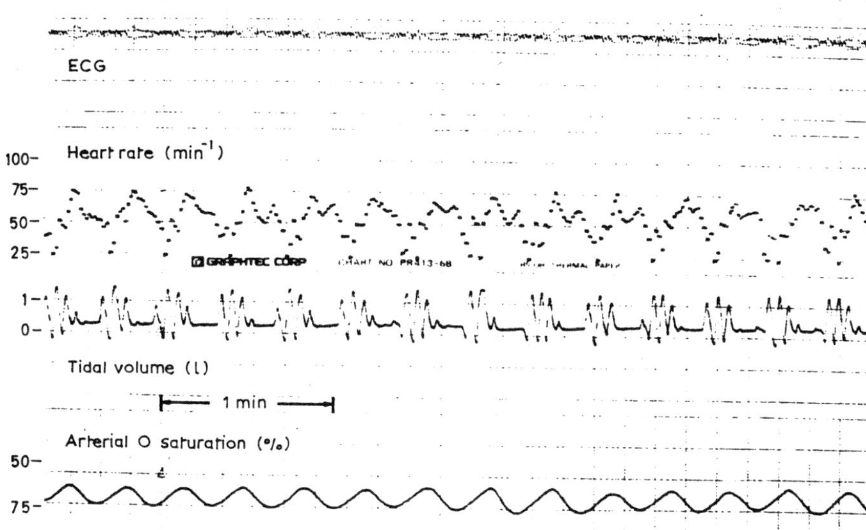

Figure 12.3 Example of periodic breathing at altitude 6300 m (P_B 351 mmHg). (From West *et al.*, 1986.)

breathing with apnoea occupied 24% of the time at 2440 m, and that the percentage increased to 40% at 4270 m. This increase in proportion of time is consistent with a theoretical model discussed below (Khoo *et al.*, 1982) and with the fact that periodic breathing is occasionally observed during sleep at sea-level but the proportion of time spent in periodic breathing is small (Goodman, 1964; Lenfant, 1967; Priban, 1963).

In the AMREE study from which Figure 12.3 is taken, we were not able to determine how much of the time the subjects were actually asleep. However other studies have shown that periodic breathing is very common during NREM sleep at high altitude, but that it is uncommon during REM periods (Reite *et al.*, 1975; Berssenbrugge *et al.*, 1983). Of course, as indicated above, REM sleep itself is uncommon at high altitude.

Table 12.1 shows that the duration of the periodic breathing cycle had a mean of 20.5 s. This was the same as the cycle length measured in a companion study at 5400 m (Lahiri *et al.*, 1983). There is evidence that cycle length decreases with increasing altitude (Waggener *et al.*, 1984) and studies at sea-level indicate a cycle period of about 30 s (Douglas and Haldane, 1909; Lugaresi *et al.*, 1978; Specht and Fruhmann, 1972). Figure 12.4 shows a plot of cycle time against altitude for several experimental studies and the theoretical model developed by Khoo *et*

Table 12.1 Features of periodic breathing at 6300 m altitude

Subject	*Age (yr)*	*Duration of study (min)*	*% of time definite periodic breathing*	*% of time uncertain periodic breathing*	*No. of periodic breathing cycles analysed*	*Cycle length of periodic breathing (s)*	*Apnoea/ cycle ratio*	*Duration of apnoea (s)*
RP	25	94	85.3	0	80	17.9	0.42	7.5
DG	30	97	61.3	12.5	61	23.4	0.38	8.8
CP	31	62	90.0	2.6	59	19.5	0.36*	7.0
CK	33	133	71.3	17.7	78	19.7	0.40	7.9
PH	33	170	57.2	13.2	54	20.1	0.38	7.6
DJ	33	210	77.7	15.8	66	24.3	0.38	9.2
FS	38	138	76.1	5.5	84	21.4	0.40	8.6
JM	51	123	61.0	15.3	79	17.7	0.35	6.2
Mean	34.3	128	72.5	10.3	70.1	20.5	0.38	7.9
SD	±7.7	±46	±12.0	±6.7	±11.4	±2.4	±0.02	±1.0

* Apnoeic periods were only seen in a small proportion of cycles in this subject

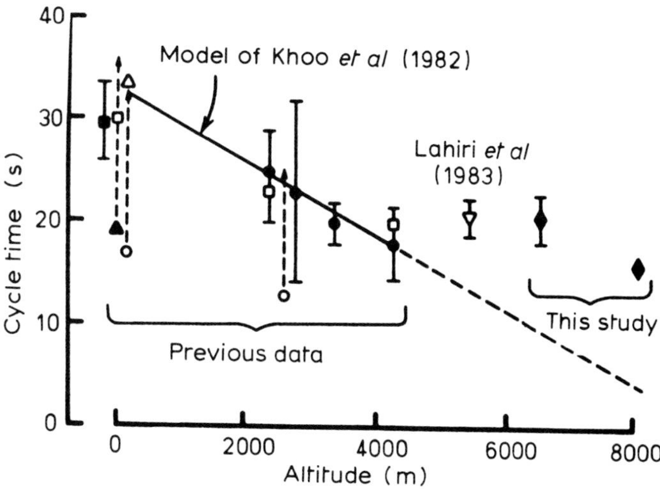

Figure 12.4 Variation of cycle time of periodic breathing with altitude. Points marked 'previous data' were originally published as Figure 8 in the paper by Khoo *et al.* (1982), the solid line being results predicted by their model (open squares). Vertical broken lines indicate differences caused by sealing between neonates and adults. For sources of data see Khoo *et al.* (1982). 'This study' refers to West *et al.* (1986). (From West *et al.*, 1986.)

al. (1982). It can be seen that the cycle times from the AMREE studies were somewhat higher than predicted by the model.

There is evidence that the apnoeic periods are of central nervous origin rather than being caused by airway obstruction. This is supported by the absence of rib cage and abdominal movements as determined from an inductance plethysmograph, a device used for detecting changes in circumference of the chest and abdomen. There was no evidence that the percentage of time during which periodic breathing was observed was altered by the duration of acclimatization. All subjects showed obvious periodic breathing but all were well acclimatized.

Changes of heart rate during the periodic breathing cycle were seen in all subjects and Figure 12.3 is a good example. In general, the maximum heart rate appeared shortly after the peak of the hyperpnoea. Cardiac rhythm abnormalities were infrequent. In one subject ventricular premature contractions occurred mainly during the apnoeic periods. However this subject had a history of occasional ventricular premature contractions at sea-level. There were no other observable changes in ECG pattern except for minor alterations that could be attributed to changes in the position of the heart caused by breathing movements.

In four subjects, evidence of periodic breathing was obtained at an

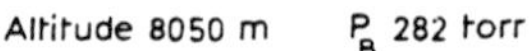

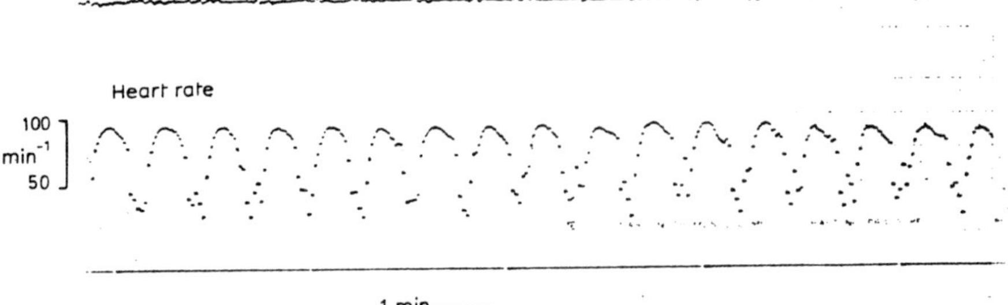

Figure 12.5 Cyclic variation of heart rate caused by periodic breathing in a climber at 8050 m altitude. P_B = 282 mmHg (torr). (From West *et al.*, 1986.)

altitude of 8050 m (P_B 282 mmHg). In these studies, breathing movements were not recorded directly because of the very remote location of the camp. However continuous ECG tracings were obtained during the night using a Holter-type monitor, and the occurrence of periodic breathing was inferred from the variations in heart rate as described by Guilleminault *et al.* (1984). An example is shown in Figure 12.5. This particular subject showed extremely regular cyclic regulation of heart rate over long periods of time (up to 40 min). It was easy to distinguish between this type of cyclic variation caused by periodic breathing and sinus arrhythmia.

12.5.2 Control of breathing

The control of breathing during sleep has been extensively studied: for a review see Phillipson *et al.* (1978). The ventilatory response to carbon dioxide is reduced, at least in NREM sleep (Bulow, 1963). However there is more uncertainty about the hypoxic ventilatory response; some studies indicate that it is increased in NREM sleep (Pappenheimer, 1977; Phillipson *et al.*, 1978). Responses to pulmonary stretch receptor stimulation appear to be intact during NREM sleep but may be decreased in REM sleep (Phillipson *et al.*, 1978).

The control of ventilation during hypoxic sleep has been less well studied and there are many unanswered questions (Dempsey, 1983). Lahiri *et al.* (1983) studied the role of added oxygen and carbon dioxide, and the importance of the hypoxic ventilatory response to periodic breathing in both well-acclimatized lowlanders and native Sherpas at an altitude of 5400 m.

Figure 12.6 shows the effect of adding oxygen to the inspired air. It can be seen that there was an immediate increase in the apnoeic period from about 10–17 s. Subsequently the apnoeic period shortened and

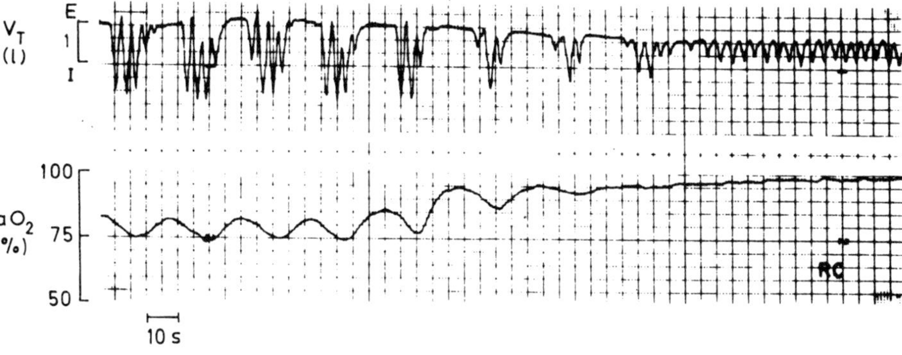

Figure 12.6 Effect of increasing the inspired P_{O_2} on periodic breathing in a lowlander during sleep at 5400 m. Note that adding the oxygen to the inspired gas raised the arterial oxygen saturation, eliminated the apnoeic periods, and reduced the strength of periodic breathing. V_T tidal volume; S_{O_2} arterial oxygen saturation. (From Lahiri and Barnard, 1983.)

shallow rhythmic breathing resumed as the arterial P_{CO_2} increased because of the fall in alveolar ventilation. In most subjects, the periodicity of breathing did not totally disappear following the addition of oxygen, but the strength of the periodic breathing was clearly greatly diminished. The changes can be partly explained by the reduction in respiratory drive from the peripheral chemoreceptors when the arterial P_{O_2} was raised.

Adding carbon dioxide to the inspired gas did not abolish the periodic breathing although it did eliminate the periods of apnoea. Withdrawal of carbon dioxide from the inspired air was followed by a prompt reappearance of apnoea, and the rapidity of the response suggested a dominant role for the peripheral chemoreceptors.

An important finding was that, although the lowlanders showed marked periodic breathing at 5400 m, the Sherpas generally did not. The only exception was one Sherpa who had spent long periods of time at low altitudes. As discussed in Chapter 4, the Sherpas generally show very low ventilatory responses to hypoxia, although the low-altitude Sherpa had an intermediate value. Figure 12.7 shows the relationship between the frequency of apnoea during sleep at 5400 m and the hypoxic ventilatory response. It is clear that a high hypoxic ventilatory response predisposes to periodic breathing.

12.5.3 Mechanism

It is profitable to discuss the mechanism of periodic breathing in terms of control theory, and a particularly useful analysis was presented by

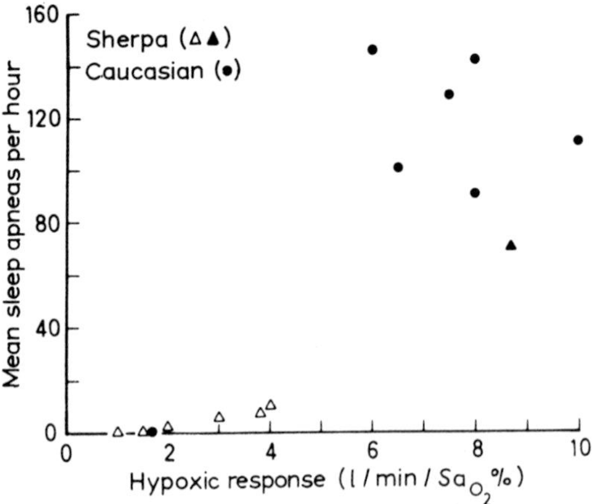

Figure 12.7 Relationship between frequency of sleep apnoea and ventilatory response to hypoxia (awake). (●), acclimatized lowlanders; (△), high-altitude Sherpas; (▲), lower-altitude Sherpa. One lowlander did not have periods of apnoea, and the low-altitude Sherpa showed periodic breathing. (From Lahiri *et al.*, 1983.)

Khoo *et al.* (1982). They pointed out that two factors are necessary for self-sustained oscillatory behaviour in a control system. In such a system we can identify a 'disturbance', for example a change in alveolar ventilation caused by some adventitious factor such as a sigh or alteration of body position. This is followed by a 'corrective action' which tends to suppress the disturbance. In the case of an increase in alveolar ventilation (caused by a sigh, for example) the corrective action would be a lowering of P_{CO_2}, which would tend to reduce ventilation by its action on central and peripheral chemoreceptors and thus constitute negative feedback. The first necessary requirement for sustained oscillatory behaviour is that the magnitude of the corrective action exceeds that of the disturbance, this ratio being known as the loop gain.

The second necessary condition is that the corrective action be presented 180° out of phase with the disturbance, so that what would otherwise inhibit the change in ventilation now augments it. This sustained oscillatory behaviour occurs when the loop gain exceeds unity at a phase difference of 180°.

This theory predicts that the higher the loop gain at a phase angle of 180°, the more likely periodic breathing is to occur, the more marked the pattern of periodic breathing, and the shorter the cycle length of the periodic breathing. The main factor increasing loop gain in acclimatized lowlanders at high altitude is the increased chemoreceptor gain, particularly the response to severe hypoxia (Chapter 4). Other contributing factors may be the hyperventilation which increases the rate of wash-out of carbon dioxide and wash-in of oxygen in the lungs, and the reduction of functional residual capacity in supine subjects.

This analysis explains why there is a difference between acclimatized lowlanders and Sherpas in periodic breathing. Because native highlanders have a blunted hypoxic ventilatory response (Severinghaus *et al.*, 1966; Milledge and Lahiri, 1967), the loop gain of the control system is reduced and the factors promoting periodicity are weak. Lahiri *et al.* (1983) have argued that this represents an important feature of the true adaptation of native highlanders such as Sherpas to high altitude. Periodic breathing is disadvantageous because of the very low levels of arterial P_{O_2} following the apnoeic periods (section 12.5.4). In addition, the reduced ventilation at high altitude lowers the oxygen cost of ventilation.

In another study of periodic breathing at high altitude, measurements were made on nine Japanese climbers who participated in an expedition to the Kunlun mountains (7167 m) in China (Masuyama *et al.*, 1989). There was a significant correlation between the degree of periodic breathing during sleep and both the hypoxic ventilatory response and hypercapnic ventilatory response measured at sea level ($P < 0.05$). Although all climbers showed desaturation during sleep, there was a negative correlation between the degree of desaturation and the hypoxic ventilation response (HVR) ($P < 0.05$). The authors concluded that the high HVR helped to maintain the arterial oxygenation during sleep, and that it was therefore advantageous.

12.5.4 Gas exchange

Periodic breathing causes marked fluctuations in the arterial P_{O_2}, which is not surprising considering the long periods of apnoea that sometimes occur. Figure 12.3 shows a typical record of fluctuations in arterial oxygen saturation as recorded by ear oximeter. Another example is seen in Figure 12.6.

In the study of nocturnal periodic breathing carried out at an altitude of 6300 m during the 1981 American Medical Research Expedition to Mt Everest (AMREE), the mean fluctuation in arterial oxygen saturation between subjects was approximately 10% (West *et al.*, 1986). In order to determine the proportion of the time during which the arterial oxygen saturation fell below a particular value, the analysis described by Slutsky and Strohl (1980) was carried out. This showed that the arterial oxygen saturation below which the subjects spent 50% of their time varied from a minimal value of 64.5% to a maximum of 74.5% with a mean of 68.8%.

Since it is not usually feasible to sample arterial blood over prolonged periods of time, most investigators of periodic breathing have relied on the arterial oxygen saturation measured by ear oximetry. However, based on spot measurements of arterial P_{O_2}, it was calculated that the maximum and minimum values of saturation of 73.0% and 63.4% from the AMREE study corresponded to arterial P_{O_2} values of approximately 39 and 33 mmHg respectively. The conclusion was that the minimal arterial P_{O_2} during sleep was approximately 6 mmHg lower than the resting daytime value, a substantial difference on this very steep part of the oxygen dissociation curve. It should be pointed out that, at high work rates, the arterial P_{O_2} falls considerably below the resting value. However climbers during their normal activity do not generally work at more than two-thirds of their maximal power (Pugh, 1958; section 10.9) so it was concluded that the most severe arterial hypoxaemia over the course of the 24 h probably occurred during sleep as a result of the periodic breathing.

Another factor which may exaggerate the effects of this arterial hypoxaemia is the augmented cardiac output during the periods when the arterial P_{O_2} is near its lowest value. As Figures 12.3 and 12.6 show, the lowest arterial oxygen saturation typically occurs just after the peak of ventilation during the periodic breathing cycle. If venous return and thus cardiac output are enhanced during this hyperpnoeic phase, this would lead to enhanced delivery of this poorly oxygenated blood. Thus it may be that the phasing of arterial P_{O_2} and cardiac output aggravate the resulting impairment of oxygen delivery.

It is possible that the severe arterial hypoxaemia during periodic breathing affects tolerance to extreme altitude. This leads to a paradox. As Figure 12.7 shows, there is a correlation between hypoxic ventilatory response and the strength of the periodic breathing, as would be expected from the control theory discussed in section 12.5.3. This would suggest that climbers with a high hypoxic ventilatory response would tolerate altitude poorly. However the opposite is generally found to be the case (Schoene *et al.*, 1984; Chapter 4). This can be explained by the better ability of these climbers to defend their alveolar P_{O_2} against the low inspired value by hyperventilation (Chapter 11). However it is clear that some elite mountain climbers have, in fact, a relatively low hypoxic ventilatory response (Milledge *et al.*, 1983; Schoene *et al.*, 1987). One possible explanation is that these climbers maintain a higher arterial P_{O_2} during the night, and this is a factor in their tolerance to extreme altitude.

12.5.5 Effects of drugs

Because of the poor quality of sleep at high altitude and the suspicion that this is sometimes related to periodic breathing, there has been

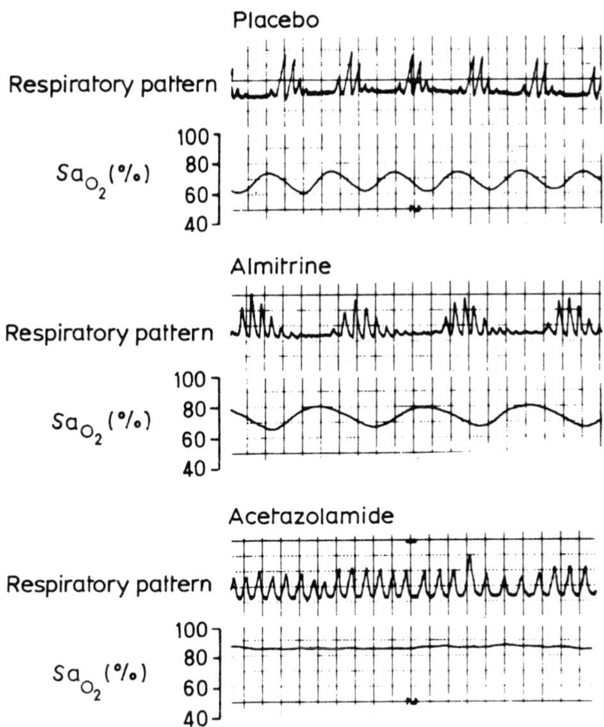

Figure 12.8 Effects of a placebo, almitrine and acetazolamide on periodic breathing and arterial oxygen saturation (Sa_{O_2}) at an altitude of 4400 m. Note that acetazolamide abolished the apnoeic periods while almitrine exaggerated them. (From Hackett *et al.*, 1987.)

considerable interest in the use of drugs to promote a normal breathing pattern. Sutton *et al.* (1979) showed that the administration of acetazolamide at a dose of 250 mg three times per day decreased the time spent in periodic breathing from 80% to 35% at an altitude of 5360 m. This was associated with an improvement in arterial P_{O_2} as judged by the arterial oxygen saturation measured by ear oximetry. Weil *et al.* (1978) used acetazolamide at an altitude of 4400 m and found that the duration of periodic breathing decreased from 35% to 18%. Hackett *et al.* (1987) found a decrease of 41% to 17% at 4400 m in four subjects with the same drug.

The mode of action of acetazolamide is not fully understood but it stimulates ventilation possibly because it induces a metabolic acidosis. At any event, its value at high altitude is now generally accepted in that it reduces the incidence of acute mountain sickness (Hackett *et al.*, 1976), maintains a higher alveolar P_{O_2} and lower P_{CO_2}, and may even prevent some of the weight loss which normally occurs as a result of muscle protein breakdown (Birmingham study, 1981).

Almitrine is another drug that stimulates ventilation, apparently through its effect on peripheral chemoreceptors. It has been shown to improve the arterial oxygenation of patients with chronic bronchitis and emphysema during sleep at sea-level (Connaughton *et al.*, 1985). Hackett *et al.* (1987) compared the effects of almitrine and acetazolamide on the respiratory pattern of four subjects at an altitude of 4400 m on Mt McKinley in a double blind, randomized, three-way crossover trial. Both almitrine and acetazolamide increased the arterial oxygen saturation during sleep but, whereas acetazolamide decreased periodic breathing, almitrine increased it (Figure 12.8). This result is consistent with the data of Figure 12.7 and the discussion in section 12.5.3 where it was pointed out that the strength of periodic breathing is related to the hypoxic ventilatory response. Since almitrine increases this response by stimulating peripheral chemoreceptors, it is not surprising that it exaggerates the periodic breathing. It should also be pointed out that almitrine tends to increase pulmonary vascular resistance by enhancing hypoxic pulmonary vasoconstriction (section 6.3.2), and since pulmonary hypertension occurs at high altitude through this mechanism, this is an undesirable side effect. Thus the use of almitrine is probably contra-indicated at high altitude.

REFERENCES

Barcroft, J. (1925) *The Respiratory Function of the Blood, Part 2, Lessons from High Altitude*, Cambridge University Press, Cambridge, p. 166.

Barcroft, J., Cooke, A., Hartridge, H., *et al.* (1920) The flow of oxygen through the pulmonary epithelium. *J. Physiol.* (*London*), **53**, 450–72.

Berssenbrugge, A., Dempsey, J., Iber, C., *et al.* (1983) Mechanisms of hypoxia-induced periodic breathing during sleep in humans. *J. Physiol.* (*London*, **343**, 507–24.

Bert, P. (1878) *La Pression Barométique*, Masson, Paris. English translation by M.A. Hitchcock and F.A. Hitchock. College Book Co., Columbus, Ohio (1943), p. 106.

Birmingham Medical Research Expeditionary Society Mountain Sickness Study Group (1981) Acetazolamide in control of acute mountain sickness. *Lancet*, **1**, 180–3.

Bulow, K. (1963) Respiration and wakefulness in man. *Acta Physiol. Scand.*, **59(suppl)**, p. 209.

Cheyne, J. (1818) A case of apoplexy in which the fleshy part of the heart was converted into fat. *Dublin Hosp. Rep.*, **2**, 216–23.

Connaughton, J.J., Douglas, N.J., Morgan, A.D., *et al.* (1985) Almitrine improves oxygenation when both awake and asleep in patients with hypoxia and carbon dioxide retention caused by chronic bronchitis and emphysema. *Am. Rev. Respir. Dis.*, **132**, 206–10.

Dempsey, J.A. (1983) Ventilatory regulation in hypoxic sleep: introduction, in

Hypoxia, Exercise and Altitude, (eds J.R. Sutton, C.S. Houston and N.L. Jones.), Liss, New York, pp. 61–3.

Douglas, C.G. and Haldane, J.S. (1909) The causes of periodic or Cheyne–Stokes breathing. *J. Physiol. (London)*, **38**, 401–19.

Douglas, C.G., Haldane, J.S., Henderson, Y. and Schneider, E.C. (1913) Physiological observations made on Pike's Peak, Colorado, with special reference to adaptation to low barometric pressures. *Phil. Trans. R. Soc. London. Ser. B.*, **203**, 185–381.

Egli-Sinclair (1894) Le mal de montagne. *Revue Scientifique (Revue Rose) Series R*, **1**, 172–80.

Goodman, L. (1964) Oscillatory behavior of ventilation in resting man. *IEEE Trans. Biomed. Eng.*, **11**, 81–93.

Guilleminault, C., Connolly, S., Winkle, R., *et al.* (1984) Cyclical variation of the heart rate in sleep apnoea syndrome. *Lancet*, **1**, 126–31.

Hackett, P.H., Rennie, D. and Levine, H.D. (1976) The incidence, importance and prophylaxis of acute mountain sickness. *Lancet*, **2**, 1149–54.

Hackett, P.H., Roach, R.C., Harrison, G.L., *et al.* (1987) Respiratory stimulants and sleep periodic breathing at high altitude. *Am. Rev. Respir. Dis.*, **135**, 896–8.

Hunter, J. (1781) *Original Cases*, Library of Royal College of Surgeons of England.

Khoo, M.C.K., Kronauer, R.E., Strohl, K.P. and Slutsky, A.S. (1982) Factors inducing periodic breathing in humans: a general model. *J. Appl. Physiol.*, **53**, 644–59.

Lahiri, S. and Barnard, P. (1983) Role of arterial chemoreflexes in breathing during sleep at high altitude, in *Hypoxia, Exercise and Altitude*, (eds J.S. Sutton, C.S. Houston and N.L. Jones), Liss, New York, pp. 75–85.

Lahiri, S., Maret, K and Sherpa, M.G. (1983) Dependence of high altitude sleep apnea on ventilatory sensitivity to hypoxia. *Respir. Physiol.*, **52**, 281–301.

Lenfant, C. (1967) Time-dependent variations of pulmonary gas exchange in normal men at rest. *J. Appl. Physiol.*, **22**, 675–84.

Lugaresi, E., Coccagna, G., Cirignotta, R., *et al.* (1978) Breathing during sleep in man in normal and pathological conditions, in *The Regulation of Respiration during Sleep and Anesthesia*, (eds R.S. Fitzgerald, H. Gautier and S. Lahirig), Plenum, New York, pp. 35–45.

Masuyama, S., Kohchiyama, S., Shinozaki, T., *et al.* (1989) Periodic breathing at high altitude and ventilatory responses to O_2 and CO_2. *Jap. J. of Physiol.*, **39**, 523–35.

Megirian, D.A., Ryan, A.T. and Sherrey, J.H. (1980) An electrophysiological analysis of sleep and respiration of rats breathing different gas mixtures.: diaphragmatic muscle function. *Electroencephalogr. Clin. Neurophysiol.*, **50**, 303–13.

Milledge, J.S. and Lahiri, S. (1967) Respiratory control in lowlanders and Sherpa highlanders at altitude. *Respir. Physiol.*, **2**, 310–22.

Milledge, J.S., Ward, M.P., Williams, E.S. and Clarke, C.R.A. (1983) Cardio-respiratory response to exercise in men repeatedly exposed to extreme altitude. *J. Appl. Physiol.*, **55**, 1379–85.

Mosso, A. (1898) *Life of Man on the High Alps*, T. Fisher Unwin, London, pp. 42–7.

Pappenheimer, J.R. (1977) Sleep and respiration of rats during hypoxia. *J. Physiol. (London)*, **266**, 191–207.

Pappenheimer, J.R. (1984) Hypoxic insomnia: effects of carbon monoxide and acclimatization. *J. Appl. Physiol.*, **57**, 1696–1703.

Phillipson, E.A., Sullivan, C.E., Read, D.J.C., *et al.* (1978) Ventilatory and waking responses to hypoxia in sleeping dogs. *J. Appl. Physiol. Respir. Environ. Exercise Physiol.*, **44**, 512–20.

Priban, I. (1963) An analysis of some short term patterns of breathing in man at rest. *J. Physiol. (London)*, **166**, 425–34.

Pugh, L.G.C.E. (1958) Muscular exercise on Mt Everest. *J. Physiol. (London)*, **141**, 233–61.

Pugh, L.G.C.E. and Ward, M.P. (1956) Some effects of high altitude on man. *Lancet*, **2**, 1115–21.

Reite, M., Jackson, D., Cahoon, R.L. and Weil, J.V. (1975) Sleep physiology at high altitude. *Electroencephalogr. Clin. Neurophysiol.*, **38**, 463–71.

Schoene, R.B., Lahiri, S., Hackett, P.H., *et al.* (1984) Relationship of hypoxic ventilatory response to exercise performance on Mount Everest. *J. Appl. Physiol.*, **56**, 1478–83.

Schoene, R.B., Hackett, P.H. and Roach, R.C. (1987) Blunted hypoxic chemosensitivity at altitude and sea level in an elite high altitude climber, in *Hypoxia and Cold*, (eds J.R. Sutton, C.S. Houston and G. Coates), Praeger, New York, p. 532 (abstract).

Severinghaus, J.W., Bainton, C.R. and Carcelen, A. (1966) Respiratory insensitivity to hypoxia in chronically hypoxic man. *Respir. Physiol.*, **1**, 308–34.

Slutsky, A.S. and Strohl, K.P. (1980). Quantification of oxygen saturation during episodic hypoxemia. *Am. Rev. Respir. Dis.*, **121**, 893–5.

Specht, H. and Fruhmann, G. (1972) Incidence of periodic breathing in 2000 subjects without pulmonary or neurological disease. *Bull. Physio-Pathol. Respir.*, **98**, 1075–83.

Stokes, W. (1854) *The Diseases of the Heart and Aorta*, Hodges and Smith, Dublin, p. 320.

Sutton, J.R., Houston, C.S., Mansell, A.L., *et al.* (1979) Effect of acetazolamide on hypoxemia during sleep at high altitude. *N. Engl. J. Med.*, **301**, 1329–31.

Tyndall, J. (1860) *The Glaciers of the Alps*, Murray, London, p. 80.

Waggener, T.B., Brusil, P.J., Kronauer, R.E., *et al.* (1984) Strength and cycle time of high-altitude ventilatory patterns in unacclimatized humans. *J. Appl. Physiol.*, **56**, 576–81.

Ward, M.P. (1973) Periodic respiration. *Ann. R. Coll. Surg. Engl.*, **52**, 330–4.

Weil, J.V., Kryger, M.H. and Scoggin, C.H. (1978) Sleep and breathing at high altitude, in *Sleep Apnea Syndromes*, (eds C. Guilleminault and W. Dement), Liss, New York, pp. 119–36.

West, J.B., Peters, R.M., Aksnes, G., *et al.* (1986) Nocturnal periodic breathing at altitudes of 6300 and 8050 m. *J. Appl. Physiol.*, **61**, 280–7.

13

Nutrition and intestinal function

Revised in collaboration with Dr S.P.L. Travis

13.1 INTRODUCTION

Anorexia and weight loss are well-known features of life at high altitude, especially extreme altitudes. The mechanism of this anorexia is not known. During the first few days after a rapid ascent, anorexia is probably part of the symptomatology of acute mountain sickness (AMS), but after this, when all other symptoms of AMS are gone, anorexia may remain. This continuing anorexia is not common below about 5000 m but is almost universal above 6000 m and becomes worse at even higher altitudes, though the severity varies considerably between individuals.

Weight loss is also common though not inevitable even at extreme altitudes (see below) and is partly due to the reduced calorie intake consequent upon the anorexia, but the possibility that it might be due also to other factors, such as malabsorption, is reviewed in this chapter. This chapter also considers diet at altitude and the evidence for the value of a high carbohydrate diet.

13.2 ENERGY BALANCE AT ALTITUDE

13.2.1 Energy output

Basal metabolism

Nair *et al.* (1971) found that after a week at 3300 m the basal metabolic rate (BMR) was elevated by about 12%. Exposure to cold as well as hypoxia (in a second group of subjects) made no difference to this effect compared with hypoxia alone. By the second week, BMR was back to control values and was below control by the third week. Cold exposure at this time resulted in elevation of BMR to above sea-level values by the fifth week and it remained elevated a week after return to sea-level. Butterfield *et al.* (1992) found BMR to be elevated by 27% on day two at Pike's Peak (4300 m). The BMR then decreased over the next few days to plateau at +17% compared with sea-level by day 10.

After acclimatization, BMR measured at 5800 m was found to be elevated by about 10% in subjects who had been at altitude for between 82 and 113 days (Gill and Pugh, 1964). It is possible that BMR rises again if subjects climb to altitudes to which they are not acclimatized.

BMR was found to be high at altitude in altitude residents (Ladakhis and Sherpas) compared with lowlanders and with predicted values (Nair *et al.*, 1971; Gill and Pugh, 1964). This elevation of BMR remained even when allowance was made for the fact that these peoples generally have less fat in their body composition. Picon-Reatequi (1961) also reported elevated BMR in Andean miners at 4540 m. The mechanism for this rise in BMR is uncertain. Faecal and urinary excretion of energy nitrogen and volatile acids are not altered in the early days at altitude (Butterfield *et al.*, 1992). There is increase in sympathetic activity at this time (section 14.6) and the finding that this increase in metabolic rate can be inhibited by a beta-blocker (Moore *et al.*, 1987) suggests it is a likely factor. Increased thyroid activity may also play a part, especially in the longer term elevation of BMR (section 14.7).

Energy expenditure due to exercise

Work in absolute terms requires the same oxygen intake at altitude as at sea-level until near maximum work rate is reached (Pugh *et al.*, 1964; West *et al.*, 1983; Wolfel *et al.*, 1991). At altitude the maximum work rate is reduced (Chapter 10) and all activity seems disproportionately fatiguing. At 8000 m, even rolling over in one's sleeping bag demands a great effort. Thus, energy expenditure for even normal activities of daily living must be reduced at extreme altitude. Another fact of life at extreme altitudes is that often the only warm place is one's sleeping bag and much of the 24 hours of the day is spent lying down. The increased work of breathing has a small opposite effect but, overall, there must be a reduction in average daily energy expenditure, especially at extreme altitude.

At intermediate altitudes (2500–4500 m) although maximum work rate is reduced, energy expenditure on normal daily activities of short duration is probably not much altered. For longer term work such as hill climbing, much will depend upon the degree of acclimatization and fitness. Pugh *et al.* (1964) found $\dot{V}_{O_2}$ intakes on climbers climbing at their 'preferred' rate to decline very little up to about 5000 m (Figure 12.1) whereas Butterfield *et al.* (1992) found a 37% reduction in energy expenditure for exercise 'more strenuous than walking'. At sea-level, daily energy expenditure was 2250 kJ d^{-1} compared with 1394 kJ d^{-1} at 4300 m.

Until recently it has been impossible to measure energy expenditure over long periods but a doubly-labelled water technique has now been developed which makes this possible. Water is labelled with both deuterium and oxygen-18. The deuterium is eliminated as water while the oxygen is eliminated as both water and CO_2. Thus CO_2 production can be calculated from the different elimination rates (Schoeller and van Santen, 1982; Coward, 1991). Using this technique, Westerterp *et al.* (1992) found average daily metabolic rates in the Alps (2500–4800 m) to be 14.7 MJ and on Mt Everest (5300–8872 m) to be not significantly different at 13.6 MJ. No data are available from this study for near sea-level climbing. Very similar daily results were obtained in the 1992 British Winter Everest Expedition of 11.7–15.4 MJ (Travis *et al.*, 1993).

13.2.2 Energy intake

Up to about 4500 m, once acclimatized, people have normal appetites and normal food intake (Consolazio *et al.*, 1968). Above 6000 m most climbers experience anorexia. This tends to become more pronounced the longer one stays at these altitudes. Climbers complain about the food available and feel that the preserved nature of food increases the anorexia and reduces their intake. There are few data on actual calorie intake under these circumstances. Those that there are rely on diary cards and estimates of portion size. On Cho Oyu in 1952 food eaten at between 5250 and 6750 m was only about 13.4 MJ a day compared with 17.6 MJ on the march out, whilst on Everest in 1953, above 7250 m, the intake was only about 6.3 MJ (Pugh and Band, 1953). On the Silver Hut expedition (1960–1961), in four climbers at 5800 m, whose living conditions were excellent and where a good variety and quantity of food was available, a daily intake of 12.6–13.4 MJ per day was estimated (Pugh, 1962). Boyer and Blume (1984) reported that on the AMREE (1981), over three days four subjects had a mean intake of 9.34 MJ at 6300 m compared with 12.5 MJ at sea-level. Dinmore *et al.* (1994) found intakes similar during the march in (1500–2000 m) and above 5500 m (10.8 and 10.3 MJ). But Westerterp *et al.* (1992) and Travis *et al.* (1993) estimated intakes high on Everest of 7.5 and 8.6 MJ respectively, indicating the expected reduction in intake above 6300 m.

Clearly, high up on major mountains (above 6000 m), when actively climbing, it is not possible to maintain caloric balance even when acclimatized. In Everest climbers studied by Westerterp *et al.* (1992) there was a daily negative balance of 5.7 MJ. They found a similar negative balance at Alpine altitudes but the two subjects were not acclimatized. Clearly more studies using this new technique are needed to answer the question of whether acclimatized subjects can maintain caloric balance at intermediate altitudes (4500–6000 m) when semi-sedentary.

13.3 WEIGHT LOSS ON ALTITUDE EXPEDITIONS

13.3.1 Weight loss on the march out

Most climbing and trekking groups experience weight loss in the initial 1–3 weeks of an expedition, even when walking below 3000 m. This is probably due to the change in life-style for most subjects from an urban semi-sedentary existence to the more active life-style of marching ten miles a day with some considerable ascents and descents. In addition, gastrointestinal infections are common.

Boyer and Blume (1984) found that 13 AMREE members, during the march out to the Everest region, lost an average of 2 kg with a range of from 0–6 kg. Those with the highest percentage of body fat to start with lost most weight, the correlation being significant; 70% of this weight loss was due to loss of fat. Two subjects with less than 13% of body fat at the start of the march out lost no weight. Dinmore *et al.* (1994) similarly found an average loss of 1.3 kg during the first week of trekking but only a further 0.5 kg in the next week.

Weight loss during this phase of an expedition or trek can be considered as shedding unnecessary fat.

13.3.2 Weight loss at altitude

On first arrival at altitude, AMS may cause anorexia and vomiting with resulting weight loss, though usually the duration is not long enough to do this. Also, fluid may be retained and subjects with AMS often gain weight (Hackett *et al.*, 1982). Consolazio *et al.* (1972) found a small gain in weight on the first day at altitude followed by a loss of weight of about 1 kg over the next five days at 4300 m.

After acclimatization, weight loss is usually seen only above about 5000 m. Dinmore *et al.* (1994) found an average loss of 3.9 kg during two weeks' climbing above 5000 m; on the 1992 British Winter Everest Expedition a mean weight loss of 5 kg was observed above 5400 m out of a total loss of 7.8 kg (Travis *et al.*, 1993). Figure 13.1 shows the crucial effect of altitude on body weight on one well-acclimatized subject. The combined effects of the march out and early residence at the Silver Hut at 5800 m, produced a weight loss of 5.3 kg. Thereafter, during time spent at the Silver Hut the subject lost weight steadily at a weekly rate of just under 400 g, but, on two occasions, when he went down to altitudes of between 4000 and 4500 m he began to gain weight. Most

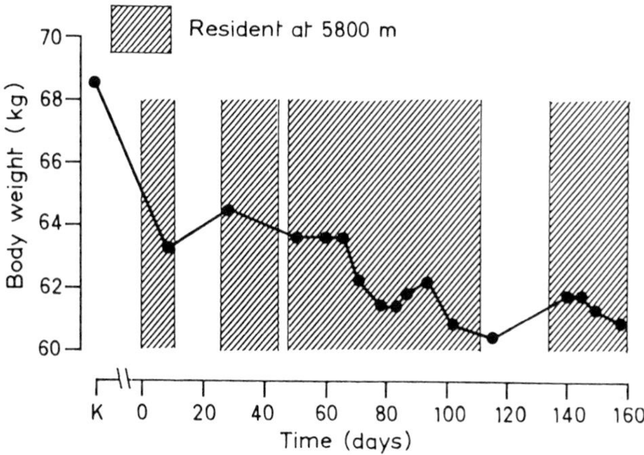

Figure 13.1 Record of body weight of one subject during the 'Silver Hut' expedition 1960–1961. After the march out from Kathmandu (K) and the initial period of preparation he was in residence at 5800 m (hatched areas) or at base camp at 4500 m. Note the loss of weight at 5800 m but weight gain during two breaks at 4500 m.

subjects in the Silver Hut lost between 0.5 and 1.5 kg a week (Pugh, 1962).

Rai *et al.* (1975) found no weight loss in their subjects living at 3500–4700 m, even though they were working quite hard at road building and digging. Indeed, on a high fat diet (232 g daily) they actually gained an average of 1.4 kg during three weeks at 4700 m. Butterfield *et al.* (1992) also found that it was possible to attenuate weight loss at 4300 m by increasing dietary intake in proportion to the increase in BMR. However, at Advanced Base Camp (6300 m) in the Western Cwm on Everest most subjects lost weight. Boyer and Blume (1984) document this weight loss as an average of 4 kg (range 0–8) over a mean of 47 days in 13 subjects. Again there was considerable individual variation in the amount of weight lost which correlated with initial percentage of body fat. Boyer and Blume also found that Sherpas who averaged only half as much body fat as the Caucasian climbers, lost no weight during the time spent above base camp, mostly at or above 6300 m.

13.3.3 Weight loss in chamber experiments

It could be argued that some of the weight loss on expeditions is due to cold, limited food supplies, and the increased energy expenditure of climbing. This may often be the case though not so in a number of the studies quoted above. Chamber studies avoid this potential criticism; most are of too short a duration to be relevant, but the two Operation Everest studies of 40 days' duration showed that, despite good environmental conditions of temperature, humidity and diet *ad libitum*, subjects lost weight (Rose *et al.*, 1988). In Operation Everest II the six subjects lost an average of 7.4 kg during the 38 days of observations as they ascended the simulated height of the summit of Everest. Caloric intake fell by 43% and, interestingly, the subjects chose a diet that resulted in a reduction of carbohydrate from 62% to 53% of the total diet. The authors considered that the weight loss could not be accounted for totally by the reduction in intake and considered that malabsorption or increase in energy expenditure must be invoked. Being a chamber study the exercise taken would probably be less than on a climbing expedition.

13.4 BODY COMPOSITION AND WEIGHT LOSS

Assuming much of the weight loss is due to negative calorie balance, a simplistic view would be that the body would use up fat stores first and then start using protein from the lean body mass, principally the muscles. However, even with a most carefully controlled diet aimed at fat reduction, it is never possible to lose fat exclusively and retain all the lean body mass (Garrow, 1987). The best that can be achieved is that, of the weight lost, 75% is fat and 25% lean body tissue. This compares with the situation during a complete fast when fat and lean body tissue are lost in roughly equal proportions (Forbes and Drenick, 1979).

Boyer and Blume (1984) used skin fold measurements to estimate body fat. There are uncertainties about the absolute results of this method, but relative changes probably can be reliable. They found that, of the average 2 kg loss during the march out to base camp, 70% was due to loss of fat, which is a figure close to the most efficient muscle sparing regimen available. However, above 5400 m, mainly at or above 6300 m, of the 4 kg average weight loss only 27% was due to loss of fat and 73% due to loss of lean body tissue, despite the fact that subjects still had at least 10% of their body weight as fat. This percentage loss of muscle, greater than that seen in starvation, suggests that at this altitude hypoxia may be interfering with protein metabolism (section 13.5).

In the Operation Everest II study (Rose *et al.*, 1988) there was loss of 2.5 kg of fat (1.6% body weight) and 4.9 kg of lean body tissue. Computerized tomographic examination of the thigh showed a 17% loss of muscle and a 34% loss of subcutaneous fat. Although loss of muscle mass must be a disadvantage, one beneficial effect is to increase the density of muscle capillaries. This is because the loss of muscle mass is achieved by reducing fibre diameter rather than number, with the number of capillaries per fibre remaining constant. Thus the inter-capillary distance decreases with an improvement in oxygenation of the muscles (Chapter 9). Evidence in support of this speculation is found in the work of Oelz *et al.* (1986), who studied muscle biopsies from six elite climbers at sea-level some months after return from altitude. It was found that their muscle fibres were smaller and the capillary density greater than controls. Another explanation for the loss of muscle mass, not mutually exclusive of the above suggestion, is that with decreased overall activity at altitude there is some disuse atrophy which would similarly reduce muscle fibre diameter. Results of muscle biopsy studies during Operation Everest II (MacDougall *et al.*, 1991) showed similar histological changes in muscle fibre size (Chapter 9 contains a fuller discussion of changes in muscle histology).

13.5 INTESTINAL ABSORPTION AND HYPOXIA

In view of the continued weight loss at altitudes above 5000 m with, in some cases, adequate intake and reduced energy output, the possibility of malabsorption and malutilization of food must be considered. Pugh (1962) reported that members of the Silver Hut expedition noted that stools tended to be greasy and bulky, suggesting possible steatorrhoea due to malabsorption of fat.

As mentioned in section 13.3, weight loss is not a feature of living at altitudes below about 5000 m, and the fact that most altitude research is conducted below this level may explain why so little work has been carried out on the topic of intestinal absorption. Other reasons for the neglect of this field may be that the methods involved are either too sophisticated for easy use in the field (e.g. absorption of radioactive materials), or are unattractive to investigators (e.g. faecal collection, liquidization and aliquot sampling etc.). Finally, few altitude physiologists have a background in gastroenterology.

13.5.1 Carbohydrate absorption and hypoxia

Milledge (1972) studied patients who were hypoxic either because of congenital heart disease or chronic obstructive lung disease. Xylose absorption decreased with decreasing arterial oxygen saturation (Figure 13.2).

On relieving the hypoxia by surgery in the cardiac cases, or by 13 h of supplementary oxygen breathing in the respiratory cases, there was improvement in xylose absorption in all patients. The xylose absorption test has a rather uncertain lower normal limit, especially in a population

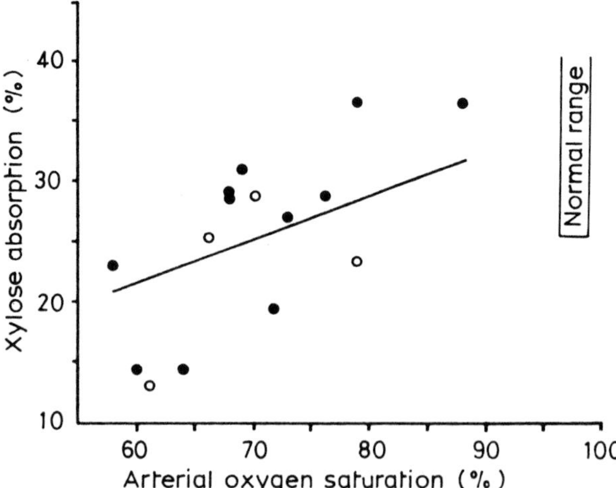

Figure 13.2 Xylose absorption in patients hypoxic because of either congenital cyanotic heart disease (○), or chronic respiratory disease (●), plotted against their arterial O_2 saturation.

where intestinal parasitic infection is common (the study was carried out in south India). However, the results suggest that, below an arterial saturation of about 70%, absorption was impaired (Figure 13.2); improvement on relief of hypoxia supports this view.

Pritchard and Lane (1974) did not find malabsorption in 26 patients with chronic obstructive lung disease, but the lowest arterial P_{O_2} was 48 mmHg, equivalent to about 78% saturation; Chesner *et al.* (1987) found no malabsorption of xylose in eleven subjects up to 4846 m, but 60-minute plasma xylose concentrations were reduced in subjects who ascended to 5600 m, confirming that absorption is not affected until hypoxia is severe. Boyer and Blume (1984), who studied subjects at 6300 m, found xylose absorption decreased by 24% in six out of seven subjects, compared with sea-level controls.

However, absorption measured by xylose has the drawback that the result is influenced by factors such as gastric emptying time, absorption area, intestinal transit and renal function. Dinmore *et al.* (1994) used a double carbohydrate test; the two non-metabolized carbohydrates used undergo different forms of mediated absorption but are otherwise subject to the same external influences which cancel out when results are expressed as a ratio (Menzies, 1984). D-xylose is absorbed by passive mediated transport whilst 3-*o*-methyl-D-glucose is absorbed by active mediated, sodium-dependant transport. They found that at 6300 m there was 34% decrease in D-xylose (Figure 13.3)

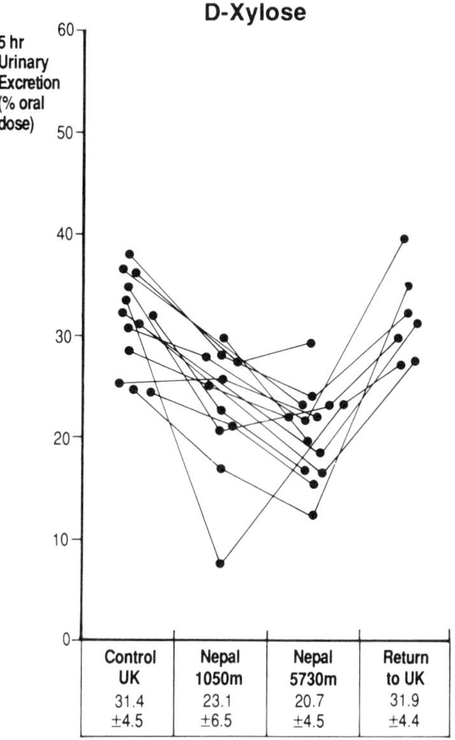

Figure 13.3 D-xylose absorption tested in a group of climbers at sea-level (UK), at altitudes indicated in Nepal and after return to UK. (Data from Dinmore *et al.*, 1994.)

and a 15% decrease in 3-*o*-methyl-D-glucose absorption. The ratio was consistently decreased at altitude and in a subsequent study the 60-minute serum xylose/3-*o*-Methyl-D-glucose ratio was 17% lower at 5400 m than at sea-level (Travis *et al.*, 1993).

13.5.2 Fat absorption and hypoxia

Rai *et al.* (1975) found no malabsorption for fat at 4700 m, neither did Chesner *et al.* (1987) at 3100 m and 4800 m. Imray *et al.* (1992), using the ^{14}C-triolein breath test, found no malabsorption of fat at 5500 m on Aconcagua, and Butterfield *et al.* (1992) found no increase in faecal excretion of volatile fatty acids at 4300 m. However, Boyer and Blume (1984) found fat absorption decreased by 49% at 6300 m compared with sea-level results in three acclimatized subjects.

13.5.3 Protein absorption and hypoxia

Kayser *et al.* (1992) measured protein absorption using urinary and faecal nitrogen-15 excretion after ingestion of nitrogen-15-labelled soya protein. They found no reduction in absorption in subjects after three weeks at 5000 m.

In summary, there is no evidence of malabsorption up to an altitude of about 5000 m and this has been confirmed by measurements of faecal energy excretion which have shown that 96% of energy intake is assimilated (Kayser *et al.*, 1992). Above 5000 m, however, there may be malabsorption of carbohydrate and fat. The mechanism of this hypoxic malabsorption is unknown. It might be due to bowel wall hypoxia, or the fat malabsorption could be due to pancreatic insufficiency and the xylose malabsorption secondary to fat malabsorption. Pappenheimer (1988) showed that the space between adjacent epithelial cells in the small intestine (zona occludens) became less with hypoxia. This may be by contraction of the actin–myosin cytoskeletal system (myoepithelial cells) which control the calibre of these pores. This would reduce sodium-coupled transport of material across the luminal cell wall.

13.6 INTESTINAL PERMEABILITY

Intestinal permeability is the facility with which molecules pass through the intestinal epithelium by passive, non-mediated transport. It can be measured by the ratio of urinary lactulose and L-rhamnose after ingestion of these test carbohydrates (Travis and Menzies, 1992). Lactulose is thought to permeate through paracellular pores of low frequency and L-rhamnose through transcellular pores at a much higher rate (Menzies, 1984). Permeability increases if the integrity of the intestinal mucosa is compromised by, for instance, mucosal damage. Dinmore *et al.* (1994) measured intestinal permeability in this way in 11 climbers. After arrival in Nepal there was an increase in permeability due possibly to 'tropical enteropathy' because of changes in gut flora. This is normally a transient phenomenon in travellers to the tropics. When the climbers ascended to altitude, studies at 5730 m showed that the ratio returned to sea-level values (Figure 13.4).

However, the transcellular permeation of the monosaccharide L-rhamnose showed a 45% decrease at 5730 m, which is a change unique to high altitude. These findings suggest that at these high altitudes the 'porosity' of the gut is unchanged but that changes may be occurring in the epithelial membranes, perhaps through a change in membrane fluidity (Travis and Menzies, 1992).

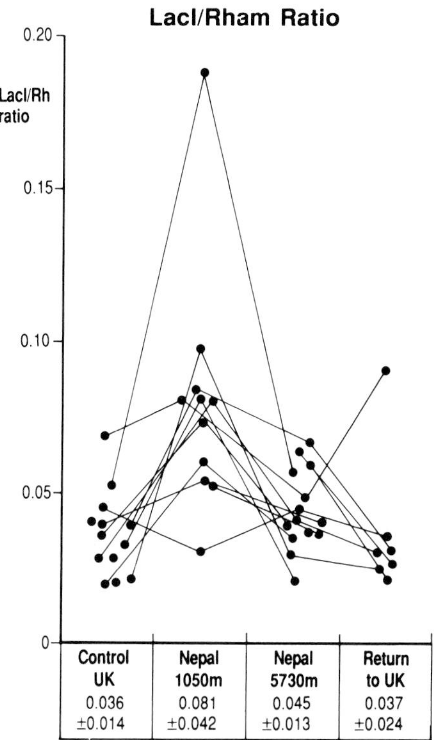

Figure 13.4 Intestinal permeability (lactose/L-rhamnose ratio) in a group of climbers tested at sea-level (UK), at altitudes indicated in Nepal and after return to UK. Results show an increase in permeability after arrival in Nepal, possibly due to a change in gut flora, but a return to sea-level values at 5730 m. (Data from Dinmore *et al.*, 1994.)

13.7 PROTEIN METABOLISM AT ALTITUDE

The obvious muscle wasting seen especially in climbers returning from extreme altitude prompts the question of whether hypoxia affects protein metabolism directly. There is very little data on this topic in man.

Consolazio *et al.* (1968) studied protein balance at altitude and found no difference between subjects there and at sea-level, but the altitude station was Pike's Peak (4300 m), below the crucial height at which continued weight loss is observed.

Rennie *et al.* (1983) studied the effect of acute hypoxia in a chamber (equivalent altitude 4550 m) on leucine metabolism in forearm muscles. They found that acute hypoxia resulted in a net loss of amino acids

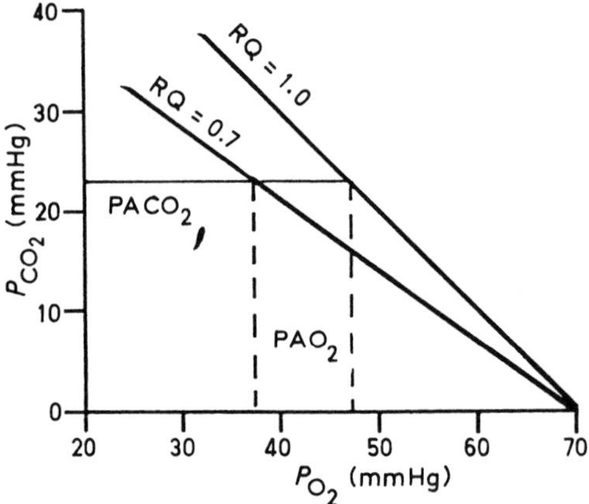

Figure 13.5 An O_2/CO_2 diagram to show the effect of the respiratory quotient (RQ) on alveolar P_{O_2} at a given PA_{CO_2}. By changing from an RQ of 0.7 (the RQ when utilizing fat) to 1.0 (the RQ when utilizing carbohydrate) the PA_{O_2} is increased from 37.2 to 47.0 mmHg.

from the muscles, probably due to a fall in muscle protein synthesis. If this finding can be extrapolated to the situation of chronic hypoxia at altitudes of above 5000–6000 m (where hypoxia in acclimatized subjects would be similar to that in the above study) then it provides a further contributing factor to the loss of muscle mass described above.

13.8 DIET FOR HIGH ALTITUDE

Views on diets (not only at altitude) are strongly held, often the strength of opinion being inversely related to the strength of scientific evidence.

13.8.1 High carbohydrate diet

There is a preference amongst climbers for a high carbohydrate, low fat diet at altitude and there are good physiological reasons for this. Figure 13.5 shows the basis for advising a high carbohydrate diet, which moves the respiratory quotient (RQ) from 0.7, if one uses fat exclusively for energy, to 1.0 when carbohydrate (or protein) is used.

The result of such a change of RQ is that for any given PA_{CO_2} the PA_{O_2} is increased. In the case illustrated in Figure 13.5, the subject is considered to be at 5800 m in the Himalayas or Andes when the barometric pressure is half that at sea-level and the PI_{O_2} is 70 mmHg. PA_{CO_2} is assumed to be 23 mmHg. With an RQ of 0.7 the PA_{O_2} would be 39.2 mmHg, whereas with an RQ of 1.0 it would be 47 mmHg; this is a very important gain in arterial oxygen saturation. This represents the extreme case of a switch from pure fat to pure carbohydrate utilization, but even a partial switch in this direction would be helpful to the climber at extreme altitudes.

Consolazio *et al.* (1969), compared a normal with a high carbohydrate diet in two groups of subjects at 4300 m. The performance of the group on a high carbohydrate diet was superior in that they had a greater endurance for heavy work, though $\dot{V}_{O_2}$ max was not significantly better; also, the symptoms of AMS were less in the high carbohydrate group.

Another reason for recommending a high carbohydrate diet is that the body becomes more dependant upon blood glucose as a fuel both at rest and on exercise after acclimatization (Brooks *et al.*, 1991).

13.8.2 Low fat diet

Most climbers find fatty foods become distasteful at altitude in contrast to the preference shown by Arctic and Antarctic travellers. Tilman, who was experienced in both Arctic and mountain travel, writes:

> If you do succeed in getting outside a richly concentrated food like pemmican a great effort of will is required to keep it down – absolute quiescence in a prone position and a little sugar are useful aids. Eating a large mug of pemmican soup at 27 200 feet as Peter Lloyd and I did in '38 is, I think, an unparalleled feat and shows what can be done by dogged greed. *(Tilman, 1975)*

There are good physiological reasons for a low fat diet at altitude; first, the effect of fat as an energy source on the RQ (as discussed above) and secondly, because of the possible effect of fat malabsorption on the absorption of sugars and amino acids. This fat intolerance is unfortunate because fat provides more calories weight for weight than carbohydrate or proteins.

13.8.3 Other dietary constituents

Iron

Since the red cell mass is increased at altitude it has been suggested that extra iron should be taken. Unless there is pre-existing iron deficiency the iron stores of the body and the iron content of a normal diet will be adequate. However, in premenopausal women there may be a degree of deficient iron stores and the addition of iron may be indicated (Richalet *et al.*, 1994). A rapid response to hypoxia is an increase in intestinal iron absorption from the gut before any change in plasma iron turnover, at least in rats and mice (Hathorn, 1971; Raja *et al.*, 1986). Thus the iron stores of the body are replenished even before they begin to be depleted.

Vitamins

It is common for expedition and trekking parties to take added vitamins, but, while such dietary supplements probably do no harm, there is no evidence that they are needed providing a normal balanced diet is taken.

13.8.4 Fresh food, flavour, variety

The appetite becomes jaded at high altitude and the most common complaints on expeditions are about the drab sameness of the flavour of preserved foods. More experienced climbers tend to adopt a policy of eating local fresh foods, supplemented as much as possible by the minimum of imported preserved foods. The sense of taste seems to be dulled at altitude and western food tastes insipid. The addition of strong flavours such as curries and herbs are increasingly appreciated. There is great individual variation in likes and dislikes, even more than at sea-level, and the wise quartermaster of an expedition will attempt to meet this by providing as wide a variety of foods and flavours as possible. However, his lot is unenviable since, whatever he provides, his fellow members will yearn for what is unavailable.

REFERENCES

Boyer, S.J. and Blume, F.D. (1984) Weight loss and changes in body composition at high altitude. *J. Appl. Physiol. Respir. Environ. Exercise Physiol.*, **57**, 1380–5.

Brooks, G.A., Butterfield, G.E., Wolfe, R.R., *et al.* (1991) Increased dependence on blood glucose after acclimatization to 4300 m. *J. Appl. Physiol.*, **70**, 919–27.

Butterfield, G.E., Gates, J., Fleming, S., *et al.* (1992) Increased energy intake minimizes weight loss in men at high altitude. *J. Appl. Physiol.*, **72**, 1741–8.

Chesner, I.M., Small, N.A. and Dykes, P.W. (1987) Intestinal absorption at high altitude. *Postgrad. Med. J.*, **63**, 173–5.

Consolazio, C.F., Matoush, L.O., Johnson, H.L. and Daws, T.A. (1968) Protein and water balances of young adults during prolonged exposure to high altitude (4300 m). *Am. J. Clin. Nutr.*, **21**, 134–61.

Consolazio, C.F., Matoush, L.O., Johnson, H.L., *et al.* (1969) Effects of high-carbohydrate diets on performance and clinical symptomatology after rapid ascent to high altitude. *Fed. Proc.*, **28**, 937–43.

Consolazio, C.F., Johnson, H.L., Krzywicki, H.J. and Daws, T.A. (1972) Metabolic aspects of acute altitude exposure (4300 m) in adequately nourished humans. *Am. J. Clin. Nutr.*, **25**, 23–9.

Coward, W.A. (1991) Measurement of energy expenditure: the doubly labelled water method in clinical practice. *Proc. Nutr. Soc.*, **50**, 227–37.

Dinmore, A.J., Edwards, J.S.A., Menzies, I.S. and Travis, S.P.L. (1994) Intestinal carbohydrate absorption and permeability at high altitude (5730 m). *J. Appl. Physiol.*, **76**, 1903–7.
Forbes, G.B. and Drenick, E.J. (1979) Loss of body nitrogen of fasting. *Am. J. Clin. Nutr.*, **32**, 1370–4.
Garrow, J.S. (1987) Are liquid diets (VLCD) safe or necessary? in *Recent Advances in Obesity Research, V*, (eds E.M. Berry, S.H. Blondheim, H.E. Eliahou and E. Shafrir), pp. 312–16.
Gill, M.B. and Pugh, L.G.C.E. (1964) Basal metabolism and respiration in men living at 5800 m (19 000 ft). *J. Appl. Physiol.*, **19**, 949–54.
Hackett, P.H., Rennie, D., Hofmeister, S.E., *et al.* (1982) Fluid retention and relative hypoventilation in acute mountain sickness. *Respiration*, **43**, 321–9.
Hathorn, M.K.S. (1971) The influence of hypoxia on iron absorption in the rat. *Gastroenterology*, **60**, 76–81.
Imray, C.H., Chesner, I., Winterbourn, M., *et al.* (1992) Fat absorption at altitude: a reappraisal (abstract). *Int. J. Sports Med.*, **13**, 87.
Kayser, B., Acheson, K., Decombaz, J., *et al.* (1992) Protein absorption and energy digestibility at high altitude. *J. Appl. Physiol.*, **73**, 2425–31.
MacDougall, J.D., Green, H., Sutton, J.R., *et al.* (1991) Operation Everest II: Structural adaptations in skeletal muscle in response to extreme altitude. *Acta Physiol. Scand.*, **142**, 421–7.
Menzies, I.S. (1984) Transmucosal passage of inert molecules in health and disease, in *Intestinal Absorption and Secretion*, Falk Symposium 36, (eds E. Skadhauge and K. Heintze), MTP Press, Lancaster, pp. 527–43.
Milledge, J.S. (1972) Arterial oxygen desaturation and intestinal absorption of xylose. *Br. Med. J.*, **2**, 557–8.
Moore, L.G., Cymerman, A., Huang, S.Y., *et al.* (1987) Propranalol blocks the metabolic rate increase but not ventilatory acclimatization to 4300 m. *Respir. Physiol.*, **70**, 195–204.
Nair, C.S., Malhotra, M.S. and Gopinarth, P.M. (1971) Effect of altitude and cold acclimatization on the basal metabolism in man. *Aerosp. Med.*, **42**, 1056–9.
Oelz, O., Howald, H., di Prampero, P.E., *et al.* (1986) Physiological profile of world-class high-altitude climbers. *J. Appl. Physiol.*, **60**, 1734–42.
Pappenheimer, J. (1988) Physiological regulation of transepithelial impedance in the intestinal mucosa of rats and hamsters. *J. Membr. Biol.*, **100**, 137–48.
Picon-Reategui, E. (1961) Basal metabolic rate and body composition at high altitudes. *J. Appl. Physiol.*, **16**, 431–4.
Pritchard, J.S. and Lane, D.J. (1974) Intestinal absorption studied in patients with chronic obstructive airways disease. *Thorax*, **29**, 609.
Pugh, L.G.C.E. and Band, G. (1953) Appendix VI: Diet, in *The Ascent of Everest*, (ed. J. Hunt) Hodder and Stoughton, London, pp. 263–9.
Pugh, L.G.C.E. (1962) Physiological and medical aspects of the Himalayan Scientific and Mountaineering Expedition, 1960–1. *Br. Med. J.*, **2**, 621–33.
Pugh, L.G.C.E., Gill, M.B., Lahiri, S., *et al.* (1964) Muscular exercise at great altitude. *J. Appl. Physiol.*, **19**, 431–40.
Rai, R.M., Malhotra, M.S., Dimri, G.P. and Sampathkumar, T. (1975) Utilization of different quantities of fat at high altitude. *Am. J. Clin. Nutr.*, **28**, 242–5.
Raja, K.B., Pippard, M.J., Simpson, R.J. and Peters, T.J. (1986) Relationship between erythropoiesis and the enhanced intestinal uptake of ferric iron in hypoxia in the mouse. *Br. J. Heamatol.*, **64**, 587–93.
Rennie, M.J., Babij, P., Sutton, J.R., *et al.* (1983) Effects of acute hypoxia on

forearm leucine metabolism, in *Hypoxia, Exercise and Altitude*, (eds J.R. Sutton, C.S. Houston and N.L. Jones), Liss, New York, pp. 317–24.

Richalet, J.-P., Souberbielle, J.-C., Antezana, A.-M., *et al.* (1993) Control of erythropoiesis in humans during prolonged exposure to the altitude of 6542 m. *Am. J. Physiol.*, **266**, R756–64.

Rose, M.S., Houston, C.S., Fulco, C.S., *et al.* (1988) Operation Everest II: nutrition and body composition. *J. Appl. Physiol.*, **65**, 2545–51.

Schoeller, D.A. and Van Santen, E. (1982) Measurement of energy expenditure in humans by doubly labelled water method. *J. Appl. Physiol.*, **53**, 955–9.

Tilman, H.W. (1975) Practical problems of nutrition, in *Mountain Medicine and Physiology*, (eds C. Clarke, M. Ward and E. Williams), Alpine Club, London, pp. 62–6.

Travis, S.P.L. and Menzies, I.S. (1992) Intestinal permeability: functional assessment and significance. *Clin. Sci.*, **82**, 471–88.

Travis, S.P.L., A'Court, C., Menzies, I.S., *et al.* (1993) Intestinal function at altitudes above 5000 m (abstract). *Gut*, **34**, T165.

West, J.B., Boyer, S.J., Graber, D.J., *et al.* (1983) Maximum exercise at extreme altitude on Mount Everest. *J. Appl. Physiol.*, **55**, 688–98.

Westerterp, K.R., Kayser, B., Brouns, F., *et al.* (1992) Energy expenditure climbing Mt Everest. *J. Appl. Physiol.*, **73**, 1815–9.

Wolfel, E.E., Groves, B.M., Brooks, G.A., *et al.* (1991) Oxygen transport during steady state submaximal exercise in chronic hypoxia. *J. Appl. Physiol.*, **70**, 1129–36.

14

The endocrine and renal systems at altitude

14.1 INTRODUCTION

Endocrinology comprises many systems controlling a great variety of bodily functions and the effect of altitude has only been studied on a fraction of these. The areas studied reflect the interests of scientists going to altitude. Thus hormones that play a part in fluid and electrolyte balance have been widely studied because of their possible relevance to acute mountain sickness (AMS) and its complications, as have thyroid hormones because of their effect on metabolic rate. Another factor in the selection of systems for study has, of course, been the availability and ease of relevant assays. This chapter surveys the principal systems studied to date but clearly there are great areas of endocrinology in which the effects of acute and chronic hypoxia have yet to be explored.

The study of endocrinology at altitude is perfectly feasible, but attention to details of sampling, such as time of day, subject's posture, diet and exercise is required in studies at sea-level. Practical aspects of collection and storage of samples are discussed in Chapter 31.

14.2 ANTIDIURETIC HORMONE

There is considerable evidence that ascent to altitude is associated with changes in body fluid compartments both in those with AMS and in asymptomatic subjects. Not surprisingly therefore, investigators have studied the role of the antidiuretic hormone (ADH) in both the normal (healthy) response to hypoxia and in AMS. Reports on the effect of hypoxia on ADH have given conflicting results.

14.2.1 Exercise and ADH

Exercise in the absence of hypoxia was studied by Williams *et al.* (1979). They studied the effect of day-long hill walking over seven consecutive days and found no alteration in ADH concentration, despite the fact that their subjects developed peripheral (exercise) oedema associated with sodium retention (section 14.3.3).

14.2.2 Acute hypoxia and ADH

Forsling and Milledge (1977) found that breathing 10–10.5% oxygen for four hours had no effect on ADH levels in samples taken at intervals of from 3 min to 4 h of hypoxia. In a chamber experiment, where subjects were taken to an equivalent altitude of 4000 m for 14 h, there was no significant change in ADH plasma concentration until subjects began to feel nauseated when levels rose markedly (Forsling and Milledge, 1980). Claybaugh *et al.* (1982) took subjects to various equivalent altitudes in a chamber and found an initial increase of urinary ADH at 8–12 h of hypoxia with subsequent return to sea-level values. In two subjects with AMS there was a rise in urinary excretion of ADH at 2–4 h of hypoxia. It would seem, therefore, that acute hypoxia alone has very little effect but nausea due to AMS is associated with a rise in ADH, analogous to that seen in motion sickness (Eversman *et al.*, 1978).

14.2.3 Chronic hypoxia and ADH

Studies conducted in the field include one by Singh *et al.* (1974), who measured a number of hormones in a group of subjects who had a history of high-altitude pulmonary oedema. In those who remained free of symptoms on going to altitude, there was no change in ADH concentration. In subjects who became sick there was a tendency to higher levels but this was mainly seen after a few days at altitude and was not statistically significant. Harber *et al.* (1981) found no significant change in urinary ADH concentration on going to altitudes up to 5400 m; nor was there any relationship with AMS. Even in a fatal case of high altitude cerebral oedema there was no significant rise in ADH. Cosby *et al.* (1988) found higher levels of ADH in five skiers with high altitude pulmonary oedema compared with controls at the same altitude, but the difference did not reach statistical significance. Ramirez *et al.* (1992) found no change in ADH with altitude.

Hackett *et al.* (1978) found normal levels in trekkers at 4300 m, including those with and without symptoms of AMS; the only exceptions were higher concentrations in two cases of high-altitude pulmonary oedema.

The conclusion from this work would seem to be that hypoxia *per se* has no significant effect on ADH concentration. High values may be associated with AMS but not all cases have high values (Claybaugh *et al.*, 1982). Where high concentrations are found they may be an effect of AMS rather than its cause.

14.2.4 Inappropriate ADH secretion at altitude

Blume *et al.* (1984) presented evidence of inappropriately low excretion of ADH at altitude. They studied 13 subjects after some weeks at 5400 m and 6300 m on Everest during the AMREE in 1981 and found ADH concentration unchanged from sea-level despite a significant increase in plasma osmolality with increasing altitude. At 6300 m the serum osmolality was 302 mOsm kg^{-1} compared with 290 mOsm kg^{-1} at sea-level (normal 280–295). An overnight dehydration test at sea-level which might produce this degree of hyperosmolality would result in ADH concentrations of about 7 μU ml^{-1}, whereas subjects on Everest had a mean value of only 0.9 μU ml^{-1}. Twelve-hour urinary ADH showed the same lack of response. Sodium, potassium, calcium and phosphate concentrations were all modestly increased compared with sea-level values. A recent study by Ramirez *et al.* (1992) confirmed these observations. They increased osmolality by intravenous sodium loading a group of subjects at sea-level and at altitude (3000 m). At sea-level there was the expected rise in ADH but at altitude there was no significant rise. Thus, at altitude, there seems to be a failure of the osmoregulatory mechanism. This is the converse of the clinical syndrome of inappropriate ADH secretion often associated with small cell carcinoma of the lung (Bayliss, 1987). In such cases serum sodium concentration and osmolality are low but ADH secretion is inappropriately high.

14.3 THE RENIN–ANGIOTENSIN–ALDOSTERONE SYSTEM

This system is depicted in Figure 14.1. Renin is released in response to a number of stimuli, including posture, exercise and, possibly, hypoxia. The mechanism common to these stimuli is sympathetic activation, and both circulating catecholamine and direct sympathetic nervous stimulation result in release of renin from the juxtaglomerular apparatus of the kidney.

Renin has no biological activity but acts on its circulating substrate (angiotensinogen), cleaving it to produce the octapeptide angiotensin I, which is also devoid of activity. Angiotensin converting enzyme (ACE) found on the luminal surface of endothelial cells converts angiotensin I to angiotensin II by cleaving the final two amino acids. The principal site of conversion is in the rich capillary network of the lung where nearly 90% of angiotensin I is converted to angiotensin II in a single passage. Angiotensin II is a powerful vasopressor and also acts on

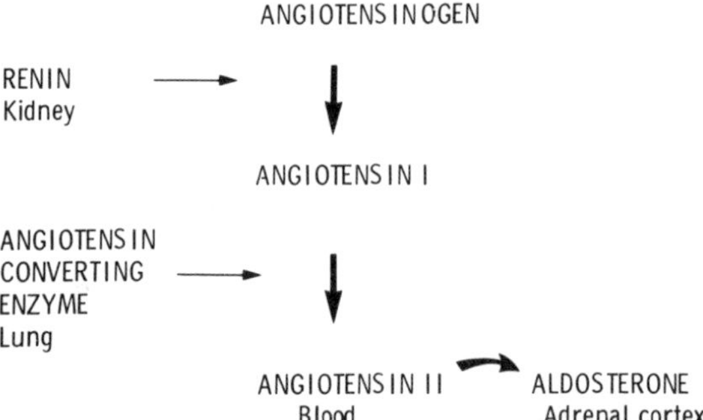

Figure 14.1 The renin–angiotensin–aldosterone system. Renin and angiotensin converting enzyme act as enzymes hydrolysing angiotensinogen and angiotensin I to angiotensin II. The latter stimulates release of aldosterone from adrenocortical cells by a receptor mechanism.

the cells of the adrenal cortex via a receptor mechanism to release aldosterone. Aldosterone acts on the renal tubules, promoting the reabsorption of sodium. In this way the system is important in the salt and water economy of the body and is the reason why it has been quite intensively studied at altitude.

14.3.1 Aldosterone and altitude

Indirect evidence of the effect of altitude on aldosterone activity was first provided by Williams (1961) who brought back samples of saliva from the Karakoram. The ratio of sodium to potassium in these samples indicated suppression of aldosterone at altitude. This has been confirmed by direct measurements of either plasma aldosterone concentration or urinary metabolites (Tuffley *et al.*, 1970; Hogan *et al.*, 1973; Frayser *et al.*, 1975; Pines *et al.*, 1977; Sutton *et al.*, 1977; Keynes *et al.*, 1982; Ramirez *et al.*, 1992); in one study the secretion rate was shown to be reduced (Slater *et al.*, 1969). Milledge *et al.* (1983a) studied the time course of the effect of altitude over a six-week stay at or above 4500 m. After initial suppression, aldosterone concentration rose to control values after 12–20 days. All these studies were made on resting subjects. In subjects who had been above 6000 m for more than ten weeks and had expanded fluid compartments (blood volume 85% above normal) the aldosterone concentration was twice normal (Anand *et al.*, 1993). These subjects were probably in incipient subacute mountain sickness (Chapter 17).

14.3.2 Renin activity and altitude

The effect of altitude on plasma renin activity (PRA) has been studied by a number of groups with conflicting results. Some have found a rise (Slater *et al.*, 1969; Tuffley *et al.*, 1970; Frayser *et al.*, 1975) and others a fall (Hogan *et al.*, 1973; Maher *et al.*, 1975a; Keynes *et al.*, 1982) and one group no change (Sutton *et al.*, 1977). However, most studies have shown a reduced response of aldosterone to renin. This is obvious where PRA has increased and aldosterone has decreased but, even where both have declined, the reduction in aldosterone has usually been greater.

It is not clear why these different studies produced different results. One possibility is that subjects, though sampled at rest, may have been more active in some studies, resulting in a rise in PRA. However, this is unlikely in view of the fact that one study showing a rise in PRA was conducted in a chamber (Tuffley *et al.*, 1970) and in another samples were taken before getting up in the morning after subjects had been flown to altitude in a helicopter (Slater *et al.*, 1969). The main stimulus to renin release is thought to be sympathetic drive and this certainly occurs with exercise but is probably also induced by altitude hypoxia alone (section 14.4) although with great individual variation. The exercise induced rise in renin can be inhibited by giving beta-blocker drugs (Bouissou *et al.*, 1989).

14.3.3 Exercise and the renin–aldosterone system

Since exercise frequently accompanies ascent to altitude, the effect of exercise needs to be considered in relation to the effect of altitude. Exercise stimulates renin release via activation of the adreno–sympathetic system. The effect can be blocked by beta-blockers (Bonelli *et al.*, 1977). After intense short term exercise (3 × 300 m sprints in 10 min) PRA, angiotensin II and aldosterone concentration were elevated at 30 min but measurable elevation was still present up to 6 h later (Kosunen and Pakarinen, 1976). The rise in PRA is also proportional to the intensity of the work, both at sea-level and at altitude (Maher *et al.*, 1975a).

Mountaineers are more concerned with day-long exercise, often continuing for a number of days. Williams *et al.* (1979) showed that this form of exercise resulted in marked sodium retention after seven days and suggested that this was due to activation of the renin–aldosterone system. There was a mean cumulative retention of 358 mmol of sodium with a modest retention of 650 ml of water. Since plasma sodium concentration did not change significantly it was argued that the extracellular space must have been expanded by 2.68 l (of which 0.68 l was in the plasma volume) mainly at the expense of the intracellular

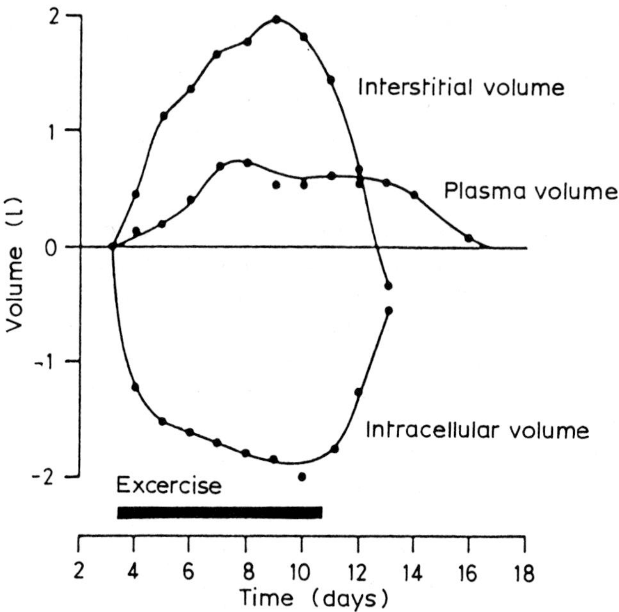

Figure 14.2 Calculated changes in body fluid compartments with exercise at sea-level. (From Williams *et al.*, 1979.)

volume. These calculated changes are shown in Figure 14.2. This increase in extracellular fluid is the probable cause of the dependent oedema frequently found after exercise of this sort.

Milledge *et al.* (1982) studied the effect of five consecutive days' hill walking on the renin–aldosterone system and on sodium and water balance, and confirmed the suggestion that the sodium retention was due to activation of the renin–aldosterone system. There was elevation of PRA and aldosterone at the conclusion of each day's exercise. This was maximal on the second or third day and was less marked on the fourth and fifth days, perhaps reflecting a training effect. Values were back to control on the second day after stopping exercise.

14.3.4 Control of aldosterone release

The control of aldosterone release via renin and angiotensin has been mentioned above and is shown in Figure 14.1, but aldosterone concentration is also controlled to an extent by ACTH and the sodium status of the subject. Salt depletion increases aldosterone release whilst salt loading inhibits it. Anderson *et al.* (1986) have shown that atrial natriuretic peptide (ANP) infusion inhibits the response of aldosterone to angiotensin II.

14.3.5 The effect of altitude on the aldosterone response to renin

Milledge and Catley (1982) showed that, if after one hour's exercise the inspired oxygen was reduced, renin activity increased while aldosterone levels decreased, indicating that the aldosterone response to renin became blunted. In the chronic situation of hill walking or climbing at altitude compared with sea-level the same phenomenon is seen. This is shown in Figure 14.3 which shows data from three studies, at sea-level, at 3100 m and on Mt Everest. This blunting has been confirmed by Shigeoka *et al.* (1985) who found the response completely abolished by hypoxia; it was also confirmed by Lawrence *et al.* (1991).

The cause of this blunting is not clear. It had been suggested that ACE activity was reduced by hypoxia, but most workers have found this not to be the case (Milledge and Catley, 1987; Bouissou *et al.*, 1988). However, one recent study has found that, while angiotensin I levels were unchanged with acute hypoxia, levels of angiotensin II were reduced (Vonmoos *et al.*, 1990). The next stage in the promotion of aldosterone release is adrenal stimulation by angiotensin II. Colice and Ramirez (1986) studied the effect of angiotensin II infusion on aldosterone release and found that hypoxia had no effect, suggesting that it did not result in an increase of inhibitors of this part of the system. However, Raff and Kohandarvish (1990) found evidence that adrenocortical cells *in vitro* were less responsive to angiotensin II under hypoxic conditions.

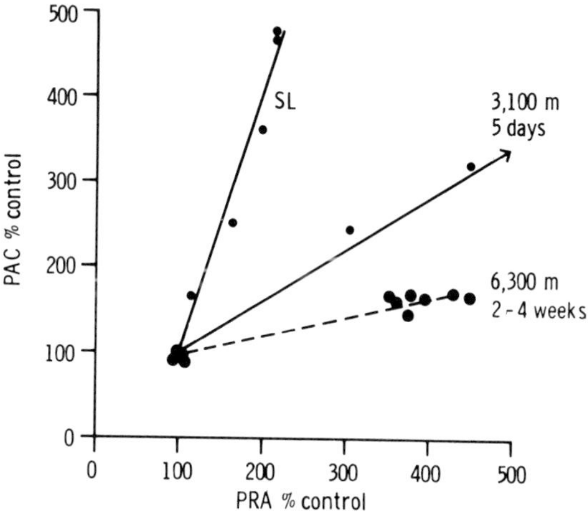

Figure 14.3 Plasma aldosterone concentration (PAC) response to plasma renin activity (PRA) from a sea-level (SL) study and from two separate altitude studies. (From Milledge *et al.*, 1983b.)

Aldosterone secretion is stimulated by ACTH as well as by angiotensin II. Ramirez *et al.* (1988) found this effect to be reduced in subjects at altitude while the ACTH-induced secretion of cortisol was unaffected. ANP has been found to inhibit aldosterone release (Elliott and Goodfriend, 1986). It is therefore possible that the rise in ANP on going to altitude (14.4.4) may be a factor in blunting this response at rest (Lawrence *et al.*, 1990) and on exercise (Lawrence and Shenker, 1991).

14.4 ALTITUDE AND ATRIAL NATRIURETIC PEPTIDE (ANP)

14.4.1 ANP release and actions

Atrial natriuretic peptide (ANP) is secreted by the atria of the heart in response to stretching. Atrial stretch is usually caused by an increase in atrial pressure. However, in the case of cardiac tamponade the pressure is high but the atrial wall is not stretched. As the tamponade is relieved the pressure falls and the atrium dilates. It has been found that relief of tamponade results in a rise in ANP plasma levels indicating that stretch rather than pressure is the stimulus for ANP synthesis and release (Au *et al.*, 1990).

Amongst its actions, ANP has the effect of increasing sodium excretion by the kidneys and thus of promoting a natriuresis and diuresis (Morice *et al.*, 1988). This provides a homeostatic mechanism for salt and water in that, if the plasma volume is increased, the raised atrial pressure results in atrial stretch and secretion of ANP, diuresis follows and vascular pressures and volume return to normal. This system is further considered in relation to the regulation of plasma volume in section 7.2.2. ANP probably also has a role as a vasodilator, countering the pressor effect of hypoxia on the pulmonary artery. It has been shown to have this effect in a dose dependent manner in the isolated rat lung (Stewart *et al.*, 1991) and in the pig (Adnot *et al.*, 1988). Liu *et al.* (1989) infused ANP (20 mg min^{-1} for 10 min) into four patients with high-altitude pulmonary edema (HAPE) and showed a reduction in pulmonary artery pressure for 1 h after the infusion.

14.4.2 ANP and hypoxia

In the last few years, since the first edition of this book, there have been numerous reports of the effect of hypoxia on the plasma levels of ANP at rest and on exercise.

Ten minutes of severe hypoxia on isolated rat and rabbit heart with constant flow perfusion caused a fourfold increase in ANP released (Baertschi *et al.*, 1986). The same group have found increases in ANP blood levels in the whole animal made hypoxic under anaesthesia.

There was great variability in the response which correlated with the baseline central venous pressure but not with any other measured variables. Winter *et al.* (1989) also found ANP levels to be increased by hypoxia in the rat after 24 h but not after only 2 h. In patients with chronic hypoxic lung disease, levels of ANP were elevated and varied inversely with the Pa_{O_2} (Winter et al., 1987).

In healthy volunteers Kawashima *et al.* (1989) studied the effect of 10 min hypoxia at two levels; 15% oxygen breathing produced no change whilst 10% oxygen breathing increased ANP levels by 15% accompanied by an increase in pulmonary artery pressure. Vonmoos *et al.* (1990) found that 60 min of 12% oxygen breathing produced a small but significant elevation of ANP, whilst Lawrence *et al.* (1990) found that the same hypoxic stimulus produced a 50% increase in ANP levels in subjects on a low salt diet and whose endogenous cortisol was suppressed with dexamethasone. Conversely, Ramirez *et al.* (1992) did not find a significant rise in ANP levels with either acute (60 min) or chronic hypoxia at 3000 m, although the ANP response to a sodium load was greater at altitude.

14.4.3 Exercise and ANP: normoxia

Somers *et al.* (1986) found that a progressive exercise test to maximum exercise resulted in an almost fourfold increase in plasma ANP with a decline to baseline after 1 h at rest. Similar results have been found for short term exercise by Schmidt *et al.* (1990) and by Lawrence and Shenker (1991). Hill walking exercise for five days also resulted in elevated ANP levels to about twice baseline values (Milledge *et al.*, 1991). It is interesting to note that during this type of exercise sodium is retained despite elevated ANP levels.

14.4.4 Exercise and ANP: hypoxia

Mountaineers and trekkers going to altitude normally have the double stimulus of exercise and hypoxia. Schmidt *et al.* (1990) studied exercise while breathing air or reduced oxygen (92 mmHg). With both maximal and submaximal exercise the ANP response to exercise was reduced under hypoxic conditions. In contrast, Lawrence and Shenker (1991), using less severe hypoxia (16% inspired) and exercise such as to give a heart rate of 70–75% of maximum for 30 min, found that hypoxia enhanced the ANP response. A third study using a decompression chamber to give a simulated altitude of 3000 m and a progressive exercise test to maximum showed a reduced response (Vuolteenaho *et al.*, 1992). The reasons for these differing results are not apparent.

Milledge *et al.* (1989) reported levels of plasma ANP in 15 subjects before and after ascent on foot from 3100 m to 4300 m. Values tended to be higher at altitude but were significantly so only in the 4 a.m. sample on the second altitude day, there being no difference on day one at altitude or in the 9 a.m. sample on either day. Bärtsch *et al.* (1991) found, in blood samples taken on the morning after the ascent to 4559 m on foot, no increase in ANP levels in a group of nine climbers who did not have AMS. Five subjects who did become sick had elevated levels. These subjects had a history of high-altitude pulmonary oedema and were shown by echocardiography to have increased atrial diameters at altitude. The increase in ANP may have been secondary to developing high pulmonary artery pressures. Kawashima *et al.* (1992) showed that, in subjects susceptible to high altitude pulmonary oedema, breathing 10% oxygen resulted in a greater rise in ANP levels than in controls, and that the rise correlated with the rise in pulmonary artery pressure.

14.4.5 ANP and acute mountain sickness (AMS)

An important motive for the study of the effect of altitude hypoxia on ANP has been the hypothesis that it may play a part in the genesis of AMS. Milledge *et al.* (1989) did not find any correlation between levels of ANP on the morning after arrival at altitude and the AMS symptom score. However Bärtsch *et al.* (1988) and Cosby *et al.* (1988) found subjects with AMS or HAPE to have higher levels than subjects without AMS. If the rise in ANP in AMS sufferers is related to high pulmonary arterial pressure, elevation would be expected mainly in AMS with pulmonary oedema and not in the milder, non-pulmonary cases. In the first-mentioned study there was no clinical evidence of pulmonary oedema.

In conclusion it seems that while both exercise and hypoxia cause an elevation of ANP, the combined stimulus does not result in very high levels at altitude. Despite its name, ANP is not a powerful natriuretic hormone. Levels of ANP are elevated in conditions where the pulmonary artery pressure is raised, including HAPE, and this rise is probably secondary. The rise in ANP is probably beneficial in that it tends to reduce the pressure by its vasodilatory function.

14.5 CORTICOSTEROIDS AND ALTITUDE

On ascent to altitude, there is stimulation of the adrenal cortex by ACTH and cortisol is secreted. Early work documented this as a rise in 17-hydroxycorticosteroids (17-OHCS) during the first few days at altitude, which fell back to control values by days 5–7 (MacKinnon *et al.*, 1963; Moncloa *et al.*, 1965). This has been confirmed by measurement of plasma cortisol by Frayser *et al.* (1975) and Sutton *et al.* (1977), who showed that with the elevation of plasma cortisol there was a decrease in its normal diurnal variation on the first day of altitude exposure. Richalet *et al.* (1989), in a chamber experiment, also found elevation of plasma cortisol with re-establishment of the diurnal variation after the first altitude day. Many of the subjects of these studies, taken rapidly to an altitude of 4300–5300 m, suffered from AMS, but even those free of symptoms showed this transitory rise in cortisol or its urinary metabolite. It is assumed that this is a non-specific stress response.

A recent interesting case report shows that there is a clinical lesson to be learnt. A 58-year-old man, who had had his pituitary removed ten years earlier for an adenoma, went trekking in Nepal. On arrival at Menang (3535 m) he complained of fatigue, abdominal pain, nausea and vomiting, but no headache. He was on regular medication with cortisone 25 mg daily and had taken his treatment. Twenty-four hours later he had deteriorated and was unable to stand. He was treated with dexamethasone 5 mg i.v. and 5 mg i.m. and oral rehydration, and his cortisone dose was quadrupled. Within 24 h all symptoms had disappeared, and the day after he successfully crossed the Thorong La (5450 m) (Westendorp *et al.*, 1993). Clearly the lesson is that subjects on corticosteroid replacement therapy should increase their dosage on going to altitude. The authors point out that this does not apply to thyroid replacement therapy since TSH is not increased by hypoxia.

The effect of prolonged stay at more extreme altitude was studied by Siri *et al.* (1969). They brought back urine samples from the 1963 Everest expedition from climbers staying at 5400 m and 6500 m. The 17-OHCS levels were not significantly different from sea-level values. They also demonstrated a normal response to injected ACTH. Mordes *et al.* (1983) collected samples from subjects who had been for some weeks at 5400 m and 6300 m and found no change from sea-level values in either morning or evening cortisol concentrations.

In animals studied after chronic hypoxia there was some hyperplasia of the adrenal cortex and of the corticotrophic cells in the pituitary. No such morphological changes have been found in man with long standing chronic bronchitis (Gosney, 1986). However, in subjects who had spent more than ten weeks above 6000 m, the cortisol level was found to be three times normal (Anand *et al.*, 1993).

14.6 THE ADRENO–SYMPATHETIC SYSTEM

14.6.1 Acute hypoxia

Acute hypoxia increases heart rate at rest and on exercise (Maher *et al.*, 1975a). This is presumed to be due to increased sympathetic activity stimulating the beta-adrenergic receptors on heart muscle cell membrane. However, measurements of plasma, epinephrine and norepinephrine after 10 min of mild isocapnic hypoxia at rest showed no increase over control values despite a rise in heart rate of 70–83 (Ind *et al.*, 1984). On light exercise, plasma catecholamine levels are increased by acute hypoxia but this is not seen after heavy exercise (75% $\dot{V}_{O_2}$ max) (Maher *et al.*, 1975a). Bouissou *et al.* (1989) also found a 32% increase in norepinephrine after 48 h at altitude but on maximal exercise the rise in catecholamines was no different from that seen at sea-level. Mazzeo *et al.* (1991) found reduced norepinephrine and raised epinephrine levels at rest. On submaximal exercise, norepinephrine levels rose as they did at sea-level. Epinephrine rose with exercise whereas at sea-level it remained unchanged.

14.6.2 Chronic hypoxia

Cunningham *et al.* (1965) reported elevated plasma and 24-hour urinary catecholamines during 17 days at 4560 m on Monte Rosa. There was no significant change in epinephrine but the increase in norepinephrine was greater on the twelfth day at altitude. Pace *et al.* (1964) found similar results at 3850 m, with urinary norepinephrine excretion rising slowly during 14 days at altitude without change in urinary epinephrine secretion. Maher *et al.* (1975a) found increased urinary catecholamines at 4300 m. Levels were increased on day one compared with sea-level and further increased on day 11. On exercise, both light and severe, the effect of chronic hypoxia compared with acute was to increase levels still further. Hoon *et al.* (1977) found no significant change in urinary catecholamine secretion in a total of 76 subjects who had no symptoms of AMS, whereas in 29 symptomatic subjects there was a small but significant rise on the first day at altitude, which was maintained through to the tenth altitude day. Mazzeo *et al.* (1991) found that, at rest, norepinephrine and epinephrine levels were higher at altitude than at sea-level. With submaximal exercise, norepinephrine rose to higher values than expected at sea-level, whilst epinephrine levels did not rise, though values remained above those at sea-level. In Operation Everest II at extreme altitude (282 mmHg) after 40 days in the chamber, resting plasma norepinephrine was raised but epinephrine was reduced. On maximum exercise, values for both catecholamines fell with increasing altitude (Young *et al.*, 1989).

In subjects who had spent more than ten weeks above 6000 m the plasma norepinephrine concentration was found to be almost three times normal (Anand *et al.*, 1993). Gosney *et al.* (1991) studied the adrenal and pituitary glands of five lifelong residents of La Paz who had lived at 3600–3800 m, and compared their glands with those of controls from sea-level. The adrenal glands were significantly bigger by about 50%. The pituitary glands were not larger but contained more corticotrophs. They surmised that greater amounts of ACTH were required to maintain adrenal function, perhaps because of hypoxic inhibition of adrenocortical sensitivity. However, Ramirez *et al.* (1988) found no such inhibition.

14.6.3 Adrenergic response and acclimatization

Acute hypoxia causes an increase in heart rate and cardiac output. However, after several days at altitude the heart rate and cardiac output fall back towards sea-level values. On exercise the maximum heart rate is limited to well below the sea-level maximum, being typically 140–150 beats per minute compared with 180–200 at sea-level (Chapter 6). This reduction in heart rate and cardiac output takes place at a time when the plasma and urinary catecholamines are higher than at sea-level.

Evidently, the heart's response to sympathetic stimulation becomes blunted. This has been demonstrated by Maher *et al.* (1975b), who showed in dogs that the cardio-acceleratory effect of an infusion of isoproterenol was reduced after 10 days' altitude acclimatization. Workers from the same institution (Maher *et al.*, 1978) found in cardiac muscle of acclimatized goats that there was a twofold rise of the enzyme *o*-methyltransferase. This enzyme inactivates cardiac norepinephrine, and its induction during acclimatization may account for the blunting of the adrenergic response to exercise. Another possibility is that there may be down regulation, that is a reduction in the density of adrenergic receptors on the heart muscle. Voelkel *et al.* (1981) have shown this to be the case in rats kept for five weeks at a simulated altitude of 4250 m. These two possible mechanisms are not mutually exclusive. Sherpa high-altitude residents do not suffer this heart rate limitation on maximal exercise. Their heart rates can go up to 190–198 a minute at 4880 m (Lahiri *et al.*, 1967).

In summary, hypoxia has no effect on epinephrine levels in the blood or urine but there is a modest rise in norepinephrine levels. This may be more marked in subjects with AMS. The response of the heart to adrenergic stimulation becomes blunted after a week or ten days at altitude and this may be due to down regulation of receptors and/or induction of the enzyme responsible for catecholamine metabolism.

14.7 THYROID FUNCTION AND THE ALTITUDE ENVIRONMENT

Hypothalamic–pituitary–thyroid axis function is affected by hypoxia and possibly by cold. The effect of cold on thyroid function is considered in Chapter 23. Iodine is essential for synthesis of thyroid hormone and is deficient in the soil and water of some mountainous regions, so that thyroid function in residents of these regions is affected.

14.7.1 Thyroid function and hypoxia

The response of the hypophyseal–thyroid axis to hypoxia seems to be quite different in man compared with animals. In animals, hypoxia results in depression of thyroid function (Heath and Williams, 1981). In the pituitary gland the number of thyrotrophs (cells that secrete thyroid stimulating hormone (TSH)) is reduced suggesting a decreased output of TSH (Gosney, 1986). In humans, however, thyroid activity is increased at altitude. Surks (1966) found elevated levels of thyroxine binding globulin (TBG) and free thyroxine (T_4) in the first two weeks at altitude (4300 m) with a peak at nine days. Kotchen *et al.* (1973), in a three-day chamber experiment (3650 m equivalent), found T_4 elevated (free and bound) but TSH to be unchanged, suggesting a shift of T_4 from extra- to intravascular compartments rather than increased pituitary activity. Westendorp *et al.* (1993) also found no increase in TSH in response to a one-hour acute hypoxia equivalent of 4115 m.

These results have been confirmed in a number of field studies (Rastogi *et al.*, 1977; Stock *et al.*, 1978b) which showed levels returning towards control in the third week at altitude. Sawhney and Malhotra (1991) studied both acclimatized lowlanders and high-altitude natives, and found levels of triiodothyronine (T_3) and T_4 to be higher than sea-level residents. T_3 concentration in erythrocytes was decreased at high altitude but there was no change in levels of reverse T_3 (rT_3), TBG, and T_4 binding capacity of TBG and thyroxine binding prealbumin. They also found no change in TSH; in L-eltroxine treated men they still found a rise in T_3 and T_4, suggesting the rise to be independent of pituitary stimulation.

Exercise increases T_3 and T_4 to a greater extent at altitude than at sea-level (Stock *et al.*, 1978b). At higher altitudes of 5400 m and 6300 m Mordes *et al.* (1983) showed elevated resting T_3, free T_4 and T_3 in subjects who had been at altitude for some weeks. In these subjects TSH was also elevated in contrast to the finding at lower altitudes.

The basal metabolic rate is elevated during the first two weeks at moderate altitude and correlates with the free T_4 (Stock *et al.*, 1978a). At higher altitudes (above 5500 m) it remains elevated for months (Gill and Pugh, 1964), as does T_4 (Mordes *et al.*, 1983). Mordes *et al.* (1983) also found evidence of impaired conversion of T_4 to T_3 at 6300 m. Perhaps there is a change in the set point for the pituitary negative feedback system, resulting in higher levels of TSH. The response of the pituitary to an injection of thyrotrophin releasing hormone was enhanced at 6300 m compared with sea-level.

14.7.2 Iodine deficiency, goitre and altitude

The frequency of goitre in mountainous areas is well known and has been discussed in Chapter 16. In England it was known as 'Derbyshire neck' and it was equally well known in the Pyrenees, the Alps, the Andes and the Himalayas, but it is not confined to the mountains.

The association of iodine deficiency and mountainous areas is mainly due to the geological factors (Chapter 16) but altitude hypoxia stimulates thyroid function (section 14.7.1). Thus the effect of iodine deficiency will result in more exaggerated hyperplasia, which contributes to the extremely high rate of goitre in resident populations at altitude.

14.8 THE CONTROL OF BLOOD GLUCOSE AT ALTITUDE

14.8.1 Acute hypoxia

On acute exposure to hypoxia there is a rise in fasting blood glucose of about 1.7 $mmol\,l^{-1}$, followed by a fall towards control values by the end of a week. At the same time insulin levels are elevated (Williams, 1975). This is presumably part of the non-specific stress response indicated by the concurrent rise in plasma cortisol levels (section 14.5).

14.8.2 Chronic hypoxia

In subjects acclimatized to high altitude, fasting blood glucose was found to be lower than at sea-level by some workers (Stock *et al.*, 1978b; Blume and Pace, 1967; Blume 1984) but unchanged by others (Sawhney *et al.*, 1986). Singh *et al.* (1974) found a persistently raised glucose level after 10 months at altitude. Resting insulin levels have also been found to be reduced (Stock *et al.*, 1978b).

Glucose loading increases both blood glucose and insulin levels at altitude as it does at sea-level, but the rise in both was found to be less than at sea-level in two studies (Stock *et al.*, 1978b; Blume, 1984) but greater in one (Sawhney *et al.*, 1986). There are a number of explanations for this blunted response. Glucose may be absorbed less rapidly, though this is probably only true above about 5500 m (section 13.5). Liver glycogen synthesis may be enhanced at altitude and some evidence for this has been found in rats injected with labelled glucose at altitude (Blume and Pace, 1971). There may be increased target organ sensitivity to insulin, presumably by up regulation (increased density) of insulin receptors on target cells. This is a feature of athletic training and may well happen as part of altitude acclimatization.

14.9 ALTITUDE AND OTHER HORMONES

14.9.1 Glucagon

Fasting glucagon levels are the same at altitude and at sea-level and are slightly depressed after glucose loading (Blume, 1984).

14.9.2 Growth hormone

Levels are unchanged in most subjects but were found to be increased fivefold in two subjects who had lost 15 kg in body weight (Blume, 1984). Although acute hypoxia causes no change in growth hormone levels, exercise under acute hypoxic conditions causes a twentyfold increase in this hormone, whereas normoxic exercise causes only a modest rise (Sutton, 1977; Raynaud *et al.*, 1981).

14.9.3 Vasoactive hormones

The levels of bradykinin, a potent vasodilator, are not changed by acute hypoxia (Ashack *et al.*, 1985), whereas endothelin, a potent vasoconstrictor, has been shown in rats to increase with increasing hypoxia (Horio *et al.*, 1991).

14.9.4 Testosterone, luteinizing hormone, follicle stimulating hormone and prolactin

Sawhney *et al.* (1985) studied levels of these hormones in lowland men after ascent to 3500 m. On day one at altitude there were no significant changes from sea-level values though luteinizing hormone (LH) and testosterone levels were already falling. By day seven, LH and testosterone levels were significantly reduced and remained so to day 18; by then prolactin levels were significantly elevated. After seven days at sea-level all values had reverted to control except for some residual depression in LH levels. These results are in accord with previous work (Guerra-Garcia, 1971) which found urinary testosterone excretion to be reduced by 50% on day three at 4300 m. Sawhney *et al.* (1985) also found a negative correlation between prolactin and testosterone levels at altitude but no correlation with LH levels. They suggested that the reduction in testosterone is due to increase in prolactin secretion rather than a reduction in LH or a direct effect of hypoxia on the testes.

In a separate experiment at sea-level Sawhney *et al.* (1985) showed a reduction in LH levels in response to daily cold exposure after one and five days, and suggested that the reduction in LH found at altitude might be due to cold rather than hypoxia. However, low levels of LH have been found in hypoxia due to chronic lung disease in hospital patients with no cold exposure (Semple, 1986); these patients also had low testosterone levels which correlated with their Pa_{O_2}.

Semple (1986) found normal testosterone levels in patients who were hypoxic because of congenital cardiac defects, presumably because of lifelong adaptation to hypoxaemia, though he suggests that an alternative mechanism may be that testosterone depression is due to dips in oxygen saturation at night, due to sleep apnoea in patients with chronic obstructive lung disease, and due to periodic breathing in lowlanders at altitude. In high-altitude residents, Bangham and Hackett (1978) found reduced levels of LH after ten days but no changes in follicle stimulating hormone, testosterone or prolactin levels.

Testosterone is increased in exercise and Bouissou *et al.* (1986) studied the effect of acute hypoxia (14% oxygen, equivalent to 3000 m) on this response. They found that when the exercise was expressed as a percentage of maximum exercise there was no effect of acute hypoxia. This is also true for the acute hypoxic effect on the exercise induced rises of lactate, epinephrine and norepinephrine.

14.10 RENAL FUNCTION AT ALTITUDE

14.10.1 General function

The kidney is remarkably resistant to altitude hypoxia. This is not surprising since it is designed to suffer quite severe reductions in blood flow and, therefore oxygen delivery, during exercise or in other situations where increased blood flow is needed elsewhere in the body. At 5800 m, after 24-hours' dehydration, the kidney concentrates urine normally and eliminates a water load as well as it does at sea-level. It also responds to ingestion of bicarbonate or ammonium chloride (metabolic alkalosis or acidosis) by producing appropriate changes in pH (Ward, reported by Pugh, 1962). Olsen *et al.* (1993) found a 10% reduction in effective renal plasma flow (ERPF) but normal glomerular filtration rate and sodium clearance in eight normal subjects at 4350 m. Dopamine infusion had less effect on ERPF than at sea-level, presumably because of increased adrenergic activity (norepinephrine was increased) and the diuretic effect of dopamine being reduced possibly because of an altitude effect on distal tubular function. High-altitude residents at 4300 m showed no evidence of deficient renal oxygenation (Rennie *et al.*, 1971a).

However, as discussed in (section 8.4.5) at extreme altitude (above

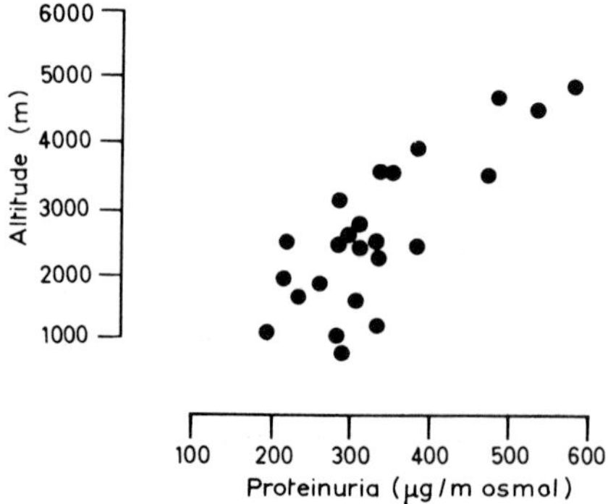

Figure 14.4 Proteinuria at altitude, the altitude being that of the subjects 24 h before urine sampling. (After Rennie 1973).

6500 m) the renal compensation for respiratory alkalosis is slow and incomplete; that is, the blood bicarbonate is very little further reduced and the blood pH becomes very alkaline as the P_{CO_2} is reduced by extreme hyperventilation. Whether this represents a degree of renal failure is debatable, since it results in a shift of the oxygen dissociation curve to the left (because of the alkaline pH) which is beneficial for oxygen transport at extreme altitude (section 8.3.6).

14.10.2 Proteinuria at altitude

Rennie and Joseph (1970) showed that proteinuria became apparent on ascent to altitude. Values rose from 290 to 578 μg mmol^{-1} as their subjects climbed to 5800 m in 12 days. There was a time lag of 1–3 days between peak altitude and peak proteinuria. Figure 14.4 shows that there is a good correlation between the degree of proteinuria and altitude, provided allowance is made for a 24-hours' time lag between ascent and its effect on the kidney.

In another study, Rennie *et al.* (1972) found no effect of acclimatization on proteinuria but Pines (1978) found less proteinuria on repeat ascents to the same altitude, and also that subjects with AMS had the greatest proteinuria. High altitude residents excrete more protein in the urine than subjects of the same race at sea-level (Rennie *et al.*, 1971b).

Patients with cyanotic heart disease who are chronically hypoxic from birth also have increased proteinuria, the severity being directly related to the degree of polycythaemia (and hypoxia) (Rennie, 1973); it is also found in patients with chronic obstructive lung disease (Wilkinson *et al.*, 1993).

The effect of acetazolamide on altitude proteinuria was studied by

Bradwell and Delamere (1982) as part of a double blind trial of the drug as a prophylactic for AMS. They found that at 5000 m albuminuria was six times greater in subjects on placebo tablets than those on acetazolamide. They found a negative linear correlation between Pa_{O_2} and percentage increase in urine albumin. The eight subjects on acetazolamide were of course less hypoxic, with $Pa_{O_2} > 42$ mmHg, than nine subjects on placebo with $Pa_{O_2} < 42$ mmHg. The authors suggest that the effect of acetazolamide on albuminuria was due to this reduction in hypoxia.

The mechanism for altitude proteinuria may be either a reduction in tubular reabsorption of protein or increased glomerular permeability to protein or both.

REFERENCES

Adnot, S., Chabrier, P.E., Brun-Buisson, C., *et al.* (1988) Atrial natriuretic factor attenuates the pulmonary pressor response to hypoxia. *J. Appl. Physiol.*, **65**, 1975–83.

Anand, I.S., Chandrashekhar, Y., Rao, S.K., *et al.* (1993) Body fluid compartments, renal blood flow, and hormones at 6000 m in normal subjects. *J. Appl. Physiol.*, **74**, 1234–9.

Anderson, J.V., Struthers, A.D., Payne, N.N., *et al.* (1986) Atrial natriuretic peptide inhibits the aldosterone response to angiotensin II in man. *Clin. Sci.*, **70**, 507–12.

Ashack, R., Farber, M.O., Weinberger, M.H., *et al.* (1985) Renal and hormonal responses to acute hypoxia in normal individuals. *J. Lab. Clin. Med.*, **106**, 12–16.

Au, J., Brown, J.E., Lee, M.R. and Boon, N.A (1990) Effect of cardiac tamponade on atrial natriuretic peptide concentrations: influence of stretch and pressure. *Clin. Sci.*, **79**, 377–80.

Baertschi, A.J., Hausmaninger, C., Walsh, R.S., *et al.* (1986) Hypoxia-induced release of atrial natriuretic factor (ANF) from isolated rat and rabbit heart. *Biochem. Biophys. Res. Commun.*, **140**, 427–33.

Bangham, C.R.M. and Hackett, P.H. (1978) Effects of high altitude on endocrine function in the Sherpas of Nepal. *J. Endocrinol.*, **79**, 147–8.

Bärtsch, P., Shaw, S., Franciolli, M., *et al.* (1988) Atrial natriuretic peptide in acute mountain sickness. *J. Appl. Physiol.*, **65**, 1929–37.

Bärtsch, P., Pfluger, N., Audetat, M.S., *et al.* (1991) Effects of slow ascent to 4559 m on fluid homeostasis. *Aviat. Space Environ. Med.*, **62**, 105–10.

Bayliss, R.I.S. (1987) Endocrine manifestations of non-endocrine disease, in *Oxford Textbook of Medicine*, 2nd edn, (eds D.J. Weatherall, J.G.G. Leadingham and D.A. Warrell), Oxford University Press, Oxford, pp. 101–19.

Blume, F.D. (1984) Metabolic and endocrine changes at altitudes, in *High Altitude and Man*, (eds J.B. West and S. Lahiri), American Physiological Society, Bethesda MD, pp. 37–45.

Blume, F.D. and Pace, N. (1967) Effect of translocation to 3800 m altitude on glycolysis in mice. *J. Appl. Physiol.*, **23**, 75–9.

Blume, F.D. and Pace, N. (1971) The utilisation of ^{14}C-labelled palmitic acid, alanine and aspartic acid at high altitude. *Environ. Physiol.*, **1**, 30–6.

Blume, F.D., Boyer, S.J., Braverman, L.E., *et al.* (1984) Impaired osmoregulation at high altitude. Studies on Mt Everest. *J. Am. Med. Assoc.*, **252**, 524–6.

Bonelli, J., Waldhausl, W., Magometschnigg, D., *et al.* (1977) Effect of exercise and of prolonged administration of propranalol on haemodynamic variables, plasma renin concentration, plasma aldosterone and c-AMP. *Eur. J. Clin. Invest.*, **7**, 337–43.

Bouissou, P., Peronnet, F., Brisson, G., *et al.* (1986) Metabolic and endocrine responses to graded exercise under acute hypoxia. *Eur. J. Appl. Physiol.*, **55**, 290–4.

Bouissou, P., Guezennec, C.Y., Galen, F.X., *et al.* (1988) Dissociated response of aldosterone from plasma renin activity during prolonged exercise under hypoxia. *Horm. Metab. Res.*, **20**, 517–21.

Bouissou, P., Richalet, J.-P., Galen, F.X., *et al.* (1989) Effect of B-adrenorecptor blockade on renin-aldosterone and a-ANF during exercise. *J. Appl. Physiol.*, **67**, 141–6.

Bradwell, A.R. and Delamere, J.P. (1982) The effect of acetazolamide on the proteinuria of altitude. *Aviat. Space Environ. Med.*, **53**, 40–3.

Claybaugh, J.R., Wade, C.E., Sato, A.K., *et al.* (1982) Antidiuretic hormone responses to eucapnic and hypocapnic hypoxia in humans. *J. Appl. Physiol. Respir. Environ. Exercise Physiol.*, **53**, 815–23.

Colice, G.L. and Ramirez, G. (1986) Aldosterone response to angiotensin II during hypoxemia. *J. Appl. Physiol.*, **61**, 150–4.

Cosby, R.L., Sophocles, A.M., Durr, J.A., *et al.* (1988) Elevated plasma atrial natriuretic factor and vasopressin in high-altitude pulmonary edema. *Ann. Intern. Med.*, **109**, 796–9.

Cunningham, W.L., Becker, E.J. and Kreuzer, F. (1965) Catecholamine in plasma and urine at high altitude. *J. Appl. Physiol.*, **20**, 607–10.

Elliott, M.E. and Goodfriend, T.L. (1986) Inhibition of aldosterone synthesis by atrial natriuretic factor. *Fed. Proc.*, **45**, 2376–81.

Eversman, T., Gottsman, M., Uhlich, E., *et al.* (1978) Increased secretion of growth hormone, prolactin, antidiuretic hormone and cortisol induced by the stress of motion sickness. *Aviat. Space Environ. Med.*, **49**, 53–7.

Forsling, M.L. and Milledge, J.S. (1977) Effect of hypoxia on vasopressin release in man. *J. Physiol.*, **267**, 22–23P.

Forsling, M.L. and Milledge, J.S. (1980) The effect of simulated altitude (4000 m) on plasma cortisol and vasopressin concentration in man. *Proc. Int. Union Physiol. Sci.*, **14**, 414.

Frayser, R., Rennie, I.D., Gray, G.W. and Houston, C.S. (1975) Hormonal and electrolyte response to exposure to 17 500 ft. *J. Appl. Physiol.*, **38**, 636–42.

Gill, M.B. and Pugh, L.G.C.E. (1964) Basal metabolism and respiration in men living at 5800 m (19 000 ft). *J. Appl. Physiol.*, **19**, 949–54.

Gosney, J. (1986) Histopathology of the endocrine organs in hypoxia, in *Aspects of Hypoxia*, (ed. D. Heath), Liverpool University Press, Liverpool, pp. 131–45.

Gosney, J., Heath, D., Williams, D. and Rios-Dalenz, J. (1991) Morphological changes in the pituitary–adrenocortical axis in natives of La Paz. *Int. J. Biometeorol.*, **35**, 1–5.

Guerra-Garcia, R. (1971) Testosterone metabolism in men exposed to high altitude. *Acta Endocrinol. Panama*, **2**, 55–9.

Hackett, P.H., Forsling, M.L., Milledge, J. and Rennie, D. (1978) Release of vasopressin in man at altitude. *Horm. Metab. Res.*, **10**, 571.

Harber, M.J., Williams, J.D. and Morton, J.J. (1981) Antidiuretic hormone excretion at high altitude. *Aviat. Space Environ. Med.*, **52**, 38–40.

Heath, D. and Williams, D.R. (1981) *Man at High Altitude*, 2nd edition, Churchill Livingstone, London, pp. 247–58.

Hogan, R.P., Kotchen, T.A., Boyd, A.E. and Hartley, L.H. (1973) Effect of altitude on renin–aldosterone system and metabolism of water and electrolytes. *J. Appl. Physiol.*, **35**, 385–90.

Hoon, R.S., Sharma, S.C., Balasubramanian, V. and Chadha, K.S. (1977) Urinary catecholamine excretion on induction to high altitude (3658 m) by air and road. *J. Appl. Physiol.*, **42**, 728–30.

Horio, T., Kohno, M., Yokokawa, K., *et al.* (1991) Effect of hypoxia on plasma immunoreactive endothelin-1 concentration in anaesthetized rats. *Metabolism*, **40**, 999–1001.

Ind, P.W., Maxwell, D.L., Causon, R.C., *et al.* (1984) Hypoxia and catecholamine secretion in normal man. *Clin. Sci.*, **67**, 58–59P.

Kawashima, A., Kubo, K., Kobayashi, T. and Sekiguchi, M. (1989) Hemodynamic response to acute hypoxia, hypobaria and exercise in subjects susceptible to high-altitude pulmonary edema. *J. Appl. Physiol.*, **67**, 1982–9.

Kawashima, A., Kubo, K., Matsuwara, Y., *et al.* (1992) Hypoxia-induced ANP secretion in subjects susceptible to high-altitude pulmonary edema. *Respir. Physiol.*, **89**, 309–17.

Keynes, R.J., Smith, G.W., Slater, J.D.H., *et al.* (1982) Renin and aldosterone at high altitude in man. *J. Endocrinol.*, **92**, 131–40.

Kosunen, K.J. and Pakarinen, A.J. (1976) Plasma renin, angiotensin II, and plasma and urinary aldosterone in running exercise. *J. Appl. Physiol.*, **41**, 26–9.

Kotchen, T.A., Mougey, E.H., Hogan, R.P., *et al.* (1973) Thyroid resönses to simulated altitude. *J. Appl. Physiol.*, **34**, 145–8.

Lahiri, S., Milledge, J.S., Chattopadhyay, H.P., *et al.* (1967) Respiration and heart rate of Sherpa highlanders during exercise. *J. Appl. Physiol.*, **23**, 545–54.

Lawrence, D.L., Skatrud, J.B. and Shenker, Y. (1990) Effect of hypoxia on atrial natriuretic factor and aldosterone regulation in humans. *Am. J. Physiol.*, **258**, E243–8.

Lawrence, D.L. and Shenker, Y. (1991) Effect of hypoxic exercise on atrial natriuretic factor and aldosterone regulation. *Am. J. Hypertens.*, **4**, 341–7.

Liu, L., Cheng, H., Chin, W., *et al.* (1989) Atrial natriuretic peptide lowers pulmonary arterial pressure in patients with high altitude disease. *Am. J. Med. Sci.*, **298**, 397–401.

MacKinnon, P.C.B., Monk-Jones, M.E. and Fotherby, K. (1963) A study of various indices of adrenocortical activity during 23 days at high altitude. *J. Endocrinol.*, **26**, 555–6.

Maher, J.T., Jones, L.G., Hartley, L.H., *et al.* (1975a) Aldosterone dynamics during graded exercise at sea level and high altitude. *J. Appl. Physiol.*, **39**, 18–22.

Maher, J.T., Manchanda, S.C., Cymerman, A., *et al.* (1975b) Cardiovascular responsiveness to B-adrenergic stimulation and blockade in chronic hypoxia. *Am. J. Physiol.*, **228**, 477–81.

Maher, J.T., Denniston, J.C., Wolfe, D.L. and Cymerman, A. (1978) Mechanism of the attenuated cardiac response to B-adrenergic stimulation in chronic hypoxia. *J. Appl. Physiol. Respir. Environ. Exercise Physiol.*, **44**, 647–51.

Mazzeo, R.S., Bender, P.R., Brooks, G.A., *et al.* (1991) Arterial catecholamine response during exercise with acute and chronic high-altitude exposure. *Am. J. Physiol.*, **261**, E419–24.

Milledge, J.S. and Catley, D.M. (1987) Angiotensin converting enzyme activity and hypoxia. *Clin. Sci.*, **72**, 149.

Milledge, J.S. and Catley, D.M. (1982) Renin, aldosterone and converting enzyme during exercise and acute hypoxia in humans. *J. Appl. Physiol.*, **52**, 320–3.

Milledge, J.S., Bryson E.I., Catley, D.M., *et al.* (1982) Sodium balance, fluid homeostasis and the renin–aldosterone system during the prolonged exercise of hill walking. *Clin. Sci.*, **62**, 595–604.

Milledge, J.S., Catley, D.M., Ward, M.P., *et al.* (1983a) Renin-aldosterone and angiotensin-converting enzyme during prolonged altitude exposure. *J. Appl. Physiol.*, **55**, 699–702.

Milledge, J.S., Catley, D.M., Blume, F.D. and West, J.B. (1983b) Renin, angiotensin-converting enzyme, and aldosterone in humans on Mount Everest. *J. Appl. Physiol.*, **55**, 1109–12.

Milledge, J.S., Beeley, J.M., McArthur, S. and Morice, A.H. (1989) Atrial natriuretic peptide, altitude and acute mountain sickness. *Clin. Sci.*, **77**, 509–14.

Milledge, J.S., McArthur, S., Morice, A., *et al.* (1991) Atrial natriuretic peptide and exercise-induced fluid retention in man. *J. Wild. Med.*, **2**, 94–101.

Moncloa, F., Donayre, J., Sobrevilla, L.A. and Guerra-Garcia, R. (1965) Endocrine studies at high altitude: I. Adrenal cortical function in sea level natives exposed to high altitudes (4300 m) for two weeks. *J. Clin. Endocrinol. Metab.*, **25**, 1640–2.

Mordes, J.P., Blume, F.D., Boyer, S., *et al.* (1983) High-altitude pituitary–thyroid dysfunction on Mount Everest. *N. Engl. J. Med.*, **308**, 1135–8.

Morice, A., Pepke-Zaba, J., Loysen, E., *et al.* (1988) Low dose infusion of atrial natriuretic peptide causes salt and water excretion in normal man. *Clin. Sci.*, **74**, 359–63.

Olsen, N.V., Hansen, J.M., Kanstrup, I., *et al.* (1993) Renal hemodynamics, tubular function, and response to low-dose dopamine during acute hypoxia in humans. *J. Appl. Physiol.*, **74**, 2166–73.

Pace, N., Griswold, R.L. and Grunbaum, B.W. (1964) Increase in urinary norepinephrine excretion during 14 days sojourn at 3800 m elevation (abstract). *Fed. Proc.*, **23**, 521.

Pines, A. (1978) High altitude acclimatization and proteinuria in East Africa. *Br. J. Dis. Chest*, **72**, 196–8.

Pines, A., Slater, J.D.H. and Jowett, T.P. (1977) The kidney and aldosterone in acclimatization at altitude. *Br. J. Dis. Chest*, **71**, 203–7.

Pugh, L.G.C.E. (1962) Physiological and medical aspects of the Himalayan scientific and mountaineering expedition 1960–61. *Br. Med. J.*, **2**, 621–33.

Raff, H. and Kohandarvish, S. (1990) The effect of oxygen on aldosterone release from bovine adrenocortical cells *in vitro*. Endocrinology, **127**, 682–7.

Ramirez, G., Bittle, P.A., Hammond, M., *et al.* (1988) Regulation of aldosterone secretion during hypoxemia at sea level and moderately high altitude. *J. Clin. Endocrinol. Metab.*, **67**, 1162–5.

Ramirez, G., Hammon, M., Agousti, S.J., *et al.* (1992) Effects of hypoxemia at sea level and high altitude on sodium excretion and hormonal levels. *Aviat. Space Environ. Med.*, **63**, 891–8.

Rastogi, G.K., Malholtra, M.S., Srivastava, M.C., *et al.* (1977) Study of the pituitary–thyroid functions at high altitude in man. *J. Clin. Endocrinol. Metab.*, **44**, 447–52.

Raynaud, J., Drouet, L., Martineaud, J.P., *et al.* (1981) Time course of plasma growth hormone during exercise in humans at altitude. *J. Appl. Physiol.*, **50**, 229–33.

Rennie, D. (1973) Field studies in hypoxia and the kidney, in *Cornell Seminars in Nephrology*, (ed. E.L. Becker), Wiley, New York, pp. 193–206.

Rennie, I.D.B. and Joseph, B.L. (1970) Urinary protein excretion in climbers at high altitude. *Lancet*, **1**, 1247–51.

Rennie, D., Lozano, R., Monge, C., *et al.* (1971a). Renal oxygenation in male Peruvian natives living permanetly at high altitude. *J. Appl. Physiol.*, **30**, 450–56.

Rennie, D., Marticorena, E., Monge, C. and Sirotzky, L. (1971b) Urinary protein excretion in high altitude residents. *J. Appl. Physiol.*, **31**, 257–9.

Rennie, D., Frazer, R., Gray, G.W. and Houston, C.S. (1972) Urine and plasma proteins in men at 5400 m *J. Appl. Physiol.*, **32**, 369–73.

Richalet, J.-P., Rutgers, V., Bouchet, P., *et al.* (1989) Diurnal variation of acute mountain sickness, colour vision, and plasma cortisol and ACTH at high altitude. *Aviat. Space Environ. Med.*, **60**, 105–11.

Sawhney, R.C. and Malhotra, A.S. (1991) Thyroid function in sojourners and acclimatized low landers at high altitude in man. *Horm. Metab. Res.*, **23**, 81–4.

Sawhney, R.C., Chabra, P.C., Malhotra, A.S., *et al.* (1985) Hormone profiles at high altitude in man. *Andrologia*, **17**, 178–84.

Sawhney, R.C., Malhotra, A.S., Singh, T., *et al.* (1986) Insulin secretion at high altitude in man. *Int. J. Biometeorol.*, **30**, 23–8.

Schmidt, W., Brabant, G., Kröger, C., *et al.* (1990) Atrial natriuretic peptide during and after maximal and submaximal exercise under normoxic and hypoxic conditions. *Eur. J. Appl. Phsyiol.*, **61**, 398–407.

Semple, P. d'A. (1986) The clinical endocrinologgy of hypoxia, in *Aspects of Hypoxia*, (ed. D. Heath), Liverpool University Press, Liverpool, pp. 147–1.

Shigeoka, J.W., Colice, G.L. and Ramirez, G. (1985) Effect of normoxemic and hypoxemic exercise on renin and aldosterone. *J. Appl. Physiol.*, **59**, 142–8.

Singh, I., Malhotra, M.S., Khanna, P.K., *et al.* (1974) Changes in plasma cortisol, blood antidiuretic hormone and urinary catecholamine in high-altitude pulmonary oedema. *Int. J. Biometeorol.*, **18**, 211–21.

Siri, W.E., Cleveland, A.S. and Blanche, P. (1969) Adrenal gland activity in Mount Everest climbers. *Fed. Proc.*, **28**, 1251–6.

Slater, J.D.H., Tuffley, R.E., Williams, E.S., *et al.* (1969) Control of aldosterone secretion during acclimatization to hypoxia in man. *Clin. Sci.*, **37**, 327–41.

Somers, V.K., Anderson, J.V., Conway, J., *et al.* (1986) Atrial natriuretic peptide is released by dynamic exercise in man. *Horm. Metab. Res.*, **18**, 871–2.

Stewart, A.G., Thompson, J.S., Rogers, T.K. and Morice, A.H. (1991) Atrial natriuretic peptide-induced relaxation of pre-constricted isolated rat perfused lungs: a comparison in control and hypoxia-adapted animals. *Clin. Sci.*, **81**, 201–8.

Stock, M.J., Norgan, N.G., Ferro-Luzzi, A. and Evans, E. (1978a) Effect of altitude on dietary-induced thermogenesis at rest and during light exercise in man. *J. Appl. Physiol. Respir. Environ. Exercise Physiol.*, **45**, 345–9.

Stock, M.J., Chapman, C., Stirling, J.L. and Campbell, I.T. (1978b) Effects of exercise, altitude, and food on blood hormone and metabolite levels. *J. Appl. Physiol: Respir. Environ. Exercise Physiol.*, **45**, 350–4.

Surks, M.I. (1966) Elevated PBI, free thyroxine, and plasma protein concentration in man at high altitude. *J. Appl. Physiol.*, **21**, 1185–90.

Sutton, J.R. (1977) Effect of acute hypoxia on the hormonal response to exercise. *J. Appl. Physiol. Respir. Environ. Exercise Physiol.*, **42**, 587–92.

Sutton, J.R., Viol, G.W., Gray, G.W., *et al.* (1977) Renin, aldosterone, electrolyte, and cortisol responses to hypoxic decompression. *J. Appl. Physiol. Respir. Environ. Exercise Physiol.*, **43**, 421–4.

Tuffley, R.E., Rubenstein, D., Slater, J.D.H. and Williams, E.S. (1970) Serum renin activity during exposure to hypoxia. *J. Endocrinol.*, **48**, 497–510.

Voelkel, N.F., Hegstrand, L., Reeves, J.T., *et al.* (1981) Effects of hypoxia on density of B-adrenergic receptors. *J. Appl. Physiol. Respir. Environ. Exercise Physiol.*, **50**, 363–6.

Vonmoos, S., Nussberger, J., Waeber, J., *et al.* (1990) Effect of metoclopramide on angiotensin, aldosterone and atrial peptide during hypoxia. *J. Appl. Physiol.*, **69**, 2072–9.

Vuolteenaho, O., Koistinen, P., Martikkala, V., *et al.* (1992) Effect of physical exercise in hypobaric conditions on atrial natriuretic peptide secretion. *Am. J. Physiol.*, **263**, R647–52.

Westendorp, R.G.J., Frölich, M. and Meinders, A.E. (1993) What to tell steroid-substituted patients about the effects of high altitude? *Lancet*, **342**, 310–11.

Wilkinson, R., Milledge, J.S. and Landon, M.J. (1993) Microalbuminuria in chronic obstructive lung disease. *Br. Med. J.*, **307**, 239–40.

Williams, E.S. (1961) Salivary electrolyte composition at high altitude. *Clin. Sci.*, **21**, 37–42.

Williams, E.S. (1975) Mountaineering and the endocrine system, in *Mountain Medicine and Physiology*, (eds C. Clarke, M. Ward and E. Williams), Proceedings of a Symposium for Mountaineers, Expedition Doctors and Physiologists, Alpine Club, London, pp. 38–44.

Williams, E.S., Ward, M.P., Milledge, J.S., *et al.* (1979) Effect of the exercise of seven consecutive days hill-walking on fluid homeostasis. *Clin. Sci.*, **56**, 305–14.

Winter, R.J.D., Davidson, A.C., Treacher, D.F., *et al.* (1987) Plasma atrial natriuretic factor in chronically hypoxaemic patients with pulmonary hypertension. *Clin. Sci.*, **73**, 51P.

Winter, R.J.D., Meleagros, L., Pervez, S., *et al.* (1989) Atrial natriuretic peptide levels in plasma and in cardiac tissues after chronic hypoxia in rats. *Clin. Sci.*, **76**, 95–101.

Young, P.M., Rose, M.S., Sutton, J.R., *et al.* (1989) Operation Everest II: plasma lipid and hormonal responses during a simulated ascent of Mt Everest. *J. Appl. Physiol.*, **66**, 1430–5.

15

Central nervous system

15.1 INTRODUCTION

Of all the parts of the body, the central nervous system (CNS) is one of the most vulnerable to hypoxia. It is not surprising therefore that people who go to high altitude often have changes in neuropsychological function including special senses such as vision, higher functions such as memory, and affective behaviour such as mood. Such changes have been observed in individuals acutely exposed to hypoxia, in lowlanders sojourning at high altitude and in high-altitude natives.

In addition to the changes in neuropsychological function seen in individuals at high altitude, there is mounting evidence that there may be persistent defects of CNS function upon return to sea-level after periods of severe hypoxia at high altitude. These findings are of special interest now because increasing numbers of climbers choose to climb at great altitudes without supplementary oxygen. Many people are concerned about the increase in morbidity and mortality on expeditions to extreme altitude and irrational decisions made by severely hypoxic climbers probably play an important role.

15.2 HISTORICAL

Changes in mood and behaviour at high altitude have been recognized from the early days of climbing high mountains. However the most extreme effects of hypoxia on the central nervous system were seen by the early balloonists where partial paralysis, difficulties with vision, mood changes, and even loss of consciousness are well documented. For example, during the famous flight of the balloon 'Zenith' by Tissandier and his two companions (Tissandier, 1875) we read, 'towards 7500 metres, the numbness one experiences is extraordinary . . . One does not suffer at all; on the contrary. One experiences inner joy, as if it were an effect of the inundating flood of light. One becomes indifferent . . .'. This lack of appreciation of the dangers of acute hypoxia is well known to aircraft pilots and is the reason why there are stringent regulations on using oxygen above certain altitudes in spite of the fact that the pilot may not feel that he needs it.

The paralysing effects of hypoxia were vividly described during the balloon ascent by Glaisher and Coxwell in 1862 (Glaisher *et al.*, 1871). At the highest altitude, Glaisher collapsed unconscious in the basket and it was left to Coxwell to vent the hydrogen from the balloon to bring it down. However Coxwell had apparently lost the use of his hands and instead had to seize the cord that controlled the valve with his teeth and dip his head two or three times. Incidentally this flight also underscored the rapid recovery from severe acute hypoxia. When the balloon landed Glaisher stated that he felt 'no inconvenience' and they both walked between seven and eight miles to the nearest village because they had come down in a remote country area.

When climbers began to reach great altitudes, neuropsychological disturbances were frequently reported. For example, there were several descriptions of bizarre changes in perception and mood on the early expeditions to Mt Everest. During the 1933 Everest expedition, Smythe gave a dramatic description of a hallucination when he saw pulsating cloud-like objects in the sky (Ruttledge, 1933). Smythe also reported a strong feeling that he was accompanied by a second person; he even divided food to give half to his non-existent companion. On occasions, the changes in CNS function suggest attacks of transient cerebral ischaemia. For example the very experienced mountaineer, Shipton, had a remarkable period of aphasia at an altitude of about 7000 m on the same expedition (Shipton, 1943). He reported that 'if I wished to say "give me a cup of tea", I would say something entirely different – maybe "tram-car, cat, put" . . . I was perfectly clear-headed . . . but my tongue just refused to perform the required movements . . .'.

In the last few years there has been increasing interest in the neuropsychological effects of high altitude. For example the Polish climber and psychiatrist Ryn found a range of psychiatric disturbances in mountaineers who had ascended to over 5500 m (Ryn, 1971). He also reported that symptoms similar to an organic brain syndrome persisted for several weeks after the expedition. Some climbers had electroencephalogram abnormalities after climbs to great altitudes. Studies made during the war between China and India in the early 1960s, when Indian troops were rapidly airlifted to high altitude, showed residual changes in psychomotor function on return to sea-level (Sharma *et al.*, 1975, 1976). Townes *et al.* (1984) made measurements on members of the American Medical Research Expedition to Everest after they had returned to sea-level following about three months at altitudes of 5400–8848 m and found residual abnormalities of neuropsychological performance. Similar results were found on Operation Everest II, including the additional interesting observation that climbers with the highest hypoxic ventilatory response were more severely affected. There have been steady improvements in the techniques of neuropsychological testing and it is becoming clear that minor changes in function are extremely common at high altitude, and that some residual impairment often remains in some climbers who return to sea-level from great altitudes.

15.3 MECHANISMS OF ACTION OF HYPOXIA

15.3.1 Hypoxia and nerve cells

In spite of a great deal of research over the last few decades, a clear understanding of the effect of hypoxia on nerve cells remains elusive (Siesjo, 1992a, 1992b; Haddad and Jiang, 1993 for recent reviews). Mild hypoxia accelerates glucose utilization by nerve cells, but utilization is depressed during severe hypoxia. Within the brain, the hippocampus, white matter, superior colliculus and lateral geniculates appear particularly sensitive to levels of oxygen. Brain lactate levels increase in early stages of hypoxia. Brain tissue concentrations of ATP, ADP and AMP apparently remain close to normal even during severe hypoxia.

Altered ion homeostasis during hypoxia clearly occurs though whether the ionic changes are primary, or whether they are due to altered oxidative or neurotransmitter metabolism, is unclear. Hypoxia interferes with calcium homeostasis. For example, very low oxygen levels diminish calcium uptake at synapses. Intracellular levels of potassium are increased during severe hypoxia. There is accumulation of free radicals which cause further injury, particularly to the capillaries. Neurotransmitter metabolism is thought to be sensitive to hypoxia although there is conflicting evidence about which transmitter or metabolic step is most sensitive. There is evidence that acetylcholine synthesis by brain is oxygen–dependent as is the biosynthesis of amino acid neurotransmitters. Brain catecholamine concentrations are apparently decreased by hypoxia though the mechanism is unclear. Much of the experimental work has been done on ischemia, and the relationship of the changes to those caused by pure hypoxia is controversial.

The effects of hypoxia on brain synapses and membrane polarization interfere with the normal electrical activity of the brain and alter the electroencephalogram (EEG). In cats in which the arterial P_{O_2} is gradually reduced from 80 to 20 mmHg, the EEG amplitude initially increases slightly and then slow waves and sharp spikes appear. Subsequently the slow waves decrease in amplitude and then disappear. Later these small spikes become sporadic and finally the EEG flattens.

The initial activation which is followed by depression may be due to the effect of hypoxia on the reticular activating system.

Evoked potentials are also altered by hypoxia. Brainstem auditory response is abolished by low levels of oxygen. Visually evoked potentials are initially increased and then abolished as the level of oxygen is reduced.

Histological changes in the brain result from severe hypoxia. The changes are indistinguishable from those due to hypotension and the greatest changes are seen in the cortex and basal ganglia. Microvacuolation of neuronal perikaryon occurs first, the H1 zone (Sommer sector) of the hippocampus being the most vulnerable region.

15.3.2 Cerebral blood flow

The levels of arterial P_{O_2} and P_{CO_2} have important effects on cerebral blood flow and since these levels are greatly altered by going to high altitude, the results are important. Arterial hypoxaemia dilates cerebral blood vessels and greatly increases cerebral blood flow. Figure 15.1 shows typical results found in anaesthetized normocapnic rats. It can be seen that cerebral blood flow was little changed until the arterial P_{O_2} fell below 60 mmHg but with lower levels of P_{O_2} there was a dramatic increase in cerebral blood flow. Note that at an arterial P_{O_2} of 25 mmHg, cerebral blood flow was approximately five times the normoxic level. As indicated in Chapter 11, the arterial P_{O_2} of a climber resting on the summit of Mt Everest is between 25 and 30 mmHg.

The results shown in Figure 15.1 were obtained in mechanically ventilated animals where P_{CO_2} was kept constant at the normoxic level. However, in conscious animals and humans, the hyperventilation caused by the hypoxaemia will cause a reduction in arterial P_{CO_2} and increase in pH which will cause cerebral vasoconstriction. Therefore the results shown in Figure 15.1 cannot be applied directly to the climber at extreme altitude.

A reduction in arterial P_{CO_2} has a strong vasoconstrictor effect on cerebral blood vessels and consequently reduces cerebral flood flow. Figure 15.2 shows typical results in mechanically ventilated anaesthetized dogs which were made hypocapnic by increasing the ventilation, or hypercapnic by adding carbon dioxide to the inspired gas. In every instance the arterial P_{O_2} was maintained at approximately the normal level. Note that when the arterial P_{CO_2} fell to about 15 mmHg, cerebral blood flow was reduced by about 40% (Harper and Glass, 1965).

In humans at high altitude, the two effects of hypoxaemia and hypocapnia will clearly have opposing effects on the cerebral circulation. There have not been systematic studies of cerebral blood flow at various altitudes partly because of the difficulties of measurement.

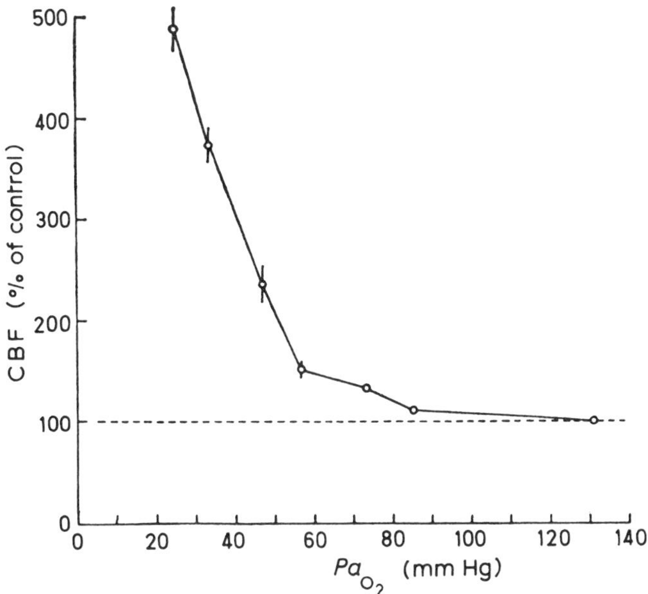

Figure 15.1 Effect of changes of arterial P_{O_2} on cerebral blood flow (CBF) in anaesthetized rats. The arterial P_{CO_2} was maintained normal. Note the very sharp rise in blood flow as the arterial P_{O_2} was reduced below 50 mmHg. (From Borgstrom *et al.*, 1975.)

However Severinghaus *et al.* (1966) measured cerebral blood flow in seven normal subjects by a nitrous oxide method at sea-level and after 6–12 h and 3–5 days at an altitude of 3810 m. The blood flow increased by an average of 24% at 6–12 h, and by 13% at 3–5 days at altitude. Acute correction of the hypoxia restored the cerebral blood flow to normal. Extrapolation of additional data suggested that if the P_{CO_2} had not been reduced at high altitude, the cerebral blood flow would have been 60% above the control.

Indirect evidence about cerebral blood flow in humans can be obtained by measuring blood flow velocity in the internal carotid artery by Doppler ultrasound. Huang *et al.* (1987) measured flow velocities in the internal carotid and vertebral arteries in six subjects within 2–4 h of arrival on Pike's Peak (4300 m), and found that the velocities in both arteries were slightly increased above sea-level values; 18–44 h later, a peak increase of 20% was observed. However, over days 4–12, velocities declined to values similar to those at sea-level. In the further study by the same group (Huang *et al.*, 1991) the effect of prolonged exercise (45 min at approximately 100 W) on blood flow velocity in the

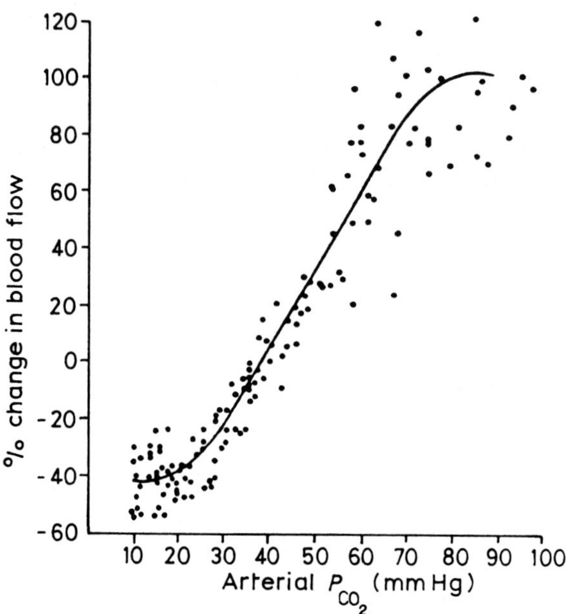

Figure 15.2 Effect of alterations in arterial P_{CO_2} on cerebral cortical blood flow in anaesthetized dogs. The zero reference line for blood flow is at an arterial P_{CO_2} of 40 mmHg. Animals were normoxic and normotensive. (From Harper and Glass, 1965.)

internal carotid artery was studied at sea-level and at 4300 m. The velocities at sea-level and high altitude were similar. In a low-pressure chamber study, Reeves *et al.* (1985) measured blood flow velocity in the internal carotid artery of 12 subjects at Denver (1600 m) and repeatedly up to 7 h at a simulated altitude of 4800 m. Their hypothesis was that an increase in blood flow velocity might be associated with the development of high-altitude headache, but no correlation was found.

Huang *et al.* (1992) measured blood flow velocity in the internal carotid arteries of 15 native Tibetans and 11 Han Chinese residents of Lhasa (3658 m) both at rest and during exercise. There were no differences at rest and during submaximal exercise. At peak exercise, the Tibetans showed an increase in flow velocity and cerebral oxygen delivery whereas the Hans did not. Frayser *et al.* (1970) measured the mean circulation time through the retina following fluorescein injection and found that the circulation time decreased from a mean of 4.9 s at base camp to 3.4 s at an altitude of 5330 m. This is consistent with an increase in cerebral blood flow.

Another possible factor at high altitude which could influence cerebral blood flow is an increased viscosity of the blood caused by polycythaemia. Although this has not been specifically studied, it is known that a blood flow of less than half the normal value can occur in severe polycythaemia vera (Kety, 1950) and that cerebral blood flow is significantly increased in severe anaemia (Heyman *et al.*, 1952; Robin and Gardner, 1953). Some drugs, including caffeine, reduce cerebral blood flow.

15.4 CENTRAL NERVOUS SYSTEM FUNCTION AT HIGH ALTITUDE

15.4.1 Moderate altitudes

There is general agreement that CNS function is impaired at altitudes over about 4500 m (approximately 15 000 ft) but an interesting question is the lowest altitude at which minor alterations in function occur. This question frequently arises in the aviation industry because it is important in selecting the cabin pressure of commercial aircraft. Many high flying commercial aircraft are pressurized to maintain the cabin pressure at or below an equivalent altitude of about 2500 m (approximately 8000 ft). This ceiling was accepted after considering the penalty of extra weight and expense which would have to be paid in order to reduce it further.

However there is some evidence that at a pressure equivalent to an altitude of 2440 m, subjects are slower to learn complex mental tasks than at sea-level. Even at the considerably lower altitude of only 1524 m (5000 ft), eight subjects were slower to learn complex tasks than a matched group breathing an enriched oxygen mixture (Denison *et al.*, 1966). The tests here involved recognizing the posture of man-like figures having different orientations and presented in random sequence on a screen. Thus it appears that even at the cabin altitudes of commercial aircraft, sensitive psychometric tests can pick up minor degrees of impairment.

Interesting problems concerning CNS function at moderate altitudes occur in relation to the operation of optical and infra-red telescopes on mountain summits. The reduction in the absorption of optical and infra-red radiation because of the reduced thickness of the earth's atmosphere at high altitude makes high mountains ideal locations for astronomical observatories. For example, several telescopes are located on the summit of Mauna Kea, altitude 4200 m (13 796 ft), on the island of Hawaii.

The barometric pressure on the summit of Mauna Kea is only about 468 mmHg, giving a moist inspired P_{O_2} of 88 mmHg. The telescope operators frequently live at sea-level and ascend rapidly by car to the summit. Forster (1986) measured arterial blood gases on 27 telescope personnel on the first day of reaching 4200 m and reported a mean arterial P_{O_2} of 42 mmHg, P_{CO_2} 29 mmHg and pH 7.49. After five days, during which time the nights were spent in dormitories at an altitude of 3000 m, the arterial blood gases at 4200 m showed a mean P_{O_2} of 44 mmHg, P_{CO_2} 27 mmHg and pH of 7.48.

A number of psychometric measurements showed no change on ascending to 4200 m, though performance of the digit symbol backwards test did deteriorate on the first day. At the end of five days, however, the scores had returned to sea-level values. Numerate memory and psychomotor ability were also reported to be impaired in commuters to Mauna Kea. Several features of acute mountain sickness were noted in shift workers particularly on their first day at the summit. Headache was the most disabling symptom but others included insomnia, lethargy, poor concentration and poor memory.

A possible solution to the problem of impaired psychomotor performance in these telescope workers would be to enrich the air in the control room by adding a small amount of oxygen to the air-conditioning system. Raising the oxygen concentration from 21% to only 24% results in a substantial fall in equivalent altitude. Oxygen could be provided by oxygen concentrators which only need electrical power and are very efficient at raising the oxygen concentration by a small percentage in large volumes of air. Calculations show that the cost of adding sufficient oxygen to increase the inspired P_{O_2} to that existing at an altitude of 3000 m would be about $30 000 per year, a relatively small price to pay for the improved efficiency of the workers. Long term oxygen enrichment of the atmosphere for people doing skilled work at high altitude has apparently never been tried but is just as reasonable as other forms of air-conditioning such as adjusting the temperature or humidity of the working environment.

15.4.2 High altitudes

A classical series of studies were carried out by MacFarland (1937a, 1937b, 1938a, 1938b) in connection with the International High Altitude Expedition to Chile which took place in 1935. In his first study, MacFarland reported on the psychophysiological effects of sudden ascents to 5000 m in unpressurized aircraft and compared the results with ascents by train and car to villages as high as 4700 m in Chile. The measurements showed that the rate of ascent was an important variable, with the rapid increase in altitude by aircraft being the most damaging. Both simple and complex psychological functions were significantly impaired at high altitudes including arithmetical tests, writing ability, and the appearance and disappearance time of after-images following exposure of the eye to a bright light. There were increased memory errors, errors in perseverance, and reductions in auditory threshold and words apprehended.

In a second study of sensory and motor responses during acclimatization, when measurements were obtained at altitudes as high as 5330 and 6100 m, significant reductions in audition, vision, and eye–hand co-ordination were seen. Measurements were made at several altitudes but in general, impairment of function was not significant below an altitude of 5330 m. Again members of the expedition with the longest periods of acclimatization appeared to suffer less deterioration.

In a further study, mental and psychosomatic tests were also administered at the same altitudes and these showed deterioration. Tests involving the quickness of recognizing the meaning of words, mental flexibility or tendency to perseveration, and immediate memory showed significant impairment. It was noted that complex mental work could be carried out if the subjects increased their concentration but in general there was increased distractibility and lethargy which tended to reduce the ability to concentrate.

In a final series of measurements, sensory and circulatory responses were measured on sulphur miners residing permanently at an altitude of 5330 m at Aucanquilcha. They were compared with a group of workmen at sea-level who were similar in age and race, and also with members of the expedition. It was found that the miners at high altitude were slower in simple and choice reaction times and less acute in auditory sensitivity than the workmen at sea-level. However MacFarland and his colleagues were impressed by the evidence for circulatory and respiratory adaptation in these permanent residents at an altitude of 5330 m.

More recently, additional studies on the deleterious effects of acute hypoxia on visual perception have been carried out, partly because of the importance of this topic in aviation. For example, Kobrick (1975) documented impaired response times in the detection of flash stimuli at equivalent altitudes of sea-level, 4000 m, 4600 m, and 5200 m during acute exposure in a low-pressure chamber. The effects of hypoxia on other peripheral stimuli have also been studied (Kobrick, 1972).

A special opportunity to study the central nervous system effects of high altitude occurred during the India–China border war in the early 1960s when large numbers of Indian troops were rapidly taken to an altitude of 4000 m and remained there for as long as two years. Sharma and his colleagues (1975) measured psychomotor efficiency in 25 young Indians ranging in age from 21 to 30 years. Psychomotor performance including speed and accuracy was determined by administering an eye–hand co-ordination test in which a stylus was moved in a narrow groove so that it did not touch the sides. The tests were performed at

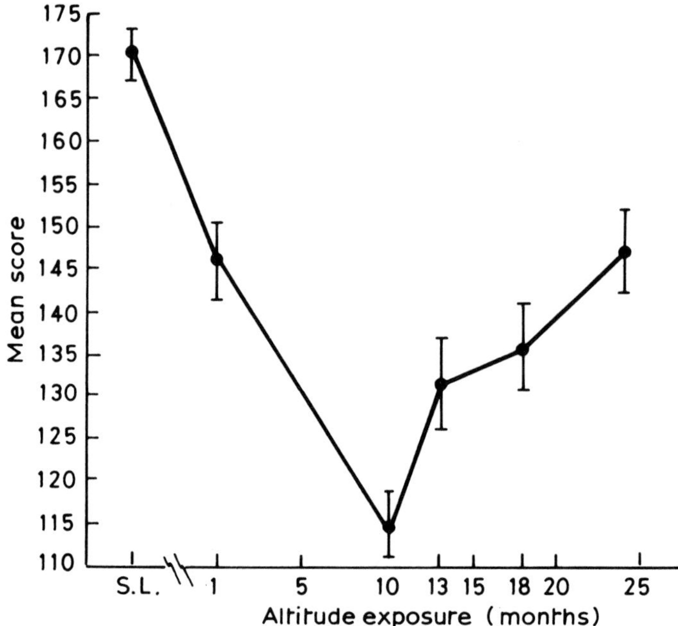

Figure 15.3 Psychomotor efficiency in young adults rapidly taken to an altitude of 4000 m where they remained for two years. Psychomotor efficiency was calculated using an eye–hand co-ordination test which included speed and accuracy. Note the deterioration in psychomotor efficiency over the first 10 months, which then gradually improved. (From Sharma *et al.*, 1975.)

sea-level and at an altitude of 4000 m after periods of 1, 10, 13, 18 and 24 months. Figure 15.3 shows how overall psychomotor efficiency declined over the first ten months of altitude exposure but then recovered somewhat over the ensuing 13 months as a result of acclimatization.

Overall psychomotor efficiency as shown in Figure 15.3 includes both the speed and accuracy scores from the test. Figure 15.4 shows a breakdown of the accuracy and speed of this test of psychomotor performance. Note that the accuracy of the measurement increased substantially after the ten-month period but there was little improvement in speed. This result is consistent with the impression given by many people who have worked at high altitude, namely that thought processes are slowed, but if one concentrates hard enough, accurate procedures can be carried out.

In a related study, Sharma and Malhotra (1976) compared the performance of three groups of Indians drawn from the Gorkha, Madrasi and Rajput areas after 10 months' stay at altitude of 4000 m. There were no differences in the scores for eye–hand co-ordination and social interac-

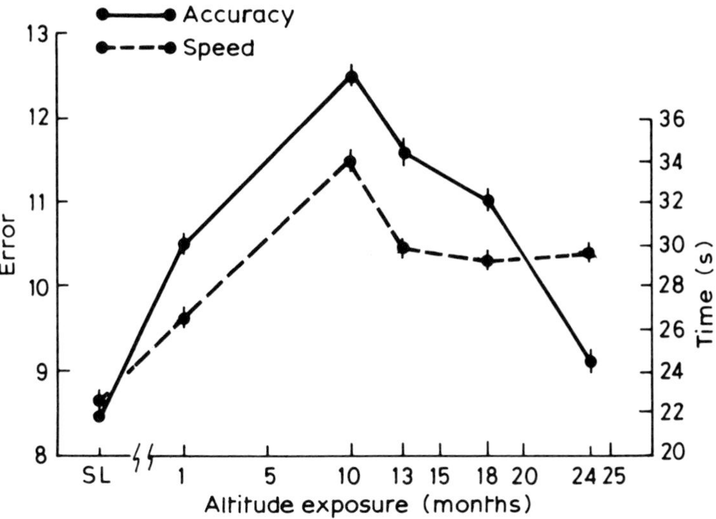

Figure 15.4 Same data as in Figure 15.3 except that psychomotor efficiency is broken down into accuracy and speed of eye–hand co-ordination. Note that the accuracy of the measurement increased after 10 months but there was relatively little improvement in speed. (From Sharma *et al.*, 1975.)

tion at altitudes for the three ethnic groups. However the Gorkhas showed a better toleration of altitude stress as evidenced by the effects on concentration, anxiety and depression.

In a study of 20 male soldiers exposed to a simulated altitude of 4700 m for 5–7 h, the relationships between symptoms and signs of acute mountain sickness, mood and psychometric performance were studied (Shukitt-Hale *et al.*, 1991). It was found that evidence of acute mountain sickness was best correlated with symptoms, then mood changes, and least with performance.

An unusual opportunity for studying the effects of very high altitude on mental performance was offered by the Himalayan Scientific and Mountaineering Expedition of 1960–1961 when several normal subjects spent up to three months at an altitude of 5800 m (19 000 ft). Mental efficiency was tested by asking the subjects to sort playing cards into bins using specially designed equipment which recorded events on magnetic tape (Gill *et al.*, 1964). It was found that the efficiency of sorting cards was less at the high altitude than at sea-level. The inefficiency took the form of a delay in placing the cards into the correct bins rather than errors of sorting. Again these results reinforce the common notion that accurate work can be done at high altitude, but it takes longer, and more effort in concentration is required. Cahoon

(1972) also showed a reduced efficiency of card sorting in eight normal subjects exposed to a simulated altitude of 4600 m (15 000 ft) for 48 h.

During the 1981 American Medical Research Expedition to Everest, a series of psychometric tests were carried out prior to the expedition, at the Base Camp (5400 m), at the Main Laboratory Camp (6300 m) and immediately after and one year after the expedition (Townes *et al.*, 1984). The main emphasis was on a comparison of CNS function before and after exposure to extreme altitude, and only a few of the measurements made at high altitude were reported. However, finger-tapping speed decreased significantly over the course of the expedition. Mean taps of the right hand were 53.7 (pretest), 52.6 (5400 m altitude), 50.8 (6300 m altitude), 48.1 (on subjects returning to 6300 m altitude from 8000 m) and 45.4 (immediately after the expedition). It is not clear from these results whether the reduction in finger-tapping speed was a function of altitude, time at high altitude, or both.

15.4.3 Electroencephalogram

Ryn (1970, 1971) reported EEG abnormalities in 11 of 30 climbers who had been over 5500 m altitude. The predominant abnormality was a decreased frequency of alpha waves and a diminution of their amplitude. He also reported paroxysmal and focal pathology in EEG records performed at high altitude.

Zhongyuan and his colleagues (1983) also reported changes in the EEG at altitudes above 5000 m in members of a Chinese expedition to Mt Everest. There was a reduced amplitude of the alpha rhythm but in this instance there was an increase in its frequency. The EEG changes were less than those observed during acute hypoxia of the same degree in a low-pressure chamber prior to the expedition. Apparently members of the expedition who tolerated the acute hypoxia well tended to show fewer EEG changes on the mountain itself.

Nevison carried out an extensive series of EEG measurements during the Himalayan Scientific and Mountaineering Expedition of 1960–1961. Although the results were not written up in the open literature, he apparently found no abnormalities in subjects living at 5800 m. Also the EEG appearances were not altered by hyperventilation or 100% oxygen breathing.

15.5 RESIDUAL CENTRAL NERVOUS SYSTEM IMPAIRMENT FOLLOWING RETURN FROM HIGH ALTITUDE

In view of the known vulnerability of the CNS to hypoxia, it is hardly surprising that neurobehavioural abnormalities can be demonstrated at high altitudes. However, there has been great interest in the possibility of residual impairment of CNS function following return to sea-level.

An extensive study was carried out by Townes *et al.* (1984) referred to in section 15.4.2. The subjects were 21 members of the 1981 American Medical Research Expedition to Everest, and all were males between 25 and 52 years of age with a mean age of 36.4 years. The general level of education was high with 15 subjects having either an MD or PhD degree. Prior to the expedition, the following psychological tests were administered at the San Diego Veterans Administration Hospital: Halstead–Reitan battery (Reitan and Davison, 1974), repeatable cognitive–perceptual–motor battery (Lewis and Rennick, 1979), selective reminding test (Buschke, 1973) and the Wechsler memory scale (Russell, 1975). These same measurements were repeated immediately after the expedition in Kathmandu, Nepal. At an expedition meeting held in Colorado one year later, the following tests were readministered: Halstead–Wepman aphasia screening test, B trials and the finger-tapping test from the Halstead–Reitan battery, the digit vigilance task from the repeatable battery, and a verbal passage from the Wechsler memory scale.

Table 15.1 shows the significant changes found between pre-expedition, post-expedition and follow-up performance on the neuropsychological tests. It can be seen that verbal learning and memory declined significantly from the beginning to the end of the expedition as measured by the Wechsler memory scale. In the Halstead–Wepman aphasia screening test, the number of expressive language errors increased significantly between pre-test and post-test after the expedition. The number of aphasic errors was significantly related to the altitude attained by the subject.

As indicated in section 15.4.2 finger-tapping speed decreased significantly over the course of the expedition. This was measured by requiring the subject to tap a lever as rapidly as possible over a period of 10 s. For a test to be acceptable, five measurements on each hand gave a difference of less than five taps between trials. Before the expedition all subjects reached this criterion. However at Kathmandu immediately after the expedition, 15 of 20 subjects could not sustain motor speed, and 13 of 16 subjects could not do so one year later.

These findings are of great interest because they provide strong objective evidence for CNS deterioration as a result of exposure to high altitude, a subject which has been debated vigorously in the past. However, other authors have reported similar or consistent findings. Ryn (1970, 1971) also found persistent abnormalities in a group of 20 male and 10 female Polish climbers several weeks after a Himalayan expedition. Half of the male climbers who ascended over 5500 m experienced symptoms similar to the acute organic brain syndrome,

Table 15.1 Wilcoxon signed-rank tests comparing performance before, immediately after (in Kathmandu), and one year after expedition to Mt Everest (From Townes *et al.*, 1984)

	Result, means ± SE			*Paired responses, z values*		
	Before	*After*	*Follow-up*	*Before and after*	*After and follow-up*	*Before and follow-up*
Improved performance						
Tactual performance test (right hand)	4.68 ± 1.56	3.86 ± 1.46		2.72*		
Category test	24.29 ± 15.46	11.05 ± 8.39		3.48†		
Decline in performance						
Finger tapping test						
Right hand	53.71 ± 4.07	45.40 ± 6.18	48.40 ± 6.60	3.39†	1.32	2.20‡
Left hand	47.65 ± 4.60	42.25 ± 5.96	41.73 ± 5.23	2.30‡	0.66	2.93*
Criterion right	1.00 ± 0	0.14 ± 0.36	0.27 ± 0.46	3.06*	0.73	2.67*
Criterion left	1.00 ± 0	0.14 ± 0.36	0.13 ± 0.35	2.93‡	0.54	2.93*
Wechsler memory scale						
Short-term verbal recall	18.12 ± 1.90	15.90 ± 2.15	17.13 ± 2.20	2.60*	2.12‡	0.98
Trials to criterion	1.24 ± 0.44	2.40 ± 1.54	2.27 ± 0.70	2.37‡	0	2.67*
Long-term verbal recall	16.35 ± 2.91	12.70 ± 3.78	14.50 ± 2.85	2.32‡	2.75	0.94
Aphasia screening test	0.59 ± 0.79	1.25 ± 1.25	0.47 ± 0.52	2.22‡	2.31‡	0.47

* $P < 0.01$
† $P < 0.001$
‡ $P < 0.05$

and for several weeks after the expedition they had changes in affect and impaired memory. Eleven of the 30 climbers had EEG abnormalities immediately after the climb. Psychological testing (Bender, Benton and Graham–Kendall tests) were reported to be normal in 13 persons, borderline in 12 persons, and indicative of organic pathology in five climbers.

Persistent cognitive impairment was described in five world-class climbers who had reached summits over 8500 m without supplementary oxygen (Regard *et al.*, 1989). The abnormalities were in the ability to concentrate, short term memory, and cognitive flexibility (the ability to shift from one learned concept to another).

In a brief report, Cavaletti *et al.* (1987) showed residual impairment of memory in seven climbers who returned to sea-level after ascending to 7075 m on Mt Satopanth without supplementary oxygen. The measurements were made before leaving Italy, at the base camp after the ascent, and 75 days after the expedition. It was shown that memory performance decreased both at base camp and, to a lesser degree, at sea-level 75 days after the climb. However tests of fluency and 'idiomotor ability' were unaffected by altitude. In a more recent study, persistent changes in memory, reaction time and concentration were reported 75 days after a single ascent over 5000 m (Cavaletti and Tredici, 1993).

One study reports cortical atrophy and brain magnetic resonance imaging (MRI) changes in 26 climbers who ascended to over 7000 m without supplementary oxygen (Garrido *et al.*, 1993). No MRI studies were performed prior to the climbs; the measurements were made 26 days to 36 months after return to sea-level. The controls were 21 normal subjects, and 46% of the climbers showed MRI abnormalities.

Not everyone has found CNS abnormalities following return after ascent to very high altitude. For example Clark *et al.* (1983) tested 22 mountaineers before and 16–221 days after Himalayan climbs above 5100 m with a battery of psychological and neurophysiological tests but found no evidence of cerebral dysfunction. This was a well designed study and it is not clear why these climbers showed no abnormalities.

Measurements from the 1985 Operation Everest II confirmed the changes in psychometric function found on the 1981 American Medical Research Expedition to Everest, and extended the observations in an interesting and unexpected direction. During Operation Everest II, eight normal subjects spent 40 days in a low-pressure chamber and were gradually decompressed, ultimately being exposed to the simulated altitude of the Everest summit. Impairments in motor speed and persistence, memory, and verbal expressive abilities were found after the simulated ascent just as with the 1981 Everest expedition (Hornbein *et al.*, 1989).

The new finding was a significant negative correlation between hypoxic ventilatory response and neurobehavioural function measured after the expedition. In other words, those climbers with the largest hypoxic ventilatory response showed the greatest decrement in neurobehavioural function. This was unexpected; indeed the prediction was that those who increased their ventilation most would protect their CNS function by preserving their alveolar and therefore arterial P_{O_2}.

A hypothesis to explain these unexpected findings was advanced by Hornbein *et al.* (1989). They argued that the subjects with the highest hypoxic ventilatory response would reduce their arterial P_{CO_2} the most and therefore develop the most cerebral vasoconstriction. This in turn would cause the most severe cerebral hypoxia even though their arterial P_{O_2} would actually be higher than that in the subjects with the smaller ventilatory responses to hypoxia.

Note that this hypothesis is not supported by the measurements of cerebral blood flow against arterial P_{CO_2} in anaesthetized dogs shown in Figure 15.2. Those data show that cerebral blood flow apparently levels off at values of P_{CO_2} below approximately 15 mmHg. However, the situation with acclimatization may be different because the arterial pH returns towards normal and this may improve cerebral blood flow. In addition the scatter in the data is such that this result may not be reliable. It should also be pointed out that the relationship between cerebral blood flow and arterial P_{CO_2} is very sensitive to the systematic arterial pressure (Harper and Glass, 1965). Hypotensive dogs show a much smaller change in cerebral blood flow for a given change in P_{CO_2} than normotensive animals. Whether changes in systemic blood pressure occur at extreme altitudes is not known although there are no obvious alterations at 5800 m (Pugh, 1964).

The correlation between hypoxic ventilatory response and residual impairment of central nervous system function leads to an interesting paradox. On the one hand, a brisk hypoxic ventilatory response is advantageous for a climber to reach extreme altitudes because otherwise the alveolar P_{O_2} cannot be maintained at the required levels. However the only way of maintaining the P_{O_2} is by extreme hyperventilation, which reduces the arterial P_{CO_2}, which in turn reduces cerebral blood flow. Thus such a climber is likely to suffer more residual central nervous impairment. In other words, the climber who is endowed by nature to go the highest is likely to suffer the most severe nervous system damage.

REFERENCES

Borgstrom, L., Johannsson, H. and Siesjo, B.K. (1975) The relationship between arterial P_{O_2} and cerebral blood flow in hypoxic hypoxia. *Acta Physiol.Scand.*, **93**, 423–32.

Buschke, H. (1973) Selective reminding for analysis of memory and learning. *J. Verb. Learn. Verb. Behav.*, **13**, 543.

Cahoon, R.L. (1972) Simple decision making at high altitude. *Ergonomics*, **15**, 157–64.

Cavaletti, G., Moroni, R., Garavaglia, P. and Tredici, G. (1987) Brain damage after high-altitude climbs without oxygen. *Lancet*, **i**, 101.

Cavaletti, G. and Tredici, G. (1993) Long-lasting neuropsychological changes after a single high altitude climb. *Acta Neurol. Scand.*, **87**, 103–5.

Clark, C.F., Heaton, R.K. and Wiens, A.N. (1983) Neuropsychological functioning after prolonged high altitude exposure in mountaineering. *Aviat. Space Environ. Med.*, **54**, 202–7.

Denison, D.M., Ledwith, F. and Poulton, E.C. (1966) Complex reaction times at simulated cabin altitudes of 5000 feet and 8000 feet. *Aerosp. Med.*, **57**, 1010–13.

Forster, P. (1986) Telescopes in high places, in *Aspects of Hypoxia*, (ed. D. Heath), Liverpool University Press, Liverpool, pp. 217–33.

Frayser, R., Houston, C.S., Bryan, A.C., *et al.* (1970) Retinal hemorrhage at high altitude. *New Engl. J. Med.*, **282**, 1183–4.

Garrido, E., Castello, A., Ventura, J.L., *et al.* (1993) Cortical atrophy and other brain magnetic resonance imaging (MRI) changes after extremely high-altitude climbs without oxygen. *Int. J. Sports Med.*, **14**, 232–4.

Gill, M.B., Poulton, E.C., Carpenter, A., *et al.* (1964) Falling efficiency at sorting cards during acclimatization at 19 000 ft. *Nature*, **203**, 436.

Glaisher, J., Flammarion, C., De Fonvielle, E. and Tissandier, G. (1871) Ascents from Wolverhampton, in *Travels in the Air*, (ed. J. Glaisher), Lippincott, Philadelphia, pp. 50–8.

Haddad, G.G. and Jiang, C. (1993) O_2 deprivation in the central nervous system. *Prog. Neurobiol.*, **40**, 277–318.

Harper, A.M. and Glass, H.I. (1965) Effect of alterations in the arterial carbon dioxide tension on the blood flow through the cerebral cortex at normal and low arterial blood pressures. *J. Neurol. Neurosurg. Psychiatry*, **28**, 449–52.

Heyman, A., Patterson, J.L. and Duke, T.W. (1952) Cerebral circulation and metabolism in sickle cell and other chronic anemias, with observations on the effects of oxygen inhalation. *J. Clin. Invest.*, **31**, 824–8.

Hornbein, T.F., Townes, B.D., Schoene, R.B., *et al.* (1989) The cost to the central nervous system of climbing to extremely high altitude. *N. Engl. J. Med.*, **321**, 1714–19.

Huang, S.Y., Moore, L.G., McCullough, R.E., *et al.* (1987) Internal carotid and vertebral arterial flow velocity in men at high altitude. *J. Appl. Physiol.*, **63**, 395–400.

Huang, S.Y., Tawney, K.W., Bender, P.R., *et al.* (1991) Internal carotid flow velocity with exercise before and after acclimatization to 4300 m. *J. Appl. Physiol.*, **71**, 1469–76.

Huang, S.Y., Sun, S., Droma, T., *et al.* (1992) Internal carotid arterial flow velocity during exercise in Tibetan and Han residents of Lhasa (3658 m). *J. Appl. Physiol.*, **73**, 2638–42.

Kety, S.S. (1950) Circulation and metabolism of the human brain in health and disease. *Am. J. Med.*, **8**, 205–17.

Kobrick, J.L. (1972) Effects of hypoxia on voluntary response time to peripheral stimuli during central target monitoring. *Ergonomics*, **15**, 147–56.

Kobrick, J.L. (1975) Effects of hypoxia on peripheral visual response to dim stimuli. *Perceptual and Motor Skills*, **41**, 467–74.

Lewis, R.F. and Rennick, P.M. (1979) *Manual for the Repeatable Cognitive–Perceptual–Motor Battery*, Axon, Grosse Pointe Park, Michigan.

MacFarland, R.A. (1937a) Psycho-physiological studies at high altitude in the Andes. I. The effects of rapid ascents by aeroplane and train. *Comp. Psychol.*, **23(1)**, 191–225.

MacFarland, R.A. (1937b) Psycho-physiological studies at high altitude in the Andes. II. Sensory and motor responses during acclimatization. *Comp. Psychol.*, **23**, 227–58.

MacFarland, R.A. (1938a) Psycho-physiological studies at high altitude in the Andes. III. Mental and psycho-somatic responses during gradual adaptation. *Comp. Psychol.*, **24**, 147–88.

MacFarland, R.A. (1938b) Psycho-physiological studies at high altitude in the Andes. IV. Sensory and circulatory responses of the Andean residents at 17 500 feet. *Comp. Psychol.*, **24**, 189–220.

Pugh, L.G.C.E. (1964) Cardiac output in muscular exercise at 5800 m (19 000 ft). *J. Appl. Physiol.*, **19**, 441–7.

Reeves, J.T., Moore, L.G., McCullough, R.E., *et al.* (1985) Headache at high altitude is not related to internal carotid arterial blood velocity. *J. Appl. Physiol.*, **59**, 909–15.

Regard, M., Oelz, O., Brugger, P. and Landis, T. (1989) Persistent cognitive impairment in climbers after repeated exposure to extreme altitude. *Neurology*, **39**, 210–13.

Reitan, R.M. and Davison, L.A. (eds) (1974) *Clinical Neuropsychology: Current Status and Applications*, Winston, Washington DC.

Robin, E.D. and Gardner, F.H. (1953) Cerebral metabolism and hemodynamics in pernicious anemia. *J. Clin. Invest.*, **32**, 598.

Russell, E. (1975) A multiple scoring method for the assessment of complex memory functions. *J. Consult. Clin. Psychol.*, **43**, 800–9.

Ruttledge, H. (1933) *Everest: The Unfinished Adventure*, Hodder and Stoughton, London, p. 212.

Ryn, Z. (1970) *Mental Disorders in Alpinists Under Conditions of Stress at High Altitudes*, Doctoral thesis, University of Cracow, Poland.

Ryn, Z. (1971) Psychopathology in alpinism. *Acta Med. Pol.*, **12**, 453–67.

Severinghaus, J.W., Chiodi, H., Eger, E.I., *et al.* (1966) Cerebral blood flow in man at high altitude. Role of cerebrospinal fluid pH in normalization of flow in chronic hypocapnia. *Circ. Res.*, **19**, 274–82.

Sharma, V.M., Malhotra, M.S. and Baskaran, A.S. (1975) Variations in psychomotor efficiency during prolonged stay at high altitude. *Ergonomics*, **18**, 511–16.

Sharma, V.M. and Malhotra, M.S. (1976) Ethnic variations in psychological performance under altitude stress. *Aviat. Space Environ. Med.*, **47**, 248–51.

Shipton, E.E. (1943) *Upon that Mountain*, Hodder and Stoughton, London, p. 129.

Shukitt-Hale, B., Banderet, L.E. and Lieberman, H.R. (1991) Relationships between symptoms, moods, performance, and acute mountain sickness at 4700 meters. *Aviat. Space Environ. Med.*, **62**, 865–9.

Siesjo, B.K. (1992a) Pathophysiology and treatment of focal cerebral ischemia. Part I. Pathophysiology. *J. Neurosurg.*, **77**, 169–84.

Siesjo, B.K. (1992b) Pathophysiology and treatment of focal cerebral ischemia. Part II. Mechanisms of damage and treatment. *J. Neurosurg.*, **77**, 337–54.

Tissandier, G. (1875) Le voyage a grande hauteur du ballon 'le Zenith'. *Nature Paris*, **3**, 337–44.

Townes, B.D., Hornbein, T.F., Schoene, R.B., *et al.* (1984) Human cerebral function at extreme altitude, in *High Altitude and Man*, (eds J.B. West and S. Lahiri), American Physiological Society, Bethesda, Maryland, pp. 32–6.

Zhongyuan, S., Deming, Z., Changming, L. and Miaoshen, Q. (1983) Changes of electroencephalogram under acute hypoxia and relationship between tolerant ability to hypoxia and adaptation ability to high altitudes. *Sci. Sin.*, **26**, 58–69.

16

High altitude populations

16.1 INTRODUCTION

This chapter considers the characteristics of people born and raised at high altitude and whose ancestors have resided at high altitude for many generations. In Chapter 3 the locations of these populations have been discussed. In general the altitude considered is above 3000 m. The duration of residence of the population is impossible to determine; it ranges from perhaps 50 000 to 100 000 years in Tibet, 20 000–40 000 years in the Andes to a few generations in the high mining towns of Colorado.

Our knowledge of the effect of lifelong residence at altitude has come from studies of particular peoples and the major problem in interpreting results is to decide whether the characteristics found to differ from lowland populations are really due to the high-altitude environment (hypoxia or cold) or due to racial, nutritional or economic factors.

Some studies have sought to eliminate racial factors by using low-altitude residents of the same ethnic background as controls. It is difficult to control for nutritional factors since high-altitude residents may well be economically disadvantaged when compared with their low-altitude controls. This seems to be the case in the Andes. The effect of poor nutrition and chronic hypoxia are similar on factors such as growth and development, thus confounding the interpretation of results. The economic advantage may be reversed, as in Ethiopia, where the highland regions are free from malaria and the residents more wealthy and better fed. The result is that studies from this part of the world do not show the differences between high and low altitude residents that are reported from the Andes. There are fewer studies from the Himalayas and Tibet than from the Andes, though this has been partially redressed in recent years with a number of studies from Lhasa.

However, if these reservations are kept in mind, some conclusions can be drawn from the many surveys about the effects of lifelong residence at high altitude, especially on birth weight and childhood development.

16.2 DEMOGRAPHIC ASPECTS OF HIGH-ALTITUDE POPULATIONS

16.2.1 Population age and sex distribution

A few high-altitude groups have been analysed in some detail and the population of the Nunoa district (4000 m) of Peru showed some differences by comparison with the total Peruvian population (Baker and Dutt, 1972). The high-altitude population was somewhat younger and the ratio of females to males was larger during infancy and childhood, but in addition there appeared to be more elderly people among the high-altitude than the general population.

The explanation seems to be that, in the high-altitude population, there was a high birth rate and high adult emigration rate. Male mortality was higher than female in infancy, childhood and early adolescence. The larger number of older individuals may have been due to the prestige associated with telling observers that they were of a great age. Claims to longevity are hard to substantiate because birth certificates and baptismal registers are seldom kept and some individuals lie outrageously about their age. In north Bhutan the oldest individuals were over 80 but not above 90 years old (Jackson *et al.*, 1966a) and some Tibetan lamas claim to have lived to a great age. There seems to be little concrete evidence for unusual longevity at high altitude.

In the Khumbu region of north-eastern Nepal, male infant mortality was higher than female. There was little permanent emigration but a higher percentage of males were involved in accidents. In north-west Nepal the number of males born relative to females was higher but mortality in male infants was increased (Baker, 1978). No figures are available for Tibet.

16.2.2 Fertility

Adaptation to the environment must include the ability of the species to reproduce. The Spanish who occupied the high altitude regions of South America in the sixteenth and seventeenth centuries found that neither their animals nor their womenfolk had live offspring for two or three generations. This was in contrast to the indigenous animals and peoples. Clegg (1978) quotes two well observed Spanish accounts of La Calancha (1639) and Cobo (1653). The former recounts the early history of the city of Potosi (4000 m) in present day Bolivia with a population of 20 000 Spaniards and 100 000 Indians. Children born to Spanish couples died either at birth or within two weeks. Pregnant Spanish women developed the habit of going down to low altitude for their pregnancy and delivery and keeping their babies there until a year old. A similar pattern is followed by Han (Chinese) women living in Tibet. The cause of failure to thrive in these infants may well have been subacute mountain sickness (Chapter 17). The Amer–Indians, of course, had no such problems nor do the indigenous Tibetans. The first Spanish child to be born and reared was after the city had been founded for 53 years. Cobo says that Jauja (3500 m), the early capital of Peru, was considered 'a sterile place' where horses, pigs, or fowls could not be raised, whereas 100 years later it was a principal pig and poultry producing area supplying Lima with these products.

Cobo also pointed out that infant survival depended upon the proportion of Indian blood in the child, with pure blooded Spanish children mostly dying, children of mixed blood faring rather better, and pure blooded Indian children having the lowest mortality, despite much poorer living conditions.

What is the cause of this lack of fertility in lowlanders at altitude? Sperm counts in lowland men fall temporarily on going to altitude but then recover. Testosterone levels also fall and then recover after a week or two (section 14.9.4). In the female, on going to altitude, there may be temporary disturbances in menstruation (Sobrevilla *et al.*, 1967). Conception rates are virtually impossible to measure, especially since chronic hypoxia may increase the frequency of early abortions. The reduced fertility may be due to a number of factors, possibly reduced conception, probably increased numbers of early abortions, stillbirths and neonatal deaths.

In altitude residents fertility is probably also reduced but the evidence is not conclusive. Hoff and Abelson (1976), using aggregate data from Peru, found that fertility measured as the number of children under five divided by the number of women aged 15–49 years, fell linearly with altitude ($P < 0.01$) but they are cautious in interpreting the data on which this is based. They also found that high-altitude women who migrate to low altitude increase their fertility.

16.3 FOETAL AND CHILDHOOD DEVELOPMENT

16.3.1 Pregnancy

Abortion

Abortion rates are notoriously difficult to measure but Clegg (1978) quotes a number of Andean studies giving incredibly low rates ranging from 0 to 1% (compared with world-wide rates of about 15%). He suggested this might be due to a high rate of very early abortions (before 2 weeks) which would be unrecognized and would help to account for the low fertility. In Ethiopian women, Harrison *et al.* (1969) reported a rather higher rate (9.1%) at 3000 m compared with less than 1% in an ethnically similar population at low altitude; however, both rates are low compared with rates in many populations.

Placental growth

Placentas are not significantly heavier at high altitude but since birth weights are low the placental/birth weight ratio is significantly increased (McClung, 1969; Mayhew, 1986), clearly an adaptation which would benefit foetal oxygenation. The number of villi and capillaries are increased in the placentas from high-altitude women; this increases the surface area for diffusion (Clegg, 1978), although Mayhew (1986) found a smaller surface area of villi but a thinner diffusion barrier, thus preserving the membrane diffusing capacity. Placental infarcts are more common in altitude placentas and more frequent in women with a European admixture of genes (McClung, 1969).

Foetal growth

The evidence suggests that, after the hazards of the first few weeks of pregnancy, growth is probably normal until the last trimester, when growth slows to produce a lighter baby at term. The cause of this growth retardation is not clear, since the evidence reviewed by Clegg (1978) suggests that the foetus at this altitude is not hypoxic compared with lowland foetuses. Possibly this is a genetic adaptive change with elimination, over generations, of genes which produce a larger baby. This would be advantageous since smaller babies are less likely to outgrow the placental capacity for oxygen transfer.

16.3.2 Birth weight and infant mortality

Results from a number of studies in the Andes and Tibet showed lower birth weight at altitude (Haas, 1976; Li, 1985). The mean weight declined from about 3.5 kg in Lima to 2.8 kg at Cerro de Pasco (4300 m) and, although there is the possibility that the nutritional status of mothers may be a factor, it is unlikely to account for more than a proportion of this difference. A similar effect of altitude has been reported from the USA (Lichty *et al.*, 1957; Grahn and Kratchman, 1963; Unger *et al.*, 1988). Women native to high altitude who descend to low altitude have heavier babies at low altitude (Hoff and Abelson, 1976). These studies include women from both indigenous high-altitude populations and low-altitude stock, and indicate that it is the high-altitude environment rather than genetics which result in low birth weights.

Infant mortality depends heavily on living standards and medical facilities and the very high infant mortality rates reported probably reflect these factors more than the effect of altitude *per se*. In Ethiopia, Harrison *et al.* (1969) reported a rate of 200 per 1000 live births at high altitude and 176 per 1000 at low altitude, while in the Andes a rate of 180 per 1000 was found in the rural area of Nunoa (4050 m) but only 73 per 1000 in urban La Paz (Baker, 1978). In Himalayan Sherpas, Lang and Lang (1971) gave a figure of 51 per 1000 at 4300 m, whilst in North Bhutan the rate was 189 per 1000 (Jackson *et al.*, 1966a). In experimental animals under controlled conditions, hypoxia increases neonatal mortality, so probably the high rates found in mountain peoples is at least partly due to the altitude. Apart from the direct effect of hypoxia an important indirect effect may be through the reduced the amount of liver glycogen present at birth, an important energy store until suckling becomes established (Clegg, 1978).

16.3.3 Growth through childhood

The high-altitude baby starts life smaller than the average low-altitude baby and its early growth is slower. Milestones, such as sitting and walking are slightly later but the difference between high- and low-altitude residents of the same race are less than those between different races or between urban and rural populations (Clegg, 1978).

In Quechua Indians in Peru, throughout childhood the high-altitude child lags behind his low-altitude counterpart in height by about two years. The adolescent growth spurt is less pronounced in high-altitude youths but their growth continues for about two years' longer and their adult stature is not reached until 22 years of age (Frisancho, 1978; Sun *et al.*, 1985). In Ethiopia, there were no such differences. Indeed, high-altitude males were taller and heavier for their age than lowlanders. In the Himalayas, a comparison of high-altitude Sherpas (3075–5050 m) with Tibetans resident at 1400 m was made by Pawson (quoted by Frisancho, 1978) who found no difference in the height of children in these populations, though other indices of maturation (skeletal and dental development and menarche) show the Sherpa children to lag behind the low-altitude Tibetans.

Investigations amongst the children of Kirghiz tribes of the Tien Shan mountains also showed delayed growth in the high-altitude children, equivalent to a lag of about one year. The altitude of residents was 2300–2800 m but in the summer months they go up to 3500 m to graze their cattle (Frisancho, 1978).

Menarche is a milestone well documented in studies from various high-altitude regions and, in girls living in the Andes, Himalayas and Tien Shan, it is 1–2 years later than in low-altitude girls (Frisancho, 1978; Jackson *et al.*, 1966b). The Ethiopian highlanders again are the exception as no difference was found (Harrison *et al.*, 1969). Adrenarche, the increase in serum androgens, also occurs one to two years later in children at altitude compared with sea-level in Peru (Goñez *et al.*, 1993).

16.4 PHYSIOLOGY OF HIGH-ALTITUDE POPULATIONS

16.4.1 Stature, lung development and function

Compared with European and North Americans, most high-altitude residents have a smaller stature and are lighter in weight, but when compared with people of similar race and living standards most of this difference disappears. The delayed growth (see above) is almost counteracted by the prolongation of active growth to beyond 20 years.

One of the most quoted aspects of lifelong adaptation to high altitude is the deep-chested development of the thorax in high-altitude residents (Barcroft, 1925). This has been documented by measurement of chest circumference and vital capacity in South American Indians living above 4500 m but is quite a small difference even in this population. Vital capacity was about 300 ml higher than predicted when corrected for body size (Velasquez, 1976). However, at 3500 m these measurements were smaller and less than the values published in the USA. High-altitude residents in the Himalayas do not have large circumference chests or bigger vital capacities than lowlanders (Frisancho, 1978) nor do younger Caucasian residents of Leadville (3100 m), but those over 50 years of age did have significantly larger vital capacities, by 440 ml, than predicted (DeGraff *et al.*, 1970). Sun *et al.* (1990) compared Tibetans and Han Chinese residents of Lhasa. Their mean ages, heights and weights were similar, but, whereas the Tibetans were lifelong residents, the Han has been resident for a mean time of eight years. The Tibetans had vital capacities significantly greater than the Han: 5080 ml compared with 4280 ml.

In Andean residents at 4540 m, the total lung capacity is about 500 ml larger than at sea-level, most of the increase being due to increased residual volume (Velasquez, 1976). Infants born at high altitude have greater thoracic compliance than infants of the same ethnic background born at low altitude (Mortola *et al.*, 1990). In adults the thoracic blood volume is increased and the residual volume/total lung capacity ratio increases from 21% to 28% in high-altitude compared with low-altitude residents. There may be some benefit from this since it would have the effect of reducing the breath-by-breath oscillations of P_{CO_2} and, hence, pH. At altitude these oscillations would otherwise be increased due to the reduction in plasma bicarbonate as part of the acclimatization process (Chapter 4). However these changes in lung volumes, even when found, are quite small and probably have little effect on performance.

The increased lung capacity may allow for an increased area of lung diffusion which, together with the increased blood volume, results in increased lung diffusing capacity. Details of studies in Andean and Caucasian residents are given in section 5.4.2. This increase in gas transfer should give the altitude resident a distinct performance advantage over the newcomer to altitude.

Vital capacity decreases with age at sea-level but this reduction is much greater at altitude, at least in Andean residents (Monge *et al.*, 1990) which may account in part for the increasing incidence of chronic mountain sickness with age (Chapter 20).

16.4.2 Ventilatory control at rest and exercise

Newcomers to high altitude find, often to their surprise, that they have to hyperventilate on the slightest exertion. They may notice that high-altitude residents seem to be relatively unaffected in this way.

Measurements of resting and exercise ventilation in high-altitude residents showed this impression to be correct. Chiodi (1957) showed resting ventilation to be higher in newcomers to altitude than in residents. At 3990 m the values were 5.3 and 4.5 $l\,min^{-1}\,m^{-2}$, and at 4515 m, 5.6 and 4.9 $l\,min^{-1}\,m^{-2}$ for newcomers and residents respectively. The Pa_{CO_2} values were in accordance with these differences. Santolaya *et al.* (1989) studied workers at the Aucanquilcha mine (5950 m). Their mean Pa_{CO_2} was 27.5 mmHg whereas lowlanders at that altitude would have a value about 5 mmHg lower, indicating a ventilation 22% higher. They also showed no respiratory alkalosis (pH 7.4), which lowlanders would have at that altitude.

On exercise, a similar distinction was found by Buskirk (1978) in Andean high-altitude residents and by Lahiri *et al.* (1967) in Sherpa subjects compared with lowlanders at altitude. It is likely that this lower ventilation in high-altitude residents is due to their low hypoxic ventilatory response (HVR) which is well documented (Chapter 4), since HVR correlates with exercise hyperventilation. As discussed in Chapter 4 this blunting of the HVR appears to take place over decades at altitude. Children resident at high altitude have normal HVR and this blunting is seen in Caucasian subjects resident in Leadville (3100 m) in Colorado, so it does not seem to be genetically determined (Lahiri *et al.*, 1976; Weil *et al.*, 1971).

Recent work by Zhuang *et al.* (1993) showed some interesting differences between lowland-born Han Chinese and highland-born Tibetans studied in Lhasa (3658 m). The Han had migrated to altitude either in childhood, adolescence or adulthood. They showed the decline in HVR with length of residence at altitude seen in Colorado altitude residents, but the Tibetans, who had a higher HVR (parameter A) than the Han, showed very little decline with age. However, Tibetans showed a paradoxical increase in ventilation on breathing 70% oxygen, a response not seen in Han subjects.

16.4.3 Haemoglobin concentration

The increase in haemoglobin concentration [Hb] at altitude is one of the best known adaptations to altitude hypoxia. It is found in both acclimatized lowlanders and lifelong residents at altitude. This is discussed in detail in Chapter 7.

In the Andes, some workers have found very high [Hb] in residents (Dill *et al.*, 1937; Talbot and Dill, 1938; Merino, 1950) and suggested that this is part of their long term adaptation to altitude. But subjects may have been included in these study populations who would now be considered to have chronic mountain sickness or Monge's disease (Chapter 20). More recent studies have not found such high levels or a significant difference between residents and acclimatized lowlanders (Penaloza *et al.*, 1971). Frisancho (1988) has reviewed the published data and showed that [Hb] values from mining areas in the Andes were higher than from non-mining areas, and that if studies from non-mining areas were compared with those from the Himalayas there was no significant difference.

In the Himalayas and on the Tibetan plateau, residents tend to have rather lower [Hb]s than acclimatized lowlanders. As discussed in Chapter 7, it is considered that, whilst a modest rise in [Hb] (to perhaps $18.0\,g\,dl^{-1}$) is advantageous, values much above this level are probably detrimental.

16.4.4 The carotid body and chemodectoma

Chronic hypoxia causes an increase in the size and weight of the carotid body. This was first reported in high-altitude Andean natives by Arias-Stella (1969). He found the weight of the two carotid bodies in residents of Lima to be just over 20 mg, whereas in altitude residents they totalled over 60 mg. Heath and co-workers found a similar increased weight of carotid bodies in patients with chronic hypoxic lung disease. They found a good correlation between carotid body and right ventricular weight, suggesting that a common correlation with hypoxia was the cause of the hyperplasia (Heath, 1986).

The principal cell involved in this hyperplasia is the sustentacular (Type II) cell with compression and obliteration of clusters of chief (Type I) cells. This type of hyperplasia is similar to that seen in systemic hypertension (Heath, 1986).

Chemodectoma, a tumour of the carotid body, is rare at sea-level, but appears to be common at high altitude. In 1973 Saldana *et al.* reported their occurrence in a higher proportion of Peruvian adults born and living at 4350 m than in those living at and above 3000 m. All were benign and the incidence was higher in females. An association between chemodectoma and thyroid carcinoma has been noted in two patients at 2380 m (Saldana *et al.*, 1973). No cases of chemodectoma have yet been reported from the Tibetan plateau or the high Himalayan valleys.

16.4.5 Cardiovascular adaptations

Andean high-altitude residents share with newcomers the raised pulmonary artery and right ventricular pressure due to the hypoxic pulmonary pressor response (Chapter 6), resulting in right ventricular hypertrophy (Recavarren and Arias-Stella, 1964). Indeed, in children at high altitude, the usual involution of the muscular coat of the pulmonary artery after birth does not take place, or does so only partially, so that the pulmonary arteries, both large and small, show far greater muscularization than is normal in sea-level residents (Saldana and Arias-Stella, 1963a,b,c).

This finding of right ventricular hypertrophy, continued muscularization of the pulmonary arteries and raised pulmonary artery pressure in residents at high altitude should be regarded as a response to high altitude rather than an adaptation, since there is no evidence that it has any physiological benefit. Indeed, it merely throws more strain on the right heart.

The purpose of the hypoxic pressor response in humans at sea-level, apart from its vital role in prenatal life, is presumably to redistribute blood away from areas of the lung that are hypoxic because of, for instance, atelectasis, and thus improve matching of ventilation and blood flow in various clinical situations. It would probably be beneficial to lose this response at altitude and the altitude-adapted yak would seem to have done this (section 16.5).

Recent studies in Tibetan highlanders suggest that they have achieved a similar adaptation to the yak and do not have raised pulmonary artery pressures at altitude even on exercise (Groves *et al.*, 1993). Neither do they develop the structural changes in their pulmonary arterial tree that are found in Andean highlanders (Gupta *et al.*, 1992).

Lifelong residents also have an increase in the number of branches to the main trunks of their coronary arteries (Arias-Stella and Topilsky, 1971).

Another adaptation of high-altitude residents is that, on exercise at altitude, their maximum heart rate does not seem to be limited as is the case for acclimatized lowlanders. This is discussed more fully in Chapter 6 and in relation to the adrenergic system, in Chapter 14.

16.4.6 Adaptation to cold

Cold is a feature of life at high altitude (section 3.8.1). Further aspects of cold adaptation are considered in Chapter 23.

16.5 ADAPTATION TO HYPOXIA OVER GENERATIONS

Most of the adaptations to hypoxia which have been shown in man appear to develop during, at most, a life time of exposure. Even the blunting of the hypoxic ventilatory response has been shown to develop in people of lowland stock over a period of decades (Weil *et al.*, 1971). The lower [Hb] in Sherpa and Tibetan subjects has been suggested as showing adaptation over many generations in Tibetan stock. However, when results from mining towns, where subjects may have lung disease, are excluded, Andean values are reduced and differences between them and Himalayan values disappear (Frisancho, 1988).

In animals, Harris (1986) has shown elegantly that, in cattle, the pulmonary pressor response, or lack of it, is genetically determined. The yak has little or no response whilst the cow has a brisk response. The cross-bred dzo has the blunted response of its yak parent while the second cross of dzo and bull produces 50% brisk and 50% low response offspring. That is, the gene responsible for a low response is dominant and the characteristic is inherited in a Mendelian way. Presumably, a low response is an advantage at altitude, a brisk response being a risk factor for brisket disease (named after the brisket, the loose skin at the animal's throat). Thus, we have a true adaptation achieved presumably by environmental pressure selecting for the low response gene. Similar adaptation has been found in the Llama.

There is evidence that in populations of Tibetan origin a similar adaptation may have taken place. Jackson (1968) found little ECG evidence of pulmonary hypertension in Bhutanese and Sherpa subjects at altitude, in that their mean frontal QRS axis differed by only 10° from healthy Edinburgh adults, in contrast to both lowlanders and Andean residents at altitude, who have marked right axis deviation due to pulmonary hypertension (Chapter 6). Recently Groves *et al.* (1993) found pulmonary artery pressures and resistances in five Tibetan subjects in Lhasa (3658 m) to be within normal sea-level values at rest and exercise. If confirmed, this would mark out the Tibetan population as showing genuine altitude adaptation, presumably by natural selection over very many generations.

16.6 DISEASES IN HIGH-ALTITUDE PEOPLES

It is clear from the biography of Yu-Thog, the elder (786–911 AD) the Physician-Saint and founder of traditional Tibetan medicine, that a number of medical conditions were known at high altitude from the earliest times. These included lung disease, leprosy, venereal disease, a 'swelling of the throat' (possibly diphtheria) and rabies, as well as urinary retention and stones in the urinary tract (Rinpoche, 1973).

Travellers to Lhasa in the eighteenth and nineteenth centuries, such as Huc and Gabet (Pelliot, 1928), reported epidemics of smallpox and in 1925 it was estimated that 7000 people died in and around Lhasa from this cause. Because of the prevalence of smallpox in Tibet, in the eighteenth century the Chinese placed a tablet in Lhasa giving instructions on how to curb the disease, and it was also reported in south Tibet and Bhutan by Saunders (1789) and in the Pamir (Forsyth, 1875). The Tibetan cure for smallpox was the skin of the ox and rhinoceros (Rinpoche, 1973), though a form of inoculation was used, apparently borrowed from China and India (Das, 1902). A kind of snuff prepared from the dried pustules of smallpox patients was inhaled, which induced a mild form of the disease, protecting the snuff taker from the severe form as described by the Pandit, A-K (Walker, 1885). These conditions (smallpox, rabies, leprosy etc.) are not, of course, *caused* by altitude.

16.6.1 Cardiovascular disease

Congenital heart disease

Congenital cardiovascular malformations are common at altitude, with patent ductus arteriosus being 15 times commoner at Cerro de Pasco (4200 m) than at sea-level in Lima (Penaloza *et al.*, 1964). Marticorena *et al.* (1959) reported an incidence of 0.72% of patent ductus arteriosus in children born around 4300 m, compared with an incidence of 0.8% for all congenital heart disease at sea-level.

In Xizang (Tibet), among the resident Tibetan population the incidence of congenital heart disease has been shown to range from 0.51% to 2.25%, with patent ductus arteriosus being the most frequently encountered abnormality (Sun, 1985). The greater the altitude the higher the prevalence; the highest documented incidence (2.50%) occurred in Chinese emigrants (Zhang, 1985). Presumably the cause of these high rates is the lack of a sudden increase in oxygen levels in the few hours after birth which normally triggers the reduction in pulmonary vascular resistance and the closure of the ductus.

Atherosclerosis

Studies of populations in the Andes suggest that both coronary artery disease and myocardial infarction are uncommon amongst high-altitude residents. No cases were found in one series of 300 necropsies carried out at 4300 m, and epidemiological studies in South America have shown that both angina of effort and ECG evidence of myocardial ischaemia are less at altitude than at sea-level (Ramos *et al.*, 1967). In the Tibetan ethnic population of north Bhutan no autopsy studies were available but angina seemed uncommon, and, as judged by ECG recordings, evidence of coronary artery disease was minimal. Studies from the Tien Shan and Pamir also suggest that degenerative cardiovascular disease is rare in these regions (Mirrakhimov, 1978).

In autopsy studies of 385 Tibetan adults living in the Lhasa area, arteriosclerosis of the aorta and its main branches occurred in 81.8% and, of the coronary artery in 65.5%. In Qinghai, coronary artery disease was common and autopsies on Tibetans showed the same incidence as in lowlanders, but the incidence of coronary infarction was low (Sun, 1985). Serum cholesterol levels were low in Andean natives and in the Bhutanese high-altitude group studied; in the latter there was no difference with age group and no progressive increase (Jackson *et al.*, 1966c).

Hypertension

Hypertension appears uncommon in high-altitude populations in South America. In a study of 300 high-altitude natives in Peru no significant rise in either systolic or diastolic pressure occurred with age. Of individuals aged between 60 and 80 years in the same area, few had a systolic pressure above 165 mmHg or a diastolic above 95 mmHg (Baker, 1978). Significant hypertension did not occur in ethnic Tibetan populations of north Bhutan, and, of 70 individuals examined, levels of blood pressure above 165/90 mmHg were found in 4%. Hypertension occurred neither in a Sherpa population studied in north-east Nepal nor in individuals studied in the Tien Shan or Pamir. In an Ethiopian group, a slightly higher systolic pressure was found in males.

By contrast, Sun reports (1985, 1986) a relatively high incidence of hypertension among indigenous Tibetans whose ancestors had lived on the plateau for 4000 years or more. He found an age associated increase in blood pressure; there was no tendency for hypertension to decline at higher altitudes and the blood pressure was higher in women than in men. The incidence was greater in the urban population around Lhasa than in rural populations. Similar observations have been made in Tibetans living in high-altitude areas of western Szechuan. However, Han (Chinese) immigrants to Tibet showed a lower incidence of hypertension than did the Tibetans. In Qinghai province (which contains the north-eastern part of the Tibetan plateau) the incidence of hypertension appears to be lower than in Xizang.

Part of the lack of age increase in blood pressure in the South American and Himalayan populations studied may be the product of food and behaviour associated with a traditional life style. The cause of hypertension among Tibetans is not clear. On the plateau, obesity is uncommon and traditionally few smoke (though this is changing). However, they do have a very high intake of salt, estimated at up to one kilo per month, much of it taken in their tea. They also add yak butter which is often slightly rancid. In the Bhutanese and Sherpa varieties of 'Tibetan' tea neither the salt nor the butter content appears, by taste, to be as high. In all houses and nomad dwellings there is a continuous supply of this tea which is offered to every visitor. Tibetans, even when they have migrated to low levels, still drink large quantities and may become very obese. The high salt and butter intake may be a factor in the high incidence of hypertension in Tibetans.

16.6.2 Infection

Direct exposure to increased solar radiation inhibits the growth of some bacteria due to the ultraviolet componant of sunlight. *Staphylcoccus* aureus is greatly inhibited yet *Escherichia coli* is more resistant (Nusshag, 1954). The number of bacteria in ambient air decreases with altitude, and a study on the Jungfraujoch (3400 m) in Switzerland showed that, despite a large number of tourists, few bacteria were present in the air.

Bacterial flora on man is not influenced by high altitudes *per se*. However, a lower incidence of many common infections of bacterial, viral and protozoal origin was observed in soldiers at altitudes up to 5538 m (Singh *et al.*, 1977). Examination of nasal swabs in a high-altitude population in north Bhutan showed that there was only a 4% carrier rate of coagulase positive staphylococci; normally the incidence is between 29–40% in western communities. A high frequency of β-haemolytic streptococci, highly sensitive to penicillin, was found in throat cultures, whereas in western communities sensitivity to penicillin would be minimal (Selkon and Gould, 1966).

In the highlanders of Peru, Colombia and Ecuador, oroya fever is found, which is caused by *Bacillus bacilliformis* becoming parasitic in the red blood cells. Various haemorrhagic fevers are described in the highlands of Bolivia. These are considered to be viral in origin, the virus belonging to the same group as lassa fever. Haemorrhagic disorders have also been described in northeastern Nepal.

Mosquitoes, which transmit malaria and yellow fever, are absent at high altitude, whilst typhus appears to be commoner than at lower levels. This may be because bathing is not usual at higher altitudes due to cold and so lice are common.

Pulmonary disease also appears common at altitude and this in part may be related to the exposure of highlanders to the smoke from open fires inside their houses or tents. In Xizang (Tibet) the incidence of chronic bronchitis was 3.7% in a low-altitude population and 22.9% in a population at 4500 m. This was complicated by emphysema in 5–12% of cases and by cor pulmonale in 0.98% (Sun, 1985). In Qinghai Province, chronic obstructive airway disease is relatively common but smoking is prevalent, particularly amongst emigrants to high altitude. In the Pamir too, respiratory infections were noted by Forsyth (1875), though they seem less common at the present time.

In Nepal, pulmonary tuberculosis seems relatively common, as it is throughout the sub-continent, whilst in Ethiopia it was rare. In Ethiopia the major communicable diseases were measles, malaria, dysentery, scabies and syphilis, and the total incidence of communicable disease was greater in the low-altitude population (Harrison *et al.*, 1969).

In northern Bhutan, respiratory infections appeared to be commoner in the younger age groups but were rare in adults; antibodies to a number of common viral infections were found. A high proportion of the population had been exposed to influenza, mumps, measles, herpes simplex and the common cold (Jackson *et al.*, 1966c), whilst in Lhasa, other parts of Tibet and the Pamir, measles epidemics with a high mortality have been reported in the past.

Leprosy occurs in Nepal and Bhutan (Ward and Jackson, 1965) and was reported in Tibet in the nineteenth, century (Das, 1902) and in the western Himalayas (Moorcroft and Trebeck, 1841a). The incidence of venereal disease appears to have been high in Lhasa (Chapman, 1938), south Tibet and Bhutan (Saunders, 1789) and in the Pamir (Forsyth, 1875). Where large flocks of sheep are found, as in Qinghai province, hydatid disease is common. Plague has also been mentioned by European travellers in Central Asia (Deasy, 1901; Grenard, 1904).

Chronic eye infections are seen in the populations of the Pamir, Himalayas and Tibetan plateau; they are exacerbated by the smoke of yak dung fires. Instruments for the treatment of cataract were available to those who practised traditional Tibetan medicine; in general, surgery was not commonly carried out.

In summary, where certain infections are common they are due to the low living standards of the people rather than to altitude *per se*.

16.6.3 Goitre

The frequency of goitre in mountainous areas has been recognized for centuries, but it is not confined to the mountains, and over 200 million people world-wide have goitre (Figure 16.1). Iodine deficiency is due to low iodine content of the soil and therefore the water. Soils poor in iodine are found where the land remained longest under quaternary glaciers. When the ice thawed, the iodine-rich soil was swept away and replaced by new soil derived from iodine-poor crystalline rocks. Seaweed, which is rich in iodine, and other folk remedies have been used since ancient times for prophylaxis and treatment (Hetzel, 1989).

Scientific proof that goitre was due to iodine deficiency was not available until a controlled trial in high-school children in Akron, Ohio, was published by Marine and Kimball (1920). They showed a reduction in the size of goitres and prevention of their development in children treated with iodine.

Iodine deficiency causes hyperplasia and retention of colloid in the thyroid, resulting in goitre and, eventually, hypothyroidism in adults. Children born to iodine deficient mothers have a range of neurological and skeletal defects known collectively as cretinism, an association noted for centuries. This term covers a range of clinical conditions which seem to vary in frequency and importance from locality to locality and includes dwarfism, goitre, facial dysmorphism, deafness, deaf mutism and intellectual impairment.

In populations with goitre, the overall work capacity of the population may be impaired, as, in addition to cretinism, there is a marked morbidity, infant mortality is raised and mental subnormality common.

Iodine deficiency may result from insufficient intake, goitrogenic substances and deficiency in intrathyroidal enzymes; an excess of calcium or fluoride in the presence of iodine deficiency may increase the incidence of goitre.

McCarrison (1908, 1913) carried out a classical study of goitre and endemic cretinism in the Gilgit Agency of Kashmir (Karakoram), and more recently Chapman *et al.* (1972) worked in the identical area.

In 1906, McCarrison found a goitre incidence of 65%, in Chapman's study it was 74%. In this study, 10 of 589 individuals examined were cretins, and hypothyroidism, excluding cretinism, was found in 24 subjects. Although the population as a whole appeared to be iodine deficient, the majority had adapted well. No evidence was found that goitre was caused by an infectious agent, a theory put forward by McCarrison.

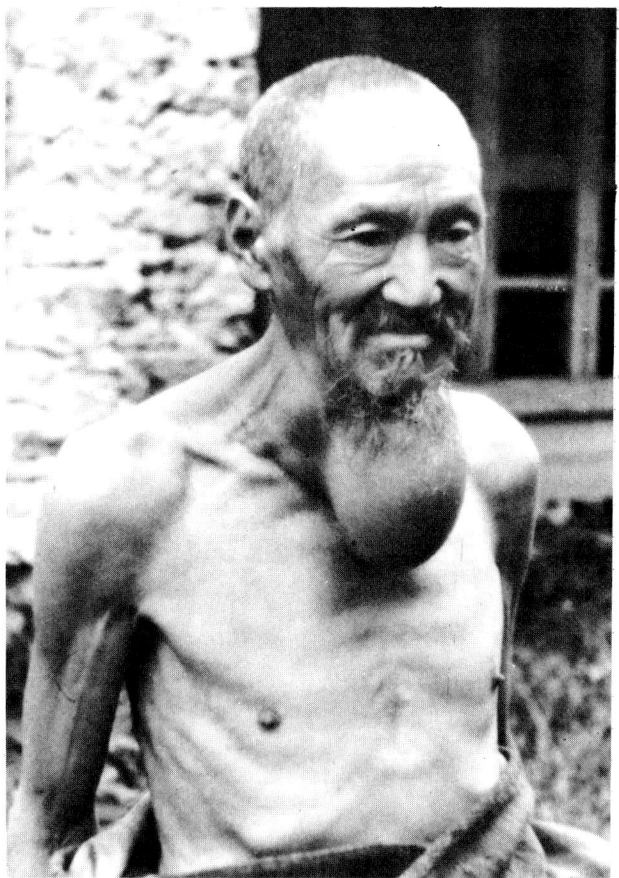

Figure 16.1 Tibetan from north Bhutan with large pendulous goitre.

The incidence of goitre may vary widely within a few miles; at some 100 miles north of the Gilgit goitre endemic, it was not observed in the semi-nomadic Kirghiz tribesmen who inhabit the Pamir plateau of southern Xinjiang. Direct questioning of the nomads revealed that they knew about goitre but they were adamant that there was no history of its occurrence amongst them (Ward, 1983), though Marco Polo noted a large population of people with goitre in Yarkand (Shache) as did Forsyth (1875). However, heresay evidence is notably unreliable. Anecdotal evidence of goitre in other regions of the Himalayas, the

Shimshall region of the Karakoram, and west Bhutan, suggests also that the incidence may vary considerably within a few miles (Saunders, 1789; Shipton, 1938).

Moorcroft and Trebeck (1841b, 1841c), whilst travelling in the western Himalayas and on the Tibetan border, comment on goitre that, 'scarcely a woman was free from it'. Later they say, 'Goitre was here very common: the water was soft whilst at Gonh it was too hard to mix with soap: but so it was at Le where goitre does not prevail.' Surgical removal is alluded to by Fraser (1820): 'We understand it (goitre) was sometimes cured when early means were taken, and these are said to consist in extirpation of the part by the knife. We saw some persons who had scars on their throat resulting from this mode of cure which had in these instances been completely successful.' Waddell (1899), in a village where goitre was prevalent writes, 'I was surprised to see that several of the goats and the domestic fowls, as well as some of the ponies, had the same large swellings.'

According to Dr Sun Sin-Fu (personal communication), in Lhasa, about 60% of Tibetan indigenous inhabitants have goitre. Das (1902) commented too that Tibetan physicians recognized six varieties of goitre. Rockhill (1891) also observed goitre, particularly in women in eastern Tibet, and other travellers noted the condition in northern Tibet (Bonavalot, 1891) and in the gorge country of south-east Tibet (Bailey, 1957).

The incidence of goitre in the Himalayan valleys is high, and in the Tibetan ethnic population of north Bhutan it was the commonest clinical condition. In subjects under 20 years old it was less marked, and younger individuals had a diffuse enlargement, whereas with age a nodular goitre was more common. No cases of cancer or thyrotoxicosis were seen, and two cretins were found in 349 individuals examined. The incidence of goitre was 60% in females and 19% in males (Jackson *et al.*, 1966b).

Ibbertson *et al.* (1972), in a survey of Sherpas (also of Tibetan ethnic origin) in the Sola Khumbu region of northeastern Nepal, found that 92% had a palpable goitre, which was visibly enlarged in 63%; 75% had below normal protein bound iodine levels in the blood and 30% were clinically hypothyroid. Classical myxoedema was present in 5.9% of the population, deaf mutism in a further 4.7% and isolated deafness in a further 3.1%. Pitt (1970) describes Nepalese babies born with goitre. In many of these areas the incidence of goitre is much lower now after various projects for giving iodine by tablets or depot injections have been carried out. A recent paper reports a survey carried out in 1980–1981 in Ethiopia where the gross goitre prevalence was found to be 30% amongst schoolchildren and 19% in household members (Wolde-Gebriel *et al.*, 1993).

16.6.4 Sickle cell disease in high-altitude populations

Adzaku *et al.* (1993) reported on 136 patients resident at about 3000 m in Saudi Arabia and compared them with 185 patients living at sea-level. Patients at both locations included those with homozygous disease (Hb SS), haemoglobin C (Hb SC) and sickle cell trait (Hb AS). The main finding was a marked increase in 2,3-diphosphoglycerate (DPG) in patients with sickle cell disease compared with normal controls at altitude and patients at sea-level. Their [Hb] was not different from sea-level patients; they were anaemic, with values around 8.0–9.0 $g\,dl^{-1}$. Sickle cell patients resident at low altitude have a high risk of crises on going to altitude (section 28.5.3). They attribute the relative well-being of their patients at altitude to their high 2,3-DPG, which, at this relatively modest altitude, would help tissue oxygenation in contrast to the situation at extreme altitude (Chapter 11).

16.6.5 Dental conditions in high-altitude populations

There is no evidence that altitude has any direct effect on the teeth but the economic conditions, dictated in part by altitude, may well affect diet and hence dental condition. Generally the diet of high-altitude populations contains less refined sugars and more fibre, giving less caries than a more 'western' diet. Green (1992) reported a much higher incidence of caries amongst Sherpa children along the popular trekking routes in Nepal (76%) than in villages off the routes (17%). The latter had not had the 'benefit' of cadging sweets from generous but misguided tourists.

REFERENCES

Adzaku, F., Mohammed, S., Annobil, S. and Addae, S. (1993) Relevant laboratory findings in patients with sickle cell disease living at high altitude. *J. Wild. Med.*, **4**, 374–83.

Arias-Stella, J. (1969) Human carotid body at high altitudes (abstract). *Am. J. Pathol.*, **55**, 82.

Arias-Stella, J. and Topilsky, M. (1971) Anatomy of the coronary circulation at high altitude, in *High Altitude Physiology*, (eds R. Porter and J. Knight), Churchill Livingstone, London, pp. 149–57.

Bailey, F.M. (1957) *No Passport to Tibet*. Hart Davis, London, p. 261.

Baker, P.T. (1978) The adaptive fitness of high-altitude populations, in *The Biology of High Altitude Peoples*, (ed. P.T. Baker), Cambridge University Press, Cambridge, pp. 317–50.

Baker, P.T. and Dutt, J.S. (1972) Demographic variables as measures of biological adaptation: a case study of high altitude population, in *The Structure of Human Populations*, (eds G.A. Harrison and A.J. Boyce), Clarendon Press, Oxford, pp. 352–78.

Barcroft, J. (1925) *The Respiratory Functions of the Blood. Part I, Lessons from High Altitudes*. Cambridge University Press, Cambridge.

Bonavalot, G. (1891) *Across Thibet*, Cassell, London, p. 116.

Buskirk, E.R. (1978) Work capacity of high-altitude natives, in *The Biology of High Altitude Peoples*, (ed. P.T. Baker), Cambridge University Press, Cambridge, pp. 173–87.

Chapman, F.S. (1938) *Lhasa. The Holy City*, Chatto and Windus, London, p. 241.

Chapman, J.A., Grant, I.S., Taylor, G., *et al.* (1972) Endemic goitre in the Gilgit Agency, West Pakistan. *Philos. Trans. R. Soc. Lond.* (*Ser. B*), **263**, 459–91.

Chiodi, H. (1957) Respiratory adaptations to chronic high altitude hypoxia. *J. Appl. Physiol.*, **10**, 81–7.

Clegg, E.J. (1978) Fertility and early growth, in *The Biology of High Altitude Peoples*, (ed. P.T. Baker), Cambridge University Press, Cambridge, pp. 65–115.

Das, S.C. (1902) *Journey to Lhasa and Central Tibet*, John Murray, London, pp. 257–60.

Deasy, H.H.P. (1901) *In Tibet and Chinese Turkestan*, T. Fisher Unwin, London, pp. 2–73.

DeGraff, A.C., Grover, R.F., Johnson, R.L., *et al.* (1970) Diffusing capacity of the lung in Caucasians native to 3100 m. *J. Appl. Physiol.*, **29**, 71–6.

Dill, D.B., Talbot, J.H. and Consolazio, W.V. (1937) Blood as a physiochemical system. XII. Man at high altitudes. *J. Biol. Chem.*, **118**, 649–66.

Forsyth, T.D. (1875) *Report of a Mission to Yarkund in 1873*, Foreign Department Press, Calcutta, pp. 66–9.

Fraser, J.B. (1820) *Journal of a Tour Through Part of the Snowy Range of the Himala Mountains and to the Sources of the Rivers Jumna and Ganges*, Rodwell and Martin, London, p. 349.

Frisancho, A.R. (1978) Human growth and development among high-altitude populations, in *The Biology of High Altitude Peoples*, (ed. P.T. Baker), Cambridge University Press, Cambridge, pp. 117–71.

Frisancho, A.R. (1988) Origins of differences in haemoglobin concentration between Himalayan and Andean populations. *Respir. Physiol.*, **72**, 13–18.

Goñez, C., Villena, A. and Gonzales, G.F. (1993) Serum levels of adrenal-androgens up to adrenarche in Peruvian children living at sea level and at high altitude. *J. Endocrinol.*, **136**, 517–23.

Grahn, D. and Kratchman, J. (1963) Variations in neonatal death rate and birth weight in the United States and possible relations to environmental radiation, geology and altitude. *Am. J. Hum. Genet.*, **15**, 329–52.

Green, S.P.T. (1992) The 1991 Everest marathon and the Namche Bazaar dental clinic. *J. R. Nav. Med. Serv.*, **78**, 165–71.

Grenard, F. (1904) *Tibet*, Hutchinson, London, p. 249.

Groves, B.M., Droma, T., Sutton, J.R., *et al.* (1993) Minimal hypoxic pulmonary hypertension in normal Tibetans at 3658 m. *J. Appl. Physiol.*, **74**, 312–8.

Gupta, M.L., Rao, K.S., Andand, I.S., *et al.* (1992) Lack of smooth muscle in the small pulmonary arteries of the native Lakakhi. *Am. Rev. Respir. Dis.*, **145**, 1201–4.

Haas, J.D. (1976) Prenatal and infant growth and development, in *Man in the Andes*, (eds P.T. Baker and M.A. Little), Dowden, Hutchinson & Ross, Stroudsburg PA, pp. 161–78.

Harris, P. (1986) Evolution, hypoxia and high altitude, in *Aspects of Hypoxia*, (ed. D. Heath), Liverpool University Press, Liverpool, pp. 207–16.

Harrison, G.A., Kuchemann, C.F., Moore, M.A.S., *et al.* (1969) The effects of altitudinal variation in Ethiopian populations. *Philos. Trans. R. Soc. Lond. (Ser. B)*, **256**, 147–82.

Heath, D. (1986) Carotid body hyperplasia, in *Aspects of Hypoxia*, (ed. D. Heath), Liverpool University Press, Liverpool, pp. 61–74.

Hetzel, B.S. (1989) *The Story of Iodine Deficiency*, Oxford Medical Publications, Oxford.

Hoff, C.J. and Abelson, A.E. (1976) Fertility, in *Man in The Andes, A Multidisciplinary Study of High-Altitude Quechua*, (eds P.T. Baker and M.A. Little), Dowden, Hutchinson & Ross, Stroudsburg PA, pp. 128–46.

Ibbertson, H.K., Tair, J.M., Pearl, M., *et al.* (1972) Himalayan cretinism. *Adv. Exp. Med. Biol.*, **30**, 51–69.

Jackson, F.S. (1968) The heart at high altitude. *Br. Heart J.*, **30**, 291–4.

Jackson, F.S., Turner, R.W.D. and Ward, M.P. (1966a) *Report on IBP Expedition to North Bhutan*, Royal Society, London, p. 99.

Jackson, F.S., Turner, R.W.D. and Ward, M.P. (1966b) *Report on IBP Expedition to North Bhutan*, Royal Society, London, pp. 40–4.

Jackson, F.S., Turner, R.W.D. and Ward, M.P. (1966c) *Report on IBP Expendition to North Bhutan*, Royal Society, London, p. 96.

Lahiri, S., Milledge, J.S., Chattopadhyay, H.P., *et al.* (1967) Respiration and heart rate of Sherpa highlanders during exercise. *J. Appl. Physiol.*, **23**, 545–54.

Lahiri, S., Delaney, R.G., Brody, J.S., *et al.* (1976) Relative role of environmental and genetic factors in respiratory adaptation to high altitude. *Nature*, **261**, 133–5.

Lang, S.D.R. and Lang, A. (1971) The Kunde Hospital and a demographic survey of the Upper Khumbu, Nepal. *N. Z. Med. J.*, **74**, 1–8.

Li, Y.Z. (1985) The birth weight, distribution of new born (in percentile) in high altitude (abstract). Second High Altitude Symposium, Qinghai, China, (unpublished proceedings).

Lichty, J.A., Ting, R.Y., Bruns, P.D. and Dyar, E. (1957) Studies of babies born at high altitude. *Am. Med. Assoc. J. Dis. Child.*, **93**, 666–7.

McCarrison, R. (1908) Observations on endemic cretinism in the Chitral and Gilgit valleys. *Lancet*, **2**, 1275–80.

McCarrison, R. (1913) *The Pathology of Endemic Goitre (Milroy Lectures 1913)*, Bale Sons and Danielson, London.

McClung, J.P. (1969) *Effects of High Altitude on Human Birth*, Harvard University Press, Cambridge MA.

Marine, D. and Kimball, O.P. (1920) Prevention of simple goiter in man. *Arch. Intern. Med.*, **25**, 661–72.

Marticorena, E., Severino, J., Penaloza, A.D. and Neuriegel, K. (1959) Influencia de las grandes alturas en la determinacion de la persistencia del canal arteral. Observaciones realizadas en 3500 escolares de altura a 4300 m. Sombre el niuel dez mar. Primeros resultados operatorios. *Revista Medica de la Provincia del Yauli* Nos 1–2, La Oroya.

Mayhew, T. (1986) Morphometric diffusing capacity for oxygen of the human term placenta at high altitude, in *Aspects of Hypoxia*, (ed. D. Heath), Liverpool University Press, Liverpool, pp. 181–90.

Merino, C.F. (1950) Studies on blood formation and destruction in the polycythemia of high altitude. *Blood*, **5**, 1–31.

Mirrakhimov, M.M. (1978) Biological and physiological characteristics of high-altitude natives of Tien Shan and the Pamirs, in *The Biology of High Altitude Peoples*, (ed. P.T. Baker), Cambridge University Press, Cambridge, p. 313.

Monge, C., Bonavia, D., Leon-Velard, F. and Arregui, A. (1990) High altitude populations in Nepal and the Andes, in *Hypoxia: the Adaptations*, (eds J.R. Sutton, G. Coates and J.E. Remmers), Decker, Toronto, pp. 53–8.

Moorcroft, W. and Trebeck, G. (1841a) Travels in the Himalayan provinces of Hindustan and the Punjab; in Ladakh and Kashmir; in Peshawar, Kabul, Kuduz and Bokhara, in *William Moorcroft, George Trebeck from 1819 to 1825*, Vol. 1, (ed. H.H. Wilson), John Murray, London, p. 180.

Moorcroft, W. and Trebeck, G. (1841b) Travels in the Himalayan provinces of Hindustan and the Punjab; in Ladakh and Kashmir; in Peshawar, Kabul, Kuduz and Bokhara, in *William Moorcroft, George Trebeck from 1819 to 1825*, Vol. 2, (ed. H.H. Wilson), John Murray, London, p. 25.

Moorcroft, W. and Trebeck, G. (1841c) Travels in the Himalayan provinces of Hindustan and the Punjab; in Ladakh and Kashmir; in Peshawar, Kabul, Kuduz and Bokhara, in *William Moorcroft, George Trebeck from 1819 to 1825*, Vol. 2, (ed. H.H. Wilson), John Murray, London, p. 30.

Mortola, J.P., Rezzonico, R., Fisher, J.T., *et al.* (1990) Compliance of the respiratory system in infants born at high altitude. *Am. Rev. Respir. Dis.*, **142**, 43–8.

Nusshag, W. (1954) *Hygiene der Haustiere*, Verlag S. Hirzel, Leipzig, p. 86.

Pelliot, P. (ed.) (1928) *Travels in Tartary, Thibet and China*, Vol. 2, Routledge, London, p. 250.

Penaloza, D., Arias-Stella, J., Sime, F., *et al.* (1964) The heart and pulmonary circulation in children at high altitude. *Pediatrics*, **34**, 568–82.

Penaloza, D., Sime, F. and Ruiz, L. (1971) Cor pulmonale in chronic mountain sickness: present concept of Monge's disease, in *High Altitude Physiology*, (eds R. Porter and J. Knight), Churchill Livingstone, London, pp. 41–60.

Pitt, P. (1970) *Surgeon in Nepal*, Murray, London, p. 135.

Ramos, D.A., Kruger, H., Muro, M. and Arias-Stella, J. (1967) Patologica del Hombre nativo de las grande alturas: investigacion de las causes de muerte en 300 autopsias. *Bon. Sanit. Panam.*, **62**, 497–507.

Recavarren, S. and Arias-Stella, J. (1964) Right ventricular hypertrophy in people born and living at high altitudes. *Br. Heart J.*, **26**, 806–12.

Rinpoche, R. (1973) *Tibetan Medicine*, Wellcome Institute of the History of Medicine, London, p. 72.

Rockhill, W.W. (1891) *The Land of the Lamas*, Longmans Green, London, p. 265.

Saldana, M. and Arias-Stella, J. (1963a) Studies on the structure of the pulmonary trunk. I. Normal changes in the elastic configuration of the human pulmonary trunk at different ages. *Circulation*, **27**, 1086–93.

Saldana, M. and Arias-Stella, J. (1963b) Studies on the structure of the pulmonary trunk. II. The evolution of the elastic configuration of the pulmonary trunk in people native to high altitudes. *Circulation*, **27**, 1094–100.

Saldana, M. and Arias-Stella, J. (1963c) Studies on the structure of the pulmonary trunk. III. The thickness of the media of the pulmonary trunk and ascending aorta in high altitude natives. *Circulation*, **27**, 1101–4.

Saldana, M.J., Salem, L.E. and Travezan, R. (1973) High altitude hypoxia and chemodectoma. *Hum. Pathol.*, **4**, 251–63.

Santolaya, R.B., Lahiri, S., Alfaro, R.T. and Schoene, R.B. (1989) Respiratory adaptation in the highest inhabitants and highest Sherpa mountaineers. *Respir. Physiol.*, **77**, 253–62.

Saunders, R. (1789) Some account of the vegetable and mineral productions of Boutan and Thibet. *Philos. Trans. R. Soc.*, **79**, 79–111.

Selkon, J. and Gould, J.C. (1966) Bacteriology, in *Report on IBP Expedition to North Bhutan*, (eds F.S. Jackson, R.W.D. Turner and M.P. Ward), Royal Society, London, pp. 88–98.

Shipton, E. (1938) *Blank on the Map*, Hodder and Stoughton, London, p. 265.

Singh, I., Chohan, J.S., Lal, M., *et al.* (1977) Effects of high altitude stay on the incidence of common diseases in man. *Int. J. Biometeorol.*, **21**, 93–122.

Sobrevilla, L.A., Romero, I., Moncloa, F., *et al.* (1967) Endocrine studies of high altitude. III. Urinary gonadotrophins in subjects native to and living at 14 000 feet and during acute exposure of men living at sea level to high altitude. *Acta Endocrinol.*, **56**, 369–75.

Sun, S.F. (1985) Epidemiology of hypertension of the Tibetan plateau (abstract). Second High Altitude Symposium, Qinghai, China, (unpublished proceedings).

Sun, S.F. (1986) Epidemiology of hypertension on the Tibetan plateau. *Hum. Biol.*, **58**, 507–15.

Sun, J.H., Lin, Z.P. and Hu, X.L. (1985) An observation on the development of normal children age between 7–17 years at three elevations (abstract). Second High Altitude Symposium, Qinghai, China, (unpublished proceedings).

Sun, S.F., Droma, T.S., Zhang, J.G., *et al.* (1990) Greater maximal O_2 uptakes and vital capacities in Tibetan than Han residents of Lhasa. *Respir. Physiol.*, **79**, 151–62

Talbot, J.H. and Dill, D.B. (1938) Clinical observations at high altitude. *Am. J. Med., Sci.*, **192**, 626–39.

Unger, C., Weiser, J.K., McCullough, R.E., *et al.* (1988) Altitude, low birth weight, and infant mortality in Colorado. *J. Am. Med. Assoc.*, **259**, 3427–32.

Velasquez, T. (1976) Pulmonary function and oxygen transport, in *Man in the Andes: A Multidisciplinary Study of High-altitude Quechua*, (eds P.T. Baker and M.A. Little), Dowden, Hutchinson & Ross, Stroudsburg PA, pp. 237–60.

Waddell, L.A. (1899) *Among the Himalayas*, Constable, London, pp. 261–2.

Walker, J.T. (1885) Four years journeyings through great Tibet by one of the trans-Himalayan explorers of the Survey of India. *Proc. R. Geogr. Soc.*, **7**, 65–92.

Ward, M.P. and Jackson, F.S. (1965) Medicine in Bhutan. *Lancet*, **1**, 811–13.

Ward, M.P. (1983) The Kongur Massif in Southern Xinjiang. *Geogr. J.*, **149**, 137–52.

Weil, J.V., Byrne-Quinn, E., Ingvar, E., *et al.* (1971) Acquired attenuation of chemoreceptor function in chronically hypoxic man at high altitude. *J. Clin. Invest.*, **50**, 186–95.

Wolde-Gebriel, Z., Demeke, T., West, C.E. and Van der Haar, F. (1993) Goitre in Ethiopia. *Br. J. Nutr.*, **69**, 257–68.

Zhang, Y.-B. (1985) *An Introduction to Medical Research in Qinghai*, High Altitude Medical Research Institute, Qinghai, China.

Zhuang, J., Droma, T., Sun, S., *et al.* (1993) Hypoxic ventilatory responsiveness in Tibetan compared with Han residents of 3658 m. *J. Appl. Physiol.*, **74**, 303–11.

17

Acute and subacute mountain sickness

17.1 INTRODUCTION

It has been known for many years that travellers to high mountains experience a variety of symptoms, an early description of which was by de Acosta (Chapter 1) and the disease has been known as Acosta's disease. But the first modern account of acute mountain sickness (AMS) was by Ravenhill (1913). He pointed out that previous descriptions by explorers and mountain climbers were complicated by fatigue, cold, lack of food, etc. He was serving as a medical officer of a mining company whose mines at 4700 m in Chile were served by a railway so that the patients he observed were suffering the uncomplicated effects of altitude alone. The local Bolivian name for AMS was 'puna' or in Peru 'soroche'. Tibetan names for AMS include 'ladrak' (poison of the pass) 'damgiri', 'duqri', 'yen chang' (from the Koko Nor region), 'chang-chi' (from Szechuan), and 'tuteck'. Ravenhill's description of simple AMS, which he calls puna of the 'normal' type can hardly be bettered. He wrote:

> It is a curious fact that the symptoms of puna do not usually evince themselves at once. The majority of newcomers have expressed themselves as being quite well on first arrival. As a rule, towards the evening, the patient begins to feel rather slack and disinclined for exertion. He goes to bed but has a restless and troubled night and wakes up next morning with a severe frontal headache.
>
> There may be vomiting, frequently there is a sense of oppression in the chest but there is rarely any respiratory distress or alteration in the normal rate of breathing so long as the patient is at rest. The patient may feel slightly giddy on rising from bed and any attempt

at exertion increases the headache, which is nearly always confined to the frontal region. *(Ravenhill, 1913)*

To this description should be added the symptoms of irritability and occasionally photophobia. Sleep is often disturbed, probably because of periodic breathing. The patient may wake with a feeling of suffocation during the apnoeic phase. Ravenhill then goes on to describe puna of the cardiac and nervous types, corresponding in our present nomenclature to acute pulmonary oedema and acute cerebral oedema of high altitude (section 17.2).

After Ravenhill, although mountain sickness was well recognized, the distinction and importance of the two complicating forms seem to have been lost, at least in the English-speaking world until rediscovered by Houston (1960) (Chapter 18).

17.2 DEFINITIONS AND NOMENCLATURE

The nomenclature of mountain sickness is summarized in Table 17.1. The terms puna and soroche are used loosely in South America, not only for the symptoms of acute mountain sickness but also for the dyspnoea normal to exertion at high altitude (Ravenhill, 1913). They are also used for chronic mountain sickness, a completely distinct clinical entity (Chapter 20). The term 'mountain sickness' needs to be qualified by the word 'acute' to distinguish it from this latter entity; the term 'acute mountain sickness' (AMS) is now well accepted for this condition or group of conditions. Finally there is the recently described subacute mountain sickness affecting either infants or adults (section 17.9).

Dickinson (1982) made the useful suggestion that the 'normal' or 'simple' AMS, which commonly affects most people going rapidly to

Table 17.1 Nomenclature of mountain sickness

Reference				
Ravenhill (1913)	Puna of the normal type	Puna of the cardiac type	Puna of the nervous type	
Dickinson (1982)	Benign AMS	Malignant pulmonary AMS	Malignant cerebral AMS	
Others	Simple AMS	High-altitude pulmonary edema (HAPE)	High-altitude cerebral edema (HACE)	Chronic mountain sickness (CMS)

high altitude and which is self limiting, be termed 'benign' while the other two forms or complications of AMS be termed 'malignant', since they are life threatening. They are thus termed 'malignant pulmonary AMS' and 'malignant cerebral AMS'.

However, this terminology, emphasizing the crucial difference between the forms of AMS, has yet to be widely adopted. The terms more commonly used for the malignant forms are: high altitude pulmonary edema (HAPE), and high altitude cerebral edema (HACE). Many cases of malignant AMS include features of both pulmonary and cerebral edema.

Benign AMS may be defined as a self limiting condition affecting previously healthy individuals on going rapidly to high altitude. After arrival there may be a period of some 6–12 h with no symptoms although Singh *et al.* (1969) say this time lag may be as long as 96 h. The symptoms described above then start gradually and peak usually on the second or third day. By the fourth or fifth day symptoms are usually gone and do not recur at that altitude.

Physical examination may reveal crackles in the chest, peripheral oedema and, occasionally, retinal haemorrhage. According to Hackett and Rennie (1979) the proportions of cases showing these signs were 23%, 18% and 4% respectively.

Later ascent to a higher altitude may precipitate a further attack. Descent and re-ascent after less than 7–10 days does not usually provoke symptoms but descent for more than about 10 days renders the subject susceptible to AMS on re-ascent, possibly more so than on the first occasion.

17.3 INCIDENCE OF BENIGN AMS

The incidence of AMS depends upon the rate at which people ascend to altitude and the height reached as well as the exact definition of the condition. The lowest altitude at which a few individuals are affected is probably about 2500 m, the height of many European climbing huts and some higher ski resorts in the Rockies. Rapid ascent to 3100 m, for instance by the railway to the Gornergrat, in Switzerland or by road to Leadville, Colorado, produces symptoms in a proportion of people by the next morning. Hackett and Rennie (1979) found an overall incidence of 43% in trekkers reaching the aid post at Pheriche (4343 m), though some affected trekkers would have dropped out before reaching this height. Among those who flew into the air strip at Lukla (2800 m), the incidence was higher than among those who walked all the way (49% versus 31%). Maggiorini *et al.* (1990) found an incidence in climbers to European alpine huts of 9% at 2850 m, 13% at 3050 m and 34% at 3650 m. A recent study of a general tourist population arriving at resorts in Colorado at altitudes of 1900–2940 m found an incidence of 25% (Honigman *et al.*, 1993). Among lowlanders who drive directly from Lima to Cerro de Pasco (4300 m) in Peru there are very few who do not have at least mild symptoms on the morning after arrival.

However if the stay at altitude is of only an hour or two the incidence of AMS is negligible. This is the case, for instance, for the great majority of tourists who drive or take the train to the summit of Pike's Peak, Colorado (4300 m).

17.4 AETIOLOGY OF AMS

17.4.1 Individual susceptibility

The aetiology of AMS is multifactorial. The most important factor is the rate of ascent and the height reached. Symptoms can be induced in almost all subjects if ascent is made rapidly to a sufficient height, but for any given altitude/time profile there is great variation in individual susceptibility.

17.4.2 AMS and fitness

There is no easy way to identify the susceptible individual as Ravenhill (1913) says:

> There is in my experience no type of man of whom one can say he will or will not suffer from puna. Most of the cases I have instanced were young men to all appearances perfectly sound. Young, strong and healthy men may be completely overcome. Stout, plethoric individuals of the chronic bronchitic type may not even have a headache. I have known several instances of this even when the persons have taken no care of themselves.
>
> *(Ravenhill, 1913)*

Certainly athletic fitness provides no immunity. A superbly fit French paratrooper on a family trek to Everest Base Camp had to be evacuated to lower altitude with severe symptoms of AMS while his mother and aunt were unaffected. A recent study found no correlation between fitness as measured by $\dot{V}_{O_2}$ max before an expedition and AMS symptom scores during the first days at altitude (Milledge *et al.*, 1991a).

17.4.3 Consistency in response to altitude

In general, individuals respond consistently, so that performance on one occasion is a reliable guide to future performance. This clinical impression has been confirmed in a study by Forster (1984), who studied workers at Mauna Kea observatory in Hawaii, situated at 4200 m. These workers alternated five days at the observatory with five days at sea-level so Forster was able to score the symptoms of AMS in 18 men on two altitude shifts. He showed that the rank order of scores correlated significantly on the two occasions. There is a tendency to acclimatize better on each subsequent trip to altitude.

Case histories do, however, show some anomalies. For instance, someone who has had little trouble on the first two trips may develop pulmonary edema on a third. Possibly a respiratory infection may be an added factor in such cases.

17.4.4 AMS, gender, age and body build

Both men and women are at risk. One study (Kayser, 1991) of trekkers going over the Thorong pass in Nepal (5400 m), found women to have a higher rate of sickness than men (69% versus 57%), but perhaps women are more ready to admit to symptoms than men. The young are probably at greater risk than the old (Hackett *et al.*, 1976) and the risk among boys seems especially high in South America (Hultgren and Marticorena, 1978).

Subjects slimmer than average (body mass index $<22\,\mathrm{kg\,m^{-2}}$) may be less susceptible to AMS than those who are standard or obese according to one study (Hirata *et al.*, 1989); Kayser (1991) also found obesity to be a risk factor in men.

17.4.5 AMS and hypoxic ventilatory response (HVR)

Beyond these factors, there is some evidence that subjects with a low HVR (Chapter 4) measured at sea-level are liable to develop AMS. The association has been shown by measurements of the response to acute hypoxia in the laboratory in studies of a few subjects (Lakshminarayan and Pierson, 1975; Hu *et al.*, 1982; Matsuzawa *et al.*, 1989). In the last study two of the ten subjects had HVRs within the normal range. Richalet *et al.* (1988) studied a large group of climbers before they went on various expeditions to the great ranges. They found that a low ventilatory and cardiac response to hypoxia were risk factors for AMS. The same group recently reported a single case of high susceptibility in a subject who had had radiation to his neck as a child and had a very low HVR (presumably because of damage to his carotid bodies). He suffered severe AMS at only 3500 m (Rathat *et al.*, 1993). However, whilst the association of AMS with relative hypoventilation seems firmly established (section 17.5.2) the correlation of AMS with a low sea-level HVR is less firm.

Two prospective studies found no correlation between HVR measured before going to altitude and symptom scores for AMS after arrival (Milledge *et al.*, 1988; Milledge *et al.*, 1991b). Selland *et al.* (1993) found that two of four subjects with a history of HAPE had HVR greater than their control subjects' mean value. Hackett *et al.* (1987) in a study of 106 climbers on Mt McKinley found that, whilst a low Sa_{O_2} predicted the likely development of AMS, there was no good correlation between HVR and Sa_{O_2} on arrival at altitude. Highlanders who generally have less AMS than lowlanders have a blunted HVR (section 4.5.2). Hackett *et al.* (1988b) found an abnormal HVR at altitude in patients with HAPE. They seemed to have hypoxic depression of ventilation which was relieved by oxygen breathing.

17.4.6 AMS and hypoxic pulmonary artery pressor response

A brisk increase in pulmonary artery pressure in response to hypoxia is probably also a risk factor (Hultgren *et al.*, 1971; Kawashima *et al.*, 1989) but it cannot be consistently predicted from a short period of acute hypoxia in a laboratory test, and clearly such tests with cardiac catheterization are not acceptable.

17.5 MECHANISMS OF AMS

17.5.1 Fluid balance and AMS

Clearly hypoxia is a crucial starting mechanism for AMS but it is not the direct cause of symptoms. Within a few minutes of exposure to high altitude P_{O_2} falls throughout the body but symptoms of acute mountain sickness are delayed for at least a few hours. This suggests that hypoxia initiates some process which requires a time course of 6–24 h before it, in turn, causes the symptoms.

Current thinking favours the hypothesis that hypoxia causes some alteration of fluid or electrolyte homeostasis with either water retention and/or shifts of water from intracellular to extracelluar compartments (Hansen *et al.*, 1970; Hackett *et al.*, 1981). This is shown in Figure 17.1 on the left. This increase in extracellular fluid in turn results in the dependent and periorbital edema often seen in patients with acute mountain sickness (Hackett and Rennie, 1979). It also causes mild cerebral edema, resulting in the symptoms of AMS. More severe cerebral edema causes the full blown malignant condition of acute cerebral edema (HACE) and pulmonary edema causes the pulmonary form (HAPE).

Evidence of fluid retention is provided by the clinical observation of lower urine output in soldiers with AMS than in soldiers free of symptoms (Singh *et al.*, 1969) and by the finding that trekkers with the

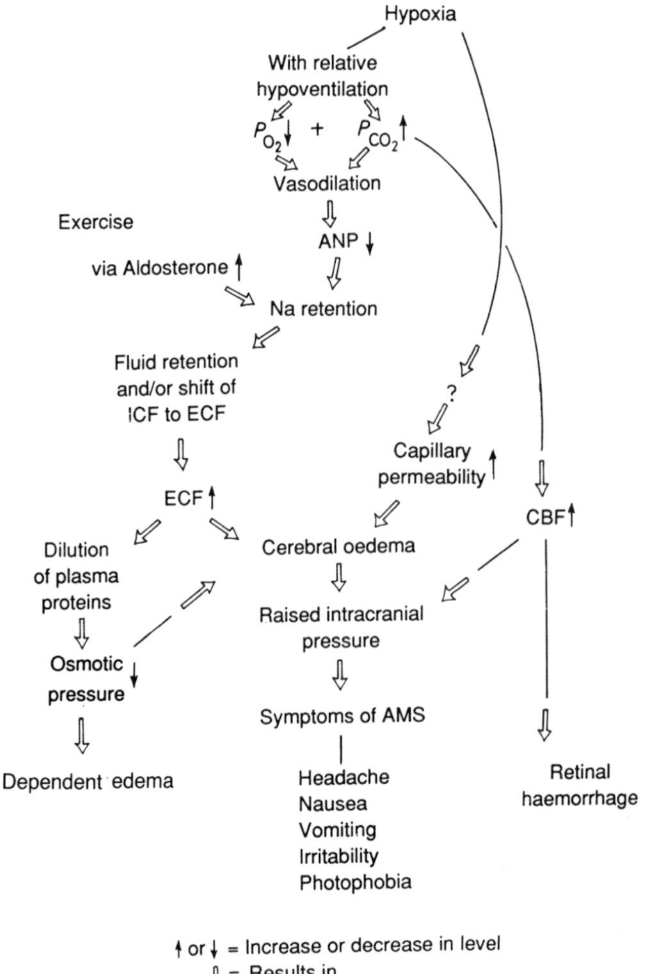

Figure 17.1 Possible mechanisms underlying acute mountain sickness (AMS). ICF, intracellular fluid; ECF, extracellular fluid; CBF, cerebral blood flow; ANP, atrial natriuretic peptide.

condition gained weight, while trekkers without AMS had lost weight by the time they reached 4243 m (Hackett *et al.*, 1982). The 'normal' response to altitude seems to be a mild diuresis, whereas subjects destined to get AMS have an antidiuresis.

Because of this antidiuresis the antidiuretic hormone (vasopressin) might be thought to underlie this mechanism but that seems not to be the case. Hackett *et al.* (1978) did find raised levels of the hormone in cases of pulmonary edema but not in benign AMS, and it was considered that when vasopressin levels were raised this was probably the result rather than the cause of malignant acute mountain sickness. Harber *et al.* (1981) found no rise in vasopressin levels in their climbers with AMS, who included one with fatal cerebral edema.

Other hormones that affect fluid balance include the renin–aldosterone system. The effect of altitude on this system is reviewed in Chapter 14. Briefly, ascent to altitude alone has a variable effect on plasma renin activity but results in lower than normal aldosterone levels at rest. Exercise stimulates the release of renin which, in turn, via angiotensin, stimulates aldosterone release and, if continued long enough, causes salt and hence water retention (Williams *et al.*, 1979; Milledge *et al.*, 1982). This may be important (Figure 17.1) especially in HAPE, in which a history of exercise is often a prominent feature (Chapter 18). AMS symptom scores were found to correlate with aldosterone levels and with reduced 24-hour urine sodium output on the first day at altitude in subjects who had ascended to 4300 m on foot on Mt Kenya (Milledge *et al.*, 1989). A similar result was reported from a study in the European alps (Bartsch *et al.*, 1988) although Hogan *et al.* (1973) in a chamber experiment, found that subjects with AMS had lower aldosterone concentrations than did asymptomatic subjects.

Atrial natriuretic peptide (ANP), which increases urinary sodium excretion and hence fluid excretion, is elevated by hypoxia in rats. (Winter *et al.*, 1987) and man (Milledge *et al.*, 1989; Bärtsch *et al.*, 1988; Cosby *et al.*, 1988). The relationship between ANP levels and AMS is variable. One study found a tendency to higher levels in subjects more resistant to AMS (Milledge *et al.*, 1989) whereas two other studies found the opposite (Bärtsch *et al.*, 1988; Cosby *et al.*, 1988). It seems that despite its name ANP is not a very powerful natriuretic hormone. Subjects hill walking at sea-level have raised ANP levels while retaining sodium vigorously (Milledge *et al.*, 1991b). ANP may have an effect by increasing capillary permeability but its significance in the aetiology of AMS remains to be established (Bärtsch *et al.*, 1988).

17.5.2 Role of P_{CO_2} in AMS and cerebral blood flow

On going to high altitude the subject experiences not only hypoxia but hypocapnea. The possibility that hypocapnea over a number of hours might be a factor in the genesis of AMS was tested by Maher *et al.* (1975). They exposed two groups of subjects to simulated altitude in a hypobaric chamber. One group had CO_2 added to the atmosphere to maintain their P_{CO_2} at control levels, the other group breathed air and became hypocapneic. Hypoxia was similar in the two groups, though to achieve this the group with CO_2 added were taken to a lower barometric pressure. Far from alleviating symptoms of AMS the added CO_2 caused more severe symptoms.

Sutton *et al.* (1976) found that in a group of subjects air lifted to a camp at 5360 m on Mt Logan, the severity of AMS correlated best with the P_{CO_2}. Forwand *et al.* (1968) found AMS symptom scores correlated well with P_{CO_2} but not with pH or P_{O_2}. In a study of 42 trekkers, Hackett *et al.* (1982) found those who gained weight on ascent to 4300 m had the highest incidence AMS and reduced their Pa_{CO_2} very little, whereas those who lost weight (presumably mainly fluid) had less frequent AMS and a low Pa_{CO_2}. Two studies of men in decompression chambers also found a correlation between AMS and hypoventilation (King and Robinson, 1972; Moore *et al.*, 1986). Maher *et al.* (1975) suggested that the mechanism connecting P_{CO_2} and AMS was the well known effect of CO_2 in increasing the cerebral blood flow.

Hypoxia also causes an increase in cerebral blood flow. In subjects with a brisk ventilatory response and low P_{CO_2} these two effects are, to a degree, counterbalanced. Whereas in subjects with little increase in ventilation and P_{CO_2} close to sea-level normal, cerebral vessels will be dilated and may contribute to cerebral edema and a rise in intracranial pressure. This is turn causes the symptoms of AMS and is shown in Figure 17.1 on the right of the diagram. Another possibility, referred to above, is that the higher P_{CO_2} and lower P_{O_2} would cause peripheral vasodilatation, which, by lowering central venous pressure, would lower the level of ANP and result in an antidiuresis. Cerebral blood flow is increased on going to altitude and falls towards sea-level values with acclimatization (Severinghaus *et al.*, 1966). However, a recent study which confirmed this general pattern found no difference in cerebral blood flow between subjects with and without AMS symptoms (Jensen *et al.*, 1990).

17.5.3 Intracranial pressure and AMS

There is a striking similarity of symptoms between AMS and the effects of high intracranial pressure due to cerebral tumours etc. The evidence for raised intracranial pressure in AMS is:

- The CSF pressure was found to be elevated by 60–210 mmH_2O during AMS compared with that after recovery (Singh *et al.*, 1969).
- In cases of malignant cerebral AMS, papilledema has been noted (Dickinson, 1979).
- In those dying with cerebral AMS, cerebral edema with flattening of the cerebral convolutions has been found (Dickinson *et al.*, 1983; Singh *et al.*, 1969).
- Computerized tomographic examination of the brain in patients with

HAPE showed diffuse low density areas in the cerebrum representing edema (Fukushima *et al.*, 1983).
- Direct measurement has been made in one unreported study (B.H. Cummings, personal communication). One of three subjects, with pressure transducers implanted in their skulls before a Himalayan expedition, was mountain sick on return from 5700 m to base camp at 4750 m. His intracranial pressure was normal at rest but elevated on the slightest exertion. Other subjects without AMS had normal pressures even on exercise.

17.5.4 Derangement of clotting mechanism

In reports on necropsy material, the presence of thromboses in lungs and brain figures prominently. No doubt parts of the pathological picture are secondary, such as the development of hyaline membrane in the alveoli and posssibly some thrombi, but there is evidence of alterations in coagulation associated with altitude (Singh and Chohan, 1972), and it has been suggested that thrombosis may form a basis for the development of both pulmonary hypertension and edema (Dickinson *et al.*, 1983). Hyers *et al.* (1979) were, however, unable to show differences in activated coagulation between those who are susceptible to pulmonary edema and more normal individuals at altitude.

Bartsch *et al.* (1987) have studied a range of clotting factors in 66 subjects presenting at the Capanna Margherita (4557 m) with varying degrees of AMS. They found that coagulation time, euglobulin lysis time and fibrin(ogen) fragment E were normal in all subject groups. Fibrinopeptide A, (FPA) a molecular marker of *in vivo* fibrin formation, was elevated in patients with HAPE. However FPA was not elevated in subjects with simple AMS even with widened (A–a) O_2 suggesting early HAPE. They conclude that the fibrin formation, which takes place in HAPE, is an epiphenomenon and not causative.

17.5.5 Microvascular permeability and AMS

Hypoxia may increase microvascular permeability directly or via mediators. Numerous animal studies have shown that hypoxia increases lymph flow with variable results on the lymph/plasma ratio for protein. The problem is to separate haemodynamic effects from permeability itself. Staub has reviewed the effect of hypoxia on microvascular permeability (1986) and concludes that, 'On best analysis . . . the change in permeability is slight, albeit statistically significant'.

However there is no really good animal model and the failure to show an important change in an animal which does not get HAPE in no way excludes the importance of permeability changes in a human patient. Three findings have served to strengthen the evidence for some effect of hypoxia on microvascular permeability:

- Larsen *et al.* (1985) have shown in rabbits that neither hypoxia alone nor the infusion of cobra venom (which activates the complement system) alone caused pulmonary edema. However, the two insults together did cause permeability-type pulmonary edema. This suggests the possibility that hypoxia, with some other factor, may increase microvascular permeability.
- Schoene *et al.* (1986) and Hackett *et al.* (1986), by analysing bronchoalveolar lavage and pulmonary edema fluid respectively, have shown conclusively that in HAPE the edema is of the high protein permeability type rather than haemodynamic. They also found significant levels of leukotriene B4 and factors chemotactic for monocytes in the lavage fluid, suggesting that the release of these and other mediators of inflammation may be involved in the mechanism of HAPE.
- Richalet *et al.* (1991) found a rise in plasma levels of most of the six eicosanoids measured in subjects taken abruptly to the Vallot observatory on Mt Blanc (4350 m). All subjects had AMS. The levels of these vasoactive mediators affecting permeability had a time course parallel to that of AMS symptoms.

These studies have concentrated on the pulmonary microvascular permeability but the same mechanism could affect microvascular permeability generally, including cerebral microvessels and thus contribute to cerebral edema as shown in Figure 17.1 (centre). Hypoxia has been shown to increase permeability of endothelial monolayers to a range of proteins *in vitro*, though quite severe hypoxia (12–19 mmHg) and incubation for 48–72 h was needed to show the effect (Gerlach *et al.*, 1992).

Proteinuria is also common during the first few days at altitude, especially in subjects with AMS (Chapter 14) and this may be due to increased microvascular permeability in the kidneys (Winterborn *et al.*, 1986).

In Chapter 18 there is further consideration of mechanisms in relation to HAPE, some of which may also apply to benign AMS.

17.6 PROPHYLAXIS OF AMS

17.6.1 Rate of ascent

A slow rate of ascent will prevent AMS, but, due to the great variation in susceptibility to AMS, it is not possible to be dogmatic in advice on rate of ascent. A suggested rule of thumb is that, above 3000 m, each night should be spent not more than 300 m above the last, with a rest day – that is two nights at the same altitude – every two to three days. In addition, anyone who experiences symptoms of AMS should go no higher until they improve.

17.6.2 Drugs for prophylaxis

Acetazolamide (Diamox)

This drug has been shown to increase ventilation and Pa_{O_2}, and decrease Pa_{CO_2} (Cain and Dunn, 1965). It has been shown to reduce the incidence and severity of AMS in a number of double blind controlled trials in the field (Forwand *et al.*, 1968; Birmingham Medical Research Group, 1981; Larsen *et al.*, 1982). All symptoms are improved, as well as general performance, as judged by peer review. Sleep was improved and the profound desaturation associated with periodic breathing (Chapter 12) was relieved (Sutton *et al.*, 1979). It has been shown to prevent patients with asthma from developing AMS (Mirrakhimov *et al.*, 1993). In these trials, the dose was 250 mg orally eight-hourly, started one day before ascent, except in the Birmingham trial where the dose was one 500 mg slow release tablet daily. This dose, or 250 mg normal release twice daily (which is cheaper), is the current recommended regimen. Treatment should be started 24–48 h before ascent to altitude.

The duration of treatment depends upon the circumstance and situation. In many treks, the exposure to conditions when AMS may be a problem is limited to a few days and obviously treatment can be discontinued when the party has descended from altitude. In situations where subjects go to altitude and stay there, the risk of AMS is limited to the first four or five days so that treatment could reasonably be stopped after that.

However, a study by the Birmingham group (Bradwell *et al.*, 1986) has shown that taking acetazolamide for three weeks at 4846 m conferred a benefit in that the group on treatment lost less weight, lost less muscle bulk and had superior exercise performance than those on placebo. Here the drug was being used not so much to prevent AMS as to reduce altitude deterioration.

The side-effects of acetazolamide consist of a mild diuresis and paraesthesiae in the hands and feet, which tend to diminish with continued use of the drug. A few people find this tingling very disturbing, some are troubled by gastric side-effects. Also, fizzy drinks taste flat; this is due to the inhibition of carbonic anhydrase in the tongue so that the conversion of CO_2 to carbonic acid fails to take place in the time available as the drink passes over the tongue, and the acid sensing buds are not stimulated. The safety of acetazolamide is assured by its widespread use in glaucoma where it is used for years at doses similar to that recommended for AMS prophylaxis.

The ethics of the use of acetazolamide (or that of any drug) especially if used throughout an expedition needs consideration but in the end is for the individual or team to decide.

The mechanism of action of acetazolamide is thought to be due to its inhibition of carbonic anhydrase rather than its diuretic action. It is quite a mild diuretic and more powerful diuretics are said to be less effective though no direct comparisons have been made in controlled trials. Interference with CO_2 transport is thought to result in intracellular acidosis, including the cells of the medullary chemoreceptor. In this way it acts as a respiratory stimulant. It has recently been shown to shift the CO_2 response curve to the left, as happens with acclimatization (section 4.12) although it does not affect the slope. The acute effect after a single dose results in a reduction in the hypoxic ventilatory response, though with a few hours administration this is restored (Swenson and Hughes, 1993).

It may also act as a respiratory stimulant by promoting the excretion of bicarbonate by the kidneys, thus correcting the respiratory alkalosis due to hypoxic induced hyperventilation. In effect the subject is given an artificial respiratory acclimatization. The importance of this renal effect is suggested by a study by Swenson *et al.* (1991), in which the drug benzolamide, a selective inhibitor of renal carbonic anhydrase, reduced high altitude periodic breathing, a feature of acetazolamide use.

Another possible mechanism is via its effect on cerebral blood flow (Vorstrup *et al.*, 1984). Acetazolamide increases cerebral blood flow, which would increase cerebral P_{O_2}. However increased P_{CO_2}, which has the same effect on cerebral blood flow, seems to increase the symptoms of AMS at the same level of hypoxia (section 17.5.2). Additionally, the dosage used in this study (1 g i.v.) was very large compared with that used in AMS prophylaxis. Jensen *et al.* (1990) found that, although 1.5 g acetazolamide caused a 22% increase in cerebral blood flow after 2 h, there was no change in AMS symptoms. Also Hackett *et al.* (1988a) found no change in CBF (as measured by trans-cranial Doppler ultrasound) in subjects with or without AMS after 0.25 g acetazolamide intravenously.

Other drugs

Spironolactone

Jain *et al.* (1986) compared spironolactone with acetazolamide and placebo. They found both drugs to be effective in ameliorating AMS, with spironolactone being possibly superior. This confirms a previous uncontrolled report (Currie *et al.*, 1976).

Dexamethasone

Dexamethasone (4 mg 6-hourly) has been tried on the grounds that it is effective in cerebral edema. In a double blind crossover chamber study it was found to be an effective prophylactic (Johnson *et al.*, 1984) and, compared with acetazolamide, was found to be superior (Ellsworth *et al.*, 1991). Rock *et al.* (1989) carried out a dose ranging chamber experiment and concluded that 4 mg 12-hourly was the minimum effective dose. The same group had previously found that, if dexamethasone was given for only 48 h after arrival at altitude, it was effective in reducing symptoms, but that, after stopping the drug, symptoms of AMS began (Rock *et al.*, 1989). The combination of acetazolamide and dexamethasone has been shown to be more effective than actetazolamide alone, especially in preventing the cerebral symptoms of AMS (Bernhard *et al.*, 1992).

17.7 TREATMENT OF AMS

Most cases of AMS will get better in 24–48 h with no treatment. If there is progression of symptoms to those of acute pulmonary edema, or serious cerebral edema, action is vital since these two disorders are frequently fatal in a matter of hours. Their treatment is discussed in Chapters 18 and 19 respectively.

Rest alone often relieves the symptoms of AMS (Bartsch *et al.*, 1993) and this fact needs to be borne in mind in trials of therapy in AMS. Acetazolamide had been shown to be an effective treatment of AMS as well as a prophylactic (Bradwell *et al.*, 1988; Grissom *et al.*, 1992). The earlier study used a single large dose (1.5 g) whereas the later study used the more conventional 250 mg 8-hourly. Pa_{O_2} as well as symptoms were improved.

Dexamethasone was shown, in a double blind trial, to be effective as an emergency treatment for acute AMS (Ferrazzini *et al.*, 1987). The dosage used was 8 mg initially followed by 4 mg every 6 h. Levine *et al.* (1989) also found it to be effective in relieving AMS symptoms compared with placebo but it had no effect on fluid shifts, oxygenation, sleep apnoea, urinary catecholamine levels, chest radiographs or perfusion scans. These findings emphasize the dictum that, in the event of HAPE or HACE, patients should be taken to lower altitude as soon as possible.

For the headache of AMS, aspirin or paracetamol is often used, but is often ineffective. An anecdotal report claims success with ibuprofen (400 mg) when aspirin had failed (Williams, 1984).

Oxygen may help, but frequently does not, and its use, besides being impractical for most cases, would impede acclimatization. Voluntary hyperventilation often helps and probably does promote acclimatization. Inhalation of 3% CO_2 in air has been claimed to alleviate symptoms in one study (Harvey *et al.*, 1988) but not in another (Bartsch *et al.*, 1990). Both found a rise in Pa_{O_2}, due presumably to hyperventilation. In the latter study most subjects given air to breathe had a reduction in symptoms, indicating the importance of the placebo effect or perhaps the beneficial effect of rest.

The place of portable inflatable pressure chambers (the Gamow bag) is considered in Chapter 18.

Table 17.2 Lake Louise consensus: scoring of AMS (From Hackett and Oelz, 1992)

(a) AMS self assessment

Symptom	*Scoring*
Headache	0 None at all 1 Mild headache 2 Moderate headache 3 Severe headache, incapacitating
Gastrointestinal symptoms	0 Good appetite 1 Poor appetite or nausea 2 Moderate nausea or vomiting 3 Severe, incapacitating nausea and vomiting
Fatigue and/or weakness	0 Not tired or weak 1 Mild fatigue/weakness 2 Moderate fatigue/weakness 3 Severe fatigue/weakness
Dizziness/lightheadedness	0 None 1 Mild 2 Moderate 3 Severe, incapacitating
Difficulty sleeping	0 Slept as well as usual 1 Did not sleep as well as usual 2 Woke many times, poor night's sleep 3 Could not sleep at all
Overall, if you had any of these symptoms, how did they affect your activities?	0 Not at all 1 Mild reduction 2 Moderate reduction 3 Severe reduction (bedrest)

Table 17.2 Continued
(b) Clinical assessment tool, all responses obtained by interview. Same questions as self assessment, plus the following:

Sign	*Scoring*
Change in mental status	0 No change 1 Lethargy/lassitude 2 Disorientated/ confused 3 Stupor/semiconscious 4 Coma
Ataxia (heel/toe walking)	0 None 1 Balancing manoeuvres 2 Steps off the line 3 Falls down 4 Unable to stand
Peripheral oedema	0 None 1 One location 2 Two or more locations

(c) Functional assessment (assigned by investigator, not self assessment)

Grade	*Assessment*
0	No symptoms
1	Symptoms, but no change in activity
2	Must reduce activities
3	Reduced to bed rest
4	Life threatening

17.8 SCORING AMS SYMPTOMS

In studies on AMS there is obviously a need to score the symptoms in some way. At its simplest, one can divide subjects into those with and those without AMS. However, in practice most people have mild or moderate AMS and it is very arbitrary to force subjects into only two categories. A better approach is to score individual symptoms and reach an overall score for AMS which reflects this continuum of severity. The most sophisticated system is the Environmental Symptom Questionnaire (ESQ) (Sampson *et al.*, 1983). This consists of 67 questions in its ESQ-III version, many of which are overlapping and of uncertain relevance to AMS. Most workers have used much more simple formats, scoring only three to five symptoms often on a 0–3 scale, with 0 for no symptoms and 1, 2 and 3 for mild, moderate and severe symptoms. The questionnaire can either be administered by one observer or self assessed; the two methods give similar results. A document was produced at the Lake Louise Symposium in 1991, which, after defining AMS, suggested a simple method of scoring along these lines shown in Table 17.2 (Hackett and Oelz, 1992).

17.9 SUBACUTE MOUNTAIN SICKNESS

Recently two forms of subacute mountain sickness have been described, one in infants born at low altitude and taken to high altitude (Sui *et al.*, 1988) and the other in adults who have spent some months or more at extreme altitude (Anand *et al.*, 1990).

17.9.1 Subacute infantile mountain sickness

The Spaniards who first colonized the Andes became well aware that their infants did not thrive if born at high altitude. They made it their practice to arrange delivery at low altitude and not to bring their babies to high altitude before one year. The lowland Han Chinese colonists of Tibet face the same environmental problem. Sui *et al.* (1988) reported the post-mortem findings on 15 infants who died in Lhasa (3600 m), of a syndrome they called subacute infantile mountain sickness. The presenting symptoms were commonly dyspnoea and cough, with often sleeplessness, irritability and signs of cyanosis, oedema of the face, oliguria, tachycardia, liver enlargement, râles in the lungs, and fever. The majority of infants had been born at low altitude but two were born at high altitude, one of Han and one of Tibetan parents. The condition was usually fatal in a matter of weeks or months. The post-mortem findings were of extreme medial hypertrophy of muscular pulmonary arteries and muscularization of pulmonary arterioles. There was massive hypertrophy and dilatation of the right ventricle and dilatation of the pulmonary trunk.

17.9.2 Adult subacute mountain sickness

Anand *et al.* (1990) described the adult form in 21 soldiers who, after a full acclimatization period, had been posted to between 5800 m and 6700 m for several months (mean 1.8 years). They presented with dyspnoea, cough and effort angina. The signs were of dependent edema. They were treated at high altitude with diuretics with improvement. When they were evacuated to low altitude by aircraft they were found to have cardiomegaly with right ventricular enlargement and, in most cases, pericardial effusion. The pulmonary artery pressure was elevated (26 mmHg) and rose significantly on mild exercise to 40 mmHg. Recovery was rapid after descent from high altitude. The mechanism includes a generalized increase in the volume of the fluid compartments of the body and total body sodium, even in subjects without overt disease at these altitudes for this length of time (Anand *et al.*, 1993). The increase in central blood volume is the probable cause of the decrease in forced vital capacity, and the radiographically engorged pulmonary vessels found in the subjects of Operation Everest II (Welsh *et al.*, 1993).

It would seem that this subacute mountain sickness is the human form of a similar condition affecting cattle taken to high altitude, and known as brisket disease (Hecht *et al.*, 1959). The brisket is the loose skin area of the cow's neck which is dependent and becomes swollen with oedema fluid in this condition.

REFERENCES

Anand, I.S., Malhotra, R.M., Chandrashekar, Y., *et al.* (1990) Adult subacute mountain sickness – a syndrome of congestive heart failure in man at very high altitude. *Lancet*, **335**, 561–5.

Anand, I.S., Chandrashekhar, Y., Rao, S.K., *et al.* (1993) Body fluid compartments, renal blood flow, and hormones at 6000 m in normal subjects. *J. Appl. Physiol.*, **74**, 1234–9.

Bärtsch, P., Waber, U., Haeberli, A., *et al.* (1987) Enhanced fibrin formation in high-altitude pulmonary oedema. *J. Appl. Physiol.*, **63**, 752–7.

Bärtsch, P., Shaw, S., Franciolli, M., *et al.* (1988) Atrial natriuretic peptide in acute mountain sickness. *J. Appl. Physiol.*, **65**, 1929–37.

Bärtsch, P., Baumgartner, R.W., Waber, U., *et al.* (1990) Comparison of carbon dioxide enriched, oxygen enriched, and normal air in treatment of acute mountain sickness. *Lancet*, **336**, 772–5.

Bärtsch, P., Merki, B., Hofsetter, D., *et al.* (1993) Treatment of acute mountain sickness by simulated descent: a randomised controlled trial. *Br. Med. J.*, **306**, 1098–101.

Bernhard, W., Miller, L., Villareal, J., *et al.* (1992) Cerebral symptoms of high altitude: Preventative effects of acetazolamide–dexamethasone versus acetazolamide alone (abstract), in *Hypoxia and Mountain Medicine*, (eds J.R. Sutton, G. Coates and C.S. Houston), Queen Printers, Burlington, p. 294.

Birmingham Medical Research Expeditionary Society Mountain Sickness Study Group. (1981) Acetazolamide in control of acute mountain sickness. *Lancet*, **1**, 180–3.

Bradwell, A.R., Dykes, P.W., Coote, J.H., *et al.* (1986) Effect of acetazolamide on exercise performance and muscle mass at high altitude. *Lancet*, **1**, 1001–5.

Bradwell, A.R., Winterbourn, M., Wright, A.D., *et al.* (1988) Acetazolamide treatment in acute mountain sickness. *Clin. Sci.*, **74(suppl 18)**, 62P.

Cain, S.M. and Dunn, J.E. (1965) Increase of arterial oxygen tension at altitude by carbonic anhydrase inhibition. *J. Appl. Physiol.*, **20**, 882–4.

Cosby, R.L., Spohocles, A.M., Durr, J.A., *et al.* (1988) Elevated plasma atrial natriuretic factor and vasopressin in high-altitude pulmonary edema. *Ann. Intern. Med.*, **109**, 796–9.

Currie, T.T., Carter, P.H., Champion, W.L., *et al.* (1976) Spironolactone and acute mountain sickness. *Med. J. Aust.*, **2**, 168–70.
Dickinson, J.G. (1979) Severe acute mountain sickness. *Postgrad. Med. J.*, **55**, 454–8.
Dickinson, J.G. (1982) Terminology and classification of acute mountain sickness. *Br. Med. J.*, **285**, 720–1.
Dickinson, J., Heath, D., Gosney, J. and Williams, D. (1983) Altitude related deaths in seven trekkers in the Himalayas. *Thorax*, **38**, 646–56.
Ellsworth, A.J., Meyer, E.F. and Larson, E.B. (1991) Acetazolamide or dexamethasone use versus placebo to prevent acute mountain sickness on Mount Rainer. *West. J. Med.*, **154**, 289–93.
Ferrazzini, G., Maggiorini, M., Kriemler, S., *et al.* (1987) Successful treatment of acute mountain sickness with dexamethasone. *Br. Med. J.*, **294**, 1380–2.
Forster, P. (1984) Reproducibility of individual response to exposure to high altitude. *Br. Med. J.*, **289**, 1269.
Forwand, S.A., Landowne, M., Follansbee, J.N. and Hansen, J.E. (1968) Effect of acetazolamide on acute mountain sickness. *N. Engl. J. Med.*, **279**, 839–45.
Fukushima, M., Yasaki, K., Shibamoto, T., *et al.* (1983) Findings of brain computed tomography in patients with high altitude pulmonary edema, in *Hypoxia, Exercise and Altitude*, (eds J.R. Sutton, C.S. Houston and N.L. Jones), Liss, New York, pp. 456–7.
Gerlach, H., Clauss, M., Ogawa, S. and Stern, D.M. (1992) Modulation of endothelial coagulant properties and barrier function by factors in the vascular microenvironment, in *Endothelial Cell Dysfunctions*, (eds N. Simoniescu and M. Simoniescu), Plenum Press, New York, pp. 525–45.
Grissom, K., Roach, R.C., Sarnquist, F.H. and Hackett, P.H. (1992) Acetazolamide in the treatment of acute mountain sickness: clinical effect on gas exchange. *Ann. Intern. Med.*, **116**, 461–5.
Hackett, P.H. and Rennie, D. (1979) Râles, peripheral edema, retinal hemorrhage and acute mountain sickness. *Am. J. Med.*, **67**, 214–8.
Hackett, P.H. and Oelz, O. (1992) The Lake Louise consensus on the definition and quantification of altitude illness, in *Hypoxia and Mountain Medicine*, (eds J.R. Sutton, G. Coates and C.S. Houston), Queen City Printers, Burlington, pp. 327–30.
Hackett, P.H., Rennie, D. and Levine, H.D. (1976) The incidence, importance and prophylaxis of acute mountain sickness. *Lancet*, **2**, 1149–54.
Hackett, P.H., Forsling, M.L., Milledge, J. and Rennie, D. (1978) Release of vasopressin in man at altitude. *Horm. Metab. Res.*, **10**, 571.
Hackett, P.H., Rennie, D., Grover, R.F. and Reeves, J.T. (1981) Acute mountain sickness and the edemas of high altitude: a common pathogenesis? *Respir. Physiol.*, **46**, 383–90.
Hackett, P.H., Rennie, D., Hofmeister, S.E., *et al.* (1982) Fluid retention and relative hypoventilation in acute mountain sickness. *Respiration*, **43**, 321–9.
Hackett, P.H., Bertman, J. and Rodriguez, G. (1986) Pulmonary edema fluid protein in high-altitude pulmonary edema. *J. Am. Med. Assoc.*, **256**, 36.
Hackett, P.H., Hollingshead, K.F., Roach, R.B., *et al.* (1987) Arterial saturation during ascent predicts subsequent acute mountain sickness (abstract), in *Cold and Hypoxia*, (eds J.R. Sutton, C.S. Houston and G. Cotes), Praeger, New York, p. 544.
Hackett, P.H., Swenson, E.R., Roach, R.C., *et al.* (1988a) 250 mg acetazolamide intravenously does not increase cerebral blood flow at high altitude (abstract), in *Hypoxia the Tolerable Limits*, (eds J.R. Sutton, C.S. Houston and G. Cotes), Benchmark Press, Indianapolis, p. 383.

Hackett, P.H., Roach, R.C., Schoene, R.B., *et al.* (1988b) Abnormal control of ventilation in high-altitude pulmonary edema. *J. Appl. Physiol.*, **64**, 1268–72.

Hansen, J.E. and Evans, W.O. (1970) A hypothesis regarding the pathophysiology of acute mountain sickness. *Arch. Environ. Health*, **21**, 666–9.

Harber, M.J., Williams, J.D. and Morton, J.J. (1981) Antidiuretic hormone excretion at high altitude. *Aviat. Space Environ. Med.*, **52**, 38–40.

Harvey, T.C., Raichle, M.E., Winterborn, M.H., *et al.* (1988) Effect of carbon dioxide in acute mountain sickness: a rediscovery. *Lancet*, **2**, 639–41.

Hecht, H.H., Lang, R.L., Carnes, W.H., *et al.* (1959) Brisket disease. I. General aspects of pulmonary hypertensive heart disease in cattle. *Trans. Assoc. Am. Physiol.*, **72**, 157–72.

Hirata, K., Matsuyama, S. and Saito, A. (1989) Obesity as a risk factor for acute mountain sickness. *Lancet*, **2**, 1040–1.

Hogan, R.P., Kotchen, T.A., Boyd, A.E. and Hartley, L.H. (1973) Effect of altitude on the renin–aldosterone system and metabolism of water and electroytes. *J. Appl. Physiol.*, **35**, 385–90.

Honigman, B., Thesis, M.K., Koziol-McLain, J., *et al.* (1993) Acute mountain sickness in a general tourist population at moderate altitude. *Ann. Intern. Med.*, **118**, 587–92.

Houston, C.S. (1960) Acute pulmonary edema of high altitude. *N. Engl. J. Med.*, **263**, 478–80.

Hu, S.T., Huang, W.Y., Chu, S.C. and Pa, C.F. (1982) Chemoreflexive ventilatory response at sea level in subjects with past history of good acclimatization and severe acute mountain sickness, in *High Altitude Physiology and Medicine*, (eds W. Brendel and R.A. Zink), Springer-Verlag, New York, pp. 28–32.

Hultgren, H.N., Grover, R.F. and Hartley, L.H. (1971) Abnormal circulatory responses to high altitude in subjects with a previous history of high-altitude pulmonary edema. *Circulation*, **44**, 759–70.

Hultgren, H.B. and Marticorena, E.A. (1978) High altitude pulmonary edema. Epidemiologic observations in Peru. *Chest*, **74**, 372–6.

Hyers, T.M., Scoggin, C.H., Will, D.H., *et al.* (1979) Accentuated hypoxemia at high altitude in subjects susceptible to high-altitude pulmonary edema. *J. Appl. Physiol.*, **46**, 41–6.

Jain, S.C., Singh, M.V., Sharma, V.M., *et al.* (1986) Amelioration of acute mountain sickness: comparative study of acetazolamide and spironolactone. *Int. J. Biometeorol.*, **30**, 293–300.

Jensen, J.B., Wright, A.D., Lassen, N.A. *et al.* (1990) Cerebral blood flow in acute mountain sickness. *J. Appl. Physiol.*, **69**, 430–3.

Johnson, T.S., Rock, P.B., Fulco, C.S., *et al.* (1984) Prevention of acute mountain sickness by dexamethasone. *N. Engl. J. Med.*, **310**, 683–6.

Kawashima, A., Kubo, K., Kobayashi, T. and Sekiguchi, M. (1989) Hemodynamic response to acute hypoxia, hypobaria and exercise in subjects susceptible to high-altitude pulmonary edema. *J. Appl. Physiol.*, **67**, 1982–9.

Kayser, B. (1991) Acute mountain sickness in western tourists around the Thorong pass (5400 m) in Nepal. *J. Wild. Med.*, **2**, 110–7.

King, A.B. and Robinson, S.M. (1972) Ventilation response to hypoxia and acute mountain sickness. *Aerospace Med.*, **43**, 419–21.

Lakshminarayan, S. and Pierson, D.J. (1975) Recurrent high altitude pulmonary edema with blunted chemosensitivity. *Am. Rev. Respir. Dis.*, **111**, 869–72.

Larsen, G.L., Webster, R.O., Worthen, G.S., *et al.* (1985) Additive effect of intravascular complement activation and brief episodes of hypoxia in producing increased permeability in the rabbit lung. *J. Clin. Invest.*, **75**, 902–10.

Larsen, E.B., Roach, R.C., Schoene, R.B. and Hornbein, T.F. (1982) Acute mountain sickness and acetazolamide. Clinical efficacy and effect on ventilation. *J. Am. Med. Assoc.*, **248**, 328–32.

Levine, B.D., Yoshimura, K., Kobayashi, T., *et al.* (1989) Dexamethazone in the treatment of acute mountain sickness. *N. Engl. J. Med.*, **321**, 1707–13.

Maggiorini, M., Buhler, B., Walter, M. and Oelz, O. (1990) Prevalence of acute mountain sickness in the Swiss Alps. *Br. Med. J.*, **301**, 853–5.

Maher, J.T., Cymerman, A., Reeves, J.T., *et al.* (1975) Acute mountain sickness: increased severity in eucapnic hypoxia. *Aviat. Space Environ. Med.*, **46**, 826–9.

Matsuzawa, Y., Fujimoto, K., Kobayashi, T., *et al.* (1989) Blunted hypoxic ventilatory drive in subjects susceptible to high-altitude pulmonary edema. *J. Appl. Physiol.*, **66**, 1152–7.

Milledge, J.S., Bryson, E.I., Catley, D.M., *et al.* (1982) Sodium balance, fluid homeostasis and the renin–aldosterone system during the prolonged exercise of hill walking. *Clin. Sci.*, **62**, 595–604.

Milledge, J.S., Thomas, P.S., Beeley, J.M. and English, J.S.C. (1988) Hypoxic ventilatory response and acute mountain sickness. *Eur. Respir. J.*, **1**, 948–51.

Milledge, J.S., Beeley, J.M., McArthur, S. and Morice, A.H. (1989) Atrial natriuretic peptide, altitude and acute mountain sickness. *Clin. Sci.*, **77**, 509–14.

Milledge, J.S., Beeley, J.M., Broom, J., *et al.* (1991a) Acute mountain sickness susceptibility, fitness and hypoxic ventilatory response. *Eur. Respir. J.*, **4**, 1000–3.

Milledge, J.S., McArthur, S., Morice, A., *et al.* (1991b) Atrial natriuretic peptide and exercise-induced fluid retention in man. *J. Wild. Med.*, **2**, 94–101.

Mirrakhimov, M., Brimkulov, N., Cieslick, J., *et al.* (1993) Effect of acetazoloamide on overnight oxygenation and acute mountain sickness in patients with asthma. *Eur. Respir. J.*, **6**, 536–40.

Moore, L.G., Harrison, G.L., McCullough, R.E., *et al.* (1986) Low acute hypoxic ventilatory response and hypoxic depression in acute mountain sickness. *J. Appl. Physiol.*, **60**, 1407–12.

Rathat, C., Richalet, J.-P., Larmignat, P. and Herry, J.-P. (1993) Neck irradiation by cobalt therapy and susceptibility to acute mountain sickness. *J. Wild. Med.*, **4**, 231–2.

Ravenhill, T.H. (1913) Some experiences of mountain sickness in the Andes. *J. Trop. Med. Hyg.*, **16**, 314–20.

Richalet, J.-P., Keromes, A., Dersch, B., *et al.* (1988) Caractéristiques physiologiques des alpinistes de haute altitude. *Sci. Sports*, **3**, 89–108.

Richalet, J.-P., Hornych, A., Rathat, C., *et al.* (1991) Plasma prostaglandins, leukotrienes and thromboxane in acute high altitude hypoxia. *Respir. Physiol.*, **85**, 205–15.

Rock, P.B., Johnson, T.S., Larsen, R.F., *et al.* (1989) Dexamethasone prophylaxis for acute mountain sickness. Effect of dose level. *Chest*, **95**, 568–73.

Sampson, J.B., Cymerman, A., Burse, R.J., *et al.* (1983) Procedures for the measurement of acute mountain sickness. *Aviat. Space Environ. Med.*, **54**, 1063–73.

Schoene, R.B., Hackett, P.H., Henderson, W.R., *et al.* (1986) High-altitude pulmonary edema. Characteristics of lung lavage fluid. *J. Am. Med. Assoc.*, **256**, 63–9.

Selland, M.A., Stelzner, T.J., Stevens, T., *et al.* (1993) Pulmonary function and hypoxic ventilatory response in subjects susceptible to high altitude pulmonay edema. *Chest*, **103**, 111–6.

Severinghaus, J.W., Chiodi, H., Eger, E.I., Brandstater, B. and Hornbein, T.F. (1966) Cerebral blood flow in man at high altitude. Role of cerebrospinal fluid pH in normalization of flow in chronic hypocapnia. *Circ. Res.*, **19**, 274–82.

Singh, I. and Chohan, I.S. (1972) Blood coagulation changes at high altitude predisposing to pulmonary hypertension. *Br. Heart J.*, **34**, 611–7.

Singh, I., Khanna, P.K., Srivastava, M.C., *et al.* (1969) Acute mountain sickness. *N. Engl. J. Med.*, **280**, 175–84.

Staub, N.C. (1986) The hemodynamics of pulmonary edema. *Clin. Respir. Physiol.*, **22**, 319–22.

Sui, G.J., Lui, Y.H., Cheng, X.S., *et al.* (1988) Subacute infantile mountain sickness. *J. Pathol.*, **155**, 161–70.

Sutton, J.R., Bryan, A.C., Gray, G.W., *et al.* (1976) Pulmonary gas exchange in acute mountain sickness. *Aviat. Space Environ. Med.*, **47**, 1032–7.

Sutton, J.R., Houston, C.S., Mansell, A.L., *et al.* (1979) Effect of acetazolamide on hypoxemia during sleep at high altitude. *N. Engl. J. Med.*, **301**, 1329–31.

Swenson, E.R., Leatham, K.L., Roach, R.C., *et al.* (1991) Renal carbonic anhydrase inhibition reduces high altitude sleep periodic breathing. *Respir. Physiol.*, **86**, 333–43.

Swenson, E.R. and Hughes, J.M.B. (1993) Effects of acute and chronic acetazolamide on resting ventilation and ventilatory responses in men. *J. Appl. Physiol.*, **74**, 230–7.

Vorstrup, S., Henriksen, L. and Paulson, O.B. (1984) Effect of acetazolmaide on cerebral blood flow and cerebral metabolic rate for oxygen. *J. Clin. Invest.*, **74**, 1634–9.

Welsh, C.H., Wagner, P.D., Reeves, J.T., *et al.* (1993) Operation Everest II: Spirometric and radiographic changes in acclimatized humans at simulated high altitudes. *Am. Rev. Respir. Dis.*, **147**, 1239–44.

Williams, E.S. (1984) Brufen and altitude headache. *Br. J. Hosp. Med.*, **31**, 318.

Williams, E.S., Ward, M.P., Willedge, J.S., *et al.* (1979) Effect of the exercise of seven consecutive days hill-walking on fluid homeostasis. *Clin. Sci.*, **56**, 305–16.

Winter, R.J.D., Melaegros, L., Pervez, S., *et al.* (1987) Plasma atrial natriuretic factor and ultrastructure of atrial specific granules following chronic hypoxia in rats. *Clin. Sci.*, **72**, 26P.

Winterborn, M., Bradwell, A.R., Chesner, I. and Jones, G. (1986) Mechanisms of proteinuria at high altitude. *Clin. Sci.*, **70**, 58P.

18

High altitude pulmonary edema

18.1 INTRODUCTION

There are a number of accounts of climbers dying of 'pneumonia' in early climbing literature. In retrospect, many if not most, of these fatalities were probably due to high altitude pulmonary edema (HAPE). One of the best known was the death of Dr Jacottet on Mt Blanc in 1891. He died in the Vallot hut (4300 m) after taking part in a rescue on the mountain. He spent a further two nights in the hut with obvious symptoms of acute mountain sickness (AMS), refusing to go down. He died during the second night. The post-mortem showed 'acute edema of the lung' (oedème considerable) (Mosso, 1898).

In 1913, Ravenhill described what he called 'puna' of the cardiac type as a lethal form or development of AMS. Though he was wrong in attributing the condition to cardiac failure, his description of three cases fits well with HAPE. However, his work was forgotten and the condition rediscovered, as far as English literature was concerned, by Houston (1960) who published his landmark paper on 'acute pulmonary edema of high altitude'. Houston said 'this single case is presented in the hope of stimulating further reports' and 'pulmonary edema of high altitude deserves further study'. Both hope and declaration have been amply fulfilled in the succeeding years by the description of hundreds of cases from all the major mountainous areas and hundreds of studies aimed at elucidating the mechanism of the condition have been conducted, some of which will be reviewed in this chapter.

18.2 CLINICAL PRESENTATION

HAPE, like AMS, affects previously healthy individuals on ascent to altitude. There is a wide range of altitude of presentation of 2000–7000 m

(Lobenhoffer *et al.*, 1982). A typical history is that the subject ascends rapidly to altitude and is very active getting there or on arrival. He suffers the symptoms of AMS after arrival, though not necessarily very severely. He then becomes more short of breath and lethargic; he may have chest pain. Physical signs are of tachycardia, tachypnoea and crackles at the lung bases. He develops a dry cough which later progresses to one productive of frothy white sputum and eventually blood-tinged sputum. Over a few hours the condition progresses with increasing respiratory distress, cyanosis, bubbling respirations, coma and death.

18.2.1 Case histories

Case 1 (Houston, 1960)

A male patient left sea-level on 18 June, reaching 16 700 ft (5090 m) by car and on foot five days later. He had no symptoms until one day later when he noted dyspnoea progressing to severe orthopnoea. Within a few hours his breathing became progressively more congested and laboured. He sounded as though he was literally drowning in his own fluid with an almost continuous loud bubbling sound as if breathing through liquid. A white froth resembling cotton candy had appeared to well up out of his mouth which was open. This was even though he was sitting up with his head tilted back. The patient died within eight hours of the onset of symptoms.

Case 2

A Sherpa on a large expedition had carried a load from 6400 m to 7000 m and returned. The following morning he complained of severe headache and malaise. He was anorexic and remained in his sleeping bag. On examination at mid-morning he was found to be breathless on the slightest exertion, cyanosed and had a dry cough. The pulse and respiratory rate were increased. Fine crackles were heard at the lung bases. At noon he started down for a lower camp at 5800 m accompanied by two expedition members. It was at once apparent that he could not carry even a light load. Every 100–200 yd he had to stop even though the route was over an easy downhill glacier. He began coughing frothy white sputum which later became blood tinged. At about 100 m above the camp he was given oxygen and was able to complete the journey then without stopping. After breathing oxygen for about three hours at the camp he declared himself well and refused any more oxygen. He descended unaided to a lower camp next day, carrying a load.

18.2.2 Incidence

It is difficult to obtain data on incidence of HAPE because of the problem of knowing the number of people at risk. As with AMS it will depend upon the rate of ascent and the height reached. Hackett and Rennie (1976) saw seven cases in 278 trekkers who passed through Pheriche (4243 m) on their way to Everest Base Camp, giving an incidence of 2.5%. The incidence of AMS in the same group was 53%. Menon (1965) found an incidence of 0.57% in Indian troops flown into the modest altitude of Leh (3500 m). Hultgren and Marticorena (1978) gave an incidence of 0.6% in adults going to La Oroya, 3750 m.

The incidence will be affected by health education of people going to altitude. It is the impression of health workers at the aid post at Pheriche (4243 m) that the incidence is less following some years of publicity about the dangers of HAPE amongst trekkers and the trekking agencies.

18.2.3 Symptoms of HAPE

Table 18.1 shows the symptoms from the largest series managed by a single physician, that of Menon (1965), who reported 101 cases. The frequency of chest pain, second only to breathlessness (66 patients), is unusually high. Only 21% of patients complained of chest pain in a German series (Lobenhoffer *et al.*, 1982). Hallucinations are not uncommon and, with confusion and irrational behaviour, may make management difficult. Nocturnal dyspnoea and the symptoms of AMS – headache, nausea and insomnia – are all common.

Table 18.1 High-altitude pulmonary edema: symptoms in 101 cases (Menon, 1965)

Symptom	*No. of cases*
Breathlessness	84
Chest pain	66
Headache	63
Nocturnal dyspnoea	59
Dry cough	51
Haemoptysis	39
Nausea	26
Insomnia	23
Dizziness	18

18.2.4 Signs

These depend upon the stage of the condition. Probably the earliest sign is of crackles at the lung bases. These may be heard in subjects with no other signs of HAPE and who do not progress to the full-blown condition. Probably mild or subclinical pulmonary edema is not uncommon early in altitude exposure. Its presence may be the cause of dry cough on exertion and of the shift to the left of the pressure/volume curve of the lung (Mansell *et al.*, 1980; Gautier *et al.*, 1982) and the reduction in forced vital capacity (Welsh *et al.*, 1993).

The pulse rate increases early and was over 120 in 70 of 101 patients in Menon's series (1965). The respiratory rate was over 30 in 69 cases; cyanosis was detected in 52 subjects. The pulmonary artery pressure is high in this condition (section 18.2.7) giving the signs of right ventricular heave and accentuated pulmonary second sound in about half the patients. Signs of right ventricular failure are not prominent but 15 of Menon's patients had raised jugular venous pressure and dependent edema is found in a number of cases. The temperature is normal in at least 25% of cases but was found to be mildly elevated (37–39°C) in 70% of Menon's cases. In only two cases was it above 39°C. The systemic blood pressure is either normal or mildly elevated (systolic 130–140 mmHg) as is found in some subjects on ascent to altitude who do not have HAPE.

Some subjects (15 in Menon's series) have mental confusion and amnesia following recovery. This may be due to hypoxia and/or cerebral edema (Chapter 19).

18.2.5 Radiology

Figure 18.1 shows a chest radiograph of a patient with HAPE and a second radiograph four days later after treatment. The typical features are of cotton wool blotches irregularly positioned in both lung fields. They are frequently asymmetrical, possibly being denser on the side which has been dependent. Very often, the right side is more densely shadowed (Menon, 1965). Quite frequently, the lower zones, especially the costo-phrenic angles, are spared as well as the apices. The pulmonary vessels may be seen to be engorged (Marticorena *et al.*, 1964). The radiographic appearance in early cases shows more pathology than would be expected from clinical examination (Menon, 1965). In patients with a second attack of HAPE there is no consistent pattern in the areas of lung involved (Hackett and Oelz, 1992). This patchy distribution of edema is even more dramatically shown in computerized tomographic scanning of the chest.

In treated cases the radiographic lesions clear rapidly (see Figure

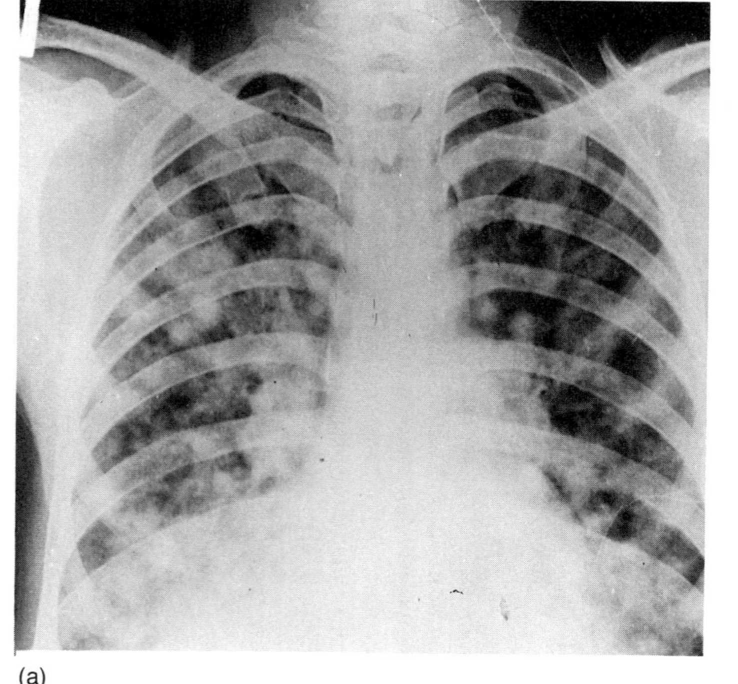

(a)

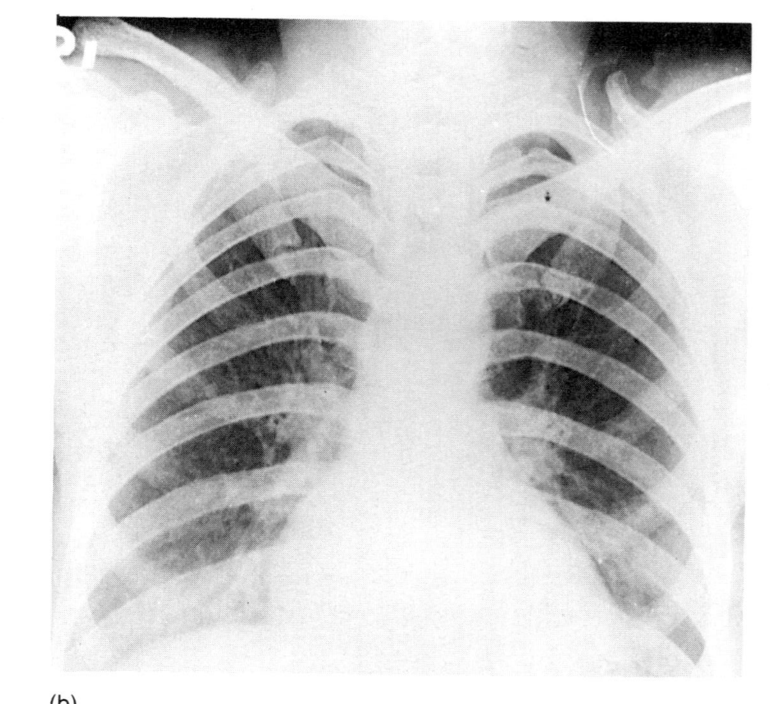

(b)

Figure 18.1 Radiograph of a patient with high-altitude pulmonary edema: (a) on admission and (b) four days later. (Reproduced with permission Dr T. Norboo of Leh, Jammu and Kashmir, India.)

18.1), often within two days (Houston, 1960), though usually lagging behind symptoms.

18.2.6 Investigations

The electrocardiograph

The ECG shows tachycardia. The P waves are often peaked (P pulmonale) and there is right axis deviation of the AQRS (mean +123°). Some patients show elevation of the S–T segment (Marticorena *et al.*, 1964). T-waves may be inverted in the precordial leads but this may be seen in asymptomatic subjects at altitude (Milledge, 1963). The ECG appearances can be attributed to the very high pulmonary artery pressure and the consequent increase in right ventricular work.

Haematology

Menon (1965) found haemoglobin concentration was $14.0–16.0\,g\,dl^{-1}$ and the sedimentation rate was normal. The white cell count was raised in 75 of 95 cases. This elevation was due to an increase in neutrophil count.

Blood gases

P_{O_2} and arterial oxygen saturation is low compared with normals for that altitude. P_{CO_2} is very variable and is not significantly different from controls (Antezana *et al.*, 1982; Schoene *et al.*, 1965).

Urine

Proteinuria was present in 4 of 101 cases (Menon, 1965), but using more sensitive tests there was an increase in urine protein in all subjects during the first few days at altitude, the degree of proteinuria correlating with severity of AMS (Pines, 1978; Chapter 14).

18.2.7 Cardiac catheter studies

There have been a number of catheter studies carried out on patients with HAPE before treatment (Penaloza and Sime, 1969; Antezana *et al.*, 1982) or soon after starting treatment (Fred *et al.*, 1962; Hultgren *et al.*, 1964; Roy *et al.*, 1969). In all these studies there was found to be a high pulmonary artery pressure compared with healthy subjects at the same altitude (Table 18.2). The wedge pressures were normal. The pulmonary artery pressure ranged up to 144 mmHg systolic (Hultgren *et*

Table 18.2 Cardiac catheter studies in HAPE (Data from Antezana *et al.*, 1982)

	n	*Pulmonary artery pressure (mmHg)*		*Wedge pressure (mmHg)*	*Cardiac output* ($l\,min^{-1}$)
		Systolic	*Diastolic*		
HAPE	5	81	49	5	5.8
Controls	50	29	13	9	6.4

al., 1964) and is usually in the 60–80 mmHg (Table 18.2). The normal wedge pressure implies normal pulmonary venous and left atrial pressures; in one subject direct measurement of left atrial pressure was made via a patent foramen ovale (Fred *et al.*, 1962). The cardiac output was within the normal range so the calculated pulmonary resistance was markedly raised. There was no evidence of left ventricular failure. Breathing 100% oxygen resulted in a fall of pulmonary artery pressure to normal values within 3 min in two of five subjects, but in the other three, pressures fell but plateaued out at 40–50 mmHg mean pulmonary artery pressure, well above the upper limit of normal at that altitude (Antezana *et al.*, 1982).

18.3 MANAGEMENT

18.3.1 Prevention

Slow ascent

It is generally considered that HAPE is a progression or complication of benign AMS. Therefore, if precautions are taken to prevent AMS by making a sufficiently slow ascent (section 17.6.1), HAPE will also be prevented. However, people often have to ascend at a rate that puts them at risk of AMS and, of course, the great majority of patients who suffer from benign AMS do not progress to the malignant forms.

Exercise

Many case histories from Houston (1960) onwards emphasize the point that patients have been very energetic while getting to high altitude or on arrival there. Ravenhill (1913) gave his opinion that physical exertion rendered a man more susceptible to AMS in general. The Indian Army, with a very large experience of HAPE since the war with China in the Himalayas in 1962, advises all inductees to altitude to take no unnecessary exertion for the first 72 h. However HAPE can occur in the absence of hard physical exertion; 66 of Menon's 101 cases had taken no exercise more strenuous than office work, travelling as a passenger in a truck or walking about on level ground (Menon, 1965). Nevertheless the anecdotal evidence is probably strong enough to advise people who have to make a rapid ascent to altitude to avoid hard physical exertion for two or three days.

Drugs

Acetazolamide (section 17.6.2), by preventing or at least reducing, AMS probably also reduces the risk of HAPE. Nifedipine has been shown in a controlled trial to reduce the risk of HAPE in susceptible subjects (Bärtsch *et al.*, 1991).

18.3.2 Treatment

The single most important manoeuvre in treating a case of HAPE is to get the patient down as fast and as far as possible. Even a descent of as little as 300 m may improve a patient's condition dramatically (report of case 2 in section 18.2). However, there are often unavoidable delays while awaiting evacuation and there are a number of therapeutic possibilities.

Oxygen

Breathing air enriched with oxygen, if available, is an obvious treatment. It relieves hypoxia and reduces pulmonary artery pressure (section 18.2.6), but, while most patients benefit, in some the relief is only partial and in a few deterioration may continue. The dosage of oxygen is usually dictated by its supply. If there is sufficient, a flow of 6–10 l min^{-1} would be indicated for the first few hours, reducing to 2–4 l min^{-1} when there is improvement.

Diuretics

Since the patient has edema, diuretics have been used in the treatment of HAPE (Singh *et al.*, 1965). However, physicians who see a lot of the condition now do not advocate their use.

Antibiotics

Antibiotics by themselves will not cure HAPE. However, many cases have mild fever and leucocytosis suggesting that infection may play a part. Therefore, it would seem prudent to add a broad spectrum antibiotic to the treatment regimen, although Menon (1965) discontinued their use in his last 44 cases with no apparent disadvantage.

Calcium channel blockers

Oelz *et al.* (1989) showed that nifedipine was of value in the treatment of HAPE. Six subjects with clinical physiological and radiographic (four subjects) evidence of HAPE were treated with 10 mg of nifedipine sublingually and 20 mg slow release orally 6-hourly thereafter. Despite continued exercise at 4559 m this treatment without oxygen resulted in clinical improvement, better oxygenation, reduced alveolar–arterial gradient and pulmonary artery pressure, and clearing of alveolar edema.

Other vasodilators

Hackett *et al.* (1992) have shown that several vasodilators are all beneficial in HAPE as indicated by a reduction in pulmonary artery pressure, pulmonary vascular resistance and improved gas exchange (Figure 18.2). Nifedipine and hydralazine were of equal benefit but rather less effective than oxygen. Phentolamine, an alpha-blocker, was more effective than oxygen and, when combined with oxygen, was even more effective.

Other drugs

Digoxin has been used. Menon (1965) observed the effect of an intravenous dose of 0.5–1.5 mg in 66 patients and claimed that the response was uniformly good in a few hours, even in patients given only $1\,l\,min^{-1}$ of added oxygen, but there was no evidence of myocardial failure nor was there atrial fibrillation, the current indications for digoxin therapy.

Morphine (15–30 mg i.v.) has been used, again with the clinical impression that this resulted in a reduction in pulmonary edema. It also makes the patient more comfortable as it does in acute left ventricular failure, possibly by causing peripheral vasodilatation and a shift of blood from central to peripheral circulations. However, its respiratory depressant effects should make for caution in its use. Corticosteroids have been used in a few cases with no clear result but the beneficial effect of dexamethasone in simple AMS shown by a controlled trial (Ferrazzini *et al.*, 1987) would justify its use in HAPE.

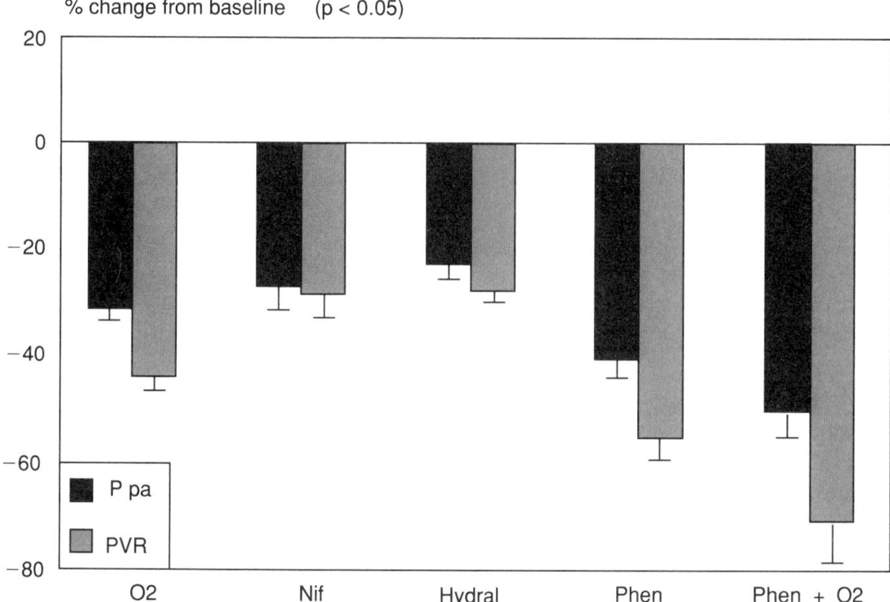

Figure 18.2 The percentage change in mean pulmonary artery pressure (Ppa) and pulmonary vascular resistance (PVR) with five different interventions in subjects with HAPE. Nif, nifedipine; Hydral, hydralazine; Phen, phentolamine. (Reproduced with permission from Hackett *et al.*, 1992.)

Expiratory positive airways pressure

Feldman and Herndon (1977) suggested that expiratory positive airways pressure might be beneficial in HAPE by analogy with its use in other forms of pulmonary edema. They proposed a simple device in which the subject exhaled through an underwater tube to achieve the desired positive pressure whilst inspiration was direct from atmosphere.

Schoene *et al.* (1985) used a commercial expiratory positive pressure mask on four patients with HAPE on Mt KcKinley. They showed that, using the mask, arterial saturation was increased with increasing positive pressure (up to 10 cm water). There was a concomitant rise in P_{CO_2} but not of heart rate. The intrathoracic pressure would be negative during inspiration so the cardiac output would probably not be reduced. A similar effect can be achieved by pursed lips expiration as used by patients with severe emphysema; this is advised by mountain guides who have presumably found it to be beneficial by experience.

Portable hyperbaric chamber: the Gamow or Certec bags

A lightweight rubberized canvas bag has been developed into which a patient can be zipped and the bag pressurized using a foot pump. There is a pressure relief valve set to 2 psi. This pressure gives the equivalent altitude reduction of almost 2000 m from a typical base camp altitude of 4000–5000 m. There are currently two commercially available bags, the Gamow from the USA and Certec from France. There have been numerous accounts of their use in HAPE and HACE, with good results (Robertson and Shlim, 1991). One report draws attention to the considerable placebo effect of the procedure. The efficacy of hyperbaric treatment has been reviewed by Roach and Hackett (1992). They conclude that both oxygen and hyperbaria are effective. There may be a rebound effect on stopping hyperbaria especially if the duration of treatment (typically 1–2 h) is too short and trials are needed to determine the optimum duration. A recent controlled trial in benign AMS has shown that 1 h in the bag at pressure (193 mbar) was significantly more effective in reducing symptoms than control (1 h at the trivial pressure of 20 mbar) (Bärtsch *et al.*, 1993).

To summarize, the treatment of HAPE is:

- Get the patient down in altitude as fast and as low as possible.
- While awaiting evacuation, or if evacuation is not possible, give oxygen or hyperbaria. Nifedipine 10 mg sublingually followed by 20 mg slow release (or possibly phentolamine) should be given and a broad spectrum antibiotic should be considered. If cerebral edema is also present give dexamethasone (Chapter 19).
- The use of expiratory positive airway pressure, with a respiratory valve device, or, failing that, by pursed lips breathing, will give some temporary improvement.

18.3.3 Outcome

In fully established cases, where evacuation to lower altitude is impossible, death within a few hours is usual. If cases are recognized early and taken down, patients usually recover completely in one or two days; but occasionally they continue to deteriorate and die even after being brought down to lower altitude, especially if there are symptoms of cerebral edema (Dickinson *et al.*, 1983). One case has been reported as progressing to adult respiratory distress syndrome (Zimmerman and Crapo, 1980). Even patients who have apparently fully recovered have been shown to have significant hypoxaemia and widened (A-a) O_2 gradients for up to 12 weeks (Guleria *et al.*, 1969). However, many climbers, after recovery at lower altitudes, have returned to climb their peaks without further trouble.

18.4 PATHOLOGY

18.4.1 Post-mortem examination

There have been a number of post-mortem studies which have shown a similar pathology in the heart and lungs (Hultgren *et al.*, 1962; Arias-Stella and Kruger, 1963; Marticorena *et al.*, 1964; Nayak *et al.*, 1964; Singh *et al.*, 1965; Dickinson *et al.*, 1983). The lungs are heavy and feel solid. The cut surface weeps edema fluid, usually blood stained, but a striking feature is the non-uniform nature of the edema. Areas of haemorrhagic edema alternate with clear edema and with areas which are virtually normal (or over-inflated). Pulmonary arterial thrombi are commonly found.

On microscopy, alveoli are filled with fluid containing red blood cells, polymorphs and macrophages, though not in great numbers. Hyaline membranes are found in the alveoli, identical with those seen in respiratory distress syndrome of the newborn. The pulmonary capillaries are congested with small arteries and veins containing thrombi and fibrin clot. Perivascular edema and haemorrhage is found. In post-mortem studies of high altitude natives from South America the pulmonary arteries are very muscular and the right ventricle is hypertrophied; in lowlanders the pulmonary vessels have normal musculature (Dickinson *et al.*, 1983).

18.4.2 The edema fluid

The hyaline membranes are probably formed by coalescence of proteins, suggesting a high protein edema. It has been shown in life that the edema fluid is rich in protein. Hackett *et al.* (1986) sampled pure edema fluid by bronchoscopy in one case and showed it to have a plasma/fluid ratio of 0.8:1.1 for total protein. Schoene *et al.* (1986) took broncho-alveolar lavage fluid from three cases of HAPE and compared it with lavage fluid from three controls at the same altitude (4400 m). The fluid from patients was rich in high molecular weight protein, red blood cells and macrophages. These findings suggest a 'large pore' leak type of edema. Further studies by the same group (Schoene *et al.*, 1988) found also that the fluid was rich in alveolar macrophages. There was evidence of activation of complement (C5a) and release of thromboxane B_2 and leukotriene B_4.

18.5 MECHANISMS OF HAPE

HAPE develops from AMS and the mechanisms that cause the symptoms of AMS (section 17.5) are already operating in these patients.

Indeed there is evidence suggesting that a degree of subclinical pulmonary edema is common during the second and third days at altitude. That is, there is a reduction in vital capacity, a shift of the pressure/volume curve of the lung (Mansell *et al.*, 1980; Gautier *et al.*, 1982) and an increase in alveolar arterial oxygen difference (Sutton *et al.*, 1976). This might simply be part of a generalized increase in extracellular fluid volume which shows itself as subcutaneous edema in the face on rising and in the ankles later in the day. In the skull, the same edema raises the intracellular pressure and gives rise to the symptoms of AMS, but the progression from this mild edema to clinical pulmonary edema requires a further mechanism or mechanisms.

18.5.1 Facts that require to be explained

Any hypothesis that seeks to explain the mechanism of HAPE must take into account the following facts:

- the edema is of the high protein type;
- the patchy distribution of the edema seen on post-mortem and radiology (Figure 18.1);
- the very high pulmonary artery pressure and normal wedge (and left atrial) pressures (Table 18.2); the improvement which follows treatment with different drugs which reduce the pulmonary artery pressure (Hackett *et al.*, 1992) indicate the importance of this factor in the mechanism of HAPE;
- the presence of vascular thrombi and fibrin clots in pulmonary vessels (section 18.4.1);
- the individual susceptibility which is associated with an increased hypoxic pulmonary pressor response (Hultgren *et al.*, 1971) and response to exercise (Kawashima *et al.*, 1989);
- the increased risk of HAPE with exercise on arrival at altitude.

18.5.2 Left ventricular failure

Although HAPE resembles left ventricular failure (LVF) clinically, which is why Ravenhill (1913) called it puna of the cardiac type, it is not now thought to be due to heart failure. Catheter studies have shown normal wedge pressures and the edema fluid is of the high protein permeability type. Also the chest radiograph and pathology are not typical of LVF.

18.5.3 Pulmonary hypertension

The extraordinarily high pulmonary artery pressure found in HAPE must, it is thought, play a role in the mechanism of the condition. High pulmonary artery pressure by itself does not cause edema (as for instance in primary pulmonary hypertension) since the resistance vessels, the arterioles, are upstream of capillaries and therefore capillary pressure should be normal. One must therefore postulate some further mechanism as well as, but related to, the pulmonary hypertension. The following have been proposed.

18.5.4 Uneven pulmonary vasoconstriction and perfusion

Hultgren (1969) suggested that the edema is caused by a very powerful, but uneven, vasoconstriction so that there is reduced blood flow in parts of the lung and torrential blood flow in other parts. He showed (Hultgren *et al.*, 1966) that if one progressively ties off more and more of the pulmonary arterial tree in a dog, thus forcing the total cardiac output through only a portion of the lung, pulmonary edema results in that part of the lung that remains perfused.

A case report by Dombret *et al.* (1987) provides confirmation in humans of Hultgren's experimental findings. The reported patient had a massive pulmonary embolus resulting in perfusion being reduced to only the left upper and middle lobes. She developed symptoms and signs of pulmonary edema which on radiograph were shown to be confined to those same perfused lobes.

Evidence in favour of this mechanism as being the cause of HAPE is provided by Viswanathan *et al.* (1979) who, at sea-level, studied 12 subjects who had recovered from HAPE. They showed that, on being given 10% oxygen to breathe, they had a greater pulmonary pressor response than controls and on lung scanning their perfusion was more uneven.

This hypothesis accounts well for the patchy distribution of the condition, and high flow through less severely constricted areas might well produce edema by capillary stress failure. Added support for this hypothesis came from a paper by Hackett *et al.* (1980), who collected four cases of HAPE occurring at very modest altitudes (2000–3000 m) in subjects who had a congenital absence of the right pulmonary artery. The edema developed in the left lung which received the total cardiac output. That four cases of HAPE developed in such an uncommon condition (only 50 cases have been described in the world literature) strongly suggests a causative rather than a coincidental association.

18.5.5 Stress failure of pulmonary capillaries

It has recently been proposed that HAPE is caused by damage to the walls of pulmonary capillaries as a result of very high wall stresses associated with increased capillary transmural pressure (West *et al.*,

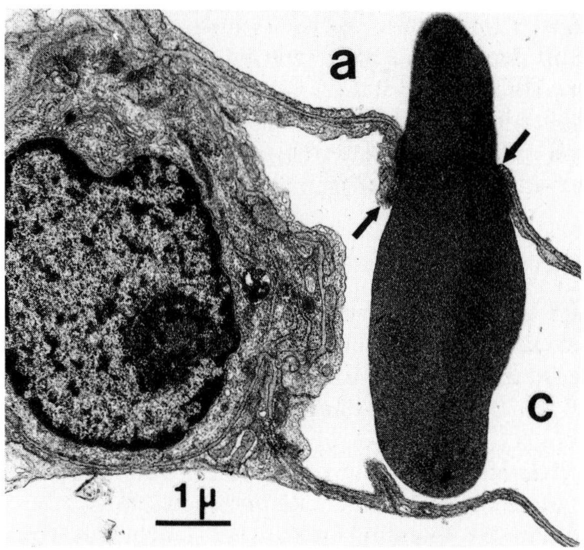

Figure 18.3 Electron micrograph of a pulmonary capillary in a rat exposed to a barometric pressure of 294 mmHg for 4 h. Note rupture of the capillary wall with a red cell moving out of the capillary lumen. (From West *et al.*, 1994.)

1991; West and Mathieu-Costello, 1992a). These high capillary pressures are the result of uneven hypoxic pulmonary vasoconstriction as originally proposed by Hultgren (Hultgren, 1969). Extensive laboratory studies have now shown that raising capillary transmural pressure causes ultrastructural damage to the capillary walls, including disruption of the capillary endothelial layer, alveolar epithelial layer, and, sometimes, all layers of the wall (West *et al.*, 1991; Tsukimoto *et al.*, 1991; Costello *et al.*, 1992; Fu *et al.*, 1992; Elliott *et al.*, 1992). The result is a high permeability form of pulmonary edema (Tsukimoto *et al.*, 1994). Figure 18.3 is an electron micrograph showing rupture of a pulmonary capillary wall in a rat exposed to a barometric pressure of 294 mmHg for 4 h. Note the red blood cell in the process of moving from the capillary lumen to the alveolar space (West *et al.*, 1994).

The work on stress failure began because of two key observations about HAPE. The first is that, as described above, there is a very strong relationship between the occurrence of HAPE and the height of the pulmonary arterial pressure. This suggests that HAPE is caused in some way by high vascular pressures in the pulmonary circulation. The second observation was that samples of alveolar fluid obtained by bronchoalveolar lavage in patients with HAPE show that the fluid is of the high permeability type with a large concentration of high molecular weight proteins and many cells. This observation strongly suggests that HAPE is associated with damage to the walls of the pulmonary capillaries by some mechanism. The problem therefore was to reconcile a hydrostatic pressure basis for the disease also accounting for the development of abnormalities in the capillary walls. As a result, extensive studies of the effects of raising pulmonary capillary pressure on the ultrastructure of pulmonary capillaries were carried out. These showed that stress failure is common in rabbit lung when the capillary transmural pressure rises to 40 mmHg, and that when it occurs it causes a high permeability type of pulmonary oedema.

It is not at all surprising that pulmonary capillaries break under these conditions because the calculated wall stress of the capillary is extremely high (West *et al.*, 1991; West and Matthieu-Costello, 1992b). The surprising thing is not that the capillaries fail, but that they do not fail more often. Stress failure is now believed to play a role in a number of lung diseases (West and Mathieu-Costello, 1992c) and is also the cause of bleeding into the lungs of racehorses, which is extremely common (West *et al.*, 1993).

Bronchoalveolar lavage studies in patients with HAPE show the presence of inflammatory markers including leukotriene B_4, other lipoxygenase products of arachidonic acid metabolism, and C5a complement fluid in the lavage fluid (Schoene *et al.*, 1988). At first sight these findings might seem to argue against stress failure of pulmonary capillaries as a mechanism. However, an important feature of the ultrastructural changes in stress failure is that the basement membranes of capillary endothelial cells are frequently exposed (Tsukimoto *et al.*, 1991). The exposed basement membrane is electrically charged and highly reactive, and can be expected to activate leucocytes and platelets. In bronchoalveolar studies of the rabbit preparation, leukotriene B_4 is seen in the lavage fluid (Tsukimoto *et al.*, 1994). Platelet activation will result in the formation of fibrin thrombi which are a feature of the pathology of HAPE (Arias-Stella and Kruger, 1963). Figure 18.4 is a diagram summarizing the mechanism of HAPE.

A striking feature of stress failure of pulmonary capillaries is that some of the breaks are rapidly reversible when the pressure is reduced. In one study carried out in rabbit lung, it was found that about 70% of both the epithelial and endothelial breaks closed within a few minutes of the pressure being reduced (Elliott *et al.*, 1992). This rapid reversibility of most of the disruptions may explain why patients with HAPE often rapidly improve when they descend to a lower altitude.

Stress failure of pulmonary capillaries has not previously been suggested as the mechanism of HAPE. However Mooi and co-workers (1978) studied the ultrastructural changes that occurred in rat lungs when the animals were exposed to acute decompression in a hyper-

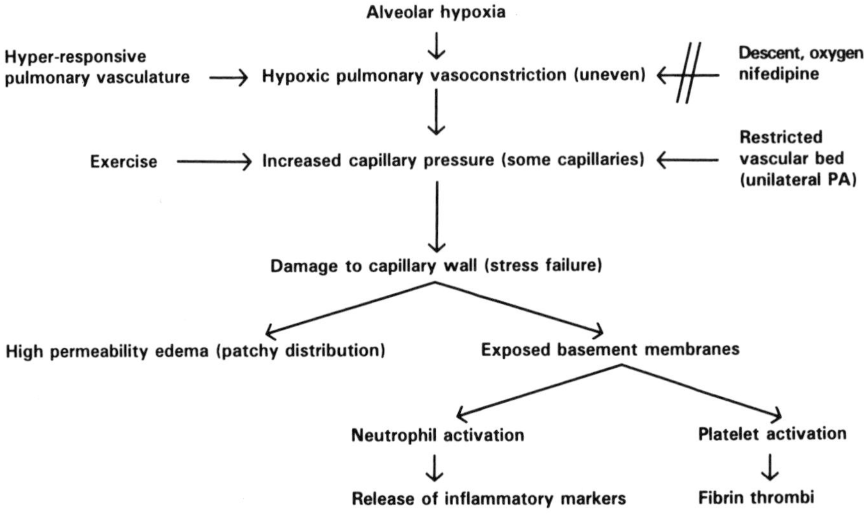

Figure 18.4 Diagram summarizing the pathogenesis of HAPE based on stress failure of pulmonary capillaries. (From West and Mathieu-Costello, 1992a.)

baric chamber. The appearances that they described are consistent with the findings seen in stress failure.

The mechanism of stress failure has clear implications for therapy. The main objective should be to reduce the pulmonary artery pressure. The pressure is high because of hypoxic pulmonary vasoconstriction, and the best way to reduce it is by rapid descent to a lower altitude which reduces the alveolar P_{O_2}. In addition, oxygen should be given if this is available. Calcium channel blockers such as nifedipine are also effective because they reduce pulmonary artery pressure (Oelz *et al.*, 1989).

18.5.6 Venular constriction

Since patients with HAPE have such a powerful arteriolar constriction in response to hypoxia, perhaps they have some degree of venular constriction as well. There is some pathological evidence for this from Wagenvoort and Wagenvoort (1976). This would not give high wedge pressures because when the catheter is wedged the blood in that segment runs off even through constricted venules and the wedge pressure reflects only the large vein and left atrial pressures, not the pressure in capillaries when the blood is flowing. To explain the patchy nature of the condition one must further postulate that the venular constriction is uneven.

18.5.7 Arterial leakage

Severinghaus (1977), impressed with the extraordinarily high pulmonary artery pressure in these patients, suggested that perhaps the fluid leak was upstream of the resistance vessels, (i.e. in the arteries). He pointed out that when there was generalized arterial vasoconstriction, Laplace's law would mean reduction in diameter of small vessels but distention of large vessels (even though their wall tension was as great or greater). Radiography frequently show distended hilar vessels (Marticorena *et al.*, 1964). These larger vessels, not designed for such high pressure, suffer minor ruptures or fenestrations which then leak high protein fluid and eventually red blood cells. The leakage is into the perivascular spaces which, when full, 'back up' to eventually cause alveolar flooding. This sequence occurs wherever the initial leak takes place since the perivascular space is the low pressure region of the lung.

Some evidence for such a mechanism was provided by two studies in animals (Whayne and Severinghaus, 1968; Milledge *et al.*, 1968) and in excised dog lungs (Iliff, 1971). This evidence was reviewed by Severinghaus (1977) who quoted Hultgren as reporting on two horses which died suddenly after running at altitude. Both were found to have a ruptured pulmonary artery. Both this and the preceding hypothesis would account for exercise as being a risk factor since it increases both flow and pressure in the pulmonary artery.

18.5.8 Multiple pulmonary emboli

Multiple scattered pulmonary emboli, even of inert substances, such as glass beads, cause a rapid profuse pulmonary oedema in animals (Saldeen, 1976) and this has been shown to be of the protein rich increased permeability type (Ohkuda *et al.*, 1978). The finding in postmortem studies of frequent vascular thrombi and fibrin clots has led to the microembolization hypothesis for HAPE on the premise that there is a derangement of the clotting system. The effect of hypoxia on coagulation has been studied by a number of workers (section 17.5.4). It seems that most clotting factors are unaffected by hypoxia; they are not disturbed in AMS. Some evidence of *in vivo* fibrin formation was found by Bartsch *et al.* (1987) in patients with HAPE but this was considered to be an epiphenomenon and not causative. If it does occur it will cause further deterioration in the patient. It is possibe that changes in the red blood cells with hypoxia might alter their rheological properties and be a factor in AMS and HAPE. Reinhart *et al.* (1991) found no difference between subjects with and without AMS with respect to a number of rheological parameters.

It has even been suggested that rapid ascent may cause bubble formation by decompression and thus air microembolization (Gray, 1983). If this were the case, HAPE should be much more common in chamber studies than in the mountains, but this is not so.

It is likely that these microemboli cause pulmonary edema through the generation of chemical mediators, so this hypothesis overlaps with the next.

18.5.9 Hypoxia and vascular permeability

Hypoxia may increase vascular permeability, either directly, or more likely, via the release of chemical mediators. Against this suggestion is evidence that, in dogs, hypoxia does not alter the threshold for edema formation at a given microvascular pressure (Homik *et al.*, 1988). However it may require some other agent acting with hypoxia to produce the effect, as suggested by the work Larsen *et al.* (1985). They showed in rabbits that neither hypoxia alone nor activation of the complement system (by infusion of cobra venom) alone caused pulmonary edema, but the two insults together did. Such a mechanism may well produce secondary intravascular coagulation which would result in further pulmonary edema.

18.5.10 Hypoventilation

Grover (1980) has pointed out that hypoventilation has two disadvantages for a subject in relation to HAPE. It will mean that the subject is more hypoxic at a given altitude than a subject with the normal altitude hyperventilation and also has a higher P_{CO_2}. The higher P_{CO_2} means that there is no peripheral vasoconstriction and reduction in plasma volume on going to altitude; hence the plasma osmotic pressure is not raised. He is therefore more susceptible to pulmonary edema. A number of studies have found subjects with a history of HAPE to have low hypoxic ventilatory responses (Hackett *et al.*, 1988; Matsuzawa *et al.*, 1989). This might lead to relative hypoventilation at altitude, although Hackett *et al.* concluded that the low HVR played a permissive rather than a causative role in the pathogenesis of HAPE, allowing hypoxia to cause depression of ventilation. They found oxygen breathing increased ventilation in some of their subjects at altitude.

18.5.11 Neurogenic pulmonary edema

In some cases of head injury, a form of acute pulmonary edema is found which can be mimicked in experimental animals by creating lesions in the fourth ventricle. High levels of catecholamines are found, and the edema can be prevented by pre-treatment with alpha-adrenergic blocking drugs. Therefore it is assumed that the edema is caused by a surge of sympathetic activity. During the first few days at altitude there is increased sympathetic activity and possibly a similar mechanism is at work. The effectiveness of the alpha-blocker, phentolamine, in HAPE (Hackett *et al.*, 1992) suggests that this may be the case.

18.5.12 Infection

Before 1960, in retrospect, many cases of HAPE were probably attributed to pneumonia. While in many cases infection plays no part in HAPE, in some it may be a factor.

18.5.13 Conclusions on mechanisms

The various mechanisms discussed are not mutually exclusive and it is probable that the genesis of HAPE is multifactorial. The importance of various factors may be different in individual cases. For example, infection may play a role in some subjects, though certainly not in the majority. Some mechanisms may be important in the initiation of the condition, others in its progression. At present it is not possible to be dogmatic about which mechanism is most important in the initiation and development of HAPE. However the mechanism of abnormally powerful pulmonary hypoxic vasoconstriction, which is uneven and may lead on to capillary stress failure, seems to have the most evidence in its favour.

REFERENCES

Antezana, G., Leguia, G., Guzman, A.M., *et al.* (1982) Hemodynamic study of high altitude pulmonary edema (12 200 ft), in *High Altitude Physiology and Medicine*, (eds W. Brendel and R.A. Zink), Springer-Verlag, New York, pp. 232–41.

Arias-Stella, J. and Kruger, H. (1963) Pathology of high altitude pulmonary edema. *Arch. Pathol.*, **76**, 147–57.

Bärtsch, P., Waber, U., Haeberli, A., *et al.* (1987) Enhanced fibrin formation in high-altitude pulmonary oedema. *J. Appl. Physiol.*, **63**, 752–7.

Bärtsch, P., Maggiorini, M., Ritter, M., *et al.* (1991) Prevention of high-altitude pulmonary edema by nifedipine. *N. Engl. J. Med.*, **325**, 1284–9.

Bärtsch, P., Merki, B., Hofsetter, D., *et al.* (1993) Treatment of acute mountain sickness by simulated descent: a randomised controlled trial. *Br. Med. J.*, **306**, 1098–101.

Costello, M.L., Mathieu-Costello, O. and West, J.B. (1992) Stress failure of alveolar epithelial cells studied by scanning electron microscopy. *Am. Rev. Respir. Dis.*, **145**, 1446–55.

Dickinson, J., Heath, D., Gosney, J. and Williams, D. (1983) Altitude related deaths in seven trekkers in the Himalayas. *Thorax*, **38**, 646–56.

Dombret, M.C., Rouby, J.J., Smeijan, J.M., *et al.* (1987) Pulmonary oedema during pulmonary embolism. *Br. J. Dis. Chest*, **81**, 407–10.

Elliott, A.R., Fu, Z., Tsukimoto, K., *et al.* (1992) Short-term reversibility of ultrastructural changes in pulmonary capillaries caused by stress failure. *J. Appl. Physiol.*, **73**, 1150–8.

Feldman, K.W. and Herndon, S.P. (1977) Positive expiratory pressure for the treatment of high altitude edema. *Lancet*, **1**, 1036–7.

Ferrazzini, G., Maggiorini, M., Kriemler, S., *et al.* (1987) Successful treatment of acute mountain sickness with dexamethasone. *Br. Med. J.*, **294**, 1380–2.

Fred, H.L., Schmidt, A.M., Bates, T. and Hecht, H.H. (1962) Acute pulmonary edema of altitude. Clinical and physiologic observations. *Circulation*, **25**, 929–7.

Fu, Z., Costello, M.L., Tsukimoto, K., *et al.* (1992) High lung volume increases stress failure in pulmonary capillaries. *J. Appl. Physiol.*, **73**, 123–33.

Gautier, H., Peslin, R., Grassino, A., *et al.* (1982) Mechanical properties of the lungs during acclimatization to altitude. *J. Appl. Physiol.*, **52**, 1407–15.

Gray, G.W. (1983) High altitude pulmonary edema. *Semin. Respir. Med.*, **5**, 141–50.

Grover, R.F. (1980) Speculations on the pathogenesis of high-altitude pulmonary edema. *Adv. Cardiol.*, **27**, 1–5.

Guleria, J.S., Pande, J.N. and Khanna, P.K. (1969) Pulmonary function in convalescents of high altitude pulmonary edema. *Dis. Chest*, **55**, 434–7.

Hackett, P.H., Bertman, J. and Rodriguez, G. (1986) Pulmonary edema fluid protein in high-altitude pulmonary edema. *J. Am. Med. Assoc.*, **256**, 36.

Hackett, P.H., Crerg, C.E., Grover, R.F., *et al.* (1980) High altitude pulmonary edema in persons without the right pulmonary artery. *N. Engl. J. Med.*, **302**, 1070–3.

Hackett, P.H. and Rennie, D. (1976) The incidence, importance and prophylaxis of acute mountain sickness. *Lancet*, **2**, 1149–54.

Hackett, P.H., Roach, R.C., Schoene, R.B., *et al.* (1988) Abnormal control of ventilation in high-altitude pulmonary edema. *J. Appl. Physiol.*, **64**, 1268–72.

Hackett, P.H., Roach, R.C., Hartig, G.S., *et al.* (1992) The effect of vasodilators on pulmonary hemodynamics in high altitude pulmonary edema: a comparison. *Int. J. Sports Med.*, **13**, S68–S71.

Homik, L.A., Bshouty, Z., Light, R.B. and Younes, M. (1988) Effect of alveolar hypoxia on pulmonary fluid filtration in *in-situ* dog lungs. *J. Appl. Physiol.*, **65**, 46–52.

Houston, C.S. (1960) Acute pulmonary edema of high altitude. *N. Engl. J. Med.*, **263**, 478–80.

Hultgren, H.N. (1969) High altitude pulmonary edema, in *Biomedicine Problems of High Terrestrial Altitude*, (ed. A.H. Hegnauer), Springer-Verlag, New York, pp. 131–41.

Hultgren, H.N. and Marticorena, E.A. (1978) High altitude pulmonary edema. Epidemiologic observations in Peru. *Chest*, **74**, 372–6.

Hultgren, H., Spickard, W. and Lopez, C. (1962) Further studies of high altitude pulmonary edema. *Br. Heart J.*, **24**, 95–102.

Hultgren, H.N., Lopez, C.E., Lundberg, E. and Miller, H. (1964) Physiologic studies of pulmonary edema at high altitude. *Circulation*, **29**, 393–408.

Hultgren, H.N., Robison, M.C. and Wuerflein, R.D. (1966) Over perfusion pulmonary edema. *Circulation*, **34(suppl 3)**, 132–3.

Hultgren, H.N., Grover, R.F. and Hartley, L.H. (1971) Abnormal circulatory responses to high altitude in subjects with a previous history of high-altitude pulmonary edema. *Circulation*, **44**, 759–70.

Iliff, L.D. (1971) Extra-alveolar vessels and edema development in excised dog lungs. *Circ. Res.*, **28**, 524–32.

Kawashima, A., Kubo, K., Kobayashi, T. and Sekiguchi, M. (1989) Hemodynamic response to acute hypoxia, hypobaria and exercise in subjects susceptible to high-altitude pulmonary edema. *J. Appl. Physiol.*, **67**, 1982–9.

Larsen, G.L., Webster, R.O., Worthen, G.S., *et al.* (1985) Additive effect of intravascular complement activation and brief episodes of hypoxia in producing increased permeability in the rabbit lung. *J. Clin. Invest.*, **75**, 902–10.

Lobenhoffer, H.P., Zink, R.A. and Brendel, W. (1982) High altitude pulmonary edema: Analysis of 166 cases, in *High Altitude Physiology and Medicine*, (eds W. Brendel and R.A. Zink), Springer-Verlag, New York, pp. 219–31.

Mansell, A., Powles, A. and Sutton, J. (1980) Changes in pulmonary PV characteristics of human subjects at an altitude of 5366 m. *J. Appl. Physiol.*, **49**, 79–83.

Marticorena, E., Tapia, F.A., Dyer, J., *et al.* (1964) Pulmonary edema by ascending to high altitudes. *Dis. Chest*, **45**, 273–83.

Matsuzawa, Y., Fujimoto, K., Kobayashi, T., *et al.* (1989) Blunted hypoxic ventilatory drive in subjects susceptible to high-altitude pulmonary edema. *J. Appl. Physiol.*, **66**, 1152–7.

Menon, N.D. (1965) High altitude pulmonary edema: a clinical study. *N. Engl. J. Med.*, **273**, 66–73.

Milledge, J.S. (1963) Electrocardiographic changes at high altitude. *Br. Heart J.*, **25**, 291–8.

Milledge, J.S., Iliff, L.D. and Severinghaus, J.W. (1968) The site of vascular leakage in hypoxic pulmonary edema, in *Proceedings of the International Union of Physiological Sciences, Abstracts, Vol. 44, International Congress*, p. 883.

Mooi, W., Smith, P. and Heath, D. (1978) The ultrastructural effects of acute decompression on the lung of rats: the influence of frusemide. *J. Pathol.*, **126**, 189–96.

Mosso, A. (1898) *Life of Man on the high Alps*, T. Fisher Unwin, London, p. 179.

Nayak, N.C., Roy, S. and Narayanan, T.K. (1964) Pathologic features of altitude sickness. *Am. J. Pathol.*, **45**, 381–7.

Oelz, O., Maggiorini, M., Ritter, M., *et al.* (1989) Nifedipine for high altitude pulmonary oedema. *Lancet*, **394**, 1241–4.

Ohkuda, K., Nakahara, K., Weidner, W.J., *et al.* (1978) Lung fluid exchange after uneven pulmonary artery obstruction in sheep. *Circ. Res.*, **43**, 152–61.

Penaloza, D. and Sime, F. (1969) Circulatory dynamics during high altitude pulmonary edema. *Am. J. Cardiol.*, **23**, 369–78.

Pines, A. (1978) High-altitude acclimatization and proteinuria in East Africa. *Br. J. Dis. Chest*, **72**, 196–8.

Ravenhill, T.H. (1913) Some experiences of mountain sickness in the Andes. *J. Trop. Med. Hyg.*, **16**, 314–20.

Reinhart, W.H., Kayser, B., Singh, A., *et al.* (1991) Blood rheology and acute mountain sickness and high-altitude pulmonary edema. *J. Appl. Physiol.*, **71**, 934–8.

Roach, R. and Hackett, P.H. (1992) *Hyperbaria and High Altitude Illness in Hypoxia and Mountain Medicine,* (eds J.R. Sutton, G. Coates and C.S. Houston), Queen City Printers, Burlington VT, pp. 266–73.

Robertson, J.A. and Shlim, D.R. (1991) Treatment of moderate acute mountain sickness with pressurization in a portable hyperbaric (Gamow) Bag. *J. Wild. Med.*, **2**, 268–73.

Roy, S.B., Guleria, J.S., Khanna, P.K., *et al.* (1969) Haemodynamic studies in high altitude pulmonary oedema. *Br. Heart J.*, **31**, 52–8.

Roy, S.B., Balasubramanian, V., Khan, M.R., *et al.* (1974) Transthoracic electrical impedance in cases of high-altitude hypoxia. *Br. Med. J.*, **3**, 771–5.

Saldeen, T. (1976) The microembolism syndrome. *Microvascular Res.*, **11**, 187–259.

Schoene, R.B., Roach, R.C., Hackett, P.H., *et al.* (1985) High altitude pulmonary edema and exercise at 4400 m on Mount McKinley. Effect of expiratory positive airway pressure. *Chest*, **87**, 330–3.

Schoene, R.B., Hackett, P.H., Henderson, W.R., *et al.* (1986) High-altitude pulmonary edema. Characteristics of lung lavage fluid. *J. Am. Med. Assoc.*, **256**, 63–9.

Schoene, R.B., Swenson, E.R., Pizzo, C.J., *et al.* (1988) The lung at high altitude: bronchoalveolar lavage in acute mountain sickness and pulmonary edema. *J. Appl. Physiol.*, **64**, 2605–13.

Severinghaus, J.W. (1977) Pulmonary vascular function. *Am. Rev. Respir. Dis.*, **115(suppl)**, 149–58.

Singh, I., Kapila, C.C., Khanna, P.K., *et al.* (1965) High-altitude pulmonary oedema. *Lancet*, **1**, 189–234.

Sutton, J.R., Bryan, A.C., Gray, G.W., *et al.* (1976) Pulmonary gas exchange in acute mountain sickness. *Aviat. Space Environ. Med.*, **47**, 1032–7.

Sutton, J.R., Houston, C.S., Mansell, A.L., *et al.* (1979) Effect of acetazolamide on hypoxemia during sleep at high altitude. *N. Engl. J. Med.*, **301**, 1329–31.

Tsukimoto, K., Mathieu-Costello, O., Prediletto, R., *et al.* (1991) Ultrastructural appearances of pulmonary capillaries at high transmural pressures. *J. Appl. Physiol.*, **71**, 573–82.

Tsukimoto, K., Yoshimura, N., Ichioka, M., *et al.* (1994) Protein, cell, and leukotriene B_4 concentrations of lung edema fluid produced by high capillary transmural pressures in rabbit. *J. Appl. Physiol.*, **76**, 321–67.

Viswanathan, R., Subramanian, S. and Radha, T.G. (1979) Effect of hypoxia on regional lung perfusion, by scanning. *Respiration*, **37**, 142–7.

Wagenvoort, C.A. and Wagenvoort, N. (1976) Pulmonary venous changes in chronic hypoxia. *Virchows Arch.* [*A*], **372**, 51–6.

Welsh, C.H., Wagner, P.D., Reeves, J.T., *et al.* (1993) Operation Everest II: Spirometric and radiographic changes in acclimatized humans at simulated high altitudes. *Am. Rev. Respir. Dis.*, **147**, 1239–44.

West, J.B. and Mathieu-Costello, O. (1992a) High altitude pulmonary edema is caused by stress failure of pulmonary capillaries. *Int. J. Sports Med.*, **13(suppl 1)**, S54–S58.

West, J.B. and Mathieu-Costello, O. (1992b) Strength of the pulmonary blood–gas barrier. *Respir. Physiol.*, **88**, 141–8.

West, J.B. and Mathieu-Costello, O. (1992c) Stress failure of pulmonary capillaries: role in lung and heart disease. *Lancet*, **340**, 762–7.

West, J.B., Tsukimoto, K., Mathieu-Costello, O. and Prediletto, R. (1991) Stress failure in pulmonary capillaries. *J. Appl. Physiol.*, **70**, 1731–42.

West, J.B., Mathieu-Costello, O., Jones, J.H., *et al.* (1993) Stress failure of pulmonary capillaries in racehorses with exercise-induced pulmonary haemorrhage. *J. Appl. Physiol.*, **75**, 1097–109.

West, J.B., Colice, G.L., Mathieu-Costello, O., *et al.* (1994) Pathogenesis of high-altitude pulmonary edema: morphological evidence of stress failure of pulmonary capillaries. *Am. J. Respir. Crit. Care Med.*, (in press).

Whayne, T.F. and Severinghaus, J.W. (1968) Experimental hypoxic pulmonary edema in the rat. *J. Appl. Physiol.*, **25**, 729–732.

Zimmerman, G.A. and Crapo, R.O. (1980) Adult respiratory distress syndrome secondary to high altitude pulmonary edema. *West. J. Med.*, **133**, 335–7.

19

High altitude cerebral edema and retinal haemorrhage

19.1 INTRODUCTION

The symptoms of benign acute mountain sickness (AMS) are probably due to mild cerebral edema, which, though unpleasant, is not serious. In a small minority of cases the condition progresses to more severe symptoms. Unmistakable signs of increased intracranial pressure become manifest and progress to coma. Death can be expected if the patient is not treated. This malignant form of AMS we call high altitude cerebral edema (HACE).

Ravenhill (1913) called the condition 'puna of a nervous type'. He describes three cases who recovered on being sent down to low altitude. As with acute pulmonary edema of high altitude, his work was forgotten and it was only during the 1960s that this serious form of acute cerebral edema of high altitude was again described (e.g. Singh *et al.*, 1969).

19.2 CLINICAL PRESENTATION

19.2.1 Symptoms and signs

Patients usually have the symptoms of benign AMS (Chapter 17). They may have headache, loss of appetite, nausea, vomiting and photophobia. Their climbing performance falls off, they may be irritable and wish only to be left alone. It can be difficult to decide the point at which these benign symptoms have progressed to malignant cerebral AMS, but the appearance of ataxia, irrationality, hallucinations or clouding of consciousness should alert one to the likelihood that the patient now has HACE. The patient may report blurring of vision which may be due to retinal haemorrhage (section 19.4) or to papilledema, which may be evident on examination of the retina. The reflexes may be brisk and later the plantars may become extensor.

There may be ocular muscle paralysis with diplopia. The pulse is often rapid and cyanosis usual.

Often there is also an element of pulmonary edema with signs and symptoms of that condition as well (sections 18.2.3; 18.2.4). As the condition progresses all symptoms and signs become more evident. The headache becomes worse, the ataxia intensifies so that the patient can no longer sit up (truncal ataxia). As coma comes on, the breathing becomes irregular. Death may come in a few hours or in a day or two in untreated cases.

19.2.2 Typical cases

Case 1 (Houston and Dickinson, 1975)

A 39-year-old Japanese female flew from 1500 m to 2750 m and during the next two days climbed to 3500 m, where she developed a severe headache. On day four at 3800 m she began to vomit. On day five at 3960 m she became dyspnoeic and weak, was vomiting and needed assistance to walk. On day six she lost consciousness and was carried down to 3350 m where she was found to be deeply unconscious and cyanosed, with a temperature of 40.6°C and a pulse of 140 beats per minute. Crepitations filled the chest. Reflexes were brisk and plantars flexor. Slight papilledema was present. She was treated with oxygen, frusemide and penicillin. On day eight she was flown to hospital at 1500 m where she was found to be in the same condition but with extensor plantar reflexes. Lumbar puncture showed a pressure of 270 mm H_2O and the CSF was normal. She slowly improved over two weeks and eventually recovered completely.

Case 2 (Dickinson et al.*, 1983)*

A 46-year-old man trekked from 1500 m to 3650 m in two days. On the way he began to feel unwell, was tired, anorexic and later began to vomit. At 3650 m he became unconscious and was evacuated to hospital at 1500 m. On examination he was deeply unconscious, responding only to pain. He was cyanosed and hyperventilating. There were crackles and wheezes in the lungs; papilledema and retinal haemorrhage were present. Respirations were 40 per minute, the pulse was 120 per minute, and the temperature 40°C. He remained unconsciousness and died after four days in hospital.

Case 3 (Houston and Dickinson, 1975)

A 42-year-old fit man reached 3600 m from sea-level in a few days. He spent two days at this altitude and on day three climbed to 4940 m, returning to sleep at 3960 m. On day four, after carrying about 25 kg to 4940 m he complained of severe headache, and went to sleep on arrival at the camp. Next morning he was confused and unable to talk coherently. He could not co-ordinate hand and foot movements and was disorientated in time and space. He was carried down to 3600 m where he became coherent and was able to walk without assistance. He was given an intramuscular steroid and by late afternoon seemed normal. The next day he was taken down to 2130 m where he was completely normal.

19.2.3 Investigations

Blood counts and blood biochemistry are usually normal. Chest radiograph may show evidence of concomitant pulmonary edema, whilst lumbar puncture usually shows raised pressure but normal CSF. Computerized tomographic scanning of the brain in 12 patients with HAPE and HACE (Koyama *et al.*, 1984) showed evidence of cerebral edema with diffuse low density of the entire cerebrum and compression of the ventricles. Recovery to normal CT findings occurred within a week in three cases but persisted for one to two weeks in two cases; one case took over a month to clear.

19.2.4 Treatment

The treatment for HACE is very similar to that for HAPE, that is, get the patient down in altitude as soon as possible. Whilst awaiting evacuation, oxygen therapy is obviously advised but often is only of marginal benefit. Dexamethasone has been shown to be of benefit in a double blind, randomized placebo controlled trial in AMS (Ferrazzini *et al.*, 1987). It is particularly the cerebral symptoms which seem to benefit by this drug, so it should certainly be tried in this situation. The dose used in the trial was 8 mg initially, followed by 4 mg six-hourly. Probably dexamethasone is to be preferred to diuretics, though, if response to the former is not adequate, they can be tried. Enthusiasm for dexamethasome should be tempered by the finding that, although symptoms are relieved, the physiological abnormalities (fluid shifts, oxygenation, sleep apnoea, urinary catecholamine levels, chest radiograph, perfusion scans and the results of psychomotor tests) were not improved (Levine *et al.*, 1989). Portable hyperbaric bags (Gamow bags) are now available. Their use in HAPE is discussed in Chapter 18. Their use in HACE is less well documented but, if available, they should certainly be used. Their use may make it possible for a patient to then descend unaided instead of having to be carried. Recovery after descent may not be as rapid as is usually the case with HAPE (Dickinson, 1979).

19.2.5 Post-mortem appearance

There have been a few reports of post-mortems in HACE (Singh *et al.*, 1969; Houston and Dickinson, 1975; Dickinson *et al.*, 1983). The usual findings in the brain are of cerebral edema with swollen, flattened gyri, and compression of the sulci. There may be herniation of the cerebellar tonsils and unci. Spongiosis, especially in the white matter, may be marked. In many cases there are widespread petechial haemorrhages; in some there are ante-mortem thrombi in the venous sinuses or there may be subarachnoid haemorrhages, but there seems to be considerable variation in the findings. It must always be remembered that the few cases that reach autopsy are highly selected and may well be very unrepresentative of the condition as seen clinically in the field.

19.2.6 Incidence and aetiology

The incidence – like that of HAPE – is difficult to determine and depends upon the rate of ascent and therefore on terrain, logistics and the pattern of movements of people from sea-level to altitude. It also depends upon definition, where the distinction between severe cases of benign AMS and mild HACE is impossible. Many cases show a mixed picture of HAPE and HACE. However, Hackett *et al.* (1976) had five cases out of 278 trekkers arriving at Pheriche (4243 m) giving an incidence of 1.8%, rather less than that for HAPE.

The age and sex distribution, like that for AMS, shows no group to be immune. Possibly the younger male is rather more at risk, perhaps because he is more likely to push on to higher altitude with symptoms, a feature of many histories in fatal cases. People native to high altitude can be victim to HACE. The impression is that the incidence in them is lower but there are no good published data.

19.3 MECHANISMS OF HACE

The mechanism for the development of cerebral edema at altitude is reviewed in Chapter 17. Hypoxia seems generally to induce an increase in extracellular fluid. It may also cause increased microvascular permeability. Hypoxia certainly increases cerebral blood flow, particularly when there is no marked reduction in P_{CO_2}. Although a recent study could find no correlation between cerebral blood flow and AMS (Jensen *et al.*, 1990). These same factors may become more pronounced to cause the symptoms of HACE but there may be others. The question of why certain individuals are susceptible while others are not is as puzzling in HACE as in other forms of AMS.

19.3.1 Venous thrombosis

This has been found on CT scan in one patient (Asaji *et al.*, 1984) and in some post-mortem studies of HACE. It may develop late in the condition as a consequence of intracranial hypertension. It will certainly exacerbate the condition.

19.3.2 Cellular oedema

In profound hypoxia, the ATP-dependent sodium pump eventually begins to fail, then sodium concentration rises in the cell and water follows to maintain osmotic equilibrium (Fishman, 1975). This may be the cause of further cerebral edema in established cases, especially with those with pulmonary edema causing further hypoxia.

19.4 RETINAL HAEMORRHAGE AT ALTITUDE

19.4.1 Clinical features

In 1970 Frayser *et al.* reported retinal haemorrhages in 35% of subjects flown to 5330 m. Since then they have been found in a proportion of climbers on a number of expeditions (Rennie and Morrissey, 1975; Clarke and Duff, 1976). The condition is almost always symptomless and self limiting. The haemorrhages are usually multiple, often flame shaped and adjacent to a vessel. If near the disc there may be some blurring of vision.

Besides haemorrhages 'cotton wool' spots have been reported in one case (Hackett and Rennie, 1982) and there may be some mild papilledema present as well. There is usually engorgement of both arteries and veins.

The haemorrhages are usually found during the first few days after ascent to altitude (the 'at risk' time for AMS) and subjects are often suffering from AMS, though the correlation with severity of AMS is not strong (Rennie and Morrissey, 1975).

19.4.2 Incidence of retinal haemorrhage

The incidence varies from zero on one ten-member expedition to Mt Kongur (7719 m), to 15 of 16 members on an expedition to Peak Communism (7495 m) (Nakashima, 1983). It seems that people going for the first time to altitude are especially liable to show this phenomenon

(Clarke and Duff, 1976) whilst experienced high-altitude climbers are relatively immune as are Sherpa residents.

19.4.3 Mechanism of retinal haemorrhage

At the time when retinal haemorrhage appears, the cerebral blood flow is increased (Severinghaus *et al.*, 1966). The blood flow through the retinal vessels is increased by 105% (Frayser *et al.*, 1970). Arterial diameter is increased by 24% and venous diameter by 19% (Rennie and Morrissey, 1975), who suggest that, in the presence of these dilated vessels, the sudden rise in vascular pressure associated with coughing and straining may cause a microvessel to rupture; cough is common and severe at altitude.

However, retinal haemorrhage has been produced in monkeys in a chamber by Sakaguchi and Yurugi (1983) when presumably cough was absent. Five monkeys in 16 exposures showed retinal haemorrhage, whereas no retinal haemorrhage was produced in 46 rabbits. The authors point out that rabbits, unlike monkeys or humans, have arteriolar–venular anastomotic vessels in their retinae which may protect them.

19.5 CORTICAL BLINDNESS AND TRANSIENT VISUAL DEFECTS

Transient blindness has been reported in otherwise healthy individuals at altitude. Six cases at an altitude of 4300 m were reported by Hackett *et al.* (1987), four on Denali and two at Pheriche near Everest. These individuals were not suffering from pulmonary edema or severe AMS. They did not have retinal haemorrhage. The blindness lasted for from 20 min to 24 h, with intermittant periods of normal vision. It was relieved by oxygen breathing. Recovery was complete. It was thought to be due to hypoxia or ischaemia of the visual cortex. Houston (1987) also reports various visual disturbances on acute exposure to altitude in chambers. There is some suggestion that subjects with a history of migraine are more susceptible and that aspirin may help prevent attacks which may be related to platelet aggregation and microemboli.

REFERENCES

Asaji, T., Sakurai, E., Tanizaki, Y., *et al.* (1984) Report on medical aspects of Mt Lhotse and Everest Expedition in 1983: with special reference to a case of cerebral venous thrombosis in the altitude. *Jpn. J. Mount. Med.*, **4**, 98.

Clarke, C. and Duff, J. (1976) Mountain sickness, retinal haemorrhages, and acclimatization on Mount Everest in 1975. *Br. Med. J.*, **2**, 495–7.

Dickinson, J.G. (1979) Severe acute mountain sickness. *Postgrad. Med. J.*, **55**, 454–8.

Dickinson, J., Heath, D., Gosney, J. and Williams, D. (1983) Altitude related deaths in seven trekkers in the Himalayas. *Thorax*, **38**, 646–56.

Ferrazzini, G., Maggiorini, M., Kriemler, S., *et al.* (1987) Successful treatment of acute mountain sickness with dexamethasone. *Br. Med. J.*, **294**, 1380–2.

Fishman, R.A. (1975) Brain edema. *N. Engl. J. Med.*, **293**, 706–11.

Frayser, R., Houston, C.S., Bryan, A.C., *et al.* (1970) Retinal haemorrhage at high altitude. *N. Engl. J. Med.*, **282**, 1183–4.

Hackett, P.H. and Rennie, D. (1982) Cotton-wool spots: a new addition to high altitude retinopathy, in *High Altitude Physiology and Medicine*, (eds W. Brendel and R.A. Zink), Springer-Verlag, New York, pp. 215–6.

Hackett, P.H., Rennie, D. and Levine, H.D. (1976) The incidence, importance and prophylaxis of acute mountain sickness. *Lancet*, **2**, 1149–54.

Hackett, P.H., Hollingshead, K.F., Roach, R.B., *et al.* (1987) Cortical blindness in high altitude climbers and trekkers – A report of six cases (abstract), in *Cold and Hypoxia*, (eds J.R. Sutton, C.S. Houston and G. Cotes), Praeger, New York, p. 536.

Houston, C.S. and Dickinson, J. (1975) Cerebral form of high-altitude illness. *Lancet*, **2**, 758–61.

Houston, C. S. (1987) Transient visual disturbance at high altitude (abstract), in *Cold and Hypoxia*, (eds J.R. Sutton, C.S. Houston and G. Cotes), Praeger, New York, p. 536.

Jensen, J.B., Wright, A.D., Lassen, N.A., *et al.* (1990) Cerebral blood flow in acute mountain sickness. *J. Appl. Physiol.*, **69**, 430–3.

Koyama, S., Kobayashi, T., Kubo, K., *et al.* (1984) Catecholamine metabolism in patients with high altitude pulmonary edema (HAPE). *Jpn. J. Mount. Med.*, **4**, 119.

Levine, B.D., Yoshimura, K., Kobayashi, T., *et al.* (1989) Dexamethazone in the treatment of acute mountain sickness. *N. Engl. J. Med.*, **321**, 1707–13.

Nakashima, M. (1983) High altitude medical research in Japan. *Jpn. J. Mount. Med.*, **3**, 19–27.

Ravenhill, T.H. (1913) Some experiences of mountain sickness in the Andes. *J. Trop. Med. Hyg.*, **16**, 314–320.

Rennie, D. and Morrissey, J. (1975) Retinal changes in Himalayan climbers. *Arch. Ophthalmol.*, **93**, 395–400.

Sakaguchi, E. and Yurugi, R. (1983) Retinal haemorrhages at simulated high altitude. *Jpn. J. Mount. Med.*, **3**, 107–8.

Severinghaus, J.W., Chiodi, H., Eger, E.I., *et al.* (1966) Cerebral blood flow in man at high altitude. Role of cerebrospinal fluid pH in normalization of flow in chronic hypocapnia. *Circ. Res.*, **19**, 274–82.

Singh, I., Khanna, P.K., Srivastava, M.C., *et al.* (1969) Acute mountain sickness. *N. Engl. J. Med.*, **280**, 175–84.

20

Chronic mountain sickness: Monge's disease

20.1 HISTORICAL

In 1925 Carlos Monge M. reported a case of polycythaemia in a patient from Cerro de Pasco (4300 m) to the Peruvian Academy of Medicine. In 1928 he reported a series of such patients with red cell counts significantly higher than normally found at altitude (Monge, C.C. and Whittembury, 1976). This condition of chronic mountain sickness (CMS) has come to be known also as Monge's disease. The 1935 international expedition led by Ancel Keys reported one case of CMS in the English literature (Talbott and Dill, 1936). In 1942 Hurtado published detailed observations of eight cases, outlining the symptomatology and haematological changes at altitude and the effect of descent to sea-level and return to altitude.

Outside South America, CMS was observed in Leadville (3100 m), a mining town in Colorado USA, by Monge M. in the late 1940s (Winslow and Monge, 1987a) and from the 1960s the condition has been studied there by Grover and, later, Weil and colleagues from Denver (section 20.3.3). Reports of CMS from the Himalayas indicate the condition to be prevalent in immigrant Han Chinese in Lhasa (3600 m) but rare in the indigenous Tibetan population (Pei *et al.*, 1989).

20.2 CLINICAL ASPECTS OF CMS

20.2.1 Symptoms of CMS

Patients typically have rather vague neuropsychological complaints including headache, dizziness, somnolence, fatigue, difficulty in concentration and loss of mental acuity. There may also be irritability, depression and even hallucinations. Dyspnoea on exertion is not commonly complained of, but poor exercise tolerance is common and patients may gain weight. The characteristic feature of the disease is that the symptoms disappear on going down to sea-level, only to reappear on return to altitude.

20.2.2 Signs

Although normal people are mildly cyanotic at an altitude of 4000 m, the patient with CMS stands out since, with a high haemoglobin concentration and lower oxygen saturation, they have a far higher concentration of reduced haemoglobin. In Andean Indians, the population with the greatest number of patients, the signs may be florid. 'The combination of virtually black lips and wine red mucosal surfaces against the olive green pigmentation of the Indian skin gives the patient with Monge's disease a striking appearance' (Heath and Williams, 1981). The conjunctivae are congested and the fingers may be clubbed. In Caucasians and at lower altitudes such as Leadville (3100 m), the appearances are rather less striking, looking similar to patients with polycythaemia secondary to hypoxic lung disease at sea-level. Some patients show very little in the way of signs.

20.2.3 Investigations

The red cell count, haemoglobin concentration and packed cell volume are raised; values as high as 28.0 g dl^{-1} [Hb] and a packed cell volume of up to 83% have been recorded (Hurtado, 1942). Like secondary poly-cythaemia at sea-level and unlike polycythaemia rubra vera there is no increase in white cell numbers. Blood gases, compared with healthy controls at the same altitude, show a higher Pa_{CO_2} and lower Pa_{O_2} and oxygen saturation (Penaloza and Sime, 1971; Kryger *et al.*, 1978a). The lower Pa_{O_2} is partly due to hypoventilation as shown by the increased Pa_{CO_2} and partly (in many cases) by an increased alveolar–arterial oxygen tension (A–a) O_2 gradient. Manier *et al.* (1988) found a mean of 10.5 mmHg in CMS patients at La Paz (3600 m) compared with the normal (A–a) O_2 of 2.9 mmHg at this altitude. Using the multiple inert gas technique, they attributed most of this to increased blood flow to poorly ventilated areas of lung rather than to true shunting. Tewari *et al.* (1991) found a reduced diffusing capacity in lowland soldiers with excessive polycythaemia which improved after descent and return to normal of the haematocrit. In some cases standard pulmonary func-tion tests show abnormalities indicating obstructive and/or restrictive defects, suggesting that patients have coexisting chronic lung disease.

20.2.4 Haemodynamics and pathology

The very high haematocrit increases the viscosity of the blood enormously. The systemic blood pressure may be moderately elevated and the pulmonary artery pressure (PAP) is significantly higher than healthy high-altitude residents. Penaloza *et al.* (1971) found a mean PAP of 64/33 mmHg in ten cases of CMS compared with 34/23 mmHg in controls. Cardiac output was not significantly different, so that calculated resistance was just over twice that of controls.

As might be expected these haemodynamic changes lead to increased right ventricular hypertrophy and associated ECG changes. There is also thickening of the pulmonary arteries to a greater degree than in normal residents at high altitude (Arias-Stella *et al.*, 1973).

20.2.5 Treatment

As already mentioned, symptoms and signs classically clear up on going down to sea-level. However, many patients want to remain at altitude for family or economic reasons. In these cases, venesection is beneficial. Venesection not only lowers the raised haematocrit but also improves many of the neuropsychological symptoms. It also improves pulmonary gas exchange (Cruz *et al.*, 1979) and exercise performance in some subjects (Winslow and Monge, 1987b). In Leadville, Colorado, with about sixty patients being regularly bled for therapeutic purposes, the blood bank has no need of any other donors! (Kryger *et al.*, 1978a).

An alternative to venesection for residents at high altitude is the long term use of respiratory stimulants. Kryger *et al.* (1978b) have reported success with medroxyprogesterone acetate. They showed a fall in [Hb] after 10 weeks' treatment in 17 patients. The drug increased ventilation and P_{O_2}, and reduced P_{CO_2} by a modest amount. Although the changes in blood gases were small they suggest that the main benefit may have been in oxygenation at night since hypoxaemia may be much greater then. The only side-effect reported was of loss of libido in four patients. In all but one, this could be overcome by lowering the dose to a level that still kept the [Hb] down. In one patient the dose had to be reduced to a point which did not hold down the [Hb].

There do not seem to have been any reported trials of other stimulants such as acectazolamide which has been shown to be effective in preventing acute mountain sickness (Chapter 17).

20.3 EPIDEMIOLOGY OF CMS

20.3.1 Andes

The condition is found most commonly in the Andes, where it was first described, mainly affecting the local American-Indian, especially the Quechuan population living on the altiplano at altitudes about 3300–

4500 m. Men are affected far more commonly than women. The average age is 40 years with a range from 22 to 51 in one reported series (Penaloza *et al.*, 1971). Occasional cases are seen in ex-patriot mining company staff. It used to be thought that CMS was virtually confined to the Andes (Heath and Williams, 1981) but this is not the case, as is discussed below.

20.3.2 Himalayas and Tibet

Until recently there have been few reported cases of CMS in the Himalayas. Winslow noted one Sherpa on the American Medical Research Expedition to Everest to have a haematocrit of 72% (Winslow and Monge, 1987c).

Pei *et al.* (1989) describe their experience of CMS in Lhasa (3600 m), Tibet. The condition is not uncommon amongst male cigarette-smoking Han Chinese. These subjects had immigrated for some years, before becoming polycythaemic and then displayed the usual signs and symptoms of CMS. In a 12-month period there were 24 patients admitted to their hospital with CMS; all were male, 23 were Han and only one Tibetan. Six were non-smokers, the rest, including the one Tibetan, were smokers. The mean duration of altitude exposure in the lowlanders was 26 years (range 9–43). However, though the incidence in Tibetans may be less than Han immigrants, CMS is now being reported in this population. Wu *et al.* (1992) reported a series of 26 cases in native born Tibetans living at between 3680 m and 4179 m with typical symptoms of CMS and [Hb] of 22.2 g dl^{-1} mean compared with 16.6 g dl^{-1} in healthy controls at the same altitude.

In Himalayan residents, haemoglobin concentration tends to be lower than the values from the Peruvian Andes, although much of this difference disappears if results from mining towns are excluded (Frisancho, 1988). It is speculated that this may be because the geography allows residents to move to lower altitudes more easily than from the altiplano of the Andes, and the way of life of the Sherpas, with seasonal migration, contributes to this movement in altitude. Like the Andes, Tibetans live on a high-altitude plain and cannot easily move up and down.

Although more evidence is needed it would seem that people of Tibetan stock are less at risk of CMS than Andean highlanders, and certainly than lowland Han subjects long resident at altitude. This may be due to genuine genetic adaptation to altitude over very many generations.

20.3.3 North America

The condition is well recognized in Leadville, Colorado (3100 m) and Kryger *et al.* (1978a) described 20 cases, all male, and mentioned that, of about 60 cases known to physicians there, only two were female. One case of apparently classical CMS in a 67-year-old woman has been reported from as low as 2000 m in California (Gronbeck, 1984).

20.4 TERMINOLOGY

20.4.1 Polycythaemia of altitude

Opinions differ about the haemoglobin value required for diagnosis of CMS. A value of 23.0 g dl^{-1} has been used, but it would seem wiser to take into account the normal value and range for that particular altitude (Chapter 7), and even then, any given value is rather arbitrary. Indeed, it has been argued that CMS does not represent a distinct entity at all and that the haemoglobin values represent merely the 'tail' of a normal distribution curve (Monge and Whittembury, 1976). For practical purposes, a value of two standard deviations above the mean for that altitude can be considered the cut-off for 'normal'. The 'tail' population may then be considered abnormal and polycythaemic for that altitude. Since at this value symptoms occur, treatment is indicated and therefore this definition has practical implications.

This concept is in line with the conclusions of a monograph on CMS by Winslow and Monge (1987d), who define it in term of a haematocrit 'above the statistical maximum for the altitude in question'. However they also draw attention to the work of Cosio who found important differences in [Hb] between two populations living in two towns at the same altitude (4600 m) (Winslow and Monge, 1987e). This illustrates the difficulty of assigning a 'normal' value for a given altitude.

20.4.2 Lung disease and polycythaemia

It is well known that hypoxic lung disease causes polycythaemia in patients even at sea-level. Many patients in the mining towns of the Andean altiplano smoke and work in dusty occupations. Is their polycythaemia simply secondary to lung disease which has greater effect because of the altitude? Arias-Stella (1971) initiated discussion at the Ciba Symposium on high altitude physiology with a paper describing a post-mortem on a woman with CMS and kyphoscoliosis. He suggested the use of the term 'Monge's syndrome' for cases like this, where there was lung or chest wall disease as a primary cause, and 'Monge's disease' proper for cases with no lung disease. The challenge was thrown out for some pathologist to report a case of polycythaemia in which lung disease had been excluded by rigorous modern pathological methods. This challenge has yet to be taken up. The usage of 'Monge's syndrome' has not been generally adopted and most workers simply refer to patients as having CMS, Monge's or polycythaemia of high altitude, with or without overt lung disease.

20.5 MECHANISMS OF CMS

20.5.1 CMS with lung disease

In cases of CMS with definite lung disease, it is easy to understand that the combination of altitude with fairly mild lung disease precipitates polycythaemia and cor pulmonale. Removal of altitude hypoxia by descent to sea-level is sufficient to reverse the process. At altitude, these patients are more hypoxic than normal people because of their lung disease, hence their stimulus to erythrocytosis via erythropoietin secretion is greater and they become abnormally polycythaemic.

20.5.2 CMS with normal lungs

The mechanism in cases with apparently normal lungs is less clear.

Hypoxic ventilatory response (HVR)

Severinghaus *et al.* (1966) found that such patients have an extremely blunted HVR compared with healthy resident controls of the same (mean) age. Maybe people at the low end of the spectrum for HVR in the population are destined to get CMS if they remain for years at altitude. The HVR decreases with age (Kronenberg and Drage, 1973) and with duration of stay at altitude (Wiel *et al.*, 1971) perhaps patients with CMS are those in whom the process is faster than average.

Kryger *et al.* (1978a), however, found no difference in HVR between patients and age matched controls in Leadville, Colorado. They did find their patients had a greater dead-space/tidal volume ratio and that their ventilation increased on breathing 100% oxygen; they therefore appeared to have hypoxic ventilatory depression. They concluded that blunted chemical drive to breathing is not the cause of CMS.

Sleep

During sleep, even in normal subjects, the ventilation is depressed. If there are frequent periods of apnoea, either central or obstructive, Sa_{O_2} will be further reduced and could contribute to the aetiology.

Gender

Women (at least before the menopause) seem to be protected from CMS as from the hypoventilation syndrome (the Pickwickian syndrome) at sea-level, possibly by the stimulating effect of female sex hormones on ventilation.

Age

Age has effects on lung function apart from its effect on HVR. The Pa_{O_2} declines with age and, while this has little effect on oxygen saturation (Sa_{O_2}) at sea-level, it has much more effect at altitude because subjects are already on the steep part of the oxygen dissociation curve. A recent study by Leon-Velarde *et al.* (1993) at 4300 m in Peru, finds an increasing incidence of CMS with age. Taking a [Hb] of above 21.3 g dl^{-1} (the mean plus 2 SD of the total population aged 20–29 years) as 'excessive erythrocytosis', the incidence at 20–29 years was 6.8% which increased to 33.7% at age 60–69 years. This study also found a decreasing vital capacity with age at altitude, in both those with and without CMS, but the reduction was significantly more marked in the CMS group. Sea-level subjects showed no reduction in vital capacity between 20–29 and 60–69 years.

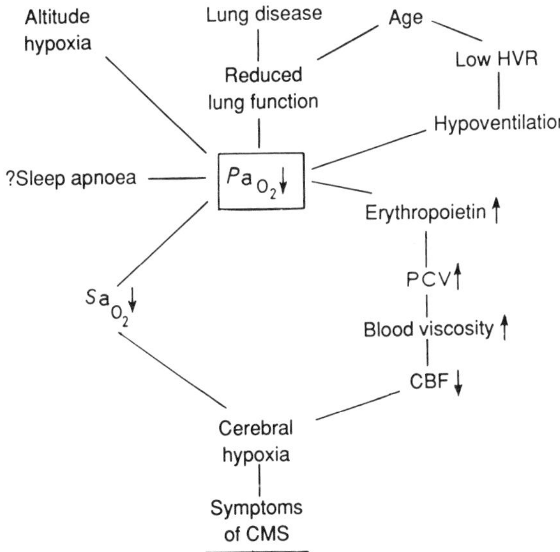

Figure 20.1 Possible mechanisms in the development of chronic mountain sickness (CMS). HVR, hypoxic ventilatory response; CBF, cerebral blood flow; PCV, packed cell volume.

Polycythaemia results in reduced cerebral blood flow (Thomas *et al.*, 1977) due to increased viscosity. There do not seem to have been studies of CBF in CMS but there is no reason to doubt the assumption that it is reduced.

Figure 20.1 shows the interaction of factors involved in CMS. Altitude hypoxia and hypoventilation will result in a low Pa_{O_2}. This hypoventilatory response may be due to a low HVR, to hypoxic depression of ventilation or some unknown cause. If lung function is also reduced by lung or chest wall disease, this will reduce Pa_{O_2} still further. Ageing results in both reduced lung function and reduced HVR, especially in a life spent at high altitude, thus further lowering the Pa_{O_2}.

The low Pa_{O_2} results in a low Sa_{O_2}. It also stimulates secretion of erythropoietin and hence an increase in packed cell volume. Although it should be noted that a study of erythropoietin levels in subjects at Cerro de Pasco (4300 m), whilst showing the expected higher mean values at altitude than sea-level, did not demonstrate any difference between subjects with and without CMS (Leon-Velarde *et al.*, 1991). The rise in packed cell volume causes a rise in blood viscosity and a fall in cerebral blood flow, which, with a low Sa_{O_2}, results in chronic severe cerebral hypoxia and symptoms of CMS.

REFERENCES

Arias-Stella, J. (1971) Chronic mountain sickness: pathology and definition, in *High Altitude Physiology: Cardiac and Respiratory Aspects*, Ciba Foundation Symposium, (eds R. Porter and J. Knight), Churchill Livingstone, Edinburgh, pp. 31–40.

Arias-Stella, J., Kruger, H. and Reavarren, S. (1973) Pathology of chronic mountain sickness. *Thorax*, **28**, 701–8.

Cruz, J.C., Diaz, C., Marticorena, E. and Hilario, V. (1979) Phlebotomy improves pulmonary gas exchange in chronic mountain polycythemia. *Respiration*, **38**, 305–13.

Frisancho, A.R. (1988) Origins of differences in haemoglobin concentration between Himalayan and Andean populations. *Respir. Physiol.*, **72**, 13–18.

Gronbeck, C. (1984) Chronic mountain sickness at an elevation of 2000 metres. *Chest*, **85**, 577–8.

Heath, D. and Williams, D.R. (1981) Monge's disease, in *Man at High Altitude*, 2nd edn, Churchill Livingstone, Edinburgh, pp. 169–79.

Hurtado, A. (1942) Chronic mountain sickness. *J. Am. Med. Assoc.*, **120**, 1278–82.

Kronenberg, R.S. and Drage, C.W. (1973) Attenuation of the ventilatory and heart rate responses to hypoxia and hypercapnia with aging in normal men. *J. Clin. Invest.*, **52**, 1812–19.

Kryger, M., McCullough, R.E., Doekel, R., *et al.* (1978a) Excessive polycythemia of high altitude: role of ventilatory drive and lung disease. *Am. Rev. Respir. Dis.*, **118**, 659–65.

Kryger, M., McCullough, R.E., Collins, D., *et al.* (1978b) Treatment of excessive polycythemia of high altitude with respiratory stimulant drugs. *Am. Rev. Respir. Dis.*, **117**, 455–64.

Leon-Velarde, F., Monge, C.C., Vidal, A., *et al.* (1991) Serum immunoreactive erythropoietin in high altitude natives with and without excessive erythrocytosis. *Exp. Hematol.*, **19**, 257–60.

Leon-Velarde, F., Arregui, A., Monge, C., Ruiz, H. (1993) Ageing at high altitude and the risk of chronic mountain sickness. *J. Wild. Med.*, **4**, 183–8.

Manier, G., Guenard, H., Castaing, Y., *et al.* (1988) Pulmonary gas exchange in Andean natives with excessive polycythemia – effect of hemodilution. *J. Appl. Physiol.*, **65**, 2107–17.

Monge, C.C. and Whittembury, J. (1976) Chronic mountain sickness. *Johns Hopkins Med. J.*, **139**, 87–9.

Pei, S.X., Chen, X.J., Si Ren, B.Z., *et al.* (1989) Chronic mountain sickness in Tibet. *Q. J. Med.*, **71**, 555–74.

Penaloza, D. and Sime, F. (1971) Chronic cor pulmonale due to loss of altitude acclimatization (chronic mountain sickness). *Am. J. Med.*, **50**, 728–43.

Penaloza, D., Sime, F. and Ruiz, L. (1971) Cor pulmonale in chronic mountain sickness: Present concept of Monge's disease, in *High Altitude Physiology: Cardiac and Respiratory Aspects*, Ciba Foundation Symposium, (eds R. Porter and J. Knight), Churchill Livingstone, Edinburgh, 41–60.

Severinghaus, J.W., Bainton, C.K. and Carcelen, A. (1966) Respiratory insensitivity to hypoxia in chronically hypoxic man. *Respir. Physiol.*, **1**, 308–34.

Talbott, J.H. and Dill, D.B. (1936) Clinical observations at high altitude: Observations on six healthy persons living at 17 500 feet and a report of one case of chronic mountain sickness. *Am. J. Med. Sci.*, **192**, 626–9.

Tewari, S.C., Jayaswal, R., Kasturi, A.S., *et al.* (1991) Excessive polycythaemia of high altitude. Pulmonary function studies including carbon monoxide diffusion capacity. *J. Assoc. Physicians India*, **39**, 453–5.

Thomas, D.J., Marshall, J., Ross Russell, R.W., *et al.* (1977) Cerebral blood-flow in polycythaemia. *Lancet*, **2**, 161–3.

Wiel, J.V., Byrne-Quinn, E., Ingvar, E., *et al.* (1971) Acquired attenuation of chemoreceptor function in chronically hypoxic man at high altitude. *J. Clin. Invest.*, **50**, 186–95.

Winslow, R.M. and Monge, C.C. (1987a) Hypoxia, polycythemia, and chronic mountain sickness. Johns Hopkins University Press, Baltimore, p. 15.

Winslow, R.M. and Monge, C.C. (1987b) Hypoxia, polycythemia, and chronic mountain sickness. Johns Hopkins University Press, Baltimore, p. 212.

Winslow, R.M. and Monge, C.C. (1987c) Hypoxia, polycythemia, and chronic mountain sickness. Johns Hopkins University Press, Baltimore, p. 17.

Winslow, R.M. and Monge, C.C. (1987d) Hypoxia, polycythemia, and chronic mountain sickness. Johns Hopkins University Press, Baltimore, p. 204.

Winslow, R.M. and Monge, C.C. (1987e) Hypoxia, polycythemia, and chronic mountain sickness. Johns Hopkins University Press, Baltimore, p. 37.

Wu, T.-Y., Zhang, Q., Jin, B., *et al.* (1992) Chronic mountain sickness (Monge's disease): an observation in Quinghai–Tibet plateau, in *High Altitude Medicine*, (eds G. Ueda, J.T. Reeves and M. Sekiguchi), Sinshu University Press, Matsumoto, pp. 314–24.

21

Vascular disorders

21.1 HISTORICAL BACKGROUND

Sporadic cases of vascular disorders have been described in the mountain and geographical literature over the last century (Table 21.1).

In 1895, whilst exploring the Anne Machin range in eastern Tibet, Roborowsky, a Russian traveller, suffered a 'stroke' whilst crossing the Mangur Pass (4300 m). He described 'a stroke of paralysis which attacked the right part of my body from head to the toes of my right foot; my tongue hardly obeyed my will. I lay in a disgusting and unbearable state for eight days'. Over the next few weeks he gradually recovered and continued his journey (Roborowsky, 1896).

Cases of hemiplegia also occurred on Everest expeditions in 1924 and 1936. One, a Gurkha soldier, died, and the other, a Sherpa porter, recovered (Norton, 1925; Tilman, 1948). A further fatal case of hemiplegia in a Sherpa was recorded by Evans (1956) on Kanchenjunga. Each of these three cases was in a fit young man who had spent a considerable period above 6000 m.

In 1954, whilst stormbound in a tent at 7465 m on K2 (Mt Godwin Austen) a young American mountaineer developed thrombophlebitis in the calf, and, after a further two days, had a haemoptysis. A provisional diagnosis of pulmonary embolus was made and he was evacuated; however, during the descent he was swept away in an avalanche (Houston and Bates, 1979).

Transient aphasia with severe headache, possibly due to migraine, has been reported by Shipton (1943), who described an episode in himself which occurred after climbing to 8565 m. Apart from severe headache he had no other symptoms and was fully recovered by the next morning (Jenzer and Bärtsch, 1993).

Coronary and cerebral thrombosis and cases of phlebitis of the limbs have been reported (Fujimaki *et al.*, 1986), as have transient ischaemic attacks and transient blindness (Wohns, 1987; Hackett *et al.*, 1987).

Table 21.1 Cerebrovascular accidents at altitude. All subjects were male adults. The two patients who died were Sherpas; the remainder were climbers from low altitude

Date	*Altitude (m)*	*Time at altitude*	*Signs*	*Outcome*	*Source*
1895	4300	?	Right hemiparesis	Recovered	Roborovsky, 1896
1924	6000	?	Hemiparesis	Died	Norton, 1925
1938	6400	?	Right hemiparesis	Recovered	Tilman, 1948
1943	6400	6 weeks	Dysphasia	Recovered	Shipton, 1943
1954	6000+	?	Hemiparesis	Died	Evans, 1956
1961	6400	7–8 weeks	Right hemiparesis	Recovered	Ward, 1968
1978	6400	?	Hemiparesis	?	Messner, 1979
1982	8200	7 weeks	Left hemiparesis	Recovered	Clarke, 1983
1983	6100	?	Semi-conscious	Recovered	Asaji *et al.*, 1984
1990	4800	9 days	Right hemiparesis	Recovered	Sharma *et al.*, 1990

21.2 PLATELETS AND CLOTTING AT ALTITUDE

In view of the frequent finding of thrombi in various organs at post-mortem in cases of AMS and its complications (Dickinson *et al.*, 1983), and cases of cerebrovascular accidents at altitude, there has been considerable interest in factors in the blood associated with clotting, and the effect of hypoxia, with and without symptoms of AMS, on these systems.

21.2.1 Platelet counts at altitude

In mice, there is a profound fall in platelet count on exposure to hypoxia. Counts are down to 36% of control by the twelfth day (Birks *et al.*, 1975). In humans, no such fall has been found. It has been reported that in the first few days there is either no change (Maher *et al.*, 1976; Sharma, 1982), or a small fall of 3% in subjects with AMS and a rise of 3% in asymptomatic subjects (Sharma, 1980). Chatterji *et al.* (1982) found a 12–26% reduction in platelet count on the second or third day at altitude in two studies at 3200 m and 3700 m. Counts increased towards control values over the next ten days. These small changes may simply reflect haemoconcentration or dilution. With more prolonged exposure Sharma (1981) found a 14% increase by 21–31 days followed by a fall to sea-level values at 180 days. At 4300 m, a rise of between 50% and 100% has been found, both on arrival and two weeks later, after climbs to higher altitude (Simon-Schnass *et al.*, 1990).

21.2.2 Platelet adhesiveness

Under a variety of conditions platelets become more sticky and this property may be important in initiating platelet thrombi. The effect of altitude on platelet adhesiveness has also been studied by Sharma (1982). On acute exposure to altitude he reported an increase in platelet adhesiveness in subjects with AMS, compared with their sea-level results. However, this was only on days two and ten of altitude exposure and not on days one and four. Also, the sea-level values for symptomatic subjects were markedly less than for the asymptomatic group. Actual values at altitude were the same for both groups. He also reported (with others) that high altitude residents had significantly higher platelet adhesiveness than lowlanders at sea-level (Sharma *et al.*, 1980).

21.2.3 Coagulation at altitude

Singh and Chohan (1972a) found an increase in fibrinogen level and fibrinolytic activity in 38 subjects at altitudes between 3670 m and 5470 m, but, in six subjects thought to have pulmonary hypertension on clinical grounds, the fibrinogen levels were lower, suggesting consumption coagulopathy. In these patients, factors V and VIII were increased, as was platelet factor III. Maher *et al.* (1976) also found a fall in fibrinogen level in eight subjects in a simulated altitude of 4400 m but no change in thrombin or prothrombin times; platelet factor III was normal. Partial thromboplastin time was shortened and factor VIII activity was reduced. Hyers *et al.* (1979) found accelerated fibrinolytic activity in subjects with and without susceptibility to AMS but no change in fibrinogen, partial prothrombin time, platelet lysis time or fibrinopeptide A. In patients with high-altitude pulmonary edema, fibrinogen levels and venous clot lysis time have been reported to be increased (Singh *et al.*, 1969; Singh and Chohan, 1972a).

Bärtsch *et al.* (1982) showed, in 20 subjects taken rapidly to 3700 m, that there were no changes in coagulation tests one hour after arrival. After strenuous exercise there was shortening of clotting time, euglobulin lysis time, increase in factor VIII activity – changes which are all found on exercise at sea-level. There was no change in fibrinopeptide A and no rise in fibrin degradation products or fibrin fragment E (i.e. no evidence of intravascular clotting). In a later project the contact phase of blood coagulation was studied in subjects who had ascended to 4559 m in three days. There was no evidence of activation of this system even in subjects who developed acute pulmonary edema of high altitude (Bärtsch *et al.*, 1989).

An extensive study of the clotting cascade during a 40-day chamber experiment, Operation Everest II, when subjects were taken in stages up to the simulated equivalent altitude of Mt Everest, showed no significant changes in clotting factors, though thrombosis round the sites of Swan–Ganz catheters was common (Andrew *et al.*, 1987).

In summary, it seems that the physiological response to hypoxia has not been shown to involve any important changes in platelet count or adhesiveness nor in other clotting factors. However, there may be changes associated with AMS and especially HAPE (Singh and Chohan, 1972b). These may include changes suggesting disseminated intravascular coagulation but this is still not proved. The changes so far demonstrated seem to appear rather too late in the course of altitude exposure to be considered causative, so, even if present, they may represent an effect or a complication of AMS rather than being essential in its genesis.

21.3 SYSTEMIC BLOOD PRESSURE

21.3.1 High-altitude native

The systemic blood pressure of high-altitude natives is low, at least in South America, Bhutan and Nepal. In populations on the Tibetan plateau, however, many cases of hypertension have been recorded (Chapter 16, for a fuller discussion and references).

21.3.2 High-altitude visitor

Bulstrode (1975) reports that, on walking to 4880 m, the systolic pressure fell but this was reversed on return to lower levels. The fall in systolic pressure was more marked in the acclimatized than the unacclimatized, and the changes in diastolic pressure were not so large as systolic pressure fluctuations. However, in recent unpublished work on Pikes Peak (4300 m), by Milledge and Ward, in eight subjects, the systolic pressure increased on ascent and remained raised (a mean systolic of 121 mmHg by comparison with the pre-ascent value of 103 mmHg). On descent, after three weeks, to Colorado Springs the systolic pressure fell to a mean of 109 mmHg within 36 h. The diastolic pressure showed no significant change. At altitude the post-exercise blood pressure was always lower than the pre-exercise and this was found at all stages of the study but it was not observed at sea-level.

Low blood pressures were recorded in individuals returning from the summit of Everest in 1953, but these may have been due to exhaustion (Pugh and Ward, 1956). Richalet (1983) also found lower blood pressures on arrival at altitude, but this was 20 mmHg higher on return to base camp after climbing to 6956 m.

21.4 SPLINTER HAEMORRHAGES AT ALTITUDE

Splinter haemorrhages may occur under the finger nails of high-altitude natives, and are more pronounced in those with CMS and in climbers at extreme altitude (English, 1987). In South American high-altitude dwellers, the incidence appears to increase with altitude, rising from 34.9% at 150 m to 57.9% at 4200 m (Heath and Williams, 1981). In over 1000 healthy Chinese children born at altitude, examination of the nails showed an increase in number of capillary loops and abnormal loops (Han *et al.*, 1985). The cause of these haemorrhages may be associated with increased capillary fragility or it may be embolic or traumatic in origin.

21.5 RISK FACTORS FOR THROMBOSIS

These include decreased physical activity, dehydration, increased haematocrit and cold.

Physical activity may be greatly decreased at altitude. Individuals may spend several days recumbent in a sleeping bag in bad weather and, even in good weather, activity can be restricted by fatigue to a shorter working period each day than at lower levels.

Dehydration is common with increased respiratory water loss due to cold and a high respiratory rate. A diminished sensation of thirst, together with the practical difficulties of melting snow to produce water, results in an inadequate fluid intake.

A haematocrit of 45–60% is normal for sea-level visitors to altitude and some high-altitude residents. When the haematocrit exceeds 50% the apparent viscosity increases steeply. Vasoconstriction further increases viscosity and thus cold will contribute (Whittaker and Winton, 1933; Pappenheimer and Maes, 1942). Cold can also damage vessel walls and by causing coronary vasoconstriction may be implicated in 'heart attacks'. Cerebral venous thrombosis has been reported (Fujimaki *et al.*, 1986; Song *et al.*, 1986).

21.6 MECHANISMS

The mechanism of vascular accidents is debatable. Short lived attacks may be due to spasm, or possibly a manifestation of migraine. Thrombosis is another possibility, due to a high haematocrit and dehydration (Ward, 1975) whilst disturbances of coagulation and platelet function may also occur. In some cases haemorrhage cannot be ruled out. As with 'stroke' at lower altitudes, there may be different causes. However, the risk of a cardiovascular accident in an otherwise fit man at altitude, though small, would appear to be greater than would be expected from such a population at sea-level.

21.7 CASE HISTORIES

Patient A

A male Caucasian, aged 32, whilst climbing at 8400 m, suddenly experienced a severe pain in the right side of his chest and collapsed. He was unable to move for 30 min and then started to cough up dark red blood. After a night at 8200 m he crawled down to a lower camp at 7800 m, continuing to complain of severe pain and coughing up blood.

Three days later, that is five days after the initial incident, he reached camp at 7800 m. He was barely conscious and his feet and hands

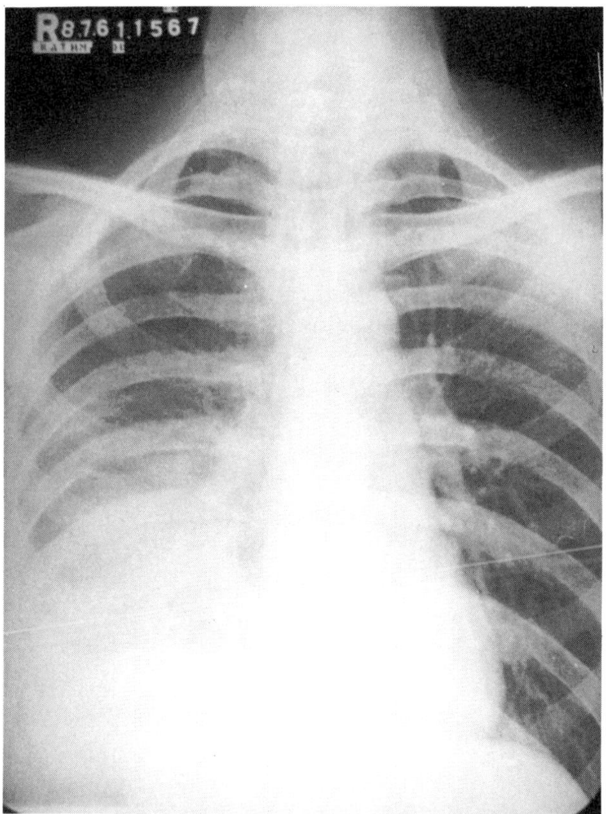

Figure 21.1 Patient A: thrombosis of the right lower lobe, which occurred at 8350 m.

were grey-white in colour and had the consistency of wood. He was evacuated to a camp at 6400 m where his general condition was poor and he was still coughing up blood. On examination, air entry at the base of the right lung was greatly diminished, and there was deep frostbite to both legs below the knees, but both popliteal and femoral arteries were palpable. Deep frost-bite was also present in the distal parts of all fingers and both thumbs.

In the next two days he was evacuated to 4600 m and then flown to hospital at 1100 m. Here a chest radiograph showed shadowing in the right lower zone, presumably an infarct. Later he developed a lung abscess in this part of the lung and then an empyema with broncho-pleural fistula. After a rib resection and drainage this resolved (Figures 21.1, 21.2, 21.3).

Eventually, bilateral below knee amputation was carried out and all finger tips on both hands were removed after mummification. There remained some scarring of the right hand with restriction of finger and thumb movement (Ward, 1968).

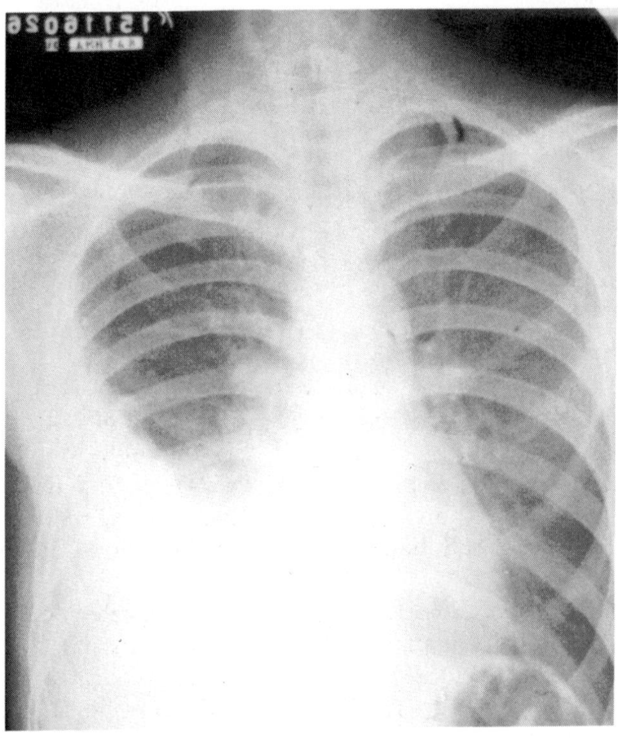

Figure 21.2 Patient A: after the development of a right pleural effusion.

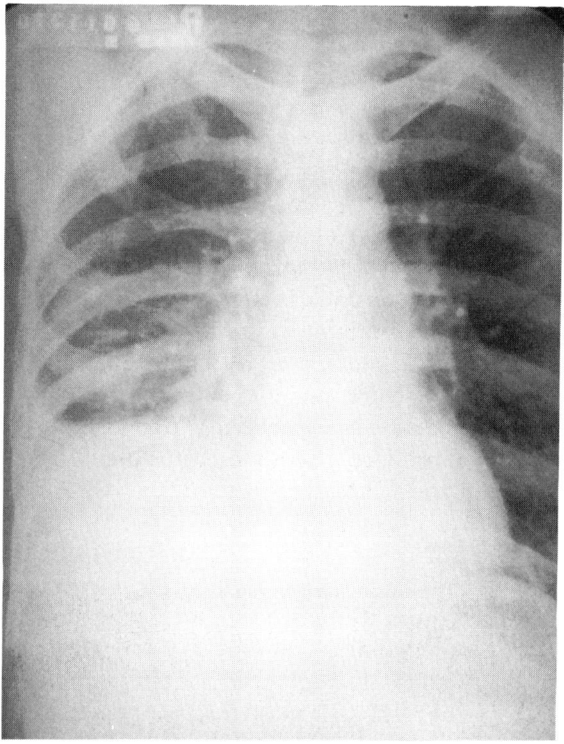

Figure 21.3 Patient A: after the development of a right pyopneumothorax and bronchopleural fistula.

Patient B

A male Caucasian climbed from 7850 m to 8750 m in 13 h using supplementary oxygen and then spent 35 min on the summit. He bivouacked for the night a few hundred metres lower. The night temperature was estimated at −30°C with winds gusting to 50–60 mph. During the night his supply of oxygen ran out and he shivered continuously. Later he estimated that he had had nothing to drink for 30 h while above 7900 m.

Next day he descended and developed a persistent cough. A day later he complained of pain in the left side of his chest and, when examined, was told that he had pneumonia and pleurisy. He continued to have chest pain and then four or five days later began coughing up blood. Eleven days after reaching the summit chest radiograph showed a left pleural effusion. Three days later he was admitted to hospital in the USA. Six weeks after the initial incident, at operation, a fibrous tissue mass occupying 50% of the lower half of the left thorax was excised. He made an uneventful recovery and postoperatively reached an altitude of 5800 m. His stamina has in no way been impaired (Wickwire, 1982).

Patient C

A male Caucasian, aged 40, complained of severe headache at 6400 m. This continued for three days being relieved by codeine tablets. By the evening of the third day he noticed that he could not speak properly. On examination he had nominal aphasia but could understand the spoken word. There was some evidence of right facial weakness with involuntary movements confined to the right side of the face. Both carotid arteries were palpable. There was loss of power in the right arm, but no loss of sensation. The lower limbs could not be examined as the patient was in a sleeping bag.

After sedation and continuous oxygen by mask for 8 hrs, he was able to descend to 5000 m, with some difficulty due to weakness of the arms and legs. For a further three days speech remained slurred, he was often at a loss for a word and individuals' names were mixed. After 15 days there were no residual signs and a note written at this time contained lucid statements and logical arguments; his writing was normal. There appeared to be no permanent after-effects (Ward, 1968).

21.8 MANAGEMENT

21.8.1 Prevention

Adequate hydration is extremely important and, as the majority of mountaineers at extreme altitudes appear to be dehydrated, the danger of thrombosis occurring probably increases with length of stay.

Posture too may be significant, particularly whilst bivouacking, when the 'foetal' position is assumed to prevent too much heat loss. As the knees, hips and arms are kept flexed there is an increased risk of thrombosis, so arm and leg stretching should be carried out regularly. Lying in a sleeping bag, particularly if the calves are constricted, may lead to the formation of 'silent' calf thrombosis. Regular movement is therefore important. Women are advised not to take oral contraceptives at altitude.

In subjects with an abnormally high haematocrit (e.g. over 0.65), after adequate hydration, venesection should be considered if the subject plans to remain at altitude. Haemodilution has been used for treating polycythaemia in mountaineers; it is considered to be a potentially hazardous manoeuvre (Sarnquist *et al.*, 1986).

21.8.2 Treatment

Treatment will depend upon the diagnosis but all patients will benefit from descent and hydration.

Oxygen may improve those who are severely shocked.

Anticoagulants are potentially dangerous and adequate laboratory facilities should be available before use. However, in exceptional circumstances in cases of thrombosis and, if the physician is experienced, small doses of a short acting anticoagulant may be given.

Return to altitude after a vascular episode should be considered with caution but some have returned with future expeditions to climb at high altitude without recurrence of symptoms.

REFERENCES

Andrew, M., O'Brodovitch, H. and Sutton, J. (1987) Operation Everest II; Coagulation system during prolonged decompression to 282 Torr. *J. Appl. Physiol.*, **63**, 1262–7.

Asaji, T., Sakurai, E., Tanizaki, Y., *et al.* (1984) Report on medical aspects of Mount Lhotse and Everest expedition in 1983: with special reference to a case of cerebral venous thrombosis in the altitude. *Jpn. J. Mount. Med.*, **4**, 98.

Bärtsch, P., Schmidt, E.K. and Straub, P.W. (1982) Fibrinopeptide A after strenuous physical exercise at high altitude. *J. Appl. Physiol.*, **53**, 40–3.

Bärtsch, P., Lammle, B., Huber, I., *et al.* (1989) Contact phase of blood coagulation is not activated in edema of high altitude. *J. Appl. Physiol.*, **67**, 1336–40.

Birks, J.W., Klassen, L.W. and Gurney, C.W. (1975) Hypoxia induced thrombocytopenia in mice. *J. Lab. Clin. Med.*, **86**, 230–8.

Bulstrode, C.J.K. (1975) A preliminary study into factors predisposing mountaineers to high altitude pulmonary oedema. *J. R. Nav. Med. Serv.*, **61**, 101–5.

Chatterji, J.C., Ohri, V.C., Das, B.K., *et al.* (1982) Platelet count, platelet aggregation and fibrinogen levels following acute induction to high altitude (3200 and 3771 metres). *Thromb. Res.*, **26**, 177–82.

Clarke, C.R.A. (1983) Cerebral infarction at extreme altitude, in *Hypoxia, Exercise and Altitude*, (eds J.R. Sutton, C.S. Houston and N.L. Jones), Liss, New York, pp. 453–4.

Dickinson, J., Heath, D., Gosney, J. and Williams, D. (1983) Altitude related deaths in seven trekkers in the Himalayas. *Thorax*, **38**, 646–56.

English, J.S.C. (1987) High altitude and the skin, in *Abstracts of the UIAA Mountain Medicine Conference*, Mountain Medicine Data Centre, St Bartholemew's Hospital, London, p. 20.

Evans, R.C. (1956) *Kanchenjunga. The Untrodden Peak*, Hodder and Stoughton, London, p. 169.

Fujimaki, T., Matsutani, M., Asai, A., *et al.* (1986) Cerebral venous thrombosis due to high altitude polycythaemia: Case report. *J. Neurosurg.*, **64**, 148–50.

Hackett, P.H., Hollingsmead, K.F., Roach, R., *et al.* (1987) Cortical blindness in high altitude climbers and trekkers. A report of six cases, in *Hypoxia and Cold*, (eds J.R. Sutton, C.S. Houston and G. Coates), Praeger, New York, p. 536.

Han, J.L., Chen, D.X. and Chen, G.J. (1985) The investigation of nail fold microcirculation in 1–13 year old healthy children at different altitudes, in *Abstracts of the Second High Altitude Medicine Symposium*, Quinghai, China, p. 44.

Heath, D. and Williams, D.R. (1981) *Man at High Altitude*, 2nd edn, Churchill Livingstone, London, pp. 323–4.

Houston, C.S. and Bätes, R. (1979) *K2, The Savage Mountain*, McGraw-Hill, New York, pp. 180–99.

Hyers, T.M., Scoggin, C.H., Will, D.H., *et al.* (1979) Accentuated hypoxemia at high altitude in subjects susceptible to high-altitude pulmonary edema. *J. Appl. Physiol. Respir. Environ. Exercise Physiol.*, **46**, 41–6.

Jenzer, G. and Bärtsch, P. (1993) Migraine with aura at high altitude: Case report. *J. Wild. Med.*, **4**, 412–15.

Maher, J.T., Levine, P.H. and Cymerman, A. (1976) Human coagulation abnormalities during acute exposure to hypobaric hypoxia. *J. Appl. Physiol.*, **41**, 702–7.

Messner, R. (1979) *Everest: Expedition to the Ultimate*, Kaye and Ward, London, p. 137.

Norton, E.F. (1925) *The Fight for Everest*, Arnold, London, p. 68.

Pappenheimer, J.R. and Maes, J.P. (1942) A quantitative measure of the vasomotor tone in the hind limb muscles of the dog. *Am. J. Physiol.*, **137**, 187–99.

Pugh, L.G.C.E. and Ward, M.P. (1956) Some effects of high altitude in man. *Lancet*, **2**, 1115–24.

Richalet, J.P. (1983) The French scientific expedition to Numbur, Autumn 1981, in *Hypoxia, Exercise and Altitude*, (eds J.R. Sutton, C.S. Houston and N.L. Jones), Liss, New York, pp. 189–95.

Roborovsky (1896) The Central Asian Expedition of Capt. Roborovsky and Lt. Kozloff. *Geogr. J.*, **8**, 161.

Sarnquist, F.H., Schoene, R.B., Hackett, P.H. and Townes, B.D. (1986) Hemodilution of polycythemic mountaineers: effect on exercise and mental function. *Aviat. Space Environ. Med.*, **57**, 313–17.

Sharma, S.C. (1980) Platelet count on acute induction to high altitude. *Thromb. Haemost.*, **43**, 24.

Sharma, S.C. (1981) Platelet adhesiveness in temporary residents of high altitude. *Thromb. Res.*, **21**, 685–7.

Sharma, S.C. (1982) Platelet count and adhesiveness on induction to high altitude by air and road. *Int. J. Biometeorol.*, **26**, 219–24.

Sharma, S.C., Balasubramanian, V. and Chadha, K.S. (1980) Platelet adhesiveness in permanent residents of high altitude. *Thromb. Haemost.*, **42**, 1508–12.

Sharma, A., Sharma, P.D., Malhotra, H.S., *et al.* (1990) Hemiplegia as a manifestation of acute mountain sickness. *J. Assoc. Physicians India*, **38**, 662–4.

Shipton, E. (1943) *Upon That Mountain*, Hodder and Stoughton, London, pp. 129–30.

Simon-Schnass, I. and Korniszewski, L. (1990) The influence of vitamin E on rheological parameters in high altitude mountaineers. *Int. J. Vit. Nutr. Res.*, **60**, 26–34.

Singh, I., Chohan, I.S. and Mathew, N.T. (1969) Fibrinolytic activity in high altitude pulmonary oedema. *Indian J. Med. Res.*, **57**, 210–17.

Singh, I. and Chohan, I.S. (1972a) Abnormalities of blood coagulation at high altitude. *Int. J. Biometerol.*, **16**, 283.

Singh, I. and Chohan, I.S. (1972b) Blood coagulation at high altitude predisposing to pulmonary hypertension. *Br Heart J.*, **34**, 611–17.

Song, S.Y., Asaji, T., Tanizaki, Y., *et al.* (1986) Cerebral thrombosis at altitude. Its pathogenesis and the problems of prevention and treatment. *Aviat. Space, Environ. Med.*, **57**, 71–6.

Tilman, H.W. (1948) *Mount Everest, 1938*, Cambridge University Press, Cambridge, pp. 93–4.

Ward, M.P. (1968) *Diseases occurring at altitudes exceeding 17 500 ft*, MD thesis, University of Cambridge, Cambridge, pp. 66–9.

Ward, M.P. (1975) Thrombosis, in *Mountain Medicine, a Clinical Study of Cold and High Altitude*, Crosby Lockwood Staples, London, pp. 289–92.

Whittaker, S.R.F. and Winton, F.R. (1933) The apparent viscosity of blood flowing in the isolated hind limb of the dog and its variation with corpuscular concentration. *J. Physiol.*, **78**, 339–69.

Wickwire, J. (1982) Pulmonary embolus and/or pneumonia on K2, in *Hypoxia, Man at Altitude*, (eds J.R. Sutton, N.L. Jones and C.S. Houston), Thieme-Stratton, New York, pp. 173–6.

Wohns, R.N.W. (1987) Transient ischaemic attacks at high altitude, in *Hypoxia and Cold*, (eds J.R. Sutton, C.S. Houston and G. Coates), Praeger, New York, p. 536.

22

Thermal balance and its regulation

22.1 GENERAL PRINCIPLES

For the past 70 million years mammals (homeotherms) have developed a system of temperature regulation which keeps the core temperature between 36°C and 38°C to maintain cell function. This enables them to be almost independent of the temperature of the environment which may vary from +40°C to −40°C, and is therefore of considerable evolutionary advantage. The price that is paid is a relatively high metabolic rate compared with poikilotherms, or cold blooded animals, whose core temperature is more closely allied to that of the environment.

To maintain cell function, the core temperature of man has to remain within a narrow band, though small variations occur during the menstrual cycle, the circadian rhythm and fever. A core temperature higher than 41°C (hyperthermia) or lower than 35°C (hypothermia) may cause death.

The relationship between heat production by the body and heat loss to the environment obeys two physical laws.

Fournier's law

This states that the rate of heat transfer between an object (or animal) and the environment is proportional to its surface area and the difference in temperature between the body and the environment. As all living organisms produce heat by metabolism and, since heat flows from a hot to a cold object, all living animals who usually have a higher body temperature than the environmental temperature will therefore lose heat to the environment.

When heat production is exactly balanced by heat loss a steady state temperature will have been achieved. As poikilotherms have no control mechanisms to alter the relationship between heat loss and heat production, their metabolic rate, body temperature and activity will be dependent on the environmental temperature.

Arrhenius's law

Put simply, this states that, as temperature increases, so does the metabolic rate and therefore the rate of heat production.

22.2 REGULATION OF CORE TEMPERATURE

Two main mechanisms regulate core temperature and keep it at 37°C. There are physiological or reflex mechanisms which are involuntary, and behavioral mechanisms which are voluntary.

22.2.1 Physiological mechanisms

Physical

These include vasomotor control, which can alter blood flow to the skin by a factor of more than 100, and sweat production. In the cold, to reduce heat loss from the periphery, blood is shunted from the surface to the deeper vessels. Conversely, as the ambient temperature rises, so more blood flows through the surface vessels to dissipate heat.

When the ambient temperature is higher than the temperature of the body surface, and heat loss by radiation, conduction and convection is not possible, then active sweat production starts and heat is lost by evaporation.

Thus by physical means alone humans can tolerate a wide range of environmental temperatures and still maintain a constant core temperature.

Chemical

These mechanisms enable adjustments of metabolism to be made by hormonal and neural methods. These come into play when physical methods have been overtaxed, for example, when maximal vasoconstriction has taken place but heat loss remains larger than heat production.

First, muscle tone is increased, then muscle tremors occur and finally shivering starts. Intense shivering can raise the metabolic rate by three to four times the basal level. Heat is produced very efficiently as no external work is done and virtually all the energy from contraction is produced as heat within the muscle. In addition, non-shivering thermogenesis can increase basal metabolism by 30–40%.

In humans, therefore, physiological mechanisms alone are capable of maintaining a constant core temperature at widely varying environmental temperatures.

22.2.2 Behavioural mechanisms

These include all voluntary actions that make the individual thermally comfortable. In hot conditions, taking cold drinks, seeking the shade and air-conditioning are common; in cold climates extra clothing is worn, exercise is increased, and the individual stays indoors and lights a fire.

These mechanisms give us the greatest independence from the environment, and, through our ingenuity and the application of modern technology, we can survive in the hottest, coldest, deepest and highest places on earth and even in space.

22.3 THERMAL BALANCE

A useful but over-simplified concept is to imagine the body as consisting of a central core at a fairly uniform temperature of 37°C, with some organs such as the liver at 1–2°C higher, and an insulating shell some degrees lower. The body is therefore continually losing heat and in a cold environment has to maintain a balance between heat production and heat loss (Burton and Edholm, 1955).

In reality there is no physical or anatomical boundary separating the central core from the insulating shell and the difference can be thought of in terms of the temperature of the tissues.

In hot weather, or during periods of increased exercise, some heat loss is necessary to maintain thermal balance, and the core is enlarged, extending into the root of the extremities. During exercise most heat production occurs in the proximal muscles of the limbs and the skin vessels are dilated to bring warm blood to the skin surface to lose heat; as a result the insulating shell is thin.

In a cold climate, or when heat production falls and it is important to conserve heat, skin vessels contract and venous return is confined to the deeper vessels. The core decreases in size and is restricted to the head, neck, thorax and abdomen, and the thickness of the insulating shell increases. As blood flow to the skin can be increased to 100 times that of normal by vasomotor activity and, as much of the transfer of heat in the body is by convection via the blood flow, this is a very important method of heat conservation.

As well as vertical temperature gradients between skin and vessels there are also longitudinal gradients down the length of the limbs where counter-current heat exchange takes place between the arteries and veins.

22.4 COLD INDUCED VASODILATATION

The object of thermal regulation is to maintain the central core temperature at 37°C and, if the environmental temperature falls, the body will 'sacrifice' the extremities to maintain the core, but it does put up a considerable fight to maintain the temperature of the extremities. To this end, under certain conditions and in some individuals only, the extremities exhibit the phenomenon of cold induced vasodilatation. When this occurs the normal response to cold, which is peripheral vasoconstriction to reduce blood flow and heat loss, is reversed, and vasodilatation occurs. Warm blood flows to the periphery and the temperature is raised. This surge is transient only and vasoconstriction then sets in. The mechanism is not certain but, whilst it could be central in origin, the neural mechanism for vasoconstriction may be inhibited by local cooling and the vessels relax.

The magnitude of the heat input to the extremity caused by cold induced vasodilatation is small and can not prevent frostbite at below zero temperatures, or non-freezing cold injury, but it may result in less finger pain when working in cold conditions (Hoffman and Wittmers, 1990).

22.5 THERMAL EXCHANGE

The body is continually losing heat to the environment and heat exchange occurs by convection, radiation, conduction and evaporation.

22.5.1 Convection

This is a molecule-to-molecule transfer of energy. The medium accepting heat is either a gas in motion or a fluid. Although the thermal conductivity and heat capacity of a gas may be low, its movement ensures a high thermal gradient between the body and the environment. The wind-chill factor describes the increased heat loss by convection due to air movement, either by wind or body movement. Convection is also an important avenue of heat exchange during immersion in water; even in still water it is 26 times that of air. Heat transfer within the body is by convection, that is by the flow of blood, which is a factor of great physiological importance.

In a cold environment warm air currents are generated adjacent to the skin and slowly rise to be replaced by cold air which in turn is heated at the expense of body temperature. The rate of convective heat exchange depends on the amount of exposed skin surface area (which is almost always less than the total body surface), and the extraneous air movement which will accelerate the movement of warm air currents; this is so-called 'forced convection'.

Posture is important and the surface area may be reduced by curling up in the foetal position, which is a behavioural response. The heat required to maintain a constant internal temperature is heavily dependent on the body mass/surface area ratio. The heat loss from a squat individual is significantly less than from a tall thin person of the same weight. Children have a particularly unfavourable ratio and easily become hypothermic.

Wind and wind-chill

An important influence on the rate of heat exchange by convection is the wind. Heat loss by forced convection, either by wind or by relative air movement (e.g. downhill skiing or riding in open vehicles), is a major cause of heat loss in a cold environment; this is known as windchill.

Wind-chill correlates the effects of wind and temperature and provides an index which corresponds to the degree of discomfort that is experienced in the field (Siple and Passel, 1945). This effect can be quantified by quoting the equivalent still air temperature produced by any given wind speed. This is shown in Table 22.1. For instance,

Table 22.1 Data redrawn from Mills (1973)

Wind speed (mph)	*Equivalent chill temperature (°C)*									
0	4	−1	−7	−12	−18	−23	−29	−34	−40	−46
5	2	−4	−9	−15	−21	−26	−32	−37	−43	−48
10	−1	−9	−15	−23	−29	−37	−34	−51	−57	−62
15	−4	−12	−21	−29	−34	−43	−51	−57	−65	−73
20	−7	−15	−23	−32	−37	−46	−54	−62	−71	−79
25	−9	−18	−26	−34	−43	−51	−59	−68	−76	−84
30	−12	−18	−29	−34	−46	−54	−62	−71	−79	−87
35	−12	−21	−29	−37	−46	−54	−62	−73	−82	−90
40	−12	−21	−29	−37	−48	−57	−65	−73	−82	−90
	Little danger			Increasing danger Flesh may freeze within 1 min			Great danger Flesh may freeze within 30 s			

10 mph = 16.1 km h^{-1}

at a temperature of −1°C the effect of a 10 mph wind on the skin is equivalent to a still air temperature of −9°C.

Under field conditions, however, the tolerance of humans to cold and wind is determined by those parts that are unprotected, often the face and hands. Exposing the face when walking into the wind is less tolerable than walking at an angle and with some protection.

The chilling power of the wind can produce extreme cooling of the skin and, without protection, frostbite of the nose, chin and cheeks is common at ambient temperatures of 0°C or above. At high altitude, because of decreased air density, the wind-chill factor for a given temperature and wind velocity is less than at sea-level, but the wind velocity is frequently very high.

Convection currents

Warm air rises and, if cooled, falls, setting up convection currents. Around the neck this produces a feeling of a draught as warm air from the skin rises around the collar to be replaced by cold air. A close fitting collar reduces heat loss by this means.

Air movement

Air in the clothes is displaced by body movement, which has a balloon effect on the trunk and a pendulum effect in moving limbs. This effect is reduced by close fitting garments. However, in so-called windproof clothing, some wind penetration and increased heat loss always occurs. With increased relative air movement as the outer layers of clothing are cooled there is an increase in the thermal gradient across the layers beneath.

22.5.2 Radiation

The transfer of heat by electromagnetic energy (i.e. movement of photons from a warm surface to a cooler one), can be a most important source of heat loss and would still take place even if the air was replaced by a vacuum. It is independent of air movement.

All objects warmer than absolute zero emit radiation and therefore lose heat, but they also gain heat from objects around them by the same process.

Heat loss by radiation can be considerable in a cold environment if the body is not covered and insulated. Exposed face and hands lose heat to the clear cold night sky by radiation, and gain heat from the bright sun even in cold conditions. The greatest source of heat gain by radiation is from the sun and, in the clear polar or mountain regions where snow forms a reflection, this effect is enhanced. An overcast sky diminishes radiation, and at night the earth loses heat by radiation to the black sky, with clear nights being cooler than those when cloud acts as a blanket and heat is retained.

The heat received by the body in full sunshine may be two or three times greater than that generated by normal metabolic processes. The amount adsorbed on the surface of clothing will depend on posture, the reflecting power of clothing surface, the absorption of radiation by dust and moisture, and reflection from the ground.

The amount of heat gained from solar radiation will vary with the degree of cloud cover and type of clothing. Black clothing adsorbs about 88% of solar radiation, khaki 57% and white clothing 30%.

In Antarctica, because of the clean air, solar radiation reaches levels which at lower latitudes are found only at high altitude. Heat gain from snow reflection – the albedo – is an important factor at high altitude and polar regions and may vary from 75–90% in snow to 25% if it is absent. Heat gain also varies with the sun's altitude in the sky, it is low at dawn and increased at midday (Chrenko and Pugh, 1961).

In Polar regions in summer, solar heat gain may be two to four times greater than in desert, and at high altitude the gain will be comparable. At extreme altitude this may be crucial to survival, as diminished oxygen uptake reduces heat output with the result that body temperature may fall, and heat from solar radiation keeps the climber in thermal balance.

22.5.3 Conduction

This involves a molecule-to-molecule transfer of energy between two solids in physical contact. Under most conditions heat exchange by this method is small because the contact surface area between individuals and the environment is small. However it may be of great importance during rescue or transporting casualties; extra insulation must be provided under the body when lying or sitting on a cold surface. Localized frost-bite may occur should the body surface come into contact with materials of a high thermal conductivity below zero temperature. Touching the cold metal of an ice-axe with bare hands or spilling liquids onto the body can result in frost-bite or hypothermia. When clothing becomes soaked one can lose up to 80% of its insulating value.

Different tissues conduct heat at different rates. Fat is a good insulator and skin over areas of fatty tissue will cool more rapidly and to lower temperatures than areas where fat deposits are scanty. For most tissues thermal conductivity is a function of fluid content and tissue blood flow in a cold climate. Prolonged vasoconstriction leads to fluid shifts and increases central blood volume, which in turn leads to a diuresis. A decrease in tissue conductivity results but this is marginal considering the total insulation required under cold conditions.

22.5.4 Evaporation

Unlike conduction, convection and radiation, where heat may be both gained and lost, with evaporation heat can only be lost.

During heavy exercise and in hot climates evaporation of sweat is essential, and in a very hot climate, where environmental temperatures exceed skin temperature, the body may be actually gaining heat by radiation, conduction and convection. Evaporation therefore is the only method of heat loss and means of preventing hyperthermia.

About 25% of the total heat loss in humans is by evaporation from the skin and respiratory tract. Significant heat loss will occur by evaporation in the process of drying clothes by body heat, particularly in a wind or at altitude where the air is dry.

Skin

As the epidermis is only slightly permeable to water, the rate of loss by passive diffusion is small. Insensible water loss and sweating account for 66% of the evaporative heat loss under normal conditions. Sweating occurs as a result of exercise and emotion, particularly fear. During exercise thermal balance is maintained by the heat of increased metabolism being balanced by the heat loss from the evaporation of sweat. However, if exercise is stopped abruptly, heat continues to be lost from evaporation of sweat on the skin and in clothing but as the metabolic rate falls the individual cools.

Large amounts of fluid, over $1\,l\,h^{-1}$, may be lost by sweating, particularly with severe exercise or in a hot environment. If the air is dry and there is a wind, heat loss by evaporation is limited only by the rate of sweat secretion. If the air is moist and still, loss is limited by the rate of water evaporated from the skin. In very cold conditions considerable loss may result from the sweat generated through exercise first evaporating, but then condensing and freezing inside the outer layers of clothing. Increased sweating therefore results in both heat and water loss.

Respiratory tract

The temperature of expired air is below body temperature and is probably not fully saturated with water even at this lower temperature (Ferrus *et al.*, 1984; Milledge, 1992). Even so, with normal ventilation, heat loss amounts to about one-third of the total loss from evaporation. At high altitude, with higher ventilation rates, this will increase particularly as the air is drier. In the cold, even at sea-level, the volume of body water lost through respiration is large enough to cause dehydration and weight loss, and may damage the upper respiratory tract.

22.6 REGULATION OF BODY TEMPERATURE

In a cold environment normal maintenance of body temperature is by balancing heat loss against heat production, the main control being a central 'thermostatic' mechanism in the hypothalamus. This regulates the body temperature within narrow limits but it is not a simple on–off device. There is a complex system of neurones linking input and output with many cross links which produces a graduated response.

Sensory input comes from central receptors along the internal carotid artery, reticular part of the mid-brain, the pre-optic region and the posterior hypothalamus. Peripheral receptors are situated in the skin and stomach, whilst there is also clinical evidence of receptors inside peripheral veins (Lloyd, 1979).

The setting of the thermostat can be altered. Diurnal variations may vary between individuals and between male and female, the lowest temperature being at 5.00 a.m. and the highest at 8.00 p.m. This may be upset when the normal day/night ratio is disturbed by prolonged daylight as in Polar travel, long underwater voyages and the Polar winter (Colquohoun, 1984). Sleep, myxoedema and mental depression lower the setting, which is also disturbed during ovulation (Crawford, 1979).

22.7 HEAT PRODUCTION

Between 27°C and 29°C, the critical air temperature, an unclothed person at rest can maintain the body temperature, as basal metabolic heat is balanced by heat loss.

Eating increases basal heat whilst malnutrition decreases it and may result in hypothermia; exercise increases heat production considerably.

22.7.1 Shivering thermogenesis

Exposure to cold increases muscle tone and metabolism and leads to shivering, which may increase oxygen uptake up to fivefold. The onset of shivering is controlled by central and peripheral stimuli working independently (Lim, 1960) and may be triggered by external stimulus. It is progressive, starting from the neck muscles, proceeding to the pectoral and abdominal musculature and then the extremities. Shivering metabolism is proportional to lowered mean skin temperature when the core temperature is constant and to the core temperature when the skin temperature is constant (Hong and Nadel, 1979).

Whilst shivering is useful for increasing metabolism in an emergency it makes co-ordinated motor tasks difficult and energy resources are depleted, hastening the onset of fatigue and hypothermia. If cold exposure continues, considerable stored glycogen is burnt and the associated water loss may be as high as 1.5 l. However, under normal conditions this should be replenished in the next 48–72 h.

22.7.2 Non-shivering thermogenesis (NST)

NST, or lipolytic thermogenesis, is the production of heat from adipose tissue, especially brown fat. There is controversy over the occurrence of non-shivering thermogenesis in adult humans (Hervey and Tobin, 1983; Rothwell and Stock, 1983), where, although brown fat persists into the sixth decade in the neck, mediastinum, kidneys and suprarenal glands and around the aorta (Heaton, 1972), it constitutes only a very small fraction of the total body fat.

The infant relies, for the most part, on NST to maintain thermal balance, brown fat accounting for 25–35% of its fat stores.

It is debatable how much noradrenaline can increase heat production in tissues other than brown fat. The breakdown and resynthesis of neutral fat is a possibility, and protein catabolism is increased on acute cold exposure (Goodenough *et al.*, 1982).

A lowered NST response has been found in post-obese individuals, while the insulation of subcutaneous fat enables obese people to withstand cold better than the lean (Jequier *et al.*, 1974).

22.7.3 Activity

Maximal physical exercise ($\dot{V}_{O_2}$ max) increases heat production by 20 times the basal rate; about five times the normal basal heat production can be maintained for several hours (Maugham, 1984). In cold conditions, additional heat may be produced through shivering, and, as this can occur during exercise, oxygen consumption will be increased.

Limitation will be imposed by altitude where oxygen uptake falls and shivering may be inhibited. In very cold conditions too, oxygen uptake may be insufficient to meet the demand imposed by both exercise and cold. Exhausted individuals and those with malnutrition cannot increase metabolism because of lack of substrate (Wang, 1978) and will be at increased risk from hypothermia.

22.8 HEAT LOSS

Overheating may at times be a problem in the mountains, particularly on glaciers in still, sunny weather. When body temperature rises due to increased exercise or too much insulation, body heat must be lost and vasodilatation occurs which raises the skin temperature. Vasodilatation also increases the transfer of heat from the core to the shell and the amount of fluid available to the sweat glands.

Sweating is an important method of heat loss which may be impaired by dehydration and drugs; there are also individual differences in regional sweating patterns (Hertzman, 1957).

22.9 HEAT CONSERVATION

Heat conservation occurs by physiological methods and by insulation of clothing and shelter.

22.9.1 Vasoconstriction

Below the critical ambient temperature of 27–29°C cold receptors in the skin initiate subcutaneous vasoconstriction which limits blood flow to the peripheral shell and this results in a decrease in skin temperature and reduced heat loss. The thermal insulation of skin varies from 0.15 CLO on vasodilatation to 0.9 CLO on vasoconstriction (Burton and Edholm, 1955). (A definition of the CLO is given in section 22.12.3.)

In the scalp there is minimal vasoconstriction and this makes the scalp less liable to cold injury by comparison with the limbs. At rest at −4°C, heat loss from the head may be half the resting heat production in a clothed subject (Froese and Burton, 1957). However, the nose, face and ears do vasoconstrict and hence are liable to frost-bite.

22.9.2 Counter-current heat exchange

Subcutaneous gradient

Subcutaneous temperature varies with the depth and location of arteriolar and venous plexuses, being highest at about 0.8 mm from the skin. A drop in temperature superficial to this is due to returning venous blood being cooler than arterial blood and heat from the arterioles being lost to the veins.

Fluctuations in temperature are controlled by arteriolar–venous anastomoses; their opening results in warm blood passing to the veins and the dissipation of heat.

Longitudinal gradient

Arterial blood loses heat in the surface capillaries and returns to cool the body. Heat lost in this manner is reduced as arteries and their accompanying veins exchange heat through their walls along the length of the limb. Thus the blood reaching the skin capillaries is pre-cooled and the temperature gradient between capillaries and the skin surface is reduced; venous blood is warmed and heat conserved.

The temperature gradient down the length of a limb may be more important in the control of insulation than the gradient from the deep tissues to the skin (Bazett and McGlone, 1927).

22.9.3 Insulation

Introduced in 1941, the CLO is a practical unit of thermal insulation for describing heat exchange in man:

$$1\ \text{CLO} = 0.18 \frac{^\circ\text{C}}{\text{kcal m}^{-2}\,\text{hr}^{-1}}$$

where °C is the difference in temperature across the clothing under consideration. For a whole suit of clothing it will be the skin temperature minus the ambient temperature.

One CLO will maintain a resting, sitting subject, whose metabolic rate is 50 kcal m^{-2} $hour^{-1}$, comfortable indefinitely in an environment of 22°C with a relative humidity less than 50% and air movement 6 m min^{-1} (20 ft min^{-1}). It will be seen therefore that the CLO is not a rigorously scientific unit of heat resistance but nevertheless is a useful working unit for the comparison of insulation.

It is equivalent to the insulation afforded by ordinary business clothing and underwear for a sedentary worker in comfortable indoor surroundings (Burton and Edholm, 1955). The value for insulation of tissues is 0.15–0.9 CLO, for air 0.8–0.2 CLO and clothing 0–6.0 CLO. The importance of the insulating values of clothes is obvious. Under certain extreme conditions, tissue insulation may be important.

22.9.4 Tissue insulation

Heat transfer in the body occurs by mass flow along the blood vessels, but, as the capillaries do not extend to the superficial parts of the epidermis, heat is transferred from the capillaries to the skin surface by conduction. This rate of heat transfer is determined by the number of capillaries and their calibre. The thermal insulation of tissues varies from 0.15 CLO on vasodilatation to 0.9 CLO on vasoconstriction; counter-current heat exchange prevents excessive heat loss. Subcutaneous fat is the most important form of natural insulation and, as fat has few blood vessels, thermal conductivity is less than in muscle. The greater the fat layer, the lower the skin temperature and the smaller the gradient between skin surface and environment (Keatinge *et al.*, 1986). Individuals with a good layer of subcutaneous fat will still shiver, as the temperature receptors are in the skin and thus superficial to the insulating layer. However, the heat produced by shivering will be retained by the subcutaneous fat and result in a smaller fall in rectal temperature and less increase in heat production. Obesity is, however, rare in indigenous people in cold climates or at altitude.

Sites where subcutaneous fat is thin or absent are more liable to local cold injury. These include the tips of the fingers, nose and ears.

22.9.5 Air insulation and wind-chill

In the cold, air density increases and loss of heat by radiation decreases, but this is almost completely compensated for by an increase in heat loss by convection. Heat loss varies with wind velocity and the loss increases up to about 10 mph. At higher speeds there is little further increase in heat loss.

22.9.6 Clothing

Insulation and protection from the wind are the most important functions of clothing in dry conditions. In wet conditions waterproofing is an important factor in maintaining insulation. Insulation depends on trapped, still air and is proportional to the volume of this air. To maintain insulation, the trapped, still air must remain immobile to prevent air currents and loss of heat by convection. A windproof outer layer should prevent a large proportion of wind penetration. Materials should maintain their thickness after compression or when wet, and the actual bulk of the material must be low to prevent heat loss by condensation. To maintain thermal balance it is as necessary to facilitate heat loss as it is to maintain heat production and preserve insulation (Adam and Goldsmith, 1965; Keighley and Steele, 1981).

A variety of clothing is necessary in order to change the amount of insulation to meet the demands of heat production and ambient temperature. If only one material, such as fur, is used, this causes difficulties; to vary insulation, clothing must be available in layers which can be put on and taken off as required to avoid overheating. Adequate and easily adjustable ventilation improves clothing adaptability and clothing should fit correctly without pressure on underlying tissues.

As wetting may decrease insulation by up to 90%, this should be prevented, whilst at the same time allowing sweat to evaporate. If a completely wind- and waterproof garment is used in freezing conditions, evaporated sweat will condense and freeze on the inner surface and clothing will become soaked, thereby reducing insulation. The outer layer should therefore be permeable to water vapour, water resistant to retard water entry and windproof to prevent excessive air movement and diminish insulation (Jackson, 1975).

Clothing assemblies may now be so effective that after many months in cold conditions there is a possibility that an individual may become heat adapted (Wilkins, 1973).

The choice of materials varies and wool and cotton are popular. Natural wool, because of its crimped fibres retains 40% of its insulating value when wet, compared with 10% for cotton. Natural down provides excellent insulation when dry but not when wet. Synthetic fibres are becoming increasingly important. Some are hydrophobic (Stephens, 1982) and do not retain moisture. These, when used as a padded jacket or trousers may not have such good insulation when dry but insulate well when wet. Clothing assemblies are very much an individual matter, but recently several equipment innovations have helped climbers at extreme altitude. Plastic boots with insulating liners have reduced weight and increased warmth and, when knee length gaiters are added, foot protection is excellent.

Underwear that absorbs sweat as well as giving some warmth under a fibre pile garment seems a thermally efficient combination, especially with an outer layer of 'breathable' fabrics like Goretex. Over the past few years a number of synthetic fibres have been developed for insulation in jackets, trousers and sleeping bags. Their qualities rival down and have the merit of not losing as much insulation when wet.

The trunk

Insulation of the trunk is relatively easy as little movement takes place and bulky garments are more acceptable than on the arms and legs. A non-irritant garment should be worn next to the skin; this will absorb sweat and skin debris. Whether this has sleeves is an individual choice. Shirts or sweaters usually form the next layer. A polo neck is often used in continuously cold conditions as it diminishes loss of heat around the neck by convection currents. If more than one layer is worn, the size must be graduated. Heat loss due to the bellows effect may be prevented by draw strings around the waist or wrists.

Padded jackets of natural down or artificial fibres, with or without sleeves, are common and they should extend over the buttocks to overlap the trousers by a wide margin. Often these have a windproof outer layer and they should open down the front and be easy to take off and put on.

Lower trunk and legs

Insulation is influenced by the amount of movement at the hip and knee and the close proximity of the skin of the inner thigh, which can cause severe chafing if garments are badly fitted. Long close fitting underpants of soft weave wool, or synthetic fibre are commonly worn. They should fit well around the ankles to prevent heat loss.

Padded trousers should not be so thick as to prevent easy leg movements. Breeches or trousers should be of hard wearing material and the fly opening should be easily operated. Gaiters are often used, which prevent snow from entering the top of the boot. Some boots have gaiters attached to the sole. One-piece padded suits may be used in extremely cold conditions, these should have convenient zips for ventilation and excretion. Salopettes, which extend up to the upper chest are increasingly worn and these provide a large overlap with the upper jacket and are very warm.

Feet

Feet remain covered all day and are not inspected as easily or as regularly as hands, and, as a result, frost-bite and non-freezing injury may remain hidden for a long period. The design of footwear for dry/cold conditions has improved markedly with the development of a boot containing a moulded plastic outer shell, including the sole, and an inner detachable boot of artificial fibre. As these are separate, the outer shell is removed when in a sleeping bag. The inner boot may be changed if it gets damp. Friction occurs between the inner and outer compartments when walking rather than between the skin of the foot and boot. Because of this blisters are less common, despite the rigidity of the outer shell.

Leather boots are seldom used now in severe dry/cold conditions, but, in World War II, the Russian Army issued leather boots several sizes too large which could be stuffed with straw or paper, whereas the German Army had well fitting boots and suffered more from cold injury of the feet.

The ideal boot has yet to be designed for wet/cold conditions and most rely on the leather boot with or without an insole, and regular changes of socks. Both Thinsulate and Goretex have been incorporated in boot design. Once the foot gets wet its temperature falls quickly due to small heat stores. An overboot or gaiters improve insulation and should extend to the knee. Crampons straps constrict the circulation of the foot in leather boots but clip-on crampons and plastic boots avoid this problem.

Socks must fit well and be kept dry, spare pairs must be available in the rucksack and feet should be inspected regularly so that incipient cold injury, blisters and infections are dealt with quickly. Meticulous care of the feet by the British Army in World War II resulted in a lower incidence of non-freezing cold injury than in any other army in the same theatre of war.

Hands

The multilayer principle is best and a mitten with four fingers in one compartment and a thumb is warmer than a glove. Individual insulation of a finger is less effective because the heat loss from the curved surface of a small cylinder is greater than from a large cylinder. As the diameter decreases to 6.5 mm, any increase in the thickness of insulation makes little or no difference to the total insulation.

Mittens or gloves should be windproof, water resistant, permeable to water vapour and robust. Dachstein mittens made of uncured wool are very effective. As metals are good conductors, contact of cold metal with a dry finger will cause a 'cold burn', whilst a wet finger freezes to the metal and tissue may be left attached. If it is necessary to use fingers for fine work, contact gloves should be worn.

It is worth noting that few indigenous mountain inhabitants wear gloves and this is partly due to local cold acclimatization, but native garments do have long fold back sleeves that can extend beyond the fingers.

The head

The head is an important avenue of heat loss. The most likely areas to freeze are the tip of the nose, and ears and cheeks. The ears are easy to protect with muffs or a hat, and a painful ear is a warning of incipient cold injury. The nose and cheeks are less easy to protect and face masks, though increasingly used, tend not to be comfortable and therefore are not popular.

A well designed anorak hood is essential for protecting the face from the wind, driving ice and snow particles. It must project well forward from the face and have a stiff but malleable wire in its leading edge. This enables the hood to be arranged so that it protects the face from whichever angle the wind comes and, if necessary, only a minute hole need be left through which the individual can see.

The use of a visor of tinted glass provides more protection than individual goggles or dark glasses. An oxygen mask may be incorporated into the visor.

Metabolic cost of clothing

Working with multilayered Arctic clothing increases the metabolic rate by 16% by comparison with carrying the weight of the clothing. This increase can be attributed to the frictional resistance of one layer sliding over the other layer during movement, and the hobbling effect which interferes with movement.

Wind, movement and wetting

If wind penetrates clothing, movement of the trapped, still air can result in a 30% fall in insulation. The magnitude of this effect depends on the degree of wind resistance of the clothes and the effectiveness of the sealing at the neck, wrist and ankle. Movement also can lower insulation to half its resting value. Exercise in the cold may cause overheating and sweating; rain may also wet clothing and as much as 50% of insulation may be lost by this means alone.

The combination of movement, wind and wetting may cause a 90% loss of insulation, as a result of which the individual is essentially unprotected from the environment.

22.9.7 Insulation and oxygen consumption

From Table 22.2 it will be apparent that at 0°C ambient temperature, to maintain a core temperature of 37°C with a total thermal insulation of 3.0 CLO it is only necessary to work at a rate equivalent to an oxygen consumption of $0.5\,l\,min^{-1}$. At sea-level this is not difficult but, at

Table 22.2 Calculated final body temperature (°C) at an ambient temperature of 0°C for a 75 kg man dependent upon the total thermal insulation (clothes plus tissue) and activity, measured as oxygen consumption (From data of Pugh, 1966)

Total thermal insulation (CLO units)	*Oxygen consumption ($l\,min^{-1}$)*					
	0.5	*1.0*	*1.5*	*2.0*	*2.5*	*3.0*
0.2	2	4	6	8	10	12
0.4	4	9	14	18	23	28
1.0	12	24	36	48	60	72
1.4	23	34	50	66	—	—
2.0	24	48	72	—	—	—
2.5	32	58	—	—	—	—
3.0	38	—	—	—	—	—
4.0	52	—	—	—	—	—

7000 m and above, a steady rate of 0.5 l min^{-1} may represent 50% of $\dot{V}_{O_2}$ max. To remain in thermal balance at an ambient temperature lower than 0°C the individual either has to work harder or wear more clothes. As neither may be possible he will become gradually hypothermic.

If insulation falls to 1 CLO, work rate has to increase threefold to 1.5 l/min to maintain thermal balance. If insulation falls even lower due to wetting, a work rate in excess of 3.0 l/min is necessary. This will not be possible for an exhausted or unfit individual who will become hypothermic.

22.9.8 Shelter

The main value of a tent is to provide protection from the wind, though some modern double skinned tents also have quite good insulating properties.

Igloos and snow caves provide good insulation by virtue of the air trapped in the snow. This is illustrated by an incident in 1902 on one of Scott's early Antarctic expeditions. One member went missing and a blizzard developed which lasted 48 h. He took shelter and was covered by snow, falling asleep for 36 h, after which he awoke and returned unscathed (Brent, 1974). Adequate ventilation is important to prevent the accumulation of carbon monoxide given off by stoves (Pugh, 1959).

22.10 FACTORS ALTERING TEMPERATURE REGULATION

22.10.1 Introduction

Trauma, haemorrhage and nausea increase heat loss, whereas exhaustion reduces heat production. Sleep, anaesthesia and alcohol also affect regulation of temperature, whilst the extremes of age are associated with increased risk of hypothermia. Abnormal thermoregulatory patterns are found in some ethnic groups living in cold environments. The core temperature of sleeping aborigines drops further than that of Europeans before causing discomfort, and natives of Tierra del Fuego maintain a high metabolic rate (Hammel, 1964). Meditation by Tibetan lamas may result in cutaneous vasodilatation and possible increased metabolic rate (Benson *et al.*, 1982).

Certain medical disorders and drugs predispose to hypothermia.

22.10.2 Malnutrition

Malnutrition, by depleting the body stores, renders the subject more liable to hypothermia. The metabolic demands of cold are similar to, though less marked, than those of exercise, and the combination of cold, fasting, exercise and altitude will impose a considerable strain on the body. As a result, mild degrees of hypothermia are probably commoner than realized at altitude (Guezennec and Pesquies, 1985).

22.10.3 Sleep

The central thermostat is set at a lower level when the individual goes to sleep, and the basal metabolic rate is reduced (Shapiro *et al.*, 1984). Heat production when asleep is 9% lower than when at rest and awake. During rapid eye movement (REM) sleep the skin temperature rises if the rectal temperature is high and falls if the rectal temperature is low (Buguet *et al.*, 1979).

In non-REM sleep, oxygen consumption and metabolic rate are at their lowest. During the night there is a gradual reduction in heat production, which rises just before wakening. The skin temperature drops during sleep which may wake the individual because of a feeling of cold. Theoretically, there is no danger from falling asleep in extreme cold since each bout of shivering would wake the person; however an exhausted individual may not shiver and thus will fall into a dangerous cooling sleep.

Mountaineers bivouacking in extreme conditions will try to keep each other awake; there seem sound physiological reasons for this as the lower body temperature set point will allow body heat content to fall before discomfort due to cold is appreciated.

22.10.4 Alcohol

It is now recognized that alcohol may be an important contributory cause of death in cold environments. Its role is complex, but even quantities which result in levels below those of legal drunkenness are dangerous prior to working in the cold.

The inhibitory action of alcohol on cerebral function can cause bravado and lessen the ability to asses risk. Prior to exercise in the cold it is associated with a decrease in blood glucose (Haight and Keatinge, 1973) which will increase the risk of exhaustion leading to hypothermia and further impairment of gluconeogenesis (Drinking and drowning, 1979). Cooling also decreases the elimination of alcohol (Krarup and Larsen, 1972); as it is also a sedative, there will be an increased tendency to sleep with resulting failure to maintain body heat. Freund *et al.* (1994) suggest that alcohol reduces central core temperature during exposure to cold and that the degree of reduction is related to the blood alcohol concentration, also hypoglycaemia increases the reduction in body temperature caused by the ingestion of alcohol.

22.10.5 Regular exposure to cold

Normal responses to cold may be modified by regular exposure. Divers regularly exposed to cold may be susceptible to progressive and symptomless hypothermia resulting in poor judgement and death (Hayward and Keatinge, 1979). During experimental cooling it is possible, by slightly raising the skin temperature at the start of shivering, to abolish both shivering and the sensation of cold without arresting the continued cooling (Keatinge *et al.*, 1980).

REFERENCES

Adam, J.M. and Goldsmith, R. (1965) Cold climates, in *Exploration Medicine*, (eds O.G. Edholm and A.L. Bacharach), Wright, Bristol, pp. 245–77.

Bazett, H.C. and McGlone, B. (1927) Temperature gradients in the tissues of man. *Am. J. Physiol.*, **82**, 415–51.

Benson, H., Lehmann, J.W., Malhotra, M.S., *et al.* (1982) Body temperature changes during the practice of G-tum-mo yoga. *Nature*, **295**, 234–6.

Brent, P. (1974) *Captain Scott and the Antarctic Tragedy*, Weidenfeld and Nicolson, London, p. 61.

Buguet, A.G.C., Livingstone, S.D. and Reed, L.D. (1979) Skin temperature changes in paradoxical sleep in man in the cold. *Aviat. Space Environ. Med.*, **50**, 567–70.

Burton, A.C. and Edholm, O.G. (1955) *Man in a Cold Environment*, Arnold, London.

Chrenko, F.A. and Pugh, L.G.C.E. (1961) The contribution of solar radiation to the thermal environment of man in Antarctica. *Proc. R. Soc. London Series B*, **155**, 243–65.

Colquohoun, W.P. (1984) Effects of personality on body temperature and mental efficiency following transmeridian flight. *Aviat. Space Environ. Med.*, **55**, 493–6.

Crawford, J.P. (1979) Endogenous anxiety and circadian rhythms. *Br. Med. J.*, **1**, 662.

Drinking and drowing (editorial). (1979) *Br. Med. J.*, **1**, 70–1.

Ferrus, L., Commenges, D., Gire, J. and Varene, P. (1984) Respiratory water loss. *Respir. Physiol.*, **56**, 11–20.

Freund, B.J., O'Brien, C. and Young, A.J. (1994) Alcohol ingestion and temperature regulation during cold exposure. *J. Wild. Med.*, **5**, 88–98.

Froese, G. and Burton, A.C. (1957) Heat loss from the human head. *J. Appl. Physiol.*, **10**, 235–41.

Goodenough, R.D., Royle, G.T., Nadel, E.R., *et al.* (1982) Leucine and urea metabolism in acute human cold exposure. *J. Appl. Physiol.*, **53**, 367–72.

Guezennec, C.Y. and Pesquies, P.C. (1985) Biochemical basis for physical exercise fatigue, in *High Altitude Deterioration*, (eds J. Rivolier, P. Cerretelli, J. Foray and P. Segantini), Karger, Basel, pp. 79–89.

Haight, J.S.J. and Keatinge, W.R. (1973) Failure of thermoregulation in the cold during hypoglycaemia induced by exercise and ethanol. *J. Physiol. (Lond).*, **229**, 87–97.

Hammel, H.T. (1964) Terrestrial animals in the cold: recent studies in primitive man, in *Handbook of Physiology, Adaptation to the Environment*, American Physiological Society, Washington DC, pp. 413–34.

Hayward, M.G. and Keatinge, W.R. (1979) Progressive symptomless hypothermia in water. Possible cause of diving accidents. *Br. Med. J.*, **1**, 1222.

Heaton, J.M. (1972) The distribution of brown adipose tissue in the human. *J. Anat.*, **112**, 35–9.

Hertzman, A.B. (1957) Individual differences in regional sweating patterns. *J. Appl. Physiol.*, **10**, 242–8.

Hervey, G.R. and Tobin, G. (1983) Luxuskonsumption. Diet-induced thermogenesis and brown fat: A critical review. *Clin. Sci.*, **64**, 7–22.

Hoffman, R.G. and Wittmers, L.E. (1990) Cold vasodilitation, pain and acclimatization in Arctic explorers. *J. Wild. Med.*, **1**, 225–34.

Hong, S.I. and Nadel, E.R. (1979) Thermogenic control during exercise in a cold environment. *J. Appl. Physiol.*, **47**, 1084–9.

Jackson, J.A. (1975) Avoidance of cold injury. Outline of basic principles, in *Mountain Medicine and Physiology*, (eds C. Clarke, M.P. Ward and E.S. Williams), Alpine Club, London, pp. 28–30.

Jequier, E., Gygax, P.-H., Pittet, P. and Vannotti, A. (1974) Increased thermal body insulation: Relationship to the development of obesity. *J. Appl. Physiol.*, **36**, 674–8.

Keatinge, W.R., Hayward, M.G. and McIver, N.K.I. (1980) Hypothermia during saturation diving in the North Sea. *Br. Med. J.*, **1**, 291.

Keatinge, W.R., Colkshaw, S.R.K., Millard, C.E. and Axelsson, J. (1986) Exceptional case of survival in cold water. *Br. Med. J.*, **292**, 171–2.

Keighley, J.H. and Steele, G. (1981) The functional and design requirements of clothing. *Alpine J.*, **86**, 138–45.

Krarup, N. and Larsen, J.A. (1972) The effect of slight hypothermia on liver function as measured by the elimination rate of ethanol, the hepatic uptake and excretion of indocyanine green and bile formation. *Acta Physiol. Scand.*, **84**, 396–407.

Lim, T.P.K. (1960) Central and peripheral control mechanisms of shivering and its effect on respiration. *J. Appl. Physiol.*, **15**, 567–74.

Lloyd, E.L. (1979) Temperature sensations in veins. *Anaesthesia*, **34**, 919.

Maugham, R.J. (1984) Temperature regulation during marathon competition. *Br. J. Sports Med.*, **22**, 257–60.

Milledge, J.S. (1992) Respiratory water loss at altitude. *Int. Soc. Mount. Med. Newsletter*, **2**, 5–6.

Mills, W.J. (1973) Frostbite and hypothermia. Current concepts. *Alaska Med.*, **15**, 26–59.

Pugh, L.G.C.E. (1959) Carbon monoxide hazard in Antarctica. *Br. Med. J.*, **1**, 192–6.

Pugh, L.G.C.E. (1966) Clothing insulation and accidental hypothermia in youth. *Nature*, **209**, 1281–6.

Rothwell, N.J. and Stock, M.J. (1983) Luxuskonsumption. Diet-induced thermogenesis and brown fat: the case in favour. *Clin. Sci.*, **64**, 19–23.

Shapiro, C.M., Goll, C.C., Cohen, G.R. and Oswald, I. (1984) Heat production during sleep. *J. Appl. Physiol.*, **56**, 671–7.

Siple, P.A. and Passel, C.F. (1945) Dry atmospheric cooling in sub-freezing temperatures. *Proc. Am. Philos. Soc.*, **89**, 177–99.

Stephens, D.H. (1982) Sleeping snugly in damp bedrooms. *J. R. Soc. Health*, **6**, 272–5.

Wang, L.C.H. (1978) Factors limiting maximum cold induced heat production. *Life Sci.*, **23**, 2089–98.

Wilkins, D.C. (1973) Acclimation to heat in the Antarctic, in *Polar Human Biology*, (eds O.G. Edholm and E.K.E. Gunderson), Heinemann Medical, London, pp. 171–81.

23

Reaction to cold

23.1 INTRODUCTION

Man reacts to cold more effectively by behavioural rather than by physiological means, and clothing and shelter enable Eskimos to live in an environmental temperature of −70°C. The opportunity to become cold tolerant is limited in Europeans as, even at Polar bases, men may be out of doors for only 10–15% of the time. Mountaineers, because they live in unheated tents or snow caves may spend longer periods exposed to cold.

Protective clothing is now so efficient that the microclimate (environment beneath the clothing) may be as warm as a temperate zone and some degree of heat acclimatization occurs. Only exposed parts, such as the hands, become cold adapted and those used to working out of doors are less liable than newcomers to frost-bite. Local acclimatization has an essentially vascular basis with an increase in blood flow, whilst improved tactile discrimination and less appreciation of pain occurs in the cold adapted (Hoffman and Wittmers, 1990).

Most people respond to cold stress by cardiovascular and metabolic changes, but not all respond equally. Some tend to raise their heat production by shivering, others adjust more by peripheral vasoconstriction.

In subjects of different body size and composition there is a wide variation in the amount of heat production resulting from shivering thermogenesis; thin men shiver more intensely than fat ones. In small to medium sized individuals, vasoconstriction with light shivering precedes heavy shivering, whilst in large men, because of their body size and subcutaneous fat, metabolic heat production is less (Strong *et al.*, 1985). Children, because of their greater surface area to weight ratio, are at greater risk of cooling than adults.

Acclimatization is a term that has been used in relation to cold by many workers and certainly changes, both short and long term, have been shown after repeated exposure (Shephard, 1985). However, the term has been used in so many different ways that it tends to confuse rather than clarify.

23.2 METABOLIC RESPONSE TO COLD

Hammel (1964) distinguishes three distinct patterns of response to moderate exposure of the whole body: those who increase their metabolic rate as body temperature falls (urban man); those whose metabolic rate falls gradually as rectal and skin temperature fall below that of urban controls (Australian aborigine); and those who start with a high metabolic rate which declines slightly and is accompanied by a fall in rectal temperature to a level no lower than that of a white control (Alaculuf Indians).

Repeated exposure to cold results in a greater sympathetic response and improved cutaneous insulation (Young *et al.*, 1986). It appears that the type of physiological response varies according to the degree, length and frequency of exposure.

23.3 SKIN AND PERIPHERAL VESSELS

The initial response to cold on the skin is the contraction of the erector pili muscles with the development of 'gooseflesh'. Constriction of the cutaneous vessels occurs and there is increased blood viscosity with decreased blood flow.

On immersion of a finger in iced water, skin temperature falls to nearly 0°C and then rises. With continued immersion, the finger temperature fluctuates, known as the 'hunting' phenomenon. This is due to reflex (cold induced) vasodilatation and increased blood flow through arteriovenous anastomoses. The temperature rise is greater in the distal than the proximal phalanges.

The explanation of 'hunting' appears to be that cold paralyses the vasoconstrictor muscle fibres, the vessels dilate, blood flow increases, the finger warms, heat is lost and the cycle repeats itself.

Pain is related to blood flow, being severe on vasoconstriction and improving on vasodilatation. With increasing cold, tissue metabolism ceases, the skin blanches and becomes waxy and pale due to continuous vasoconstriction. The bloodless region cools to the environmental temperature and frost-bite may occur.

The general thermal state affects the peripheral circulation and local vasodilatation is greatly increased when the individual is warm and reduced when cold. The extent of peripheral vasodilatation depends too on the area heated. Heating the face is far more effective than the chest or leg in varying skin temperature and blood flow to the hand.

Cooling of one part of the body surface results in diminished blood flow to other regions also. When the whole body surface is cooled there is a general cutaneous vasoconstriction with diminished blood flow to peripheral tissues (Burton and Edholm, 1955).

Both cold phlebitis and cold arteritis may occur on prolonged exposure. Those with varicose veins should consider treatment prior to long periods in the cold.

23.4 NERVES

Exposure of the hands to cold, even above freezing, impairs nerve function after a period of about 15 minutes, and this is not immediately reversed by warming and may occasionally persist for more than 4–5 days (Marshall and Goldman, 1976). There is diminished skin sensation followed by a lessening of manual dexterity. The critical air temperature for tactile sensitivity is 8°C and for manual dexterity it is 12°C (Fox, 1967). Above these temperatures performance is little affected though the hands may feel cold, but at lower temperatures performance falls markedly. Not all tasks are equally affected and impairment may persist after the hands have been rewarmed to normal temperatures. Many climbers returning from high altitude have some loss of sensation in their finger tips which may last several weeks.

23.5 MUSCLE

Cold also decreases the power and direction of muscle contraction and this seems to have a direct effect on the muscle fibre, as blood flow is not decreased (Guttman and Gross, 1956). Hand grip diminishes considerably when the forearm is immersed in water at 10°C (Coppin *et al.*, 1978).

Increasing failure of muscle function may be due to a combination of failure of nerve conduction, neuromuscular function and the direct action of cold on muscle fibres. Cold muscles are notoriously liable to rupture and the more explosive the activity the greater the risk, hence the need for a warm-up before taking exercise. Muscle is more vulnerable to cold than skin or bone (Kayser *et al.*, 1993).

23.6 JOINTS

The temperature of the joints falls faster than that of muscles, and cold joints are stiff joints (Hunter *et al.*, 1952). Cold increases the viscosity of synovial fluid and, by reducing its lubricating qualities, it increases the resistance of joints to movements, increasing the risk of tearing tendons and muscles.

23.7 CARDIOVASCULAR SYSTEM

A number of thermoregulatory systems designed to reduce heat loss are brought into play immediately on exposure to cold; these affect the cardiovascular system with an increase in cardiac output, blood pressure and pulse rate (Hayward *et al.*, 1984). Initially, catecholamine excretion increases but, as core temperature falls from 31–29°C, this decreases (Chernow *et al.*, 1983).

23.7.1 Blood pressure

In normal people and untreated hypertensives, the blood pressure is higher in the winter. This rise in systemic blood pressure increases with age and in thin people (Brennan *et al.*, 1982). Exercise in the cold usually decreases diastolic pressure but this may be countered by the inhalation of cold air (Horvath, 1981) and may precipitate angina because, with the associated increase in ventricular pressure, the oxygen needs of the myocardium increase (Gorlin, 1966).

On cold exposure, constriction of the peripheral vessels shunts a large volume of blood into the capacitance vessels causing an increase in cardiac load. With the same volume of blood restricted to a smaller vascular bed a rise in blood pressure occurs and angina or cardiac failure may be precipitated as a result. A rise in systemic blood pressure is associated with a risk of cerebral haemorrhage; the incidence of stroke is increased in the UK in winter (Haberman *et al.*, 1981).

23.7.2 Intravascular changes

Subjects exposed to cold for 6 h show an increase in packed cell volume, circulating platelets and blood viscosity. These increase the risk of thrombosis and also the incidence of myocardial infarction, which often occurs within 24 h of the onset of a cold spell, as a house takes approximately this time to cool (Keatinge *et al.*, 1984). Mortality from ischaemic heart disease increases in direct proportion to a fall in environmental temperature and the rate rises after a few cold days especially in the elderly (Blows from the winter wind, 1980).

Both the factors of cold stress and hypoxia, should therefore be taken into account in cases of vascular disorders in fit young men at altitude (Ward, 1975) (Chapter 21).

23.8 PULMONARY ARTERY

Acute exposure to cold is known to cause pulmonary hypertension in sheep and cattle and this involves peripheral sensory stimulation and the efferent innervation of the pulmonary vessels (Bligh and Chauca, 1978, 1982; Will *et al.*, 1978). At altitude this may be added to the rise in pressure produced by hypoxia which is a local effect on these vessels. However, Yanagidaira *et al.* (1994) found that rats exposed to cold over a long period had no right ventricular hypertrophy.

In the Arctic many middle-aged and elderly Inuit Eskimo develop progressive pulmonary hypertension resulting in right heart failure, or 'Eskimo lung'. These Inuits had been hunters and trappers when young, which involved hard physical work in very cold conditions. Similar respiratory problems have been noted in white trappers and in native and immigrant Russian workers exposed to extreme conditions in Siberia. Inuit women and men who did little or no winter hunting were relatively free of pulmonary hypertension due to cold (Schaefer *et al.*, 1980).

23.9 FLUID BALANCE

Exposure to cold causes peripheral vasoconstriction with shunting of blood into the deep capacitance vessels. This results in an increased circulating volume in a diminished vascular bed and an increased arterial pressure. The body responds to this excess volume of fluid by a diuresis (Hervey, 1973), initially caused by the release of atrial natriuretic peptide (Atrial natriuretic peptide, 1986). With further body cooling, diuresis results from the failure of tubular reabsorption of sodium and/or water and occurs despite diminished renal blood flow and glomerular filtration (Tansey, 1973). The often severe weight loss experienced by people exposed to cold over a long period is due to fluid loss (Rogers, 1971).

Complicating factors are numerous. Respiratory fluid loss occurs during exercise in the cold and at altitude (Hamlet, 1983). Vigorous exercise in the cold can also produce marked fluid loss due to sweating, which the individual may not notice because the air is dry and evaporation rapid. This loss may amount to $1-2\,l\,day^{-1}$ or between 0.74% and 3.4% of total body mass in 24 h (Budd, 1984). Cold also has a tendency to depress the sensation of thirst as does hypoxia and, as water may not be easily available to mountaineers at altitude, dehydration is common.

The severity of fluid shifts is directly related to the time exposed to cold. Another complicating feature is that the type of exercise associated with hill walking results in appreciable sodium retention and expansion of the extracellular fluid at the expense of the intracellular fluid; this may result in overt clinical oedema of the face and ankles due to activation of the renin–aldosterone system (Williams *et al.*, 1979; Milledge *et al.*, 1982).

During re-warming the circulating blood volume may increase up to 130% of its value prior to cooling. This is probably due to a reversal of fluid shifts and the volume of fluid available for return will depend on the duration of cooling. If rewarming is too rapid, therefore, fluid overload may cause either cerebral or pulmonary oedema (Lloyd, 1973).

23.10 RESPIRATORY TRACT

It is generally believed that the mechanisms available in the upper respiratory tract for warming cold inspired air remove the possibility of cold injury to the lungs, and certainly there has been no evidence of damage to the lungs in those working at the South Pole, in winter joggers or cross-country skiers (Buskirk, 1977). The inhalation of cold dry air can, however, damage the epithelium of the upper respiratory tract in man and dogs (Houk, 1959) and Somervell, a surgeon, at 7500 m on Everest nearly suffocated from the sloughing of the mucosa of his nasopharynx. He gives a graphic account:

> when darkness was gathering I had one of my fits of coughing and dislodged something in my throat which stuck so that I could breathe neither in nor out. I could not of course make a sign to Norton or stop him for the rope was off now; so I sat in the snow to die whilst he walked on . . . I made one or two attempts to breathe but nothing happened. Finally, I pressed my chest with both hands gave one last almighty push – and the obstruction came up. *(Somervell, 1936)*

Because the environmental air is never fully saturated there is a net loss of heat and water when air is exhaled and as much as 50–60% of the heat transferred to inhaled air may be lost on expiration.

If the individual is breathing quietly and at rest the inspired air is equilibrated with body temperature and has achieved full saturation by the time it has reached the tracheal bifurcation. As the tracheal temperature falls during hyperventilation, the mucosa shrinks and becomes pale in the same way as skin; this will prevent the temperature of the upper airways from rising and provide a thermal gradient for the recovery of heat and moisture during expiration.

Exercise may induce bronchospasm in patients with asthma. Its severity is directly related to the rate of respiratory heat loss and can be prevented by inhaling warm humid air (Strauss *et al.*, 1978). However, asthmatic subjects seem to do well in general on high-altitude expeditions, possibly because the beneficial effects of removal from their usual allergens more than outweighs any detrimental effects of inhaling cold air.

Exercise in a cold environment can cause bronchoconstriction. During severe exercise in extremely cold conditions horses may develop frosting of the lungs and sled dogs show evidence of pulmonary oedema

(Schaefer *et al.*, 1980). There are also anecdotal reports of Arctic hunters having 'freezing of the lung'.

23.11 ALIMENTARY TRACT

Cold stress can significantly delay gastric emptying and acid secretion. The initial reduction in both gastric secretion and pancreatic trypsin output is followed in the post-stress period by an increase. This appears to be a non-specific response, as normal postprandial function of the upper gastrointestinal tract can be disturbed by other stressful stimuli (Thompson *et al.*, 1983).

23.12 HORMONAL RESPONSES

23.12.1 Adrenocortical function

In those with no prior exposure to cold, a rise in 17-OHCS levels has been found. This may reflect the nature and severity of the stress, that is disturbance of sleep and shivering together with the painful sensation of cold. Cold adapted invididuals showed no increase in 17-OHCS activity (Radomski and Boutelier, 1982).

23.12.2 Adrenomedullary function

Norepinephrine secretion increases in the non-adapted and remains raised (Weeke and Gundersen, 1983), whilst the well adapted showed no such increase.

Epinephrine secretion increased in both the non-adapted and adapted individuals (Radomski and Boutelier, 1982).

23.12.3 Thyroid function and growth hormone

In rats and some other animals T_3 secretion increases in response to cold exposure but there is also evidence that the main stimulus to non-shivering thermogenesis is a hypothalamic activity via the sympathetic system (Galton, 1978).

In man, the possibility of an increased metabolic rate due to thyroid activity has been considered but there is little evidence that it takes place in response to cold exposure. Korean women divers have a higher BMR in winter, greater utilization of T_4, increased thermal insulation and changes in peripheral blood flow (Hong, 1973), but most studies designed to show increased thyroid activity in response to cold have failed to show any change that could not be accounted for by increased physical activity (Galton, 1978).

On acute exposure to cold there is inhibition of growth hormone secretion (Weeke and Gundersen, 1983).

23.13 MENTAL FUNCTION

The decrease in cerebral blood flow associated with hypothermia results from a drop in metabolism (Hernandez, 1983). There is an ideal level of temperature and humidity at which mental tasks may be carried out, and an increase in cold stress decreases the standard of performance, as well as decreasing the rate of work (Enander, 1984). Cold causes apathy and distracts individuals from their tasks. Performance in the cold depends on familiarity; well motivated subjects can complete given tasks even if the central core temperature has dropped (Baddeley *et al.*, 1975).

Individuals, when exposed to both fatigue and cold stress, adjust their performance so that they maintain as steady a core temperature as possible and limit their heart rate to about 120 beats per minute. To maintain maximum 'comfort' between various stresses, a physiological compromise is reached, and, rather than increase work output so that anaerobic exercise is performed, a lowered core temperature is accepted (Cabanac and LeBlanc, 1983).

Accidents show an increase with low environmental temperature possibly, due to loss of manual dexterity (Goldsmith and Minard, 1976). Workers in cold stores have a reduction in the ability to concentrate and personal irritability increases (Andrew, 1963). Silly errors (verbal, mechanical and clerical) may occur as a result of the inability to concentrate. Subjects may not be aware of the drop in performance and consider that they had done particularly well when, in fact, they had the greatest impairment in function. The individual developing hypothermia is not aware of any mental impairment, and may totally lack insight (Hamilton, 1980).

Exposure to cold produces mental stress, and changes in personality and hallucinations are a sign of incipient or actual hypothermia (Ogilvie, 1977). There are many accounts in the mountain literature of people seeing and talking to a non-existent presence, feeling abnormal fear or pleasure and hearing footsteps or sounds when none exist. In the majority of cases cold, hypoxia, fatigue, starvation or a combination have been present.

Hallucinations are said to occur when the core temperature drops below 32°C, but they often occur above this level (Hirvonen, 1982). Although mountaineers at great altitude report hallucinations, similar findings have been recorded at sea-level in mountain country and elsewhere. Acute hypoxia is not usually associated with hallucinations (Hatcher, 1965), which seem to occur when cerebral hypoxia has been present for some time, suggesting that this may be the result of the biochemical changes resulting from hypoxia rather than the hypoxia *per se*. Some individuals respond to hallucinations, by paradoxical undressing, going beserk and attempting to kill their companions (Wedin *et al.*, 1979). Even on reaching safety, a hypothermic hypoxic patient may be unable to identify exactly where he has been.

REFERENCES

Andrew, H.G. (1963) Work in extreme cold. *Trans. Assoc. Indust. Med. Off.*, **13**, 16–19.

Atrial natriuretic peptide (editorial). (1986) *Lancet*, **2**, 371–2.

Baddeley, A.D., Cuccaro, W.J., Egstrom, G.H., *et al.* (1975) Cognitive efficiency of divers working in cold water. *Hum. Factors*, **17**, 446–54.

Bligh, J. and Chauca, D. (1978) The effects of intracerebroventricular injections of carbachol and noradrenaline in cold induced pulmonary artery hypertension in sheep. *J. Physiol.*, **284**, 53P.

Bligh, J. and Chauca, D. (1982) Effects of hypoxia, cold exposure and fever on pulmonary artery pressure and their significance for Arctic residents, in *Circum Polar Health 1981*, (eds B. Harvald and J.B. Hart Hansen), Nordic Council for Arctic Medical Research, Report 32, Copenhagen, pp. 606–7.

Blows from the winter wind (editorial). (1980) *Br. Med. J.*, **1**, 137–8.

Brennan, P.J., Greenberg, G., Miall, W.E. and Thompson, S.G. (1982) Seasonal variation in arterial blood pressure. *Br. Med. J.*, **2**, 919–23.

Budd, G.M. (1984) Daily Fluid Balance. International Biomedical Expedition to the Antarctic. *6th International Symposium on Circum Polar Health*, Anchorage, May 1984, pp. 59–60.

Burton, A.C. and Edholm, O.G. (1955) *Man in a Cold Environment*, Arnold, London, pp. 140–1.

Buskirk, E.R. (1977) Temperature regulation with exercise. *Exercise Sports Sci. Rev.*, **5**, 45–88.

Cabanac, M. and LeBlanc, J. (1983) Physiological confliction in humans: Fatigue vs cold discomfort. *Am. J. Physiol.*, **244**, 621–8.

Chernow, B., Lake, C.R., Zaritsky, A., *et al.* (1983) Sympathetic nervous system 'switch off' with severe hypothermia. *Crit. Care Med.*, **11**, 677–80.

Coppin, E.G., Livingstone, S.P. and Kuehn, L.A. (1978) Effects on hand grip strength due to arm immersion in a 10°C water bath. *Aviat. Space Environ. Med.*, **49**, 1319–26.

Enander, A. (1984) Performance and sensory aspects of work in cold environments – a review. *Ergonomics*, **27**, 365–78.

Fox, V.F. (1967) Human performance in the cold. *Hum. Factors*, **9**, 203–90.

Galton, V.A. (1978) Environmental effects, in *The Thyroid*, 4th edn, (eds S.C. Werner and S.H. Ingbar), Harper Row, New York, pp. 247–52.

Goldsmith, R. and Minard, D. (1976) Cold, cold work, in *Occupational Health and Safety*, vol. 1, International Labour Office, Geneva, pp. 319–20.

Gorlin, R. (1966) Physiology of the coronary circulation, in *The Heart*, (eds J.W. Hurst and R.B. Logan), McGraw-Hill, New York, pp. 653–8.

Guttman, R. and Gross, M.M. (1956) Relationship between electrical and mechanical changes in muscle caused by cooling. *J. Coll. Comp. Physiol.*, **48**, 421–30.

Haberman, S., Capildeo, R. and Rose, F. (1981) The seasonal variation in mortality from cerebro-vascular disease. *J. Neurol. Sci.*, **52**, 25–36.

Hammel, H.T. (1964) Terrestrial animals in the cold. Recent studies in primitive man, in *Handbook of Physiology: Adaptation to the Environment*, American Physiological Society Washington DC, pp. 413–34.

Hamilton, S.J.C. (1980) Hypothermia and unawareness of mental impairment. *Br. Med. J.*, **1**, 565.

Hamlet, M.P. (1983) Fluid shifts in hypothermia, in *The Nature and Treatment of Hypothermia*, (eds R.S. Pozos and L.E. Wittmers), Croom Helm, London/ University of Minnesota Press, Minneapolis, pp. 94–9.

Hatcher, J.D. (1965) Acute anoxic anoxia, in *The Physiology of Human Survival*, (eds O.G. Edholm and A.L. Bacharach), Academic Press, London, pp. 81–120.

Hayward, J.S., Eckerson, J.D. and Kemna, D. (1984) Thermal and cardiovascular changes during three methods of resuscitation from mild hypothermia. *Resuscitation*, **11**, 21–33.

Hernandez, M.J. (1983) Cerebral circulation during hypothermia, in *The Nature and Treatment of Hypothermia*, (eds R.S. Pozos and L.E. Wittmers), Croom Helm, London/University of Minnesota, Minneapolis, pp. 61–8.

Hervey, G.R. (1973) Physiological changes encountered in hypothermia. *Proc. R. Soc. Med.*, **66**, 1053–7.

Hirvonen, J. (1982) *Accidental Hypothermia*, Nordic Council Arctic Medical Research Report, No. 30, pp. 15–19.

Hoffman, R.G. and Wittmers, L.E. (1990) Cold vasodilatation, pain and acclimatization in Arctic explorers. *J. Wild. Med.*, **1**, 225–34.

Hong, S.K. (1973) Pattern of cold adaptation in women divers of Korea. *Fed. Proc.*, **32**, 1414–22.

Horvath, S.M. (1981) Exercise in a cold environment. *Exercise Sports Sci. Rev.*, **9**, 191–263.

Houk, V.N. (1959) Transient pulmonary insufficiency caused by cold. *US Armed Forces Med. J.*, **10**, 1354–7.

Hunter, J., Kerr, E.H. and Whillans, M.G. (1952) The relation between joint stiffness upon exposure to cold and the characteristics of synovial fluid. *J. Can. Med. Sci.*, **39**, 367–77.

Kayser, B., Binzoni, T., Hoppeler, H., *et al.* (1993) A case of severe frostbite on Mt Blanc: A multi-technique approach. *J. Wild. Med.*, **4**, 167–74.

Keatinge, W.R., Coleshaw, S.R.K., Cotter, F., *et al.* (1984) Increases in platelet and red cell counts, blood viscosity and arterial pressure during mild surface cooling: Factors in mortality from coronary and cerebral thrombosis in winter. *Br. Med. J.*, **2**, 1405–8.

Lloyd, E.L. (1973) Accidental hypothermia treated by central re-warming via the airway. *Br. J. Anaesth.*, **45**, 41–8.

Marshall, H.C. and Goldman, R.F. (1976) Electrical response of nerve to freezing injury, in *Circumpolar Health*, (eds R.J. Shephard and S. Itoh), University Press, Toronto, p. 77.

Milledge, J.S., Bryson E.I., Catley, D.M., *et al.* (1982) Sodium balance, fluid homeostasis, and the renin–aldosterone system during the prolonged exercise of hill walking. *Clin. Sci.*, **62**, 598–604.

Ogilvie, J. (1977) Exhaustion and exposure. *Climber and Rambler*, Sept., pp. 34–9, Oct., pp. 52–5.

Radomski, M.N. and Boutelier, C. (1982) Hormone response of normal and intermittent cold pre-adapted humans to continuous cold. *J. Appl. Physiol.*, **53**, 610–16.

Rogers, T.A. (1971) The clinical course of survival in the Arctic. *Hawaii Med. J.*, **30**, 31–4.

Schaefer, O., Eaton, R.D.P., Timmermans, F.J.W. and Hildes, J.A. (1980) Respiratory function impairment and cardiopulmonary consequences in long term residents of the Canadian Arctic. *Can. Med. Assoc. J.*, **119**, 997–1004.

Shephard, R.J. (1985) Adaptation to exercise in the cold. *Sports Med.*, **2**, 59–71.

Somervell, T.H. (1936) *After Everest*, Hodder and Stoughton, London, p. 132.

Strauss, R.H., McFadden, E.R., Ingram, R.H., *et al.* (1978) Influence of heat and humidity on the airway obstruction induced by exercise in asthma. *J. Clin. Invest.*, **61**, 433–40.

Strong, L.H., Gin, G.K. and Goldman, R.F. (1985) Metabolic and vasomotor insulative responses occurring on immersion in cold water. *J. Appl. Physiol.*, **58**, 964–77.

Tansey, W.A. (1973) *Medical Aspects of Cold Water Immersion: A review.* US Navy Submarine Medical Research Laboratory Report NSMRL 763, NTIS Document AD-775-687.

Thompson, D.G., Richelson, E. and Malagelada, J.R. (1983) A perturbation of upper gastro-intestinal function by cold stress. *Gut*, **24**, 277–83.

Ward, M.P. (1975) *Mountain Medicine, A Clinical Study of Cold and High Altitude*, Crosby Lockwood Staples, London, pp. 289–92.

Wedin, B., Vanggaard, L. and Hirvonen, J. (1979) 'Paradoxical undressing' in fatal hypothermia. *J. Forensic Sci.*, **24**, 543–53.

Weeke, J. and Gundersen, H.J.G. (1983) The effect of heating and cold cooling on serum T.S.H., G.H., and norepinephrine in resting normal man. *Acta Physiol. Scand.*, **47**, 33–9.

Will, D.H., McMurty, I.F., Reeves, T.J., *et al.* (1978) Cold-induced pulmonary hypertension in cattle. *J. Appl. Physiol.*, **45**, 469–73.

Williams, E.S., Ward, M.P., Milledge, J.S., *et al.* (1979) Effect of the exercise of seven consecutive days hill-walking on fluid homeostasis. *Clin. Sci.*, **56**, 306–16.

Yanagidaira, Y., Sakai, A., Kashimura, O., *et al.* (1994) The effects of prolonged exposure to cold on hypoxic pulmonary hypertension in rats. *J. Wild. Med.*, **5**, 11–19.

Young, A.J., Muza, S.R., Sawka, M.N., *et al.* (1986) Human thermo-regulatory responses to cold air are altered by repeated cold water immersion. *J. Appl. Physiol.*, **60**, 1542–8.

24

Hypothermia

24.1 INTRODUCTION

Populations of 100 million or more may be at risk due to cold injury, yet in civilian life the condition is less common than in wartime. In all campaigns carried out at an environmental temperature around freezing point cold injury is common and environmental hazard is now a major factor with armies in the field.

Hippocrates wrote on the climate of different lands and the influence of the climate on their inhabitants. He made many observations on cold injury, including the occurrence of blisters, blackening of the skin and tingling in the hands. Many observers since then have described the effects of cold and Napoleon's army suffered severely on their retreat from Russia.

Considerable casualties also occurred in the American Civil War, in World Wars I and II and in Korea, whilst, more recently, in the Falkland Islands campaign (1982), 13.6% of casualties were due to non-freezing cold injury (Marsh, 1983).

In peacetime, cold injury occurs particularly after natural disasters, such as earthquakes during the winter months. Polar travellers, mountaineers and skiers also are at risk, despite improvements in clothing, technique and equipment. Cavers, divers, fishermen and swimmers are also exposed to cold injury (Washburn, 1962). The elderly and the young may both also be liable, especially if they are in poor nutrition or are ill.

Accidental hypothermia has been reported in many tropical countries. In the Sahara, where there are peaks up to 3010 m in the Hoggar, the temperature may fall to near freezing point at night (Pierre and Aulard, 1985). Even in Kampala, where the environmental temperature never falls below 16°C cases have occurred (Sadikali and Owor, 1974; Barber, 1978).

Hypothermia is defined as lowering of the central core temperature below 35°C (RCP, 1966). Exposure is a non-medical term used in relation to cold to describe a serious chilling of the body surface, usually associated with exhaustion, leading to a progressive fall in body temperature with the risk of death from hypothermia. Cold stress is the term used to describe the stimulus which initiates the physiological thermoregulatory response to cold.

24.2 CLASSIFICATION

Hypothermia may be classified according to central core temperature:

- mild: central core temperature 35–32°C
- severe: central core temperature 32°C and below.

It may also be classified according to length of exposure:

- Acute: the cold stress is so great and sudden that the body's resistance to cold is overridden despite heat production being at or near maximum. Hypothermia occurs before exhaustion develops.
- Subacute: a critical factor is exhaustion and depletion of the body's food store. Normally cold stress is combated by peripheral vasoconstriction and increase in heat production which maintains normal body temperature until exhaustion supervenes and core temperature falls. This is the type of hypothermia from which trekkers, hill walkers and mountaineers suffer.
- Chronic: usually there is prolonged exposure to a mild degree of cold stress and while the thermoregulatory response is not overwhelmed it is insufficient to counteract the cold. The core temperature will fall over days or weeks. This form of hypothermia is commonly seen in the elderly.

24.3 CLINICAL FEATURES

24.3.1 Mild hypothermia

The individual, if a mountaineer, complains of feeling cold and loses interest in any activity except getting warmer. They also develop a negative attitude towards the aims of the party, and as cooling continues, become inco-ordinate, is unable to keep up with the rest of the party and then starts to stumble. There may be attacks of violent shivering.

24.3.2 Severe hypothermia

At core temperatures below 32°C there is altered mental function and the patient becomes careless about self-protection from the cold.

Thinking becomes slow, decision making difficult and often wrong, and memory deteriorates. There may be a strong desire for sleep and eventually the will to survive collapses with the individual becoming progressively unresponsive and lapsing into coma. Slurred speech and ataxia may be confused with a stroke. Gastrointestinal mobility may slow or cease, and gastric dilatation and ileus are common (Paton, 1983).

Individuals show a great range of response to cold and loss of consciousness may occur with a core temperature as high as 33°C or as low as 27°C, depending on the rate of cooling. Consciousness is usually lost around 30°C but patients have been reported to be conscious though confused at lower temperatures than this (Paton, 1983; Lloyd, 1972).

Though shivering usually stops as the temperature drops below 30°C, it has been observed at a core temperature of 24°C (Alexander, 1945). Some cases have been reported to cool without shivering (Marcus, 1979) (Chapter 22).

When the temperature drops to below 30°C, ventricular fibrillation may supervene. Survival depends on sufficient cardiac function to

Table 24.1 Clinical features of hypothermia (Adapted from Lloyd, 1986a)

Temperature (°C)	*Clinical features*
37.6	Normal rectal temperature
37	Normal oral temperature
35	Maximal shivering/delayed cerebration
34	Lowest temperature compatible with continuous exercise
33–31	Retrograde amnesia, clouded consciousness Blood pressure difficult to obtain
30–28	Progressive loss of consciousness Muscular rigidity Slow respiration and pulse Ventricular fibrillation may develop if heart irritated
27	Appears dead Voluntary movement lost Deep tendon reflex and pupil reflex absent
25	Ventricular fibrillation may develop spontaneously
24–21	Pulmonary edema develops
20	Heart stopped
14	Lowest temperature in accidental hypothermia patient with recovery (MacIntyre, 1994)
9	Lowest temperature in cooled hypothermic patient with recovery
1–7	Rats and hamsters revived successfully

maintain output adequate for brain and heart perfusion. Cardiac function is more relevant to survival than brain temperature.

The patient with profound hypothermia may be indistinguishable from one who is dead. The skin is ice cold to touch and the muscles and joints are stiff and simulate rigor mortis. Respiration may be difficult or impossible to register, the peripheral pulses absent and blood pressure unmeasurable. In profound hypothermia pupils do not react to light and other reflexes are absent.

The ECG shows a slow rhythm with multifocal extrasystoles, broad complexes, and atrial flutter (Jessen and Hagelstein, 1978). There may also be 'J' waves present (Osborne, 1953).

Both haemoglobin and white cell count will be raised due to a shift of fluid from plasma to the interstitial space. Thrombocytopenia has been reported (Vella *et al.*, 1988).

Even when there is evidence of a total stoppage of cardiorespiratory function, survival is possible (Siebhke *et al.*, 1975); a flat EEG is not a certain indicator of death in hypothermia. The only certain diagnosis is failure to recover on rewarming (Lilja, 1983; Golden, 1973). Before brain death can be diagnosed the core temperature must be normal (NHS, 1974); however, brain death may be a cause of hypothermia (Table 24.1).

24.4 MANAGEMENT

The principles of management are to prevent further heat loss, to restore body temperature to normal and to maintain life whilst doing so.

Choice of technique will depend upon circumstances, facilities available and the experience and skill of the doctor. In mildly hypothermic patients a slow rewarming technique is acceptable, but for severe hypothermia rapid, active rewarming should be carried out. If there is no circulation the patient should be transferred to a unit where rewarming by heat exchange is possible.

A summary of the technique is as follows:

- Mild hypothermia 35–32°C
  - Surface rewarming
  - Warm i.v. fluids
  - Warm inspired oxygen
- Severe hypothermia 32°C and below
  - Warm i.v. fluids
  - Airway warming via endotracheal tube
  - Warm bath immersion
  - Peritoneal dialysis
  - Gastric lavage

- If circulatory arrest occurs
  Cardiopulmonary resuscitation
  Airway rewarming
  Peritoneal dialysis
  Gastric lavage
  Central rewarming via heat exchanger.

24.4.1 In the field

Mild hypothermia

The individual should be stopped from walking and placed in shelter out of the wind, rain or snow. They should be protected from further cooling and warmed by any method available.

Ideally, wet clothing should be replaced by dry, but if dry clothing is not available wet clothing should be wrung out and put back on. If wet clothing, which has some insulating value, is left on it should be covered by an impermeable material to prevent further heat loss by evaporation. As large amounts of heat may be lost from the head it should be covered. Warm fluids should be given but never alcohol.

A patient with mild hypothermia can recover with these simple procedures, but recovery will be hastened if external heat is added (e.g. getting into a sleeping bag with another person). Central re-warming methods have been described (Lloyd, 1973; Foray and Salon, 1985) using warmed inhaled air which can be applied in the field with suitable apparatus.

Severe hypothermia

The management of severe hypothermia in the field will depend upon the local situation, possibilities for evacuation and access to specialist medical facilities. Where these are good, as in the mountains of Europe and North America, patients should be evacuated as soon as possible with the minimum of treatment in the field. However, active treatment in the field has been successful (Fischer *et al.*, 1991). Aluminium foil 'blankets' and suits provide good thermal protection in rescue situations (Ennemoser *et al.*, 1988). When bad weather delays evacuation the patient should be rewarmed slowly and treated as gently as possible to try and avoid ventricular fibrillation.

If there is cardiac arrest it is reasonable to attempt external cardiac massage, however the difficulty is to be certain of the diagnosis of cardiac arrest in a case of profound hypothermia. The peripheral pulse may be absent but the heart may still be beating slowly. Misguided attempts at cardiac massage may then precipitate ventricular fibrillation

(Mills, 1983). The mortality rate of hypothermia in the field is of the order of 50% but with increasing expertise in management this figure should improve.

It must be emphasized that the diagnosis of death in hypothermia should be made with caution because profound hypothermia can simulate death. Strictly, the diagnosis of death can only be made when the patient fails to revive after the core temperature has been brought to normal.

24.4.2 In hospital (Bohn, 1987)

Those patients with mild hypothermia (32–35°C) can be allowed to rewarm slowly on a general ward and warm humidified oxygen can be given by mask. Those with severe hypothermia (32°C and below) should be admitted to an intensive care unit.

Intubation and ventilation should be carried out by a skilled anaesthetist with adequate preoxygenation to prevent cardiac arrhythmia, if there is:

- absence of vital signs;
- coma;
- apnoea;
- hypoxaemia not corrected by oxygen by mask;
- cardiac arrhythmia;
- aspiration pneumonia;
- hypercarbia.

If there is no pulse or respiration then full cardiorespiratory resuscitation should be carried out, regardless of ECG activity. Between 30°C and 28°C the heart may fibrillate spontaneously but the presence of sinus rhythm does not mean that there is a useful cardiac output, so immediate external cardiac massage should be started.

Below 28°C the fibrillating heart will not convert to sinus rhythm, so there is little point in using shock therapy until the core temperature is above this value. Cardiac pacing and atropine seem of little benefit; dopamine can improve cardiac output. An increase in filling pressure can be achieved by using pneumatic trousers to decrease peripheral volume.

24.5 METHODS OF REWARMING

Even in hospital with perfect insulation, the rate of warming varies greatly at between 0.14°C to 0.5°C per hour, and failure to rewarm may occur. Too rapid rewarming may result in fluid shifts with pulmonary and cerebral edema. Young people, particularly those in whom acute hypothermia was precipitated by drug overdose, have a high survival rate when allowed to warm spontaneously (Tolman and Cohen, 1970). In the elderly with chronic hypothermia, there is a high mortality rate (Treating accidental hypothermia, 1978) unless treatment is carried out in an intensive care unit (Ledingham and Mone, 1980).

In severe hypothermia, when the patient no longer shivers, some method of active rewarming is necessary as metabolic heat production is so low.

24.5.1 Peripheral (surface) rewarming

This may be carried out either rapidly or at a slow to moderate rate; it is only advisable for conscious patients suffering from acute accidental hypothermia.

Rapid rewarming

The conscious patient should be placed in a bath which is then heated to 40–42°C, hand hot, as rapidly as possible. The advantages are that it is the fastest way of transferring heat, needs unsophisticated equipment, suppresses shivering and speeds the feeling of well-being.

The disadvantages are that, by dilating the peripheral circulation before the body temperature has been fully restored, there is a danger of 'rewarming shock' (Golden, 1983). Also, because of the problem of maintaining the airway, this method of treatment is not advocated in an unconscious patient.

Slow to moderate rewarming

This includes the use of hotwater bottles, blankets, hot water packs, temperature controlled cabinets and cradles and hot water sarongs (Paton, 1983). This method requires an effective peripheral circulation and most, but not all, patients do rewarm (Ledingham and Mone, 1980).

Superficial burns are an important hazard associated with all forms of surface heating, and may occur even when the temperature is quite low (e.g. hand-warm hot water bottles) (de Pay, 1982). Another disadvantage is that, with peripheral vasodilatation, heat is further dissipated and cold blood returns to the heart causing irregularities of rhythm (Anderson *et al.*, 1970).

Shivering is abolished by surface hot water warming and oxygen demand is reduced. However, not all methods of surface rewarming provide enough heat and abolition of shivering may put the patient further at risk.

24.5.2 Central rewarming via the airways

Heat is supplied to the body via the airways by giving the patient warmed, moist air or oxygen from a suitable apparatus via a mask or endotracheal tube (Lloyd, 1973). The main value of airway warming is due to the prevention of heat and moisture loss from the respiratory tract rather than by the additional heat supplied, which is quite modest. Other methods of central rewarming supply heat more rapidly. The advantage of this method is that it is relatively non-invasive.

It has also been claimed that the incidence of cardiac irregularities are less common with airway rewarming. Heat flow through the airways and mediastinal structures warms the heart from the pericardium inwards and warm blood from the lungs will heat the endocardium and myocardium via the coronary arteries (Lloyd and Mitchell, 1974). In addition, more rapid warming of the brain will occur, reducing the cold-induced depression of the respiratory centre, and giving a selective improvement of cerebral function.

Airway warming reduces shivering in hypothermic patients and during rescue this can be important as it will reduce oxygen requirement and blood flow to the limbs; thus, heat loss, cardiac load and metabolic demand will be less.

Various types of equipment are available:

- condenser-humidifier, which traps heat and moisture during expiration returning both on the next inspiration;
- electrically powered humidifier;
- a closed circuit consisting of a soda-lime canister and oxygen cylinder. The reaction between soda-lime and expired CO_2 produces heat and moisture (Lloyd, 1986a).

24.5.3 Central warming via a heat exchanger

In open heart surgery total body cooling and rewarming is routine. From experience gained by this method it was natural to suggest that similar methods be used in severe hypothermia.

Blood is removed from the femoral vein, warmed in a heat exchanger and returned by the femoral artery. Heat may be supplied very rapidly by this method and the body temperature raised by 10°C in one hour.

The heart is perfused directly with warm blood and cardiac irritability is reduced. If hypovolaemic shock due to peripheral vasodilatation occurs, then a warm heart can compensate better than a cold or irritable one. A definite indication for extracorporeal rewarming is ventricular fibrillation associated with hypothermia (Braun, 1985), and patients who are 'frozen solid and dead' with a core temperature as low as 17.5°C have been resuscitated by this means. The method is safe in experienced hands and is becoming more popular in centres where open heart surgery is routine.

24.5.4 Irrigation of body cavities

Mediastinal

Thoracotomy and mediastinal irrigation has been successful, but it is an open, invasive method requiring a sophisticated team. It causes more trauma to the patient, there is a risk of infection, and it is doubtful if it is more effective than central warming by heat exchange (Paton, 1983).

Peritoneal

Peritoneal lavage is an efficient method of heat transfer. The temperature gradients throughout the body are more normal than with surface rewarming. The inferior vena cava is warmed directly and thus venous blood returning to the heart is selectively warmed. Additional heat to the heart and lungs is transferred via the diaphragm, and cardiac, liver and renal functions are improved. It is a simple method not requiring highly trained personnel and sophisticated equipment (Patton and Doolittle, 1972; Pickering *et al.*, 1977).

Problems include peritonitis which are related to perforation of the bowel and respiratory insufficiency due to the pressure of fluid in the peritoneal cavity. Recent abdominal surgery is a contra-indication because of the possibility of adhesions.

24.5.5 Other methods

Intragastric balloons have been used, in which a double lumen tube transports the warm fluid to and from the balloon. A double lumen oesophageal tube with a thermostat controlled pump has also been tried (Kristensen *et al.*, 1986). These offer some promise as a method of warming the central core without the sterile precautions needed for peritoneal lavage. A technique using a modified Sengstaken tube through which Ringer's lactate solution is circulated at 41°C has been described (Ledingham, 1983). Enemas and gastric lavage have been described but require larger amounts of fluid. Intracolonic balloons may also be used.

Diathermy requires sophisticated and expensive equipment, but it has considerable potential for delivering significant amounts of heat by transmitting energy through the superficial tissues to the deeper ones where it is converted to heat. Three main types are considered by

Harnett *et al.* (1983): ultrasonic, shortwave and microwave. There are a considerable number of hazards and disadvantages (Lehmann, 1971).

24.6 ASSOCIATED THERAPY

24.6.1 Drugs

There is controversy over the use of corticosteroids in hypothermia. Some recommend their use from clinical experience and steroids have been given as a last resort to apparently moribund mountaineers with some success (MacInnes, 1971).

24.6.2 Electrolyte abnormalities

These may be found in hypothermic patients but the pattern is completely inconsistent. Hypokalaemia should be treated by giving potassium; calcium will protect against the effects of hypokalaemia on the myocardium.

24.6.3 Glucose

Hypoglycaemia was an important factor in one series of hypothermic patients (Fitzgerald and Jessop, 1982), but a high blood sugar may be found in cases of hypothermia (non-diabetic) probably due to non-utilization of glucose by cold muscles; on rewarming, the glucose level will fall. Hypoglycaemia may precipitate hypothermia and the centre controlling heat production may be impaired. In cases of exhaustion hypothermia, glucose may be given to provide metabolic substrate for rewarming (MacInnes, 1979).

24.6.4 Oxygen

Hypothermia will have the effect of shifting the oxygen dissociation curve to the left (i.e. increasing the haemoglobin affinity for oxygen) (Chapter 8). This means that there may be difficulty in giving up oxygen in the tissues, which may then be hypoxic. Therefore, there is a theoretical advantage in the use of oxygen (which should be warmed) in cases of hypothermia, though this has not been demonstrated. Bohn (1987) considers that all hypothermic patients should be considered hypoxaemic until proved otherwise.

24.7 AFTER DROP

The core temperature continues to fall before rising after the individual has been removed from cold water; this has been termed the 'after drop'. As many deaths have occurred after removal from cold water and because this collapse coincided with the time that the rectal temperature was at its lowest (Golden, 1983), it was assumed that death and the after drop were connected, and that ventricular fibrillation had been precipitated by the continued cooling of the heart.

However, the belief that the after drop is caused by cold blood returning to the core from the cooled peripheral circulation has now been challenged by Golden and Hervey (1981). In fact, if the rate of heat production from core to periphery is high enough to balance heat flow there is no after drop (Golden and Hervey, 1981). The way that heat flows through the body tissues can explain the rectal temperature fall (Webb, 1986). Savard *et al.* (1985) have shown that the 'after drop' in core temperature *precedes* peripheral vasodilatation in human volunteers exposed to hypothermia. Moreover, at the time of maximum peripheral vasodilatation, core temperatures had already started to rise. Slow passive rewarming may therefore be used in mild hypothermia and rapid active rewarming is only indicated for severe hypothermia.

24.8 VENTRICULAR FIBRILLATION

The exact mechanism involved in the production of ventricular fibrillation due to cold has so far not been defined. Changes in electrolyte concentration occur but there is no general agreement on their interpretation. Hypoxia of the myocardium might be a cause but, in hypothermia, oxygen carried in the blood is adequate for the reduced myocardial work, though sudden hypoxia may precipitate ventricular fibrillation in hypothermia.

Cardiac temperature may be very low without ventricular fibrillation (Laufmann, 1951) and the direct effect of cold is often asystole. However, it seems probable that the effect of cold blood on the Purkinje fibres selectively cools them relative to the cardiac muscle. This could result in ventricular fibrillation following cardiac irritation (Lloyd and Mitchell, 1974).

Defibrillation below 28°C is unlikely to be successful although there are some exceptions. Ideally one should manage such patients in a cardiac surgical unit. The circulation should be maintained artificially until cardiac temperatures exceed 28°C before attempting defibrillation, as too many attempts are likely to burn the pericardium. However, with direct core rewarming, a heart in asystole has started spontaneously at 24°C, and defibrillation has been successful at 22.5°C. Bretylium tosylate is a most effective antifibrillatory drug at low temperature and can be used prophylactically (Paton, 1991).

24.9 INTRAVASCULAR VOLUME

This is depleted in all hypothermia patients, especially when associated with septicaemia and trauma. Incidents of cardiovascular collapse and cardiac arrest during rewarming may be due to vasodilatation in a volume-depleted patient and not to 'after drop', the toxic effects of metabolites or the effect of cold blood on the heart.

Death may therefore be due to hypovolaemia. During cooling, there is a shift in body fluids from the intravascular to the interstitial compartment, causing overt oedema, which is increased on rewarming. The severity of the shifts is directly related to the duration of cold exposure.

During rewarming, reversal of fluid shifts occur most rapidly in the peripheral vascular bed, causing a rise in central venous pressure.

Survival from hypothermia depends, therefore, on a balance between the size of the vascular bed controlled by vasomotor tone and the circulating blood volume dependent on the extent of dehydration. It is also dependent on the extent and rate of reversal of the fluid shifts that occur during cooling. If vasomotor tone is poor, death from hypovolaemia may occur, whilst fluid overload may cause heart failure; dehydration may affect either.

The only sure method of distinguishing these is by central venous pressure monitoring; this should be done routinely in hospital. If the blood pressure falls, a rapid infusion of 500 ml of warmed fluid will, if hypovolaemia is present, raise the blood pressure temporarily (Lloyd, 1986b).

24.10 COMPLICATIONS

For the previously healthy hypothermic patient the risk of serious complications is low. Many of those listed below result from pre-existing conditions, chronic disease, malnutrition and alcoholism (Wilkerson *et al.*, 1986) (Table 24.2).

Table 24.2 Complications of profound hypothermia (Adapted from Wilkerson *et al.*, 1986.)

Pneumonia and pulmonary edema
Gastric erosion or ulcer
Acute pancreatitis
Haemolysis and disseminated intravascular coagulation
Acute renal failure and haematuria
Myoglobinuria
Temporary adrenal insufficiency

REFERENCES

Alexander, L. (1945) *The Treatment of Shock from Prolonged Exposure to Cold Especially in Water*, Combined Intelligence Objective Sub-Committee, Item No. 24, File No. 24-37.

Anderson, S., Herbring, B.G. and Widman, B. (1970) Accidental profound hypothermia (case report). *Br. J. Anaesth.*, **42**, 653–5.

Barber, S.G. (1978) Drugs and doctoring for trans-Saharan travellers. *Br. Med. J.*, **2**, 404–6.

Bohn, D.J. (1987) Treatment of hypothermia in hospital, in *Hypothermia and Cold*, (eds J.R. Sutton, C.S. Houston and G. Coates), Prager, New York, pp. 286–305.

Braun, P. (1985) Pathophysiology and treatment of hypothermia, in *High Altitude Deterioration*, (eds J. Rivolier, P. Cerretelli, J. Foray and P. Segantini), Karger, Basel, pp. 140–8.

De Pay, A.W. (1982) Medical treatment of hypothermic victims, in *Unterkuhlung im Seenotfall*, 2nd Symposium Deutsche Gesellschaft zur Rettung Schiffbruchiger, (eds P. Koch and M. Kohfahl), Cuxhaven, Germany, pp. 146–53.

Ennemoser, O., Ambach, W. and Flora, G. (1988) Physical assessment of heat insulation of rescue foils. *Int. J. Sports Med.*, **9**, 179–82.

Fischer, A.P., Stumpe, F. and Vallotton, J. (1991) Hypothermia in an avalanche: A case report, in *A Colour Atlas of Mountain Medicine*, (eds J. Vallotton and F. Du Bas), Wolfe, London, pp. 96–7.

Fitzgerald, F.T. and Jessop, C. (1982) Accidental hypothermia. A report of 22 cases and review of the literature. *Adv. Intern. Med.*, **27**, 127–50.

Foray, J. and Salon, F. (1985) Casualties with cold injuries: Primary treatment, in *High Altitude Deterioration*, (eds J. Rivolier, P. Cerretelli, J. Foray and P. Segantini), Karger, Basel, pp. 149–58.

Golden, F. St C. (1973) Recognition and treatment of immersion hypothermia. *Proc. R. Soc. Med.*, **66**, 1058–61.

Golden, F. St C. (1983) Rewarming, in *The Nature and Treatment of Hypothermia*, (eds R.S. Pozos and L.E. Wittmers), Croom Helm, London/University of Minnesota Press, Minneapolis, pp. 194–208.

Golden, F. St C. and Hervey, G.R. (1981) The 'after drop' and death after rescue from immersion in cold water, in *Hypothermia Ashore and Afloat*, (ed. J.N. Adams), Aberdeen University Press, Aberdeen, pp. 37–56.

Harnett, R.M., Pruitt, J.R. and Sias, F.R. (1983) A review of the literature concerning resuscitation from hypothermia, Part II. Selected rewarming protocols. *Aviat. Space Environ. Med.*, **54**, 487–95.

Jessen, K. and Hagelstein, J.O. (1978) Peritoneal dialysis in the treatment of profound accidental hypothermia. *Aviat. Space Environ. Med.*, **49**, 424–9.

Kristensen, G., Drenk, N.E. and Jordening, H. (1986) Simple system for central rewarming of hypothermic patients. *Lancet*, **2**, 1467–8.

Laufmann, H. (1951) Profound accidental hypothermia. *J. Am. Med. Assoc.*, **147**, 1201–12.

Ledingham, I. McA. (1983) Clinical management of elderly hypothermic patients, in *The Nature and Treatment of Hypothermia*, (eds R.S. Pozos and L.E. Wittmers), Croom Helm, London/University of Minnesota Press, Minneapolis, pp. 165–81.

Ledingham, I. McA. and Mone, J.G. (1980) Treatment of accidental hypothermia: A prospective clinical study. *Br. Med. J.*, **1**, 1102–5.

Lehmann, J.F. (1971) Diathermia, in *Handbook of Physical Medicine and Rehabilitation*, 2nd edn, Saunders, Philadelphia, pp. 1397–442.

Lilja, G.P. (1983) Emergency treatment of hypothermia, in *The Nature and*

Treatment of Hypothermia, (eds R.S. Pozos and L.E. Wittmers), Croom Helm, London/University of Minnesota Press, Minneapolis, pp. 143–51.

Lloyd, E. Ll. (1972) Diagnostic problems and hypothermia. *Br. Med. J.*, **3**, 417.

Lloyd, E. Ll. (1973) Accidental hypothermia treated by central re-warming through the airway. *Br. J. Anaesth.*, **45**, 41–8.

Lloyd, E. Ll. (1986a) *Hypothermia and Cold Stress*, Croom Helm, London, pp. 199–203.

Lloyd, E. Ll. (1986b) *Hypothermia and Cold Stress*, Croom Helm, London, p. 74.

Lloyd, E. Ll. and Mitchell, B. (1974) Factors affecting the onset of ventricular fibrillation in hypothermia: A hypothesis. *Lancet*, **2**, 1294–6.

MacInnes, C. (1971) Steroids in mountain rescue. *Lancet*, **1**, 599.

MacInnes, C. (1979) Treatment of accidental hypothermia. *Br. Med. J.*, **1**, 130–1.

MacIntyre, B. (1994) Ice-cream comforts girl who survived big freeze. *The Times*, March 4, p. 15.

Marcus, P. (1979) The treatment of acute accidental hypothermia. Proceedings of a Symposium held at the RAF Institute of Aviation Medicine. *Aviat. Space Environ. Med.*, **50**, 834–43.

Marsh, A.R. (1983) A short but distant war: The Falklands campaign. *J. R. Soc. Med.*, **76**, 972–82.

Mills, W.J. (1983) General hypothermia. *Alaska Med.*, **25**, 29–32.

NHS. (1974) *Accidental Hypothermia*. N.H.S. Memorandum No. 1974 (Gen.) 7, Scottish Home and Health Department.

Osborne, J.J. (1953) Experimental hypothermia: Respiratory and blood pH changes in relation to cardiac function. *Am. J. Physiol.*, **175**, 389–98.

Paton, B.C. (1983) Accidental hypothermia. *Pharmacol. Ther.*, **22**, 331–77.

Paton, B.C. (1991) Hypothermia, in *A Colour Atlas of Mountain Medicine*, (eds J. Vallotton and F. Dubas, Wolfe, London, pp. 92–6.

Patton, J.F. and Doolittle, W.H. (1972) Core rewarming by peritoneal dialysis following induced hypothermia in the dog. *J. Appl. Physiol.*, **33**, 800–4.

Pickering, B.G., Bristow, G.K. and Craig, D.B. (1977) Core rewarming by peritoneal irrigation in accidental hypothermia. *Anaesth. Analg.*, **56**, 574–7.

Pierre, B. and Aulard, C. (1985) *Escalades et Randonnés du Hoggar et dans les Tassilis*, Arthaud, Paris, p. 153.

RCP. (1966) *Report of Committee on Accidental Hypothermia*, Royal College of Physicians, London.

Sadikali, F. and Owor, R. (1974) Hypothermia in the tropics. A review of 24 cases. *Trop. Geogr. Med.*, **26**, 265–70.

Savard, G.K., Cooper, K.E., Veal, W.L. and Malkinson, T.J. (1985) Peripheral blood flow during rewarming from mild hypothermia in humans. *J. Appl. Physiol.*, **58**, 4–13.

Siebkhe, H., Breivik, H., Rod, T. and Lind, B. (1975) Survival after 40 minutes' submersion without cerebral sequelae. *Lancet*, **1**, 1275–9.

Tolman, K.G. and Cohen, A. (1970) Accidental hypothermia. *Can. Med. Assoc. J.*, **103**, 1357–61.

Treating accidental hypothermia (editorial). (1978) *Br. Med. J.*, **2**, 1383–4.

Vella, M.A., Jenner, C., Betteridge, D.J. and Jowett, N.I. (1988) Hypothermia induced thrombocytopenia. *J. R. Soc. Med.*, **81**, 228–9.

Webb, P. (1986) After drop of body temperature during re-warming – an alternative explanation. *J. Appl. Physiol.*, **60**, 385–90.

Washburn, B. (1962) Frostbite. What it is – and how to prevent it – emergency treatment. *N. Engl. J. Med.*, **266**, 974–89.

Wilkerson, J.A., Bangs, C.C. and Hayward, J.S. (1986) *Hypothermia, Frostbite and Other Cold Injuries*, The Mountaineers, Seattle, p. 45.

25

Local cold injury

25.1 INTRODUCTION

Many are cold, yet few are frozen and frost-bite is not common. However both non-freezing injury (immersion injury, trench foot) and freezing cold injury (frost-bite) may be present in the same limb and both may be associated with hypothermia.

Non-freezing cold injury normally occurs between 0–15°C, though the upper limits are not precisely known and feet exposed for some time in water at 26°C may become swollen, hyperaemic and painful. Freezing cold injury (frost-bite) occurs at temperatures below 0°C in dry/cold conditions, especially if there is a wind. Frost-bite may occur in fully clothed individuals at extreme altitude at subzero temperatures if oxygen uptake is insufficient for adequate heat production, when the tissues cool to the environmental temperature.

25.2 FROST-BITE

Many clinical factors may precipitate local cold injury. These are shown in Table 25.1.

25.2.1 Clinical features

Distribution of frost-bite

Any area may be affected but some are more prone to cold injury because of pressure, position, lack of insulating fat or liability to wetting. These include:

- face: bridge of nose (due to spectacles), tip of nose, chin (double chin especially), ear lobes, cheeks, lips, tongue (due to drinking or sucking snow or ice);

Table 25.1 Factors which may precipitate frost-bite

Excessive reaction to cold i.e. Raynaud's syndrome
Diabetes
Endarteritis – local – result of previous cold injury
Endarteritis obliterans
Vascular damage due to trauma or infection
Arteriosclerosis
Thyroid hypofunction
Hyperhidrosis – congenital or acquired
Hypovolaemia – loss of blood or through shock
Dehydration due to gastrointestinal disease or exercise
Nicotine
Metal spectacle frames or seats

- upper limb: fingers (particularly the index finger in rifle shooting), head of radius, lower end of ulnar, olecranon, medial and lateral epicondyle of humerus;
- lower limb: patella, head of fibula, subcutaneous border of tibia, medial condyle of tibia, lower end of fibula, lateral edge of foot, planter aspect of toes, dorsal surface of foot joints, soles of feet, heels;
- male genitalia: penis and testicles (difficulty in fastening zip; wetting due to overflow incontinence); jogging in conditions of severe wind chill (Hershkowitz, 1977);
- buttocks and perineum (sitting on metallic seats).

Cultural patterns may influence the site of frost-bite. With long hair frost-bite of the ears is unusual, whilst short hair is associated with frozen ears. Some activity at low temperatures associated with inadequate foot gear (e.g. running shoes) may also predispose to the development of cold injury; a similar type of shoe is used for cross-country skiing.

Drug abuse may also contribute to cold injury, as nasal 'snorting' of cocaine causes vasoconstriction, and this makes the nose more prone to cooling in a cold environment.

Although a number of classifications have been proposed it is simpler to consider frost-bite as being either superficial, involving skin and subcutaneous tissue, or deep involving muscle and bone as well.

Superficial frost-bite

In frost-nip, the exposed skin (often of the tip of the nose, cheeks or ears which have been painful), blanches and loses sensation, but re-

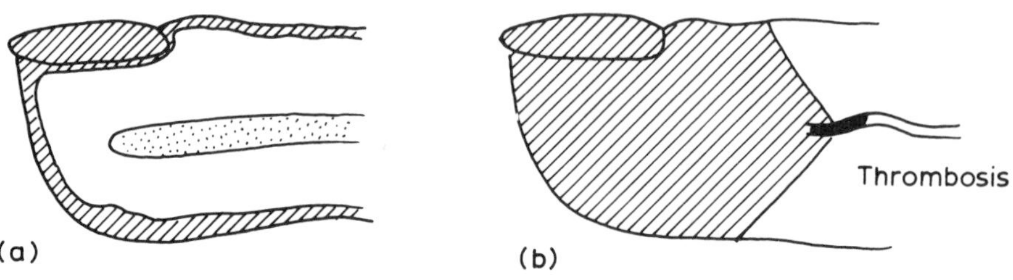

Figure 25.1 (a) Superficial frost-bite: gangrene is limited to the superficial 2–3 mm of tissue. (b) Arterial thrombosis: gangrene extends through all tissues.

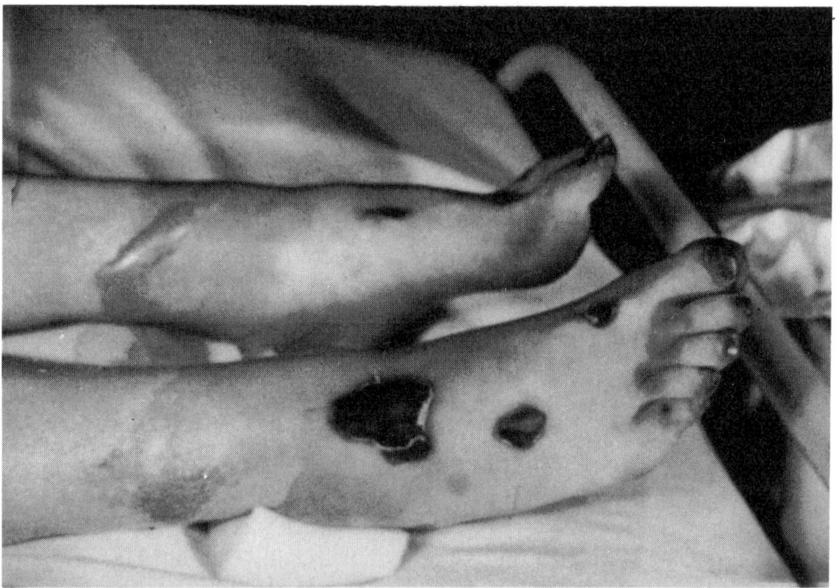

Figure 25.2 Blister formation, swelling and gangrene on feet and ankles several days after freezing cold injury.

mains pliable. On rewarming, the part tingles, becomes hyperaemic and may have some skin desquamation several days later.

In superficial frost-bite (Figure 25.1a), skin and subcutaneous tissues are affected; the skin becomes white and frozen, with the deep underlying tissues remaining fairly pliable. On rewarming the skin becomes mottled, and blue or purple and will swell. Paraesthesiae are common.

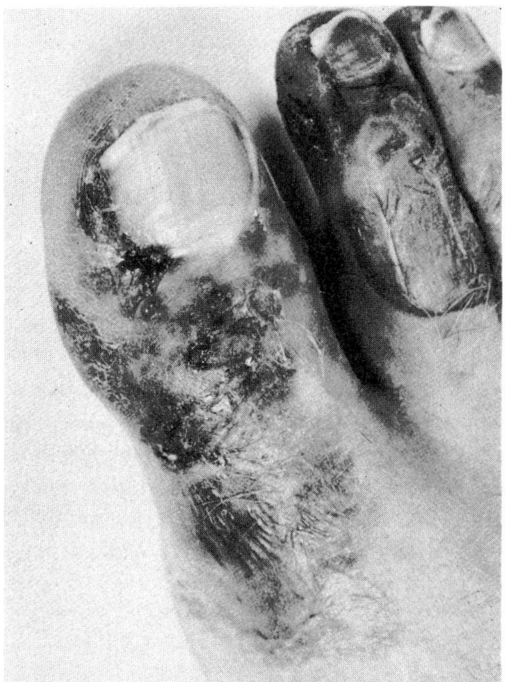

Figure 25.3 Superficial frost-bite showing black carapace developing after collapse of blisters on the toes.

Within 25–48 h, blebs, initially fill with colourless serum, appear; they are more usually found where the skin is lax, such as the backs of the hands or dorsum of the feet (Figure 25.2). Later they may be filled with serosanguineous fluid which is absorbed and a black carapace forms (Figure 25.3). Often white frost-bitten tissue may become black without the formation of blisters.

The gangrene of frost-bite is superficial, not more than a few millimetres thick (Figure 25.1a) in contrast to that seen commonly in hospital due to arterial thrombosis (Figure 25.1b), where the gangrene involves all tissue layers. This means that the surgical approach is more conservative in the case of frost-bite (section 25.2.4).

The carapace is insensitive and fits like a lead glove over the underlying tissue. If the contour of the blackened tissue corresponds to the original part, tissue loss is unlikely but if contour is lost, loss of tissue is almost certain.

After some weeks, the blackened carapace begins to separate at the

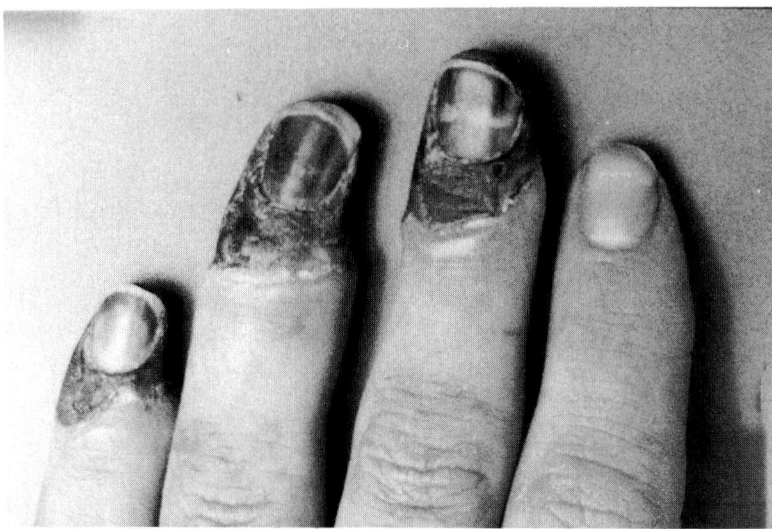

Figure 25.4 Frost-bitten finger tips showing blackened carapace and line of demarcation.

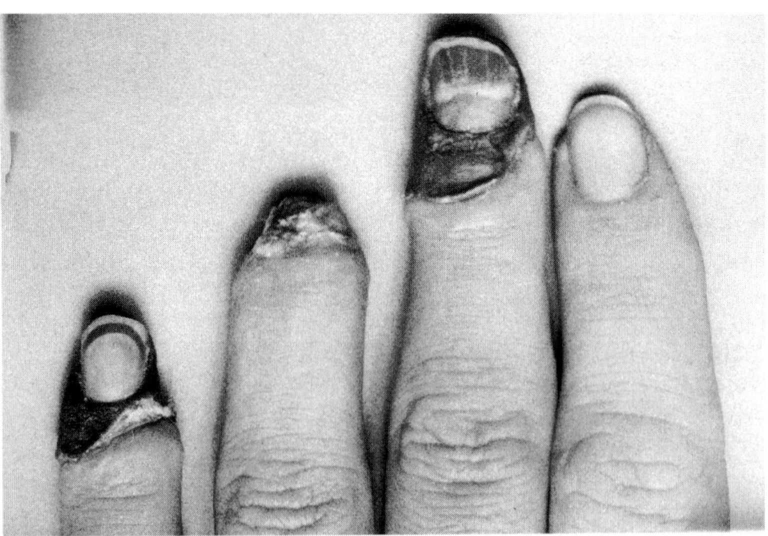

Figure 25.5 Same fingers as in Figure 25.4, now showing separation of carapace from the ring finger leaving, a conical stump.

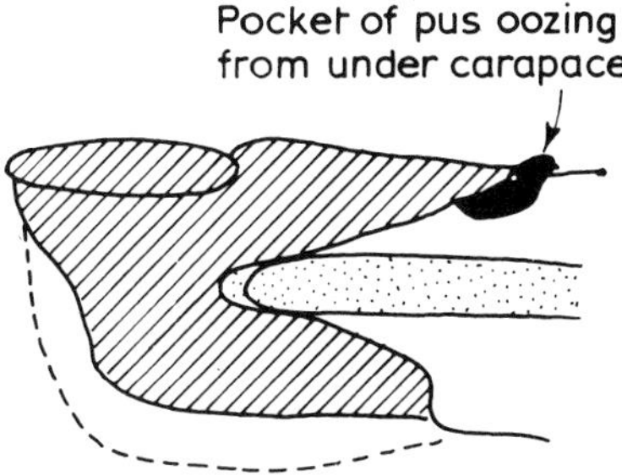

Figure 25.6 Deep frost-bite showing loss of contour and mummification with development of a pocket of pus.

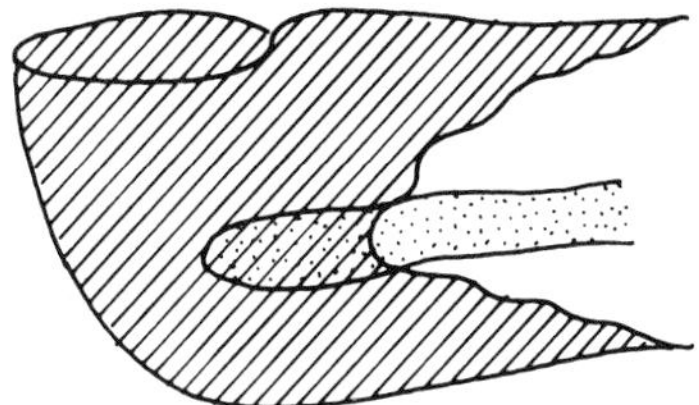

Figure 25.7 Deep frost-bite showing profile of tissue loss (cf. Figure 25.1(b)).

line of demarcation, and a black, mummified cast of tissue peels off like a glove or sock (Figures 25.4, 25.5). Hidden pockets of infection or pus may lead to tissue loss (Figure 25.6).

The underlying tissue is pink, unduly sensitive 'baby-skin' and there may be abnormal sweating. In 2–3 months it will take on a normal appearance.

Deep frost-bite

This involves the deeper structures (muscle, bone and tendons), as well as the skin and subcutaneous tissues (Figure 25.7). The part is insensitive, wooden and grey-purple or white marble in colour. Because tendons are less sensitive to cold and the associated muscle groups are distant from the injury, the part can be moved (Figure 25.8). Blisters filled with dark purple fluid may appear after some weeks. Eventually dry gangrene and mummification occurs and a cast of the affected tissued separates.

Permanent loss of tissue is almost inevitable with deep frost-bite, however the limbs may return to normal over a period of months, and amputation should never be carried out precipitately.

A deep boring pain may be present throughout much of the period.

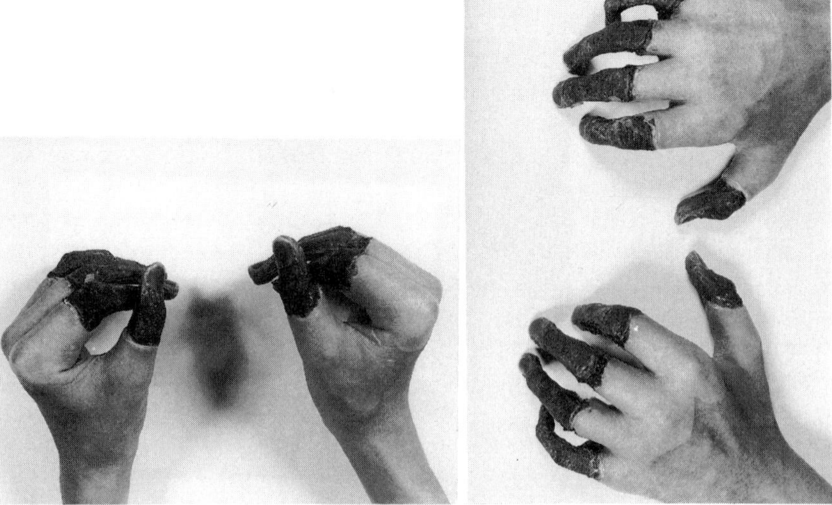

Figure 25.8 Deep frost-bite of fingers with mummification showing that movement is possible because muscles are unaffected and tendons are still intact.

25.2.2 Pathophysiology

The cells remain in a 'metabolic icebox' whilst frozen, but, on rewarming, perfusion restarts and a number of biochemical reactions come into play. The part swells and ischaemia may increase as a result of sludging of red cells and thrombosis. Frost-bite could therefore be considered as an injury both of freezing and of rewarming (Paton, 1987).

Skin

Skin freezes at −0.53°C but, provided the period is short, this causes no lasting injury. After 11 min at −1.9°C it becomes red and tender for days, whilst repeated exposures for 20 min or more at this level causes blistering (Keatinge and Cannon, 1960).

Cold injury is associated with hyperkeratosis of the skin and atrophy of elastic fibres. The sebaceous glands and hair follicles also show change; there is atrophy of the root sheaths of hair and the nails become brittle, thick and cracked.

Blood vessels

Normally, following intense vasoconstriction, the skin temperature equilibrates with environmental temperature, the stagnant plasma cools and viscosity increases. On rewarming, vasodilatation occurs and there is immediate recovery of microvascular perfusion, provided no thrombosis is present. If pathological vasodilatation occurs with release of histamine or other tissue metabolites, this results in blood with a high haematocrit reaching the capillaries and the velocity of the blood flow is decreased, red cell aggregates appear and an increase in viscosity occurs. This may trigger further retardation of blood flow and further aggregation leading to complete occlusion of microvessels with complete stasis and gangrene.

Damage to blood vessels depends on the duration of freezing with resulting plasma leakage and blister formation. The blisters contain tissue breakdown products associated with vasoconstriction, increased leucocyte sticking and platelet aggregation. Analysis of the blister fluid shows prostaglandins and high levels of thromboxane to be present (Heggers *et al.*, 1990). Due to the action of precapillary sphincters, arteriovenous shunts open and close in cycles and blood bypasses the frozen area. Complete closure of the a–v shunts renders the part avascular and protects the body core from cooled blood and the patient from hypothermia (Greene, 1943; Washburn, 1962; Schmid-Schonbein and Neumann, 1985). Both phlebitis and arteritis may occur as a result of frost-bite.

Ice crystal formation

If freezing is slow, interstitial ice crystals form which enlarge at the expense of intracellular water, osmotic pressure rises, and enzyme mechanisms are disturbed, with resulting cell death. If freezing is rapid ice crystals form everywhere and rupture of cell membranes is the result.

Nerves

Increasing cold and nerve malfunction are matched by severe morphological changes to peripheral nerves.

The main findings are an immediate increase in the mean diameter of myelinated and non-myelinated fibres, marked oedema, axon degeneration, and infrequent, segmented and paranodal demyelination. There is selective vulnerability to cold, based on nerve fibre diameter with myelinated fibres being more susceptible than non-myelinated. Degeneration of nerve fibres is probably due to increased permeability of endoneural vessels which leads to diffuse oedema, toxin production, changes in osomolarity and increase in endoneural pressure. Whilst there is clear evidence of ischaemia in freezing cold injury this is less clear in non-freezing injury, though some changes in vascular endothelium occur.

Once the temperature falls below freezing for more than a few seconds degeneration occurs affecting all nerve fibres equally. There is complete necrosis of all structures within the perineurium, except the endothelial lining of the blood vessels (Peyronnard *et al.*, 1977; Nukada *et al.*, 1981).

Muscle

In freezing cold injury to muscle, the degree of injury depends on the amount of exposure. The superficial, coldest layer shows coagulation necrosis, slow necrosis occurs in the intermediate zone and muscle atrophy alone in the deepest layer; repair is by fibrous tissue (Lewis and Moen, 1952). Biopsy and ultrastructural analysis has shown vascular damage and damage to membrane structure, contractile elements and mitochondria (Kayser *et al.*, 1993).

Oedema

Primary

Normally cold is associated with tissue dehydration, however, the longer the limbs take to cool the more likely is oedema to occur, possibly as the result of changes in tissue pH.

Secondary

This is the result of rewarming and vasodilatation and forms within 12–25 h. Plasma passes through the cold damaged capillaries into the interstitial tissue. Associated exercise may cause swelling of the feet, so-called exercise edema (Williams *et al.*, 1979).

Bones and joints

Bone cells are more sensitive to cold than overlying skin. A clear line of demarcation occurs, but the damage extends proximal to this. Epiphyseal cartilage is more sensitive than bone, and periosteal new bone formation can occur. The direct action of cold, or microvascular changes with end artery thrombosis, or both, may be the cause of the damage (Hunter *et al.*, 1952; McKendry, 1981).

Eye disorders

The eye and optic nerve are protected from cold by the paranasal sinuses. Impairment of vision occurs only in hypothermia and not with local cooling. Conjunctivitis due to cold has been observed, along with cold injury to the cornea in downhill skiers and ice skaters unprotected by goggles.

25.2.3 Frost-bite and altitude

Though few statistics are available, frost-bite at great altitudes appears to be commoner for comparable environmental temperatures than at lower altitudes. Both cold and altitude raise the packed cell volume and viscosity and slow the peripheral blood flow, whilst cold injury to capillary walls leads to plasma leakage and intravascular sludging. This local haemoconcentration will be increased at altitude and impaired tissue nutrition and necrosis may occur more rapidly. Dehydration, from whatever cause, will also increase viscosity of the blood, and thrombosis may be encouraged due to relative inactivity.

Maximal oxygen uptake is progressively lowered and, with it, the ability to increase heat production through exercise and probably the ability to shiver are decreased (Gautier *et al.*, 1987). Hypoxia also blunts mental function and precautions taken against cold injury may be inadequate. Poor appetite will lower calorie intake and loss of insulating subcutaneous fat will occur (Ward, 1974).

The effect of altitude hypoxia on the tone of the peripheral microvasculature is important in determining the risk of frost-bite at altitude. However studies of this effect have given conflicting results (Durand and Martineaud, 1971; Durand and Raynaud, 1987).

25.2.4 Prevention

Different parts of the body may be subjected to widely varying temperatures at any one time. For example, the foot may be at below freezing in deep powder snow with the environmental temperature many degrees above freezing. Temperature variation throughout the day is considerable and both feet and hands should be kept as dry as possible.

Footwear has to perform many functions other than the prevention of cold injury, and there is no footgear available at present which will prevent local cold injury under all circumstances.

The most useful preventative measures are to limit the period exposed to the possibility of cold injury, keep warm, maintain hydration, and keep the part dry and free from abrasion. In many situations, particularly wartime, these measures are not always practicable.

The 'buddy' system is valuable for preventing frost-bite, especially in large groups. The party is paired off and each member of a pair is responsible for keeping a close rather than a casual watch on his companion. This is done at regular intervals to note early signs and is the most effective form of early detection.

25.2.5 Treatment

Introduction

Both superficial and deep frost-bite may be associated with hypothermia, which has priority in treatment. In any event few patients present with simple frost-bite and the temperature gradient down the affected limbs ensures that, if frost-bite is present in the extremities, some degree of non-freezing cold injury will be present proximally. In addition, many patients will have been exposed to a freeze–thaw–freeze sequence with potentially disastrous results whatever the treatment; if there is skin loss the tissues will have frozen solid. Associated fractures may interfere with blood supply. At high altitude, dehydration, raised haematocrit, and exhaustion with poor heat output will enhance cold injury.

The ten principles of management are:

- buddy system (see above);
- avoid further trauma;
- avoid freeze–thaw–freeze;
- avoid infection;
- keep clean;
- rewarm;
- maintain morale;
- delay surgery;
- treat associated conditions;
- avoid subsequent frostbite.

In the field

Frost-nip

The part should be warmed out of the wind by the gloved hand or by placing the affected part in the arm pit or under clothing. It should not be rubbed. Within a few minutes sensation is restored and normal working can be resumed.

Frost-bite

Under no circumstance should the part be beaten, rubbed or overheated. Excessive heat from wood fires, heat from exhaust pipes of cars or from stoves car give disastrous results and the part will become burnt or baked because of cold anaesthesia (Flora, 1985). Rubbing with ice or snow does not rewarm and causes tissue damage. Thawing in the field is contra-indicated as this will immediately be followed by freezing and the catastrophic freeze–thaw–freeze sequence precipitated.

Before thawing, the frozen part should be protected to avoid trauma, but during mountain rescue this may not be possible. Once thawing has started it must continue and refreezing be avoided. It is better to walk on frozen feet (Mills and Rau, 1983) to a low camp from which evacuation is possible than to start warming and have to be carried, or walk on partially rethawed feet.

In hospital

Patients should be kept in pleasant surroundings and given a high calorie, high protein diet and anti-tetanus serum. Broad spectrum antibiotics should be given if there is any likelihood of infection; because of devitalized tissue this may take hold very rapidly causing considerable tissue loss. The affected part should be inspected daily. Morale must be maintained.

Investigations

Tissue viability should be assessed by clinical examination and Doppler ultrasound. Tissue and bone scintigraphy allows perfusion to be assessed more accurately than Doppler ultrasound (Salimi, 1985; Shih *et al.*, 1988; Ikawa *et al.*, 1986). Other research methods include: thermal clearance and measures of skin blood flow (Roussel *et al.*, 1982), ^{133}Xe muscle blood flow (Nugent and Rogers, 1980; Sumner *et al.*, 1971), muscle biopsy (Kayser *et al.*, 1993), and thermography. The temperature of the deeper tissues can be measured by means of a special probe, thus distinguishing between superficial and deep frost-bite (Hamlet *et al.*, 1977). ^{31}P NMR scans and be used daily to follow the state of the tissue with time (Kayser *et al.*, 1993).

Thawing

Various methods of thawing have been used but, at present, rapid rewarming is the most favoured, as greatest tissue preservation seems to occur and the results in deep frost-bite are reasonably good (Foray and Salon, 1985; Mills, 1983). Gradual rewarming gives satisfactory results with superficial frost-bite but variable results with deep frost-bite. Thawing should be carried out in warm water, containing an antiseptic (e.g. Phisohex) in a whirlpool bath or tub at 37–41°C. The temperature should be continuously monitored and warmed; intravenous fluids can be used. Analgesics are usually required.

After thawing, the extremities should be elevated, and enclosed in a 'burns' bag which has the advantage of protecting from infection. Protection by cradles avoids further trauma or pressure. Treatment in whirlpool baths containing an antiseptic is continued twice daily; in this way necrotic and infected tissue is gently removed.

Minor surgery

Blebs are left intact if the contents are sterile or, if infected, they are drained but the tissue left as a cover. However, as the fluid contains tissue breakdown products which can cause continued vasospasm, some advise repeated aspiration.

A thickened eschar, which may limit joint movement or even constrict normal tissue, can be split or removed (Mills, 1983). Debridement or amputation should be delayed for up to 90 days so that mummification is complete. Fasciotomy to release pressure due to oedema in tissue compartments has been advocated (Franz *et al.*, 1978). Fractures should be treated conservatively by closed rather than open methods. Dislocations should be reduced immediately to prevent tissue pressure.

Other methods

The majority of patients are dehydrated, so rehydration with warmed fluids is important. To decrease blood viscosity with a plasma expander after blood has been removed from the patient may be effective. Dextran (or newer colloids) can also be given. Pain in the lower limbs may be controlled with epidural bupivacaine.

Sympathectomy reduces pain and decreases oedema. After this, the line of tissue demarcation is said to appear more rapidly, and become more proximal. However increased tissue preservation does not necessarily occur and possibly the non-sympathectomized limb does better. Medical sympathectomy using intra-arterial reserpine and intravenous blockade by the Bier technique has been used with some success. Evidence in this area is still anecdotal and there is need for good clinical trials.

Hyperbaric oxygen appears to have been discarded though it may be of value in the post-thaw period.

Unless infection is present, there is no indication for antibiotics, but infection can take hold very rapidly in devitalized tissue, causing considerable tissue loss. The affected part should be inspected daily for signs of infection and, if there is any doubt, a broad spectrum antibiotic should be started.

Thrombolytic enzymes are being evaluated (Flora, 1985), but there is a risk, especially if intracranial injuries are present.

Both anticoagulants and vasodilators have been used but there is disagreement about their effectiveness. Tobacco should be prohibited. Biofeedback training has been tried (Kappes and Mills, 1984).

Fractures should be treated conservatively and dislocations should be reduced immediately to prevent tissue pressure.

Amputation

Premature surgery is a most potent cause of morbidity and surgical intervention should be minimal. When amputation is necessary (Figure 25.9) closure should, if possible, be by skin flaps rather than grafts, and sufficient deep tissue should be removed to achieve this. However, skin grafts have been successful. If infection is present a modified guillotine procedure is recommended with secondary closure. Irrigation of the infected stump is often successful. Necrosis of the stump is a hazard because of cold endarteritis and trophic changes may also occur. Active movements of the fingers after amputation must be encouraged to avoid stiffness and the development of a claw hand. Isolated ulcers of the stump may develop due to deep-seated bone necrosis, or osteomyelitis.

Patients should be mentally prepared for treatment that can last months and involve many amputations and reconstructive surgery. They may need much psychological support.

Trauma

The risk of frost-bite in exposed subdermal tissue is considerable. Devitalized flesh freezes in 1 min at 0°C if wind speeds rise above 2 m sec^{-1}. As exposed wet tissues rapidly become frozen, tissue necrosis, wound sepsis and delayed healing are common. Immediate thermal protection by suture or a wound dressing is necessary. The patient should then be evacuated. Routine wound debridement should be carried out and secondary suture performed as circumstances dictate (Butson, 1975).

If hypotension or haemorrhagic hypovolaemia are present the normal signs of hypothermia may be masked. The risk of hypothermia is also increased when partially perfused exposed tissue is at subzero temperatures. When warmed, these hypothermic patients may start to bleed profusely from injured tissues. The analgesic protection afforded by cold will also be lost on rewarming (Pearn, 1982).

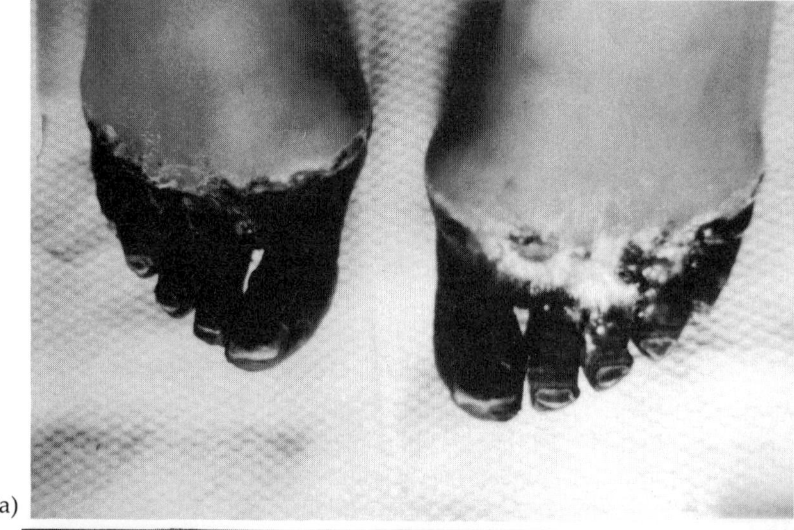

(a)

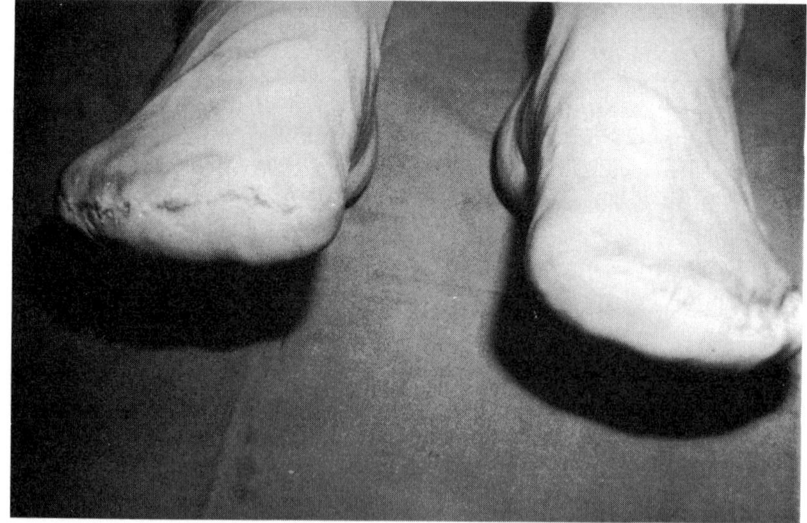

(b)

Figure 25.9 Deep frost-bite of forefeet (a) before and (b) after surgery. The operation was disarticulation at the metatarso-phalangeal joints. (Reproduced with permission C.J.C. Renton.)

25.2.6 After-effects

Both short and long term sequelae of local cold injury have been reported. Even at normal temperatures skin may crack, causing painful fissures and ulceration. Fungating and ulcerating squamous cell carcinomas of the heel have been reported 40 years after frost-bite. These were well differentiated, of low malignancy and with no evidence of spread. Treatment was by local excision and skin grafting. Unstable scar tissue, chronic irritation and pressure were factors in aetiology (Rossis *et al.*, 1982).

Fibrosis follows cold injury to muscle. There may be persistent vasomotor paralysis, analgesia, and paraesthesia; both early anhidrosis and late hyperhidrosis have been reported. Axon regeneration in both myelinated and non-myelinated fibres, with full return of nerve function, may take nine months or longer. A burning sensation in the feet has been noted in 61% after full recovery and intractable pain may be present for upto 35 years (Suri *et al.*, 1978; Kumar, 1982).

There may be persistent and marked vasospasm to cold stimuli which continues long after the initial stimulus has been removed. Re-exposure to cold is likely to cause a relapse since a high incidence of non-freezing cold injury occurs in those with a history of local cold injury.

Problems with rigidity of the feet, fallen arches and osteoporosis are reported. New bone formation usually restores the normal radiographic appearance (Francis and Golden, 1985). Changes in the epiphyses of children with frost-bite can lead to cartilage and bone abnormalities due either to the direct action of cold on chondrocytes or microvascular changes with end artery thrombosis, or both (McKendry, 1981).

Renal failure

Following severe frost-bite of both lower limbs and in non-freezing cold injury of the feet in children rhabdomyolysis with incipient renal failure has been recorded. Severe, long continued exercise may also be a factor in muscle breakdown (Raifman *et al.*, 1978; Ross and Attwood, 1984).

25.3 NON-FREEZING COLD INJURY

Prolonged exposure of tissue to temperatures below 15°C, or to marginally higher temperatures in water, will result in non-freezing cold injury, often with lasting damage to muscles and nerves.

'Trench foot' is the commonest form of this condition and is a significant cause of injury in military operations when, for combat reasons, long periods have to be spent with feet in water or in deep snow. Water both increases and accelerates the risk of injury, as does any factor that impedes circulation to the extremities, such as a cramped position, immobility, tight clothing, tight boots and tight socks. Mountaineers are at risk when powder snow gets into their boots by the ankle or is melted by foot warmth; damp socks will increase cooling.

Exactly the same sequence occurs with the hands in mittens or gloves made sodden by water or snow. However because the hands are easier to inspect and keep dry and warm, 'trench hand' is uncommon.

Non-freezing cold injury, though initially reversible, becomes irreversible if cooling is prolonged. It often occurs in tissues immediately proximal to frost-bite.

25.3.1 Clinical features

It is convenient to classify these into mild, moderate and severe (Table 25.2).

When first seen, the affected part will be pale and sensation and movement poor. The pulse may be absent, but freezing has not occurred. If these features do not improve on warming, non-freezing cold injury is present.

After a few hours the part becomes swollen, numb, blotchy pink-purple and heavy. After 24–36 h a vigorous hyperaemia develops with a bounding pulse and burning pain proximally but not distally. Oedema with 'blood blisters' appears and, if the skin is poorly perfused, it will become gangrenous and slough.

In severe cases there is a progressive reduction in sensation. The joints become stiff and muscles cease to function. To maintain balance the legs are kept apart and the sensation of movement has been likened to walking to cotton wool (Ungley *et al.*, 1945). Repeated minor trauma, such as running, associated with the neuropathy encountered in non-freezing cold injury, may result in severe blister formation with partial thickness skin loss (Reichl, 1987).

Hyperaemia appears to be due to vasomotor paralysis with paleness on elevation and redness when the part is dependent. This phase may last from days to weeks, as may changes in sensation. Persistent anaesthesia suggests neurone degeneration with the prospect of long term symptoms (Burr, 1993).

A late feature is hyperhidrosis; this may lead to blistering, maceration

Table 25.2 Clinical classification of non-freezing cold injury

Mild	*Moderate*	*Severe*
Erythema	Edema	'Blood' blisters
Edema	Hyperaemia	Gangrene
Temporary sensory change	Blisters	Permanent disability
	Persistent sensory change	

of the skin and infection. After some months sensation and blood flow return to normal but gangrene may also occur. Severe changes occur more commonly and are more extensive in dependent, immobile tissues, whilst poor nutrition, fatigue, stress, injury and associated illness exacerbate the condition.

25.3.2 Pathophysiology

Because water is such a good conductor of heat, stored heat is lost rapidly and the deeper tissues, nerves, muscles, blood vessels and bones, may be affected before there is any recognizable skin change. Changes in nerve conduction and sensation are common as are changes in vessel permeability, which result in oedema, blistering, and compression of peripheral vessels (Francis and Golden, 1985).

Initially, there is vasoconstriction followed by vasodilatation. Limb arteries exposed to non-freezing cold injury are not normally thrombosed but this may occur in injured limbs. Muscle damage may occur due to direct cooling, as may fat necrosis and atrophy (Friedman, 1945). Infected wet gangrene may result but dry gangrene and mummification can also occur.

After weeks or months, blood flow returns to normal but limbs may remain very sensitive to temperature changes, with cooling causing intense vasoconstriction and warming intense vasodilatation. Profuse sweating, sensory loss and loss of muscle power may persist. Amputation may have to be carried out.

25.3.3 Prevention

Some degree of non-freezing cold injury is much commoner than normally recognized and the majority who spend long periods in cold conditions or at high altitude have some minor symptoms, usually paraesthesiae, that persist over a few months and then disappear.

If the risk of non-freezing cold injury is recognized then common sense measures are normally adequate to prevent its occurrence. Particularly at risk are the feet as they remain covered throughout the day.

By rigorous and simple measures in World War I the British army reduced the incidence of trench foot from 29 172 cases in 1915 to 443 cases in 1916–1918. In 1988 the incidence in one USA marine unit of 355 soldiers was 11%. Tobacco smoking (but not race) was associated with a higher incidence of trench foot (Tek and Mackey, 1993).

Preventive measures include the following.

- Heavy socks should be worn in well fitting boots.

- Clothes should be loose fitting, and the trunk kept warm.
- Boots and socks should be removed twice a day. Feet should be washed, dried, massaged and warmed.
- Those at risk should sleep with dry feet. Wet socks and boots should be removed and dried.
- Keep feet out of water, snow and mud when bivouacking; elevate them if possible and keep toes and feet moving.
- Numbness and tingling are signs of 'trench foot'; warm the feet immediately.
- Always carry a spare pair of socks (dry). They can double as gloves.
- Modern mountaineering boots with a plastic outer shell and inner detachable boot of artificial fibre are better for high altitudes than leather boots.

25.3.4 Treatment

The patient should be removed from the cold; whole body warming should be started (Lahti, 1982) and dehydration corrected. Rapid warming of the part has been advocated but not universally adopted. Because of pain, analgesics should be given, the patient rested and the part raised. Blisters that develop should be left unless infected, when drainage should be carried out. Sympathectomy does not appear to be very effective as hyperaemia occurs naturally.

Gangrene may occur later, and this may be more widespread and affect deeper tissues more extensively than freezing cold injury. Conservative management should be adopted and surgical procedures kept to the minimum. In the long term, non-freezing cold injury may be more serious than freezing cold injury because of the unrecognized cooling effect on deeper and more proximal structures.

25.4 CONDITIONS ASSOCIATED WITH COLD STRESS

25.4.1 Cold allergy

The clinical features of this condition, described by Horton and Brown (1929) and Wanderer (1979), are malaise, shivering, aching joints and generalized urticaria. Susceptibility is transmitted as a genetic dominant (Eady *et al.*, 1978). Sensitized mast cells are found in the skin; exposure to cold causes degranulation with release of mediators causing hypersensitivity both generally and locally. Wheals occur at the sites of local cooling, and even inside the mouth on taking cold drinks. Swimming may produce familial cold urticaria. It has been suggested that cases of sudden death within a few minutes of entering the water are due to undiagnosed cold urticaria (Cold hypersensitivity, 1975; Ting, 1984).

25.4.2 Chilblains

These are local inflammatory conditions developing as a result of exposure to cold and are more frequent in humid conditions than in a cold dry climate, probably because humidity increases local thermal conductivity. Women are more affected than men, and inadequate clothing with subsequent cooling is an important predisposing factor. Central heating reduces the incidence of chilblains (Lahti, 1982; Cold hypersensitivity, 1975).

25.4.3 Raynaud's syndrome

This may be defined as intermittent vasospasm of the arterioles of the distal part of the limbs following exposure to cold or emotion. The extremities first become pale, then cyanosed and then red.

The commonest identifiable disorder underlying Raynaud's phenomenon is scleroderma; the vasospastic elements may be the presenting features. Trophic changes are common. Underlying disorders are other collagen diseases, neurogenic lesions, occupational trauma, occlusive arterial disease, cryoglobulinaemia and cold agglutinin.

True Raynaud's disease occurs mainly in young females, who have intermittent bilateral and symmetrical attacks in the absence of organic arterial occlusion. Trophic changes occur in fingers or toes. It is most common in the upper limbs, though the lower limbs may be affected.

25.4.4 Acrocyanosis

Acrocyanosis occurs virtually only in women and is characterized by cold and blue extremities. It is worse in cold weather but is also present in warm weather. All peripheral pulses are present and the symptoms are symmetrical and constant.

25.4.5 Livedo reticularis

This condition is characterized by persistent patchy red-blue mottling of the legs, and occasionally the arms, which is worse in cold weather. Chronic ulceration may occur. It is due to intermittent and random spasm of cutaneous arterioles with secondary dilatation of capillaries and vessels.

25.4.6 Cold hypersensitivity following trauma and cold exposure

A number of conditions with a vasospastic component follow frost-bite and trauma. Pain is a prominent feature, and the limb is pale and cold and may show evidence of disuse atrophy.

REFERENCES

Burr, R.E. (1993) Trench foot. *J. Wild. Med.*, **4**, 348–52.

Butson, A.R.C. (1975) Effects and prevention of frostbite in wound healing. *Can. J. Surg.*, **18**, 145–8.

Cold hypersensitivity (editorial). (1975) *Br. Med. J.*, **1**, 643–4.

Durand, J. and Martineaud, J.P. (1971) Resistance and capacitance vessels of the skin in permanent and temporary residents at high altitude, in *High Altitude Physiology: Cardiac and Respiratory Aspects*, Ciba Foundation, (eds R. Porter and J. Knight), Churchill Livingstone, London, pp. 159–70.

Durand, J. and Raynaud, J. (1987) Limb blood and heat exchange at altitude, in *Hypoxia and Cold*, (eds J.R. Sutton, C.S. Houston and G. Coates), Praeger, New York, pp. 100–13.

Eady, R.A.J., Bentley-Phillips, C.B., Keahey, T.M. and Greaves, M.W. (1978) Cold urticaria vasculitis. *Br. J. Dermatol.*, **99(suppl 16)**, 9–10.

Flora, G. (1985) Secondary treatment of frostbite, in *High Altitude Deterioration*, (eds J. Rivolier, P. Cerretelli, J. Foray and P. Segantini), Karger, Basel, pp. 159–69.

Foray, J. and Salon, F. (1985) Casualties with cold injury: Primary treatment, in *High Altitude Deterioration*, (eds J. Rivolier, P. Cerretelli, J. Foray and P. Segantini), Karger, Basel, pp. 149–58.

Francis, T.J.R. and Golden, F. St C. (1985) Non-freezing cold injury: The pathogenesis. *J. R. Navy Med. Serv.*, **71**, 3–8.

Franz, D.R., Berberich, J.J., Blake, S. and Mills, W.J. (1978) Evaluation of fasciotomy and vasodilators for the treatment of frostbite in the dog. *Cryobiology*, **15**, 659–69.

Friedman, N.B. (1945) The pathology of trench foot. *Am. J. Pathol.*, **21**, 387–433.

Gautier, H., Bonora, M., Schultz, S.A. and Remmers, J.E. (1987) Hypoxia induced changes in shivering and body temperature. *J. Appl. Physiol.*, **62**, 2577–81.

Greene, R. (1943) The immediate vascular changes in true frostbite. *J. Pathol. Bacteriol.*, **55**, 259–68.

Hamlet, M.P., Veghte, J., Bowers, W.D. and Boyce, J. (1977) Thermographic evaluation of experimentally produced frostbite of rabbit feet. *Cryobiology*, **14**, 197–204.

Heggers, J.P., Phillips, L.G., McAuley, R.L. and Robson, M.C. (1990) Frostbite: Experimental and clinical evaluation of treatment. *J. Wild. Med.*, **1**, 27–32.

Herschkowitz, M. (1977) Penile frostbite: An unforseen hazard of jogging (letter). *N. Engl. J. Med.*, Jan. 20, vol 296, 178.

Horton, B.T. and Brown, G.E. (1929) Systemic histamine like reactions in allergy due to cold. *Am. J. Med. Sci.*, **198**, 191–202.

Hunter, J., Kerr, E.H. and Whillans, M.G. (1952) The relation between joint stiffness upon exposure to cold and the characteristics of synovial fluid. *J. Can. Med. Sci.*, **39**, 367–77.

Ikawa, G., Dos Santos, P.A.L., Yamaguchi, K.T., *et al.* (1986) Frostbite and bone scanning: The use of ^{99}m-labelled phosphates in demarcating the line of viability in frostbite victims. *Orthopaedics*, **9**, 1257–61.

Kappes, B.W. and Mills, W.J. (1984) Thermal biofeedback training with frostbite patients (abstract). *Sixth International Symposium on Circumpolar Health*, May 13–18, Anchorage, Alaska, p. 100.

Kayser, B., Binzoni, T., Hoppeler, H., *et al.* (1993) A case of severe frostbite on Mt Blanc: A multi-technique approach. *J. Wild. Med.*, **4**, 167–74.

Keatinge, W.R. and Cannon, P. (1960) Freezing point of human skin. *Lancet*, **1**, 11–14.

Kumar, V.N. (1982) Intractable foot pain following frostbite. *Arch. Phys. Med. Rehab.*, **63**, 284–5.

Lahti, A. (1982) Cutaneous reactions to cold. *Nordic Council Arctic Med. Res.* **No. 30**, pp. 32–5.

Lewis, R.B. and Moen, P.W. (1952) Further studies on the pathogenesis of cold induced muscle necrosis. *Surg. Gynecol. Obstet.*, **95**, 543–51.

McKendry, R.J.R. (1981) Frostbite arthritis. *Can. Med. Assoc. J.*, **125**, 1128–30.

Mills, W.J. (1983) Frostbite. *Alaska Med.*, **25**, 33–8.

Mills, W.J. and Rau, D. (1983) University of Alaska, Anchorage. Section of high latitude study, and the Mount McKinley Project. *Alaska Med.*, **25**, 21–8.

Nugent, S.K. and Rogers, M.C. (1980) Resuscitation and intensive care monitoring following immersion hypothermia. *J. Trauma*, **20**, 814–15.

Nukada, H., Pollock, M. and Allpress, S. (1981) Experimental cold injury to nerve. *Brain*, **104**, 779–813.

Paton, B.C. (1987) Pathophysiology of frostbite, in *Hypoxia and Cold*, (eds J.R. Sutton, C.S. Houston and G. Coates), Praeger, New York, pp. 329–39.

Pearn, J.H. (1982) Cold injury complicating trauma in sub-zero environments. *Med. J. Aust.*, **1**, 505–7.

Peyronnard, J.M., Pednault, M. and Aquayo, A.J. (1977) Neuropathies due to cold. Quantitative studies of structural changes in human and animal nerves, in *Proceedings of 11th World Congress of Neurology*, Amsterdam, pp. 308–29.

Raifman, M.A., Berant, M. and Levarsky, C. (1978) Cold weather and rhabdomyolysis. *J. Paediatr.*, **93**, 970–1.

Reichl, M. (1987) Neuropathy of the feet due to running on cold surfaces. *Br. Med. J.*, **294**, 348–9.

Ross, J.H. and Attwood, E.C. (1984) Severe repetitive exercise and haematological status. *Postgrad. Med. J.*, **60**, 454–7.

Rossis, C.G., Yiacoumettis, A.M. and Elemenoglou, J. (1982) Squamous cell carcinoma of the heel developing at site of previous frostbite. *J. R. Soc. Med.*, **75**, 715–18.

Roussel, B., Dittmar, A., Delhomm, C., *et al.* (1982) Normal and pathological aspects of skin blood flow measurements by thermal clearance method, in *Biomedical Thermology*, (eds M. Guthrie, E. Albert and R. Alar), Liss, New York, pp. 421–9.

Salimi, Z. (1985) Assessment of tissue viability by scintigraphy. *Postgrad. Med.*, **17**, 133–4.

Schmid-Schonbein, H. and Neumann, F.J. (1985) Pathophysiology of cutaneous frost injury: Disturbed microcirculation as a consequence of abnormal flow behaviour of the blood. Application of new concepts of blood rheology, in *High Altitude Deterioration*, (eds J. Rivolier, P. Cerretelli, J. Foray and P. Segantini), Karger, Basel, pp. 20–38.

Shih, W.-J., Riley, C., Magoun, S. and Ryo, U.Y. (1988) Intense bone imaging agent uptake in the soft tissues of the lower legs and feet relating to ischemia and cold exposure. *Eur. J. Nucl. Med.*, **14**, 419–21.

Sumner, D.S., Boswick, J.A. and Doolittle, W.H. (1971) Prediction of tissue loss in human frostbite with xenon-133. *Surgery*, **69**, 899–903.
Suri, M.L., Vijayan, G.P., Puri, H.C., *et al.* (1978) Neurological manifestations of frostbite. *Indian J. Med. Res.*, **67**, 292–9.
Tek, D. and Mackey, S. (1993) Non-freezing cold injury in a marine infantry battalion. *J. Wild. Med.*, **4**, 353–7.
Ting, S. (1984) Cold induced urticaria in infancy. *Pediatrics*, **73**, 105–6.
Ungley, G.G., Channell, G.D. and Richards, R.L. (1945) The immersion foot syndrome. *Br. J. Surg.*, **33**, 17–31.
Wanderer, A.A. (1979) An 'allergy' to cold. *Hosp. Pract.*, **14**, 136–7.
Ward, M.P. (1974) Frostbite. *Br. Med. J.*, **1**, 67–70.
Washburn, B. (1962) Frostbite. What it is – how to prevent it – emergency treatment. *N. Engl. J. Med.*, **266**, 974–89.
Williams, E.S., Ward, M.P., Milledge, J.S., *et al.* (1979) Effect of the exercise of seven consecutive days hill-walking on fluid homeostasis. *Clin. Sci.*, **56**, 305–16.

26

Accidents, surgical emergencies and anaesthesia

26.1 MOUNTAINEERING

Statistics for the incidence of accidents and emergencies, and their morbidity and mortality, are seldom accurate or readily available. The numbers at risk are hardly ever known but certain trends are apparent. Cold injury, both general and local, is liable to complicate any accident or illness in mountain country at whatever altitude. With increasing numbers of visitors to the mountains, accidents and mortality will inevitably increase.

26.1.1 United Kingdom

Although the mountains of the UK reach only 1400 m, they can provide a hostile environment, especially in Scotland in winter, where winds of 150 mph are recorded.

It is only recently that reasonably accurate records have become available in the UK. These show that between 1959 and 1968 the total number of accidents was 1521, with 254, or about 20%, being fatal (Hartley, 1970). Hill walkers and climbers accounted for 98%, with cavers and others accounting for the remainder. Since then the number of accidents and deaths has increased in line with the numbers of those who hill walk and climb.

The commonest site of injury was the legs, with head injuries the second most common. Despite the use of helmets many head injuries were fatal. Injuries to the trunk, arms and shoulders were equal in third place.

An unusual feature was the number of heart attacks, a high percentage of which were fatal. Exercise in the cold can decrease exercise tolerance in patients with angina, and breathing cold air (−20°C) for a short period may produce angina in some patients with coronary artery disease (Horvath, 1981).

Because of the easy access to hill country, many people take vigorous exercise with little physical conditioning. The chilling effect of wind and rain is underestimated, as is the extreme rapidity with which the weather changes.

Cases of exhaustion and hypothermia are also due to the miscalculation of the severity of weather conditions, particularly in Scotland. Here, on the highest peak, Ben Nevis (1400 m) the average daily temperature throughout the year is only a little above freezing point. In winter the weather and wind approach Polar dimensions and, despite the low altitude, it is 'big country' and long distances have to be covered on foot either over soft snow or bog (Mountain Rescue Committee, 1977–1984; Scottish Mountain Accidents, 1984, 1985, 1986).

The number of reported cases of hypothermia is broadly similar to those reported from North America, which emphasizes the effect of wind and rain at low altitude.

26.1.2 European and New Zealand Alps and Japan

Accident statistics for the European Alps dating back to 1859 are available from alpine journals.

In the Swiss Alps, the number of accidents had doubled between 1956 and 1968, and between 1964 and 1968 there was an average of 125 deaths each year. Accurate figures are not available for the years up to 1981, but an average yearly mortality rate appears to be of the order of 250–350. Figures published by the IKAR for the European Alps between 1981 and 1983 show an annual mortality of between 850 and 950. In the years 1984–1985 the number killed by avalanche was 232. (IKAR Reports, 1982–1984). At the present time there are about 3000 accidents each year in the Swiss Alps (Durrer, 1993); 90% are rescued by helicopter.

Accidents from both avoidable and unavoidable causes are common in the Alps and, since the first ascent of Mt Blanc (4807 m) in 1786, it is estimated that there have been about 8000 deaths on this peak alone in the last 200 years.

The mountains of New Zealand rise to just under 4000 m, and Mt Cook, the highest, is 3800 m. Some glaciers extend to sea-level so that the extent of ice covered terrain is greater than in Europe where glaciers extend to about 1500 m. The dangers in both Europe and New Zealand are similar, with altitude playing a lesser role than in Asia and South America. Figures from New Zealand over the last ten years show little or no increase in the number of incidents for which rescue was carried out or the number of deaths recorded, despite an assumed increase in numbers at risk. This suggests a reduction in incidence (Federated Mountain Club of New Zealand, 1986).

In the Japanese Alps, with peaks up to 3800 m, the average number of accidents each year has been about 500, with between 100–150 deaths per annum. In 1990, 571 accidents occurred involving 729 climbers. The majority of accidents occur in the months of July and August, and the commonest causes are slips or falls in climbers in their twenties.

In 1990, a total of 7253 policemen and over 17 000 private rescue personnel were involved. Helicopter search and rescue operations were much the most efficient method of evacuation (Omori, 1992).

26.1.3 North America

Since 1951, accidents occurring in the mountains of mainland USA and Canada have been reported annually in the *American Alpine Journal*, though, like the UK and European Alps, the numbers at risk are not usually known. From 1951 to 1986 there have been a total of 3032 injured and 1049 killed. The majority of accidents occurred in the age group 15 to 25, and were due to a slip or fall. The commonest injury was a fracture. Cold injury occurred more often than acute mountain sickness and its complications.

Figures from Alaska are among the few which give the numbers of climbers at risk. They show that, between the years 1903 and 1982 on Mt McKinley and Mt Foraker, there were 6080 mountaineers of whom 40 (0.8%) were killed. The causes of death were falls (25%), avalanche (26%), exposure (22%), mountain sickness and its complications (12%) and falls into a crevasse (10%) (Wilson, 1983). Mills *et al.* (1987) commented that the annual casualty rate on Mt McKinley for the few years previous to 1987 had been 12% to 16%, with a fatality rate of 4.3 per 1000 climbers (Lattimore, 1993).

A survey of accidents in the Grand Teton National Park USA, between 1981 and 1986 showed that the accident incidence was 2.5 accidents per 1000 climbers per year, or 5.6 accidents per 10 000 climber hours. In all 43 631 climbers were at risk. There were 108 accidents and 28 fatalities. The total cost of rescue in this period was $148 614, all of which was borne by the National Park Service. The injured made up two different groups: climbers climbing at the limit of their capabilities, and inexperienced mountaineers (Schussman *et al.*, 1990). A retrospective survey of Australian rock climbers suggested that there was a relatively low injury rate (Humphries, 1993).

26.1.4 South America

Little information is available from Central and South America, but the effects of altitude would be expected to become of greater importance since the peaks are higher, rising to over 7000 m.

26.1.5 Himalayas and Central Asia

A retrospective survey (Brendel *et al.*, 1985) of 3200 mountaineers who took part in 402 expeditions to the Hindu Kush, Karakoram and Himalayas between 1940 and 1978 showed a mortality of nearly 3%. Nearly a quarter, 24%, had their health or life put at risk. The causes of morbidity and mortality were intercurrent disease, mountain sickness and its complications, cold injury and accidents. Of 277 climbers who suffered from high-altitude complaints, five died from acute pulmonary edema, two of cerebral edema and two from vascular episodes, giving an overall mortality rate of 0.3% due to the effects of altitude alone.

As far as accidents were concerned, the highest mortality was due to climbers falling, followed by avalanche, crevasse accidents and rock falls.

Respiratory disease, often pneumonia, and gastrointestinal complaints were common and exhaustion occurred more often above than below 6000 m. Cold injury was commoner than mountain sickness and pulmonary edema was commoner than cerebral edema, retinal haemorrhage or vascular disorders.

A broadly similar pattern of mortality (6–7%) and morbidity was found among Europeans on expeditions to the world's ten highest peaks up to and including the first ascent (Ward, 1975) (Table 26.1). The fatality rate in Himalayas mountaineers is 29 per 1000 climbers (Shlim and Houston, 1989).

Between 1895 and 1980 there were 266 expeditions to peaks over 8000 m, with 188 deaths. Deaths on Everest between 1921 and 1982 numbered 62 (Ward, 1984). Town (1986) quotes a morbidity rate

Table 26.1 Mortality* on the world's ten highest peaks up to their first ascent (From Ward, 1975)

Cause	*Number*
Avalanche and accident	36
Exhaustion and sequelae	15
High altitude edema	3
Frost-bite	2
Cerebrovascular accident	2
Enteric fever	1
Unknown	5
Total	64

*Mortality rate 6–7%

of 3.4% on peaks over 8000 m; the highest mortality occurred on Annapurna (8%), then Nanga Parbat (5%) and Everest (3%). Pollard and Clarke (1988), in a review of British expeditions to peaks over 7000 m in the Greater Himalayas between 1968 and 1987, quote a figure of 23 deaths out of 533 mountaineers at risk (i.e. 4.3%). The most frequently visited peak was Everest (8848 m) where there were seven deaths out of 121 individuals at risk, a mortality rate of 5.8%. On K2, the world's second highest mountain, there were three deaths out of 28 individuals at risk (11%). Of all deaths, 70% were due to accidents and avalanche. Some of the remainder were due to cerebral or pulmonary edema, whilst the cause in a number was unknown. The higher the altitude of the expedition, the greater the risk of fatality; the contribution of hypoxia cannot be ignored.

By the end of 1992, Everest had been climbed 485 times by 422 people, and since 1922 there have been 115 deaths (Gillman, 1993). In these deaths the element of hypoxia was a major factor, often in the form of pulmonary and cerebral edema and hypothermia (Ward, 1987; Oelz, 1990). Over 51 mountaineers have now climbed Everest without supplementary oxygen.

Between 1968 and 1982, 24 UK expeditions with more than four lead climbers went to the Himalayas. There were 12 deaths in the UK personnel involved, and one in two expeditions lost a member. There was an overall mortality of 5%. Between 1975 and 1983, 20 UK expeditions with less than four lead climbers took place in the Himalayas. There were four deaths in the 70 UK personnel at risk (mortality 5%). About one in five expeditions lost a member (Mountain Medicine Data Centre, 1986).

Over 8000 m, the cause of death, according to Town (1986), was due to objective dangers in 60% of cases. Whilst bad weather is responsible for a significant number of deaths, the combination of hypoxia and hypothermia with associated mental effects, particularly lack of judgement, plays a major role. The rate of success in reaching the summit on peaks above 8000 m is 47%, whilst on Everest it is a little lower at 41%. There is a general feeling, but few accurate statistics, that the mortality rate is higher in those attempting to climb Everest without supplementary oxygen (Oelz, 1990).

26.2 MANAGEMENT OF MOUNTAINEERING ACCIDENTS

26.2.1 Introduction

Accidents in the mountains may often be complicated by the subsequent development of cold injury. The detailed management of injury in the mountains is covered in numerous books and articles (e.g.

Wilkerson, 1985; Steel, 1988; Bollen, 1989). The general principles only will be discussed in the following pages.

The peaks of the Himalayas and Central Asia are not just a larger equivalent of the European Alps or the Rockies; the highest are always dangerous by virtue of hypoxia, cold and weather, which can convert a minor illness or accident into a major disaster. The highest priority should always be given to getting ill or injured individuals down to lower altitudes as soon as possible.

At altitudes exceeding 7000 m it is rare for every member of a party to be continuously fit, and for this reason expeditions with a small number may be at greater risk of failure to climb their peak because of lack of reserves. There is a growing tendency for expeditions of four members or fewer to attempt the more difficult and highest peaks in the world by hard routes, often in winter; this puts a great strain on even the fittest and hardiest mountaineer. Solo ascents of these highest peaks are also becoming commoner. Team selection is of great importance as members should be compatible both physically and mentally. A 'weak' individual may indirectly cause 'stress' to climbing companions and thereby increase the liability to illness and accidents.

Over an altitude of 8000 m, fancifully but often accurately called 'the death zone', the stresses are extreme, particularly if supplementary oxygen is not used. Cases of pulmonary edema have been reported at extreme altitude, some despite the use of acetazolamide (Oelz, 1987) and too rapid an ascent is probably a factor. Judgement is impaired, hallucinations common and individual variation is marked.

Ambition should not override caution, particularly as fixity of purpose is a feature of hypoxia. Long term mental effects of oxygen lack following weeks of high altitudes have been reported.

The chances of a successful rescue are likely to be increased if the ill or injured climber can move 'under his own steam' for even short periods. It may be necessary to ignore factors which make any medical conditions worse in order to get off the mountain. Mobility of the victim may be life saving and, if analgesia in large doses can increase mobility, the patient should be given large doses. Patients with head injuries travel well and, even if dazed or with a compound fracture of the skull, should be persuaded to move. Desperate situations need desperate remedies.

26.2.2 General principles

The medical and surgical problems that mountaineers encounter at altitude are as much a problem of the mountain, cold and altitude as they are of the medical and surgical conditions. The principles of first aid are the same anywhere – namely to save life, prevent further injury and to maintain the victim in good physical and mental condition during evacuation.

The immediate objective is to maintain **airway**, **breathing** and **circulation** and **donate heat** to the central core to prevent **death** from cold injury.

A critical factor is time, and the 'rules of four' apply. Death due to acute oxygen lack takes 4–6 min, due to cold and shock 4–6 h, due to dehydration 4–6 days and due to complete starvation 40 days.

Shelter from the wind is vital to prevent rapid cooling and hypothermia. Snow is a good insulator, so a snow hole, cave or slot should be made. Always insulate the victim **from** the snow. Always make a continuous record of the patient's condition; Simple notes are adequate. Always shelter from falling rocks, avalanche etc.

Evacuation depends on the type of injury, strength of the party, weather and communication.

26.2.3 Falls

Owing to the increasing popularity of extreme rock climbing over the past few years and of the harder routes being done at altitude, there has been an increase in the number of falls as individuals climb nearer their limit. Most mountaineers wear a seat harness that fits around the pelvis. However, these do not prevent fractures of the spine or a head injury unless a 'controlled fall' is undertaken. In a controlled fall the rope close to the body is held by one or both hands. This prevents the climber 'turning over', hyperextending his spine, and causing a whiplash injury and fracture or rupture of the spinal cord. In addition, the falling climber may turn upside down and the head may be hit against the rock causing concussion and a possible fracture of the skull.

If a chest harness is used these injuries are less likely to happen, but the combination of chest and pelvic harness is not popular as it tends to restrict free movement. It is therefore seldom worn.

26.2.4 Airway blockage and cardiac arrest

Complete blockage causes coma in 4 min and death in 6 min. The treatment is to unblock the airway and use mouth to mouth resuscitation if breathing has stopped, and make sure that the **airway always remains clear**.

The commonest cause of cardiac arrest is myocardial infarction, followed by severe hypothermia, trauma or being struck by lightning. In the mountains, cardiac arrest is normally fatal. The pupils are dilated, and there is no carotid pulsation (radial artery pulsation may be absent due to cold), and there is no respiration. Cardiopulmonary resuscitation should be attempted but it is hard work and 30 min is the longest period most can manage alone.

26.2.5 Haemorrhage

All bleeding, whether arterial, venous or capillary can be stopped by pressure. Primary haemorrhage occurs at the time of injury. Reactionary haemorrhage occurs within 24 hours and is due to dislodgement of a clot as the result of a rise in blood pressure, restlessness, coughing or movement. Secondary haemorrhage due to infection occurs within 7–10 days and is preceded by 'warning' haemorrhages.

External bleeding may be controlled by putting a clean thumb on the bleeding point and maintaining pressure for at least 10 min by the clock. Venous bleeding may be stopped by raising the bleeding point above the level of the heart or by pressure. Capillary oozing may be stopped by pressure.

Internal bleeding can be life threatening and evacuation is mandatory. All fractures cause considerable bleeding into the tissues, usually more than is generally realized.

26.2.6 Shock

'Shock' is an imprecise term used to describe the effect of a sudden reduction in the circulating blood volume, the result of bleeding, burning, major trauma and overwhelming infection.

The patient feels cold, has a clammy skin, a rapid, 'thready' pulse and a low blood pressure. This is the result of peripheral vasoconstriction, which endeavours to maintain an adequate central blood volume.

Management is by restoring blood volume and removing the cause of the shock, which may cause death within 4–6 h. If the blood pressure remains too low for too long, irreversible renal damage may occur.

26.2.7 Head injury

Serious head injuries may be prevented by wearing helmets. In general, patients with severe head injuries get worse and die, whilst the less serious improve and live.

The Hippocratic maxim that 'no head injury is too minor to be neglected nor too great to be despaired of' is as true today as it was in his time. Head injuries do travel well.

In every head injury it is important to make certain that there is no neck injury, or injury of the chest, abdomen or limbs. The level of consciousness should be assessed and written down, scalp bleeding

Table 26.2 The Glasgow coma scale

Response	*Score*
Eye opening [e]	
Spontaneous	4
To command	3
To pain	2
Nil	1
Motor response [m]	
Obeys command	6
Localizes pain	5
Withdraws from pain	4
Abnormal flexion to pain	3
Extensor response to pain	2
Nil	1
Verbal response [v]	
Orientated and converses	5
Disorientated and converses	4
Inappropriate words	3
Incomprehensible	2
Nil	1
Total score [e+m+v] gives prognosis	
Will probably survive	7–8
Doubtful outcome	6
Will almost certainly die	4–5
Nearly dead	3

should be stopped by pressure, and the individual protected from further injury. If the brain is exposed, cover the wound with a clean dressing and give antibiotics.

Management of the unconscious patient includes maintaining the airway and dealing with a full bladder. Semiconscious patients may remember comments made about their condition so rescuers should be careful of what they say.

Each case should be assessed according to the Glasgow coma scale or similar index. The Glascow coma scale (Table 26.2) is used internationally to estimate the level of consciousness and replaces vague confusing terms such as 'stupor' and 'black-out'. Noting the scale over several hours will show any change in the level of consciousness. It will indicate if the patient is becoming 'lighter' and approaching normal consciousness or 'deepening' due to increasing intracranial pressure because of oedema or haemorrhage.

26.2.8 Neck and spinal injury

About 20% of head injuries are associated with some form of cervical injury. Usually in these cases the paraspinal cervical muscles go into spasm, preventing further complications.

If a patient is unable to move the head or it gives great pain, the neck should be splinted. When transported, the whole spine including the neck should be moved in one piece to prevent further dislocation and injury to the spinal cord.

Any possibility of injury to the thoracic or lumbar spine should be dealt with as if a cord injury did exist. Urinary retention may be a problem.

26.2.9 Chest injury

Fractured ribs are very painful, as movement occurs with each breath. They should be strapped and local anaesthetic infiltrated around the fracture site. Fractured ribs or a penetrating injury may cause a pneumothorax. If the patient is unduly breathless this should be considered, and given urgent attention.

26.2.10 Abdominal injury

Abdominal injuries may be closed or open and should be treated with the utmost suspicion, as either can be associated with the rupture of an abdominal viscus. Associated chest injury can occur.

Closed injuries that are potentially serious often have bruising of the abdominal wall. Intestine may be involved in both open and closed injuries; it may be ruptured or bruised.

Rupture of the spleen and kidney is associated with haemorrhage into the peritoneal cavity and profound shock; similarly a ruptured bladder, when urine floods the peritoneal caverty.

26.2.11 Dislocations and fractures

The sooner a dislocation is reduced or a fracture realigned and rendered immobile the more comfortable and stable the accident victim will be, and the more easily evacuated (Serra, 1991).

Dislocations

Dislocations are incapacitating and easily identified by comparing the joints on the two sides of the body. Reduction is easier immediately after the injury, before muscle spasm and swelling have developed, and results in dramatic relief of pain. It also reduces the risk of vascular and neurological complications, makes transport of the patient easier, and improves the safety of the whole party. It is important always to check for vascular and neurological involvment.

Fractures

Fractures may be open and potentially infected, or closed. There is always loss of blood into the tissues due to vascular involvement. This may be considerable and associated nerve lesions are not uncommon. Deformities should be reduced and realigned as soon as possible; pain and swelling can be reduced by the application of snow. The fracture should be stabilized by whatever means are available.

Various commercial splits are available, including air splints, but differences in barometric pressure should be taken into account and the circulation of the limb must be checked frequently.

26.2.12 Wounds and soft tissue injuries

To prevent infection, all wounds should be covered or the edges approximated by tape or sutures. Abrasions should be cleaned, and, if left open, the formation of a clot will provide protection. Delayed primary suture should be used with infected wounds.

Blisters should be prevented by well fitting footgear and the application of plaster to the area that may be blistered **before** the boot is worn. A blister, once formed, may contain serum, blood or pus. This should be aspirated and the devitalized skin left in place as it protects the raw area, which should be covered with a dressing that absorbs fluid.

Puncture wounds are all potentially serious, especially of the abdomen, when a viscus may be pierced, or the chest, when the lung or heart may be affected. In addition bacteria are driven deep into the wound. The patient should be given antibiotics.

Wounds over a fracture site should either be covered or sutured to prevent infection of the bone. Potentially infected wounds require antibiotic cover and the tetanus immunization status should be checked.

Bruising of the soft tissues due to trauma may be extensive. The possibility of infection is high, particularly if there is any break in the continuity of the skin, and prophylactic antibiotics should be considered.

Wound healing at altitude

Landon (1905) observed during the British Mission to Tibet 1904–1905 that:

> wounds and scratches took an abnormal time to heal owing to the oxygen less state of the air. Colonel Wadell (The Principal Medical Officer) did indeed try to obtain a cylinder of oxygen for certain medical purposes but they were found impossible to transport.
>
> *(Landon, 1905)*

On the American Medical Research Expedition to Everest 1981, four expedition members, including two Sherpas, had minor wounds on feet and hands which failed to heal at base camp (5400 m), but healed promptly when they decended to 4300 m (West, 1985).

An adequate tissue P_{O_2} is a crucial factor in wound healing (Kuhne *et al.*, 1985). In the early stage of healing, 'physiological' hypoxia occurs; without this, capillary budding is scanty (Knighton *et al.*, 1981). In the later stages, the rate of healing is proportional to tissue P_{O_2}. The critical level for wound healing appears to be between 10–20 mmHg and below this level healing is delayed and infection more common (Knighton *et al.*, 1984).

26.2.13 Muscle injuries

Muscle problems are common and vary from stiffness to rupture.

Stiffness is common and appears a few hours after unaccustomed exercise, such as prolonged 'negative work' (i.e. walking or running downhill when not in training). The histology shows an injury in the myofibrillae, especially at the level of the Z-band. This disappears with training.

Strain occurs when the muscle is stretched beyond its normal physiological capabilities, but there is no sign of macroscopic injury. It is the result of imbalance of exercising muscles due to old injuries or an inadequate 'warm-up' period.

Microscopic rupture of muscle fibres may occur with some interstitial damage. This may show up on ultrasound examination. It presents as sudden pain; the treatment is conservative.

Macroscopic rupture of muscle presents with sudden pain, a snapping sound and a 'tearing' sensation at the site of injury. Examination reveals a 'hole' with a 'lump', which is the retracted muscle. Ultrasound confirms the diagnosis as does MRI examination. Treatment is either conservative or surgical repair, depending on the extent and severity of the injury and the experience of the surgeon.

Bruising of the muscle may occur as a result of direct injury, with the formation of an intramuscular haematoma. The treatment of all soft tissue lesions should include immediate immersion in cold water or the application of snow; a crepe bandage will minimize swelling. Further management depends on the severity and type of injury.

Injury of the tendinous insertions of muscles, particularly the tendo Achilles, may occur. Repeated minor trauma to untrained muscle causes muscle haemorrhages, and produces localized pain and swelling. Ultrasound confirms the clinical diagnosis. Rupture of the tendo Achilles is not uncommon and presents with a sudden sharp pain in the calf as though the individual has been kicked. Walking becomes impossible. Treatment is by suture of the tendon which is often very ragged (Lanzetta and Seratoni, 1991; Rostan and Gobelet, 1991).

A stress fracture of the 3rd and 4th metatarsals can be caused by a long uphill walk carried out over several days carrying a heavy load. Occult fractures and injury to the insertions of ligaments and tendous to bones (enthesopathy) may also occur. Bone scintigraphy may reveal unsuspected damage to bone (Orr and Taylor, 1993).

26.2.14 Burns and scalds

Burns are caused by dry heat, scalds by wet heat. They may be due to rope friction, lightning, stove explosion, fat or boiling water.

The surface area of a burn has a bearing on treatment and survival. The palm of the patient's hand represents 1% of the patient's surface area. Minor burns are under 15% and usually heal unaided. Major burns are over 15% in adults, but over 10% in children, as the surface to weight ratio is higher. They are a threat to life. To assess the surface area of the burn, the 'rule of nines' is a useful approximation.

Partial thickness burns leave some epithelial tissue for regeneration; clinically there is response to pinprick. In full thickness burns all the epithelial elements are destroyed, healing is by granulation tissue and skin grafting will be necessary; there is no response to pinprick.

Damage to capillary walls results in loss of plasma and occasionally blood. This can lead to shock.

Treatment is by immersion in snow or cold water, and removal of all charred clothing and dead tissue. The extent (rule of nines) and depths (pinpick) of the burn should be recorded and it should be covered with an absorbent pad which is kept in place by a bandage. Blisters should be left alone, but if they burst they must be covered. Parenteral antibiotics should be given. Burns of the face should be cleaned and left exposed. Corneal burns are uncommon; the eye should be irrigated, and antibiotic ointment and homatropine instilled. Burns of the hand should be covered with antibiotic cream and covered in a plastic bag, with a mitten for protection.

After major burns (>15% surface area), fluid must be replaced, ideally by the intravenous route. In mountaineers this is not usually possible, so 3 l day^{-1} should be given by mouth, using the WHO formula; if this is not available, plain water may be substituted. Rectal fluids are another possibility.

To make up the WHO formula, in 1 l of water put:

- Glucose 20 g = 1.5 teaspoon honey, corn syrup;
- Sodium chloride 3.5 g = 0.5 teaspoon table salt;
- Sodium bicarbonate 2.5 g = 0.5 teaspoon baking powder;
- Potassium chloride 1.5 g = 0.5 teaspoon of orange or other fruit juice.

26.3 SPORT CLIMBING

Sport climbing, which began in the USA in the 1970s, has developed greatly over the last 20 years. It is a competitive development of the techniques of rock climbing to an extremely high standard, with a high degree of protection. The use of artificial walls is standard and a high degree of neuromuscular co-ordination with a high strength to weight ratio is an advantage. Inevitably the developments in this sport will be applied to mountaineering in the world's high mountain ranges. The most common injuries are due to over-use, particularly in the upper limb, and accidents.

Over-use injuries are due to excessive muscle development over a relatively short period rather than slowly over longer time, irregular and over-training, and an inadequate warm-up period before competing. Good technical supervision is necessary to develop a sound technique which does not overstrain certain muscle groups and the relatively fragile tendon and pulley mechanism of the finger and hands.

About 70% of injuries affect the upper limbs, mainly the fingers, in particular the third and fourth fingers. The reason for this is that the diameter of the fourth finger is smaller than that of the second and third fingers and is therefore more often used as the sole support on very small holds. The most common condition is a tendonitis of the common flexor tendons. It is important to treat this immediately otherwise the condition can become chronic and the individual unable to take part in any further competition.

Prevention includes an adequate warm-up period and adequate training procedures aimed at strengthening the relevant muscles. Above all, long term planning is necessary and should extend over several months or years, as for any competitive sport carried out to Olympic standard.

Accidents are due to falls and usually involve the foot and ankle.

Fracture of the talus is one of the commonest and is to be feared because of the development of avascular necrosis (Leal and Rané, 1991).

26.4 ANAESTHESIA AT ALTITUDE

John F. Nunn

A considerable number of major medical centres are at altitudes between 1500 m and 2000 m. General anaesthetics are administered there safely and with only minor modifications of techniques. Above 2000 m, increasing attention must be paid to the effects of decreased pressure. Anaesthetics are not normally administered above 4000 m, and the response to general anaesthesia has not been documented. Anaesthesia above this altitude might, however, be required in an emergency and is potentially very dangerous.

26.4.1 Avoidance of hypoxia

During anaesthesia with spontaneous ventilation, breathing is almost always depressed and alveolar ventilation may be reduced to half the value appropriate to the metabolic rate. Whether breathing is spontaneous or artificial, there is usually an increase in the alveolar/arterial P_{O_2} gradient, equivalant to a shunt of about 10% of pulmonary arterial blood flow. For these reasons maintenance of a normal arterial P_{O_2} requires, at sea-level, an increase in the inspired oxygen concentration to 35–40%. The inspired P_{O_2} is thus about 300 mmHg and this should be maintained regardless of barometric pressure. The concentration of oxygen breathed by the anaesthetized patient should therefore be increased in accordance with altitude as shown in Table 26.3.

Nitrous oxide is an effective anaesthetic at an alveolar partial pressure of about 750 mmHg (70% nitrous oxide at sea-level is only a partial anaesthetic). It will be clear from Table 26.3 that it cannot make a very effective contribution to anaesthesia above 2000 m, at which altitude

Table 26.3 Minimal concentration of oxygen in the inspired gas required to maintain a normal arterial P_{O_2} in the anaesthetized patient

Altitude (m)	*O_2 concentration (%)*
Sea-level	40
2000	54
4000	72
6000	100

only 46% of the inspired gas is available for nitrous oxide. It is contra-indicated at any higher level and general anaesthesia must then be based on potent volatile anaesthetic agents vaporized in oxygen en-riched mixtures. Intravenous anaesthetics should only be used with oxygen enrichment of the inspired gas according to Table 26.3.

26.4.2 Hypoxic ventilatory drive

Survival at altitudes much in excess of 5000 m depends upon hyper-ventilation in response to hypoxic drive, although this is counteracted by negative feedback, resulting from reduction of the P_{CO_2}. It is now established that anaesthesia (and even subanaesthetic concentrations of anaesthetics) will totally abolish the peripheral chemorecptor response to hypoxia (Knill and Gelb, 1978). It is therefore possible to envisage a situation in which a patient at 6000 m, who would normally have an arterial P_{O_2} of 45 mmHg and a P_{CO_2} of 23 mmHg might perhaps be anaesthetized with chloroform and air. There would be rapid inacti-vation of peripheral chemoreceptors with decrease of P_{O_2} to about 23 mmHg, which would threaten life. An increased oxygen concen-tration is therefore essential, not only during anaesthesia, but in the postoperative period, because the peripheral chemoreceptors are severely depressed by as little as one-tenth of the anaesthetic concen-tration of volatile anaesthetic agents.

26.4.3 Performance of vaporizers

Calibrated vaporizers depend upon known dilution of saturation con-centrations of volatile anaesthetics. The saturation concentration equals the vapour pressure divided by the barometric pressure. Vapour pressure depends only on temperature. Thus, if the barometric pressure is halved, the saturation concentration will be doubled. If the dilution ratio of the vaporizer is unaffected by the reduction in barometric pressure (a reasonable assumption), it may be expected that the vaporizer will then deliver twice the concentration shown on the dial. However, the pharmacological effect depends on partial pressure. Twice the concentration at half the barometric pressure gives the same partial pressure as at sea-level. Therefore, as a first approximation, probably adequate for clinical purposes, a temperature controlled calibrated vaporizer may be expected to produce the same effect for the same dial setting at altitude as at sea-level.

These concepts have never been tested at altitude. However, one of the authors (MPW) and I anaesthetized one another and Professor Woolmer at a chamber pressure of 375 mmHg in 1961, in preparation for the Himalayan Scientific and Mountaineering Expedition (Silver Hut) 1960–1961. The apparatus was based on equipment designed for use in Antarctica (Nunn, 1961). With a carrier gas of 60% oxygen in nitrogen, obtained with oxygen flow through an injector, and a standard halothane vaporizer (Fluotec Mark 2), uneventful anaesthesia was easily obtained in all three subjects and recovery was rapid and uneventful. In view of the subsequent discovery of the effect of anaesthetics on the peripheral chemoreceptors, we would now favour 100% oxygen at this simulated altitude of nearly 6000 m.

26.4.4 Practical considerations

The greater the altitude, the lower is the possibility of a trained anaesthetist and appropriate equipment being available. Dangers are multiplied by anaesthesia being attempted in this very hostile environment by someone who is untrained. The first rule must be to avoid anaesthesia above 4000 m if at all possible and to evacuate rather than attempt surgical intervention on the spot.

If anaesthesia is essential, then oxygen enrichment of the inspired gas is essential for both patient and anaesthetist throughout the perioperative period. The safest technique is probably a non-irritant volatile anaesthetic (halothane, enflurane or isoflurane) vaporized in oxygen enriched air according to Table 26.3. It was demonstrated that this technique could be accomplished at sea-level by medical officers without special training in anaesthesia who were destined for the Antarctic (Nunn, 1961). Transport of sufficient oxygen, the vaporizer and the gas delivery system would clearly present logistic difficulties. Use of the open mask is not recommended because of the difficulty in controlling the inspired oxygen concentration. Ruttledge (1934) described a near disaster when chloroform was administered on an open mask at 4300 m on the Tibetan plateau during the march in on the 1933 Everest expedition. This would be expected on present understanding.

Intravenous anaesthesia should not be attempted at altitude by those without experience because of the dangers of respiratory obstruction and depression. However, ketamine (2–4 $mg\,kg^{-1}$) might well be satisfactory because the patient's airway and respiratory drive are well maintained with this drug. This is logistically very attractive for major disasters, mass casualties and warfare. There is good analgesia, and duration is sufficient for any procedure likely to be considered. Hallucinations may occur but would be the least of the patient's problems. Ketamine should only be administered with oxygen enrichment. The author is, however, unaware of any trial of ketamine at altitude and its use should therefore be regarded as experimental. Reliance on injectable solutions must be tempered by the hazard of freezing and breakage of ampoules.

Local anaesthetic techniques are obviously safer and should be used if at all possible in preference to general anaesthesia at altitude.

26.4.5 Postanaesthetic period

In the postanaesthetic period, after a general anaesthetic, the hazard of hypoxia due to respiratory depression discussed above is still very real. Indeed, in the hours after the operation, the danger may be greater since the patient may not be so closely watched as during anaesthesia.

It should be remembered that, even at sea-level, patients are normally mildly hypoxic during this stage. Hypoxia may cause restlessness, irritability and confusion, which may be misinterpreted as being due to pain. Additional analgesics may then be administered which further depress respiraton and the patient may die from hypoxic cardiac arrest. This was probably the sequence of events in a Sherpa operated upon for debridement of frost-bitten fingers at an altitude of 4300 m. Clearly, supplementary oxygen should be given during the postanaesthetic period if available. The patient must be closely watched and stimulated to breathe either by verbal encouragement or, possibly, by the use of a respiratory stimulant such as doxapram.

REFERENCES

Bollen, S. (1989) *First Aid on Mountains*, British Mountaineering Council, Manchester.

Brendel, W., Weingart, J.R. and Haas, L.R. (1985) Medical statement analysis of 3200 high altitude climbers, in *High Altitude Deterioration*, (eds J. Rivolier, P. Cerretelli, J. Foray and P. Seganatini), Karger, Basel, pp. 180–91.

Durrer, B. (1993) Rescue operations in the Swiss Alps in 1990 and 1991. *J. Wild. Med.*, **4**, 363–73.

Federated Mountain Club of New Zealand. (1986) *Reports 1976–1986*.

Gillman, P. (1993) *Everest*. Little, Brown, Boston MA.

Hartley, A.K. (1970) Accidents and rescue. *Alpine J.*, **75**, 265–7.

Horvath, S.M. (1981) Exercise in a cold environment. *Exercise Sport Sci. Rev.*, **9**, 221–63.

Humphries, D. (1993) Injury rate in rock climbers. *J. Wild. Med.*, **4**, 281–5.

IKAR Reports, (1982–1984) (Available from Alpine Club, London).

Knighton, D.R., Silver, I.A. and Hunt, T.K. (1981) Regulation of wound healing angiogenesis. Effect of oxygen gradients and inspired oxygen concentration. *Surgery*, **90**, 262–70.

Knighton, D.R., Halliday, B. and Hunt, T.K. (1984) Oxygen as an antibiotic. The effect of inspired oxygen on infection. *Arch. Surg.*, **119**, 199–204.

Knill, R.L. and Gelb, A.W. (1978) Ventilatory responses to hypoxia and hypercapnia during halothane sedation and anaesthesia in man. *Anaesthesiology*, **49**, 244–51.

Kuhne, H.H., Ullmann, U. and Kuhne, F.W. (1985) New aspects on the pathophysiology of wound infection and wound healing – the problem of lowered oxygen tension in the tissue. *Infection*, **13**, 52–6.

Landon, P. (1905) *Lhasa*, Vol. 2, Hurst and Blackett, London, p. 383.

Lanzetta, A. and Seratoni, R. (1991) Injuries related to hiking and trekking, in *A Colour Atlas of Mountain Medicine*, (eds J. Vallatton and F. Dubas), Wolfe, London, pp. 123–7.

Lattimore, C. (1993) Mountaineering emergencies on Denali. *J. Wild. Med.*, **4**, 358–62.

Leal, C. and Rané, A. (1991) Injuries in sport climbing, in *A Colour Atlas of Mountain Medicine*, (eds J. Vallatton and F. Dubas), Wolfe, London, pp. 176–82.

Mills, W.J., Gower, R., Hackett, P.H., *et al.* (1987) Cold injury, dehydration, and multiple system trauma, in *Hypoxia and Cold*, (eds J.R. Sutton, C.S. Houston and G. Coates), Praeger, New York, pp. 340–62.

Mountain Rescue Committee. (1977–1984) *Mountain and Cave Rescue. Annual Reports of Mountain Incidents in England and Wales*, Alpine Club, London.

Mountain Medicine Data Centre. (1986) *Accident data*, UIAA St Bartholomew's Hospital, London.

Nunn, J.F. (1961) Portable anaesthetic apparatus for use in the Antarctic. *Br. Med. J.*, **1**, 1139–43.

Oelz, O. (1987) A case of high-altitude pulmonary edema treated with nifedipine (letter). *J. Am. Med. Assoc.*, **257**, 780.

Oelz, O. (1990) Death at extreme altitude. *J. Wild. Med.*, **1**, 141–3.

Omori, S. (1992) Mountaineering accident rescue conditions in Japan, in *High Altitude Medicine*, (eds G. Ueda, J.T. Reeves and M. Sekiguchi), Shinsu University, Japan, pp. 441–6.

Orr, L. and Taylor, A. (1993) Wilderness-related musculo-skeletal injury: Role of bone scintigraphy. *J. Wild. Med.*, **4**, 407–11.

Pollard, A. and Clarke, C.R.A. (1988) Deaths during mountaineering at extreme altitude (letter). *Lancet*, **1**, 1277.

Rostan, A. and Gobelet, C. (1991) Muscular lesions, in *A Colour Atlas of Mountain Medicine*, (eds J. Vallaton and F. Dubas), Wolfe, London, pp. 128–34.

Ruttledge, H. (1934) *Everest 1933*. Hodder and Stoughton, London, p. 78.

Shlim, O.R. and Houston, R. (1989) Helicopter rescues and deaths among trekkers in Nepal. *J. Am. Med. Assoc.*, **261**, 1017–19.

Schussman, L.C., Lutz, L.J., Shaw, R.R. and Bohnn, C.R. (1990) The epidemiology of mountaineering and rock climbing accidents. *J. Wild. Med.*, **1**, 235–48.

Scottish Mountain Accidents. (1984) Twenty-year table, 1964–1983, *Scottish Mountaineering Club J.*, pp. 77–9.

Scottish Mountain Accidents. (1985) *Scottish Mountaineering Club J.*, pp. 202–4.

Scottish Mountain Accidents. (1986) *Scottish Mountaineering Club J.*, pp. 356–7.

Serra, J.B. (1991) Management of dislocations and fractures in the wilderness environment, in *Proceedings of the 1st World Congress on Wilderness Medicine*, Wilderness Medical Society, California, pp. 269–77.

Steel, P. (1988) *Medical Handbook for Mountaineers*, Constable, London.

Town, J. (1986) Death and the art of database maintenance. *Mountain*, **10**, 42–5.

Ward, M. (1975) Accidents in *Mountain Medicine*, Crosby Lockwood Staples, London, pp. 335–47.

Ward, M.P. (1984) Accidents and death at altitude, in *Lightweight Expeditions to the Great Ranges*, (eds C. Clarke and A. Salkeld), Alpine Club, London, pp. 38–43.

Ward, M.P. (1987) Cold, hypothermia and dehydration, in *Hypoxia and Cold*, (eds J.R. Sutton, C.S. Houston and G. Coates), Praeger, New York, pp. 475–86.

West, J.B. (1985) *Everest: The Testing Place*, McGraw-Hill, New York, p. 64.

Wilkerson, J.A. (ed.) (1985) *Medicine for Mountaineers*, The Mountaineers, Seattle.

Wilson, R. (1983) Deaths amongst climbers on Mt McKinley and Mt Foraker. *Jpn. J. Mount. Med.*, **3**, 1–16.

27

Skiing injuries and rescue in the mountains; heat injury and solar radiation

27.1 SKIING INJURIES

27.1.1 Piste

Downhill skiing on prepared pistes attracts large numbers of people to the mountains and because of this many injuries and a few deaths occur each year.

27.1.2 Cross country

The hazards of cross country skiing and ski mountaineering are broadly similar to those of mountaineering. For centuries in Scandinavia and the mountain regions of Russia the normal method of movement in winter has been by ski, it is only recently that this has developed into an increasingly popular sport.

Prepared trails

In the USA it is estimated that there are at least 4 million cross-country skiers, whilst in Canada about 4 million people over the age of 12, representing 20% of the population, ski across country by comparison with 2.4 million who piste ski. Figures for Japan and Europe must be more than double this figure.

Equipment differs from that used by piste skiers in that the toes are fixed, leaving the heel free. Shoes are flexible and the skis light enough to minimize fatigue.

Figures show that the average age of the cross-country skier is 35 years, and the overall injury rate for two seasons in one series was 0.72 per 1000 skiers. About 25% were beginners and 47% were intermediate, whilst 23% were expert. Injuries included hip fractures and dislocations, fractures of the femoral shaft and ankle, and injuries to the knee ligaments. About 10% of injuries were to the face and trunk, 41% to the upper limbs and 49% to the lower limbs. Half the injuries were serious, with either a dislocation or fracture (Johnson, 1982).

Wilderness skiing

In cross-country skiing on unprepared tracks ('wilderness skiing'), the risks of injury and of getting lost are higher and cold injury is common. The proficient wilderness skier must be knowledgeable about winter survival, have an understanding of the country and hazards such as avalanche, and be able to read the weather and a map.

Ski marathons

Ski marathons have become popular in Nordic countries attracting up to 10 000 participants. Even in cold weather (−15°C or less) surprisingly light clothing, with an insulation value of not more than 1 CLO, may be adequate. A high level of heat production dominates the thermal sensation despite low skin temperature and low thermal insulation. However, if heat production were to stop suddenly due to an accident, exhaustion or bad weather, hypothermia would rapidly supervene (Smolander *et al.*, 1986).

27.1.3 Ski mountaineering

This term is used for those who cross mountain country and climb peaks on skis, usually in winter. It was pioneered in the European Alps over 100 years ago. In the Himalayas skis were used on Mt Kamet at 7200 m in 1925 (Smythe, 1932) and some Central Asian peaks have now been descended on skis (Cleare, 1983). A ski traverse of the European Alps in winter has been carried out on more than one occasion (Cliff, 1973). Ski mountaineers are exposed to all the risks of the mountain environment and especially to avalanche danger because of the time of year when they take to the mountains (i.e. the winter and spring).

27.1.4 Injuries

Skiing injuries are conditioned by the environment, the skiers capabilities and his equipment. Injuries are becoming more severe.

The size of the problem is indicated by statistics from one hospital in Grenoble, at the centre of a large French ski area. Between 1968 and

1988 the accident and orthopaedic department treated 17200 people involved in ski accidents. The figures are now running at 1000 cases a year and increasing. Ninety per cent of the injuries occurred in the lower limbs and 10% in the upper. Recent developments in mono-skiing and snow surfing are changing the pattern of these statistics (Bezes *et al.*, 1991).

Every type of injury is encountered; cuts due to ski edges and impalement on ski sticks and slalom poles, and head, spinal, chest, facial and abdominal injuries are all reported. The improvement in ski equipment has resulted in injuries occurring at higher speeds than formerly, with an increasing proportion of injuries to the upper limbs.

Two injuries will be discussed, partly because they are common, and partly because one component of each injury, or even the severity of the injury, may be missed or disregarded.

Skier's thumb

A common injury, whose severity is often ignored, but, as the thumb is 'half the hand', even the smallest injury has considerable consequences. Skier's thumb is the rupture, or partial rupture, of the collateral ligament of the metacarpophalangeal joint of the thumb. It usually results from a fall on the outstretched hand when holding a ski stick and the thumb becomes forcibly abducted and hyperflexed. Because of the importance of the thumb gripping, this injury should always be taken seriously. Surgery should be considered for primary suture of ligaments if they are torn or if a chip fracture is found on X-ray examination (Cantero and Vallotton, 1991).

Skier's knee

This is rupture of the medial collateral ligament, a torn medial meniscus and rupture of the anterior cruciate ligament. In recent years injuries to the lower limb have changed because of the introduction of new ski equipment. Initially, ankle injures were common as the short legged boot was used. The high legged boot protects the ankle and work is performed by the thigh muscles. There is also an increased incidence of knee injuries and fractures of the tibia at the level of the boot top, which is an area of the tibia where delayed or non-union is relatively common.

The knee joint is the most vulnerable of all joints because its stability depends on the muscles and ligaments, not its shape. Active muscle strength protects the passive ligamentous integrity, and, if for any reason the muscles are not developed enough for the task they are asked to perform, or they are fatigued, then the ligaments alone maintain the joint stability. All degrees of ligamentous injury up to complete rupture are recorded; the attachments of the menisci may be affected.

The commonest severe injury is a rupture of the medial collateral ligament, tearing of the medial meniscus, to which it is attached, and partial or complete rupture of the anterior cruciate ligament, the so-called 'unhappy triad of O'Donoghue'. In the past the injury to the anterior cruciate ligament was often missed with a resulting unstable knee joint. Endoscopic surgery with suture of the ligaments has much improved the prognosis in all injuries of the knee joint.

All knee injuries due to skiing may have long term consequences and treatment should be carried out by those well versed in their management (Leyvraz, 1991).

27.1.5 Prevention

Most ski injuries are the skier's own fault. Physical fitness is of paramount importance; the skier should be fit enough to ski, not ski to get fit.

To prevent injury, ski bindings have become very sophisticated and are of great importance. They must always be adjusted to suit the skier's build, age, height and ability. A constant check on their adjustment should be made, particularly in children. The length of the skis and adequate 'ski stoppers' that work are also very important.

27.2 AVALANCHES

About 80% of avalanche victims survive if they remain on the surface. In those buried to a mean depth of 1.06 m, 30–40% are alive after 1 h, but only 10% after 4 h. The victim should therefore be located as quickly as possible (Dubas *et al.*, 1991a; Flann, 1991). The main injuries caused by an avalanche are asphyxia, hypothermia, frost-bite and blast injury.

The main cause of death is asphyxia. This may be due to inhalation of snow, rupture of the lungs, compression of the thorax, airway obstruction in an unconscious patient, brain damage resulting in depression of ventilation, or the air around the victim's face may get used up. Gray (1987) records a woman who survived after 20 min in a wet snow avalanche where she was unable to breathe. He suggested that the 'diving reflex', which causes bradycardia, was triggered by the direct contact of the snow with the face, and this, together with the relatively rapid onset of hypothermia, was an important factor in survival.

Because there is variable permeability of air and carbon dioxide according to the type of snow, a victim completely covered by snow must not be assumed to have asphyxiated. It is because of this permeability that dogs are able to scent buried victims. People have been known to survive for several days if an air pocket is created.

The development of hypothermia is not inevitable after being buried, because of the low heat conductivity of snow and because the individual is protected from the wind. If clothing insulation is good and it remains dry the individual is likely to remain normothermic (Dubas, 1980). Removal from the protection of avalanche snow will increase heat loss in a wind and the rate of cooling may be as much as $9° h^{-1}$. If the victim is unconscious, mouth to mouth respiration or intubation and ventilation should be tried.

27.3 CREVASSES

A fall into a crevasse can be fatal but if not, the weight of the victim's body can leave him wedged with compression of the thorax. This is often associated with multiple injuries. The victim's body heat will melt the ice and the climber will sink deeper and deeper. The body will cool rapidly and many instances are recorded where the victim has been found dead from hypothermia.

The only way to unwedge the individual is to remove the ice by a drill or ice axe, although a thawing liquid can be very effective. A tripod leaning over the crevasse is the best method of extraction. A method of airway warming which can be carried out whilst the victim is still trapped has been developed (Foray and Cahen, 1981; Dubas *et al.*, 1991b).

27.4 BIVOUACS AND TENTS

Crevasses, snow caves and snow slots make good bivouacs because of the low thermal conductivity of snow. They should be out of the line of stone fall or avalanche, and provide protection from wind, fatiguing wind noise and heat loss. In both Himalayan and Alpine crevasses temperatures of 0°C at 3 m from the surface have been recorded when the outside air temperature was well below this. A constant day and night temperature of −7°C was noted in a snow cave at 5800 m when the outside temperature dropped to −20°C at night; it was used for sleeping throughout the Silver Hut Expedition in the Everest resion in the winter of 1960–1961.

The temperature inside a tent is more liable to considerable variation. At 6000 m in the Western Cwm on the 1953 Everest Expedition, the temperature inside a tent dropped from 30°C to 0°C in 4 min as the tent went into the shade at dusk. In contrast, the temperature rose from −5°C to 30°C in 2 h as the sun struck the tent at dawn (Pugh, 1955).

Individuals, when bivouacking or sleeping on snow, must always protect themselves from the snow with which their bodies are in contact. They should huddle together and be enclosed as much as possible so that exhaled warm air heats the body. The foetal position exposes only 60% of the body surface to cooling and therefore should be adopted. Occasional movement will diminish the possibility of thrombosis. Crampons should always be removed as metal conducts heat away from the foot. If boots and socks are tight they must also be removed; a rise of up to 8°C in skin temperature has been observed on removing a tight sock (Pugh, 1950).

Attempts should be made to stay awake and not slip into sleep with subsequent body cooling and hypothermia. At extreme altitude, oxygen even at low flow rates, will counter exhaustion and cold injury.

27.5 RESCUE: THE USE OF DOGS

A working dog probably smells the scent generated by bacteria attached to regularly shed epidermal flakes, perspiration and skin oils of an individual human. Gas exhaled from the lungs and from the gastro-intestinal tract also contribute a smell unique to each person.

About 12% of a dog's brain is concerned with smell. Man has about 5 million olfactory cells whilst a German shepherd dog has over 200 million, with the result that a dog's sensitivity to scent is about 100 times that of humans. In addition, a dog's hearing is much better than a human's, and they are able to locate a sound with amazing accuracy. This is a learned ability and not totally instinctive (Fenton, 1992).

27.6 CASUALTY TRANSPORT

In inaccessible places, if an injured climber can help themselves by any means at all, crawling, hopping, or using ski sticks or an ice axe, survival is more likely than if they have to be transported.

27.6.1 Man carrying

A victim can be carried by an individual climber using a specially designed pack frame or a coiled rope. The carrier should be roped to two good climbers for belay protection, but only very fit and experienced climbers should undertake this. Up to eight persons may be necessary to carry one victim on a stretcher.

27.6.2 Air rescue

This is the most efficient method of transport and has developed greatly in all the mountainous regions of the world over the last few years.

In Switzerland each year there are about 3000 helicopter rescue missions and 3000 hospital transfer flights, with about 1200 missions for road accidents. In British Columbia, an extremely rugged province of western Canada with an extensive wilderness and many mountain ranges and the 3.5 million inhabitants concentrated in the south-west corner, about 6200 helicopter/fixed wing rescue evacuations are made annually.

About 90% of mountain rescues in the Swiss Alps are by air, usually helicopter, 5% are by ground/air and 5% are pure ground rescues. In over 80% of the helicopter missions it is possible to land close to the victim, 15% are winch evacuations, and in 5% the patient is taken aboard whilst the helicopter hovers, a very dangerous method of evacuation. In 1990, 600–700 climbers were rescued by winch evacuation and it is now possible to reach every part of the north face of the Eiger by this method. Many injured climbers have severe head and trunk injuries; if this is likely a medically qualified individual should be aboard the helicopter, who may if necessary start treatment before the injured person is winched aboard. Some members of rescue teams are both medically qualified and are qualified mountain guides.

Some winch rescues are extraordinarily dangerous, needing up to 70 m of line. Precision may be obtained by the helicopter pilot having a transparent 'bubble' in the floor of the cockpit so that the rescuer can be seen at the end of the line underneath the helicopter. Walkie-talkie communication is also much commoner now (Durrer and Henzelin, 1991; Durrer, 1993).

27.7 HEAT INJURY

This occurs when heat production is greater than heat loss and the combination of high temperature and high humidity blocks the mechanisms for heat loss and predisposes to heat injury.

Basal metabolism alone can produce heat at 65–85 kcal h^{-1}, enough to raise core temperatures 1°C h^{-1}, were it not for the various mechanisms for heat removal. Moderate work done can increase this fivefold (300–600 kcal h^{-1}) and solar radiation may increase heat gain by 150 kcal h^{-1}. Raised body temperature, of itself, increases cell metabolism and therefore heat production (Arrhenius's Law).

As long as the air temperature is lower than body temperature, 65% of cooling occurs by radiation or the transfer of heat from the body to the environment.

Above an environmental temperature of about 37°C, evaporation is the only method of heat loss and, if humidity exceeds 75%, heat loss by this method falls and sweating exacerbates dehydration without cooling.

Overheating can be a problem at altitude because very high solar temperatures are common on enclosed glaciers and snow fields such as the Western Cwm of Everest. Climbing at night or before dawn should be considered under these circumstances.

Temperatures inside a tent may be as high as 30°C and a sun temperature of 59°C measured with a black bulb radiation thermometer has been recorded on Everest (Pugh, 1955).

27.7.1 Predisposition to heat injury

The elderly are less able to maintain cardiac output and dissipate heat and may be dehydrated. A previous myocardial infarct may also limit the ability for vasodilatation. Obese individuals have more insulation and less relative surface area from which to lose heat, hyperthyroidism increases heat production, and large areas of skin affected by disease may interfere with heat loss by sweating. Various drugs may predispose to heat illness, such as beta-blockers inhibiting a compensatory increased cardiac output.

27.7.2 Acclimatization to heat

In contrast to cold, some general acclimatization to heat does occur. It takes about ten days to reach its maximum benefit and requires up to $2\,h\,day^{-1}$ of daily exercise.

The mechanisms, though poorly understood, are associated with increased aldosterone production and sodium conservation. Sweating occurs at a lower core temperature and may be more than double the normal amount. An increased cardiac output results in the increased delivery of heated blood from core to periphery and, in addition, there is increased density of mitochondria per unit of muscle which allows for increased oxygen usage (Weiss, 1991).

27.7.3 Clinical features of heat injury

There are three main clinical stages, heat exhaustion preceded by 'glacier lassitude' and heat stroke.

- Glacier lassitude has been well recorded since the start of mountaineering over 150 years ago. It is associated with extreme lethargy and dehydration, and loss of salt. It occurs when heat uptake from solar radiation is considerable, and is described particularly when climbing in a 'bowl of snow'.
- Heat exhaustion is a further stage, but the core temperature remains normal. There may be 'flu-like symptoms with faintness, anorexia, nausea, vomiting and muscle cramps. Sweating is usually present but diminished. The central nervous system is usually normal.

- Heat stroke is a true medical emergency. It is not common amongst mountaineers but its possibility should be recognized during an approach to the mountain across hot desert. Sweating stops and characteristically the core temperature is above normal. Onset is rapid with the victim becoming confused and unco-ordinated; hypotension, tachycardia and tachypnoea are common. All untreated cases die with brain damage. The degree of residual cerebral damage in treated cases is directly related to the time that has elapsed before treatment. The mortality rate is high, between 30–80%.

27.7.4 Treatment

For heat exhaustion, the patient must be taken out of the sun and given fluids and salt.

For heat stroke, treatment must start immediately. The body must be cooled as rapidly as possible. Cooling must be promoted by any means, and fluid (even urine) does not have to be cold to provide heat loss by evaporation. Packs of snow or ice should be placed on the body where the large blood vessels come to the surface: at the neck, axilla or groin. The limbs should be gently massaged to prevent peripheral stagnation and accelerate cooling. This technique avoids generalized vasoconstriction and shivering. Cooling rates of $0.1°C\,min^{-1}$ have been recorded. No fluids should be given by mouth and patients should be taken to hospital as soon as possible and cooled rapidly.

In hospital the optimum treatment is controversial and includes peritoneal lavage, water spray and fans, cold water baths and gastric lavage. One or more methods may be used. Evaporation techniques to keep the skin at about 20°C, together with ice packs to the axilla and groin is practical in that monitoring is easy to manage. Most patients can be cooled to a core temperature of 38°C in under 40 min by this method. Cooling should be stopped at 37°C to prevent overcompensation and hypothermia. Intravenous fluids should be started if nessesary.

27.7.5 Complications of heat stroke

- Decreased renal perfusion can lead to tubular necrosis and renal failure.
- Muscle damage and rhabdomyolysis can produce myoglobulinuria and exacerbate renal failure.
- Hypoglycaemia and hypocalcaemia may occur.
- Total body potassium usually decreases.
- Liver enzymes may be raised.
- Thermal damage to vessel endothelial cells can occur with disorders of blood coagulation (Weiss, 1991).

27.8 INJURY FROM SOLAR RADIATION

Light from the sun includes radiation of wavelengths of 290–1850 nm; the proportion reaching the earth's surface varies with the season and atmospheric conditions. Much solar radiation is filtered out by smoke or fog, but less by cloud. At high altitude these screens are less effective and reflection from the earth's surface, especially where there is snow, increases exposure.

27.8.1 Snow blindness (photophthalmia)

This is an inflammation of the cornea and conjunctiva due to ultraviolet light of wavelength 200–400 nm. At altitude this makes up 5–6% of solar radiation compared with 1–2% at sea-level. Snow reflects 85% of light waves and the eyes are particularly vulnerable.

Acute

Within a few hours the epithelial cells of the cornea die. There is loss of surface adhesion and the cells are brushed off the cornea by the mechanical act of blinking. The corneal nerve endings are then exposed. Within about 4 h, symptoms are felt that range from a feeling of 'grit in the eye' to excruciating pain and sensitivity to light. The slightest eye movement causes spasm of the eyelids, pupillary vasoconstriction, eye pain and headache. There is conjunctival inflammation, the eyelids are swollen and the secretion of tears profuse. The condition lasts 6–8 h and disappears in 48 h.

Treatment includes cold compresses, hydrocortisone eye ointment, an eye patch to exclude light, and the avoidance of light. The pupils should be dilated with atropine and an ocular antibiotic used in case corneal ulceration occurs. Analgesics may be necessary.

Chronic

This occurs in those inhabitants of mountainous and snowy regions over a long period. Visual disturbances, with sensitivity to light and chronic conjunctival inflammation, are reported.

Prevention

Inhabitants of mountainous regions have used primitive methods for centuries. These include yak wool and hair pulled forward over the eyes, slits in wood, or cardboard strapped to the head.

Glasses or goggles with lenses that cut out radiation of wavelength 250–400 nm are normally used for protection. The quality of the lens is important, and they can be made either of plastic or glass. The main advantage of plastic is that it is of light weight and unbreakable, but it does not filter out all the ultraviolet light, whilst glass is heavier but filters out most of the ultraviolet light. Ideally, the external surface is mirror finished to reflect light, whilst the internal surface should not reflect light onto the cornea. The upper and lower parts of the lens should be darker than the central part, through which the wearer is able to see clearly. Frames should have side and nasal shields for protection against sun, and a safety cord must always be firmly attached. A spare pair of glasses or goggles should always be carried. Goggles should have adequate ventilation to stop them steaming up (Lomax *et al.*, 1991; Petetin, 1991).

27.8.2 Sunburn

Overexposure to ultraviolet radiation of wavelengths 200–400 nm can damage the skin. Ultraviolet B (UVB) (290–320 nm) is primarily responsible for burning, tanning and the formation of skin cancer. Ultraviolet A (UVA) (320–400 nm) contributes to skin ageing. Melanin is the ideal sun screen and burning, ageing and skin cancer are decreased in blacks, whilst blondes and redheads are particularly susceptible.

Seasonal variation is striking. The intensity of UVA doubles in the summer, whilst that of UVB increases tenfold in the same period.

Certain drugs make the skin sensitive to the effects of solar radiation. These include sulphonamides, phenothiazines, dimethylchlortetracycline and thiazide diuretics. Visual reactions to sunlight can occur in those suffering from lupus erythematosus, porphyria and albinism. In patients with abnormal sensitivity, prolonged use of antimalarial drugs such as chloroquine may suppress or reduce this sensitivity. Cold sores may be exacerbated by prolonged exposure to stray sunlight (Lomax *et al.*, 1991).

Acute

Clinical features of acute sunburn, which vary from slight erythema to considerable blistering, appear within a few hours. The severity of the patient's condition varies with the surface area involved. Treatment should include removal from the sun, cold compresses, and corticosteroid cream. Secondary infection should be treated with antibiotics. Following exposure to ultraviolet radiation the rate of melanin formation increases and protects the skin from further damage.

Chronic

Recurrent exposure over many years causes atrophy of the skin and loss of elastic tissue with scattered pigmented areas (liver spots). Most of the skin characteristics attributed to ageing are due to exposure to the sun, as skin on protected sites such as the buttocks appears 'young' even the elderly.

27.9 SKIN CANCER

Ultraviolet radiation causes skin cancer in mice, and the epidemiological evidence for sunlight causing skin cancer in man is overwhelming. It is one of the common cancers in the US. The possible depletion of the ozone layer may cause a further increase in skin cancer.

27.9.1 Prevention

Sunburn is preventable and exposure should be graded so that skin can become pigmented. Clothes protect better than sun screens; dark, dry fabrics are more effective than white, wet garments. The under surface of the nose and the chin, also the lips and ears, are susceptible to reflected ultraviolet light. Sun screens that contain molecules that absorb ultraviolet radiation are now commonly used.

Dibenzoylmethanes absorb UVA and, in combination with screening agents against UVB, provide effective sun protection over a broad range of wave lengths.

It is important that children and young people get into the habit of using sun screens as this will decrease the incidence of sunburn, photo-ageing and skin cancer (Kaplan, 1992).

27.10 LIGHTNING

Lightning is a visible electrical discharge caused when the increased electrical charge within a cloud overcomes the insulating effect of the surrounding air. The initial, rarely visible discharge travels from cloud to ground and is followed by a highly visible return strike from ground to cloud. The strike may be eight miles long and be up to 15 million volts.

About 80% of those struck by lightning lose consciousness, and cardiac and neurological symptoms of varying severity occur. Burns of the skin are most common at the entry and exit points. Death may occur if the electrical discharge traverses the heart or if a climber falls as a result of being struck.

Prevention is by not climbing when weather conditions are unstable.

In storms, summits and ridges should be avoided and metal gear and ice axes should be kept at a distance. Ground currents are dangerous, especially when there are streams of water. The climber should if possible avoid cracks, overhanging rocks and direct contact with the rock face. To avoid ground discharge, sit on a rope or rucksac, as far as possible from a rock face, with hands placed on the knees. As the current can spread along a rope, particularly if wet, discard the rope and do not abseil (Baptiste *et al.*, 1991).

REFERENCES

Baptiste, O., Girer, A. and Foray, J. (1991) Lightning, in *A Colour Atlas of Mountain Medicine*, (eds J. Vallotton and F. Dubas), Wolfe, London, pp. 117–19.

Bezes, H., Massart, P. and Guyot, C. (1991) The management of skiing accidents, in *A Colour Atlas of Mountain Medicine*, (eds J. Vallotton and F. Dubas), Wolfe, London, pp. 141–51.

Cantero, J. and Vallotton, J. (1991) Capsulo-ligamentary injuries to the metacarpophalangeal joint of the thumb (skier's thumb), in *A Colour Atlas of Mountain Medicine*, (eds J. Vallotton and F. Dubas), Wolfe, London, pp. 155–9.

Cleare, J. (1983) Ski-mountaineering in China. The ascent of Mustagh Ata. *Alpine J.*, **88**, 29–36.

Cliff, P. (1973) Ski traverse of the Alps. *Alpine J.*, **78**, 13–22.

Dubas, F. (1980) Aspects médicaux de l'accident par avalanche hypothermie et gelure. *Z. Unfallmed. Berufskr.*, **73**, 164–7.

Dubas, F., Henzelin, R. and Michelet, J. (1991a) Avalanches: prevention and rescue, in *A Colour Atlas of Mountain Medicine*, (eds J. Vallotton and F. Dubas), Wolfe, London, pp. 104–12.

Dubas, F., Henzelin, R. and Michelet, J. (1991b) Rescue in crevasses, in *A Colour Atlas of Mountain Medicine*, (eds J. Vallotton and F. Dubas), Wolfe, London, pp. 112–16.

Durrer, B. (1993) Rescue operations in the Swiss Alps in 1990 and 1991. *J. Wild. Med.*, **4**, 363–73.

Durrer, B. and Henzelin, R. (1991) Mountain rescue: Modern strategies and technical aspects, in *A Colour Atlas of Mountain Medicine*, (eds J. Vallotton and F. Dubas), Wolfe, London, pp. 18–33.

Fenton, V. (1992) The use of dogs in search, rescue and recovery. *J. Wild. Med.*, **3**, 292–300.

Flann, A.W. (1991) Search, dog, probe and beacon techniques, in *Proceedings of the First World Congress on Wilderness Medicine*, Wilderness Medical Society, Point Reyes Station Ca pp. 383–8.

Foray, J. and Cahen, C. (1981) Les hypothermies de montagne. *Chirurgie*, **107**, 255–310.

Gray, D. (1987) Survival after burial in an avalanche. *Br. Med. J.*, **294**, 611–12.

Johnson, R.J. (1982) Symposium on skiing injuries. *Clin. Sports Med.*, **1**, (2).

Kaplan, L.A. (1992) Suntan, sunburn and sun protection. *J. Wild. Med.*, **3**, 173–96.

Leyvraz, P.G. (1991) Injuries to the ligaments of the knee, in *A Colour Atlas of Mountain Medicine*, (eds J. Vallotton and F. Dubas), Wolfe, London, pp. 152–5.

Lomax, P., Thinney, R. and Mondino, B.J. (1991) The effects of solar radiation, in *A Colour Atlas of Mountain Medicine*, (eds J. Vallotton and F. Dubas), Wolfe, London, pp. 67–71.

Petetin, D. (1991) Eye protection at high altitude, in *A Colour Atlas of Mountain Medicine*, (eds J. Vallotton and F. Dubas), Wolfe, London, pp. 71–2.

Pugh, L.G.C.E. (1950) *Physiological studies on HMS Vengeance: Royal Naval cold weather cruise 1949*, MRC Royal Naval Personnel Research Committee, RNP 49/561.

Pugh, L.G.C.E. (1955) *Report on Cho Oyu 1952, and Everest 1953 Expeditions* (unpublished archival material).

Smolander, J., Louhevarra, V. and Ahonen, M. (1986) Clothing, hypothermia and long distance ski-ing (letter). *Lancet*, **2**, 226–7.

Smythe, F.S. (1932) Kamet conquered. Gollancz, London, p. 216.

Weiss, E.A. (1991) Environmental heat illness, in *Proceedings of the First World Congress on Wilderness Medicine*, Wilderness Medical Society, Point Reyes Station Ca, pp. 347–57.

28

Medical conditions at altitude: leisure and commercial activities

28.1 INTRODUCTION

With more and more people going to altitude for adventure holidays, expeditions and skiing, doctors are more frequently being asked to counsel patients on the advisability of their trip. People are also continuing these pursuits into later life (including the authors of this book) and thus are increasingly likely to be suffering from chronic diseases which may prompt questions about their fitness for altitude. There is not much hard data on which to base one's advice to such people, but such as there is will be reviewed in this chapter. Although most lowlanders going to altitude do so for pleasure there are substantial numbers of high-altitude miners and construction workers whose jobs necessitate frequent ascents to altitude. Problems in this area are also considered here.

The effect of any condition that interferes with oxygen transport will be increased by altitude. As a general rule individuals should be as fit as possible before they leave for a holiday at altitude, though fitness is not protective of acute mountain sickness.

Those who have problems with their health should find out as much as possible about their condition before setting out. The action of specific medicines they use must be understood and an adequate supply taken, particularly when regular doses are necessary, as with diabetes mellitus or asthma (Rennie and Wilson, 1982).

28.2 AGE

All bodily functions deteriorate with age; this includes the maximum oxygen uptake both at sea-level and at altitude (Pugh *et al.*, 1964). However, the effect of age on $\dot{V}_{O_2}$ max is very variable (Dill *et al.*, 1964). West *et al.* (1983) reported the results of measurements of $\dot{V}_{O_2}$

max on two subjects. There was only a moderate deterioration in performance over a 20-year period (aged 31–51 years). Ability to go to altitude will depend more on an individual's degree of fitness than his age. Fit men of 75 years who normally live at sea-level have spent months at 5000 m without difficulty and a peak of 6000 m has been climbed by an 80-year old mountaineer (Alpine Club Newsletter, 1992). However, the ability to carry loads is reduced with increasing age. No one should be discouraged from going to altitude on grounds of age alone, but rapid ascent and undue exertion will place more strain on those in the older age group than on those who are younger. However, their greater experience will enable them to pace themselves so that, given time, they can often achieve worthwhile objectives.

Increasing numbers of middle-aged and elderly people are visiting high altitudes to ski, trek, climb and attend conferences. The effects of altitude on cardiovascular and pulmonary problems is being increasingly studied and a recent survey of over 1900 visitors to Keystone, Colorado (2783 m) revealed that 48% were between 40 and 60 years and 15% were aged over 60. Approximately 10% of trekkers in Nepal were 50 years of age or older (Hultgren, 1992) and a few mountaineers of this age have climbed Everest using supplementary oxygen (Gillman, 1993).

Infants and young children born at sea-level do not appear to tolerate altitude well and are susceptible to mountain sickness and cerebral and pulmonary oedema. Adolescents are at risk in stressful situations because of emotional lability; they use up energy inefficiently and become exhausted. As a result, hypothermia and frost-bite are more common and considerable caution should be exercised in taking adolescents to the high mountains.

Infants and young children born at high altitude regularly cross the Nangpa La, a pass just under 6000 m on the borders between Tibet and Nepal, except during the winter months. Tibetans and Sherpa children carry considerable loads from a young age and herd yak, sheep and goats at 5500 m during the summer months.

28.3 CARDIOVASCULAR DISORDERS

28.3.1 Coronary artery disease

Coronary artery disease is one of the major causes of death in men and women aged over 40. If angina of effort is present at sea-level it is likely that ascent to altitude will increase symptoms. If exercise is limited by pain and the exercise capacity reduced, it is likely that symptoms will occur at altitude and the risk of cardiac irregularities and infarction will be increased.

A recent cardiac infarction is a contra-indication to ascent but, after a mild infarct, providing the patient has been symptom free for several months there is probably little risk in going to altitude (Halhuber *et al.*, 1985). A patient (known to the author) with auricular fibrillation and good left ventricular function has been to moderate altitudes, 4000 m, with no problem.

Patients with poorly controlled heart failure due to coronary artery disease should obviously be advised not to go to high altitude. Those with well controlled disease who can manage a high level of exercise such as hill walking at low altitude may well be able to cope with the added strain of altitude but clearly will be at some risk.

It must be remembered that cold tends to make the platelets more sticky and theoretically could increase the possibility of infarction. Cold also is thought to predispose to coronary artery spasm.

Patients who have had successful coronary bypass surgery without any history of myocardial infarction and have a good exercise tolerance can certainly enjoy an altitude holiday. One such patient was the subject of correspondence in the *Journal of the American Medical Association* and a subsequent editorial (Rennie, 1989). He enjoyed a trek to 5760 m with no adverse effect. Another was a 67-year-old climber who enjoyed two Himalayan expeditions after his operation, although, on the second expedition, his altitude ceiling was limited to 4700 m. Ambulatory monitoring of his ECG when climbing and asleep at 4700 m did not show any evidence of ischaemia. Patients can be warned that their condition may limit their performance and accept that, but their fear, and that of their companions, centres on the risk of sudden death due to cardiac causes. Clearly there is a risk that the graft may block at any time but there is no evidence that altitude may precipitate this event.

In the wider context of cardiac disease, Halhuber *et al.* (1985) found negligible morbidity in 1273 'cardiac patients' who ascended to 1500–3000 m. These patients included 434 with coronary artery disease of whom 141 had had myocardial infarction. Only one of these had a new infarct at altitude.

A larger question is that of occult coronary artery disease, especially in those with known risk factors such as a family or smoking history, obesity, a sedentary life style etc. Risk factors which can be modified should obviously be attended to, although there will be little benefit in the short term. Beyond that, should doctors carry out 'check-ups' and tests to identify any patients at risk? Is altitude a significant risk factor for sudden cardiac death?

Shlim and Houston (1989) reviewed deaths amongst trekkers in Nepal. By obtaining the number of trekking permits issued, they were able to give a number for the denominator as well. Out of 148 000 trekkers in three and a half years there were eight deaths, none of which were known to be cardiac in origin, although two were of unknown cause. There were six helicopter evacuations for cardiac reasons out of a total of 111 evacuations. Two were men in their late 50s with severe known cardiac disease, one was a young man with persistent ectopic beats and three had chest pain thought eventually to be non-cardiac. These reports suggest that if altitude is a risk factor for sudden cardiac death it is a minor one.

Should a symptomless subject be advised to have an exercise ECG test before undertaking an altitude trip? In view of the apparent low risk and the known poor sensitivity of the test (50%) the answer should be 'no'. Rennie (1989) argues that the predictive value of such a test might be 0.001%, and would therefore have identified only one patient with silent disease who would have a fatal event during a trip for every 100 000 tests carried out. Furthermore, since the specificity of the test is only 90%, the great majority of positive tests will be false positives.

So what should the general practitioner do when asked for advice from someone proposing to go on an adventure holiday to altitude? They should take a history including coronary disease risk factors, advise on these and encourage the patient to get fit. Weight and blood pressure should also be checked. In the absence of any evidence of disease no further tests are indicated. It should be pointed out that 'getting away from it all' also involves getting away from easy access to medical treatment and that people going on such holidays must take a greater responsibility for their own health than on a standard package holiday.

28.3.2 Hypertension

Acute hypoxia has a variable effect on blood pressure in hypertensive subjects but there is a tendency to elevation both at rest and at exercise at 3460 m (Savonitto *et al.*, 1992), however, Halhuber *et al.* (1985) found that mild hypertensives who ascended and lived at up to 3000 m had few symptoms and both systolic and diastolic pressures fell. No cases of cerebrovascular accident or cardiac failure were noted in 935 patients. This improvement was continued for 4–8 months after returning to lower levels. Those with well controlled hypertension may go to altitude; in two such treated hypertensives, a six-week stay at altitudes of 3500–5000 m produced little change in either systolic or diastolic pressures.

28.3.3 Other cardiac conditions

Patients who have had valve replacements should, in general, not take hard physical exercise. Poor lung function is more often associated with mitral than aortic valve replacement. The risks of going to moderate altitude, provided anticoagulants are taken and hard exercise avoided, are probably acceptable.

After repair of a ventricular septal defect, residual pulmonary hypertension is not uncommon, and patients who have had a correction of Fallot's tetralogy may often have some residual strain on the right ventricle due to obstruction of the pulmonary outflow tract. Ascent to altitude in both will increase pulmonary artery pressure and will put the individual at risk.

Following operation for coarctation of the aorta, some residual cerebral hypertension may be present and, in theory, cerebral oedema may be more common. Providing cardiac pressures are normal, the ascent to altitude following repair of a patent ductus arteriosus and atrial septal defect is probably acceptable.

28.4 LUNG DISEASE

28.4.1 Asthma

Asthma is very common and sufferers are often young and active, so the question of the advisability of an asthmatic individual undertaking an altitude trip is a common one. An attack of asthma may be provoked by cold air and exercise but in fact many asthmatic patients have less trouble at altitude than at home, possibly because the freedom from inhaled allergens is of greater importance than the effect of hyperventilation in cold air. Also the increased sympathetic and adrenocortical activity will counter the bronchoconstriction of asthma in the first few days at altitude. The importance of taking a sufficient supply of medication and using it regularly must be stressed. There is no evidence that asthmatics are at greater risk of acute mountain sickness than non-asthmatics, though it must be presumed that poorly controlled patients must be at some risk. Acetazolamide helps to prevent acute mountain sickness in asthmatic patients (Mirrakhimov *et al.*, 1993).

28.4.2 Chronic obstructive lung disease

Under this heading is included chronic bronchitis and emphysema. Ventilatory capacity is reduced and oxygen uptake impaired. If patients are short of breath on exercise at sea-level they will certainly be worse at altitude. Even mild sufferers will find their performance markedly diminished at altitude. The reserve capacity of the lung may be further diminished by infection and antibiotics should be started at the first sign of an infective exacerbation. Such patients should probably be advised to select holidays which avoid altitude.

28.4.3 Interstitial lung disease

This includes pulmonary fibrosis from whatever cause, such as sarcoidosis. In these conditions there is both restriction of the lung and interference with gas exchange. Altitude has a marked effect on this aspect of lung function and patients will find themselves much more short of breath. Cystic fibrosis patients with bronchiectasis have problems of both airways obstruction and gas exchange. A recent paper describes two patients where an altitude holiday appeared to tip them into cor pulmonale (Speechley-Dick *et al.*, 1992). In all but the mildest cases they should be advised against going to altitude.

Cystic fibrosis patients with stable disease who are proposing to go to altitude or indeed to fly in commercial aircraft can be tested in the laboratory by breathing a hypoxic gas mixture (15% oxygen in nitrogen) for ten minutes. The arterial oxygen saturation measured by a finger pulse oxymeter gives a good indication of how they will fare at altitude (Oades *et al.*, 1994). Other patients with stable lung disease might also benefit from the test.

28.4.4 High-altitude pulmonary edema

A previous attack of high altitude pulmonary edema indicates susceptibility and the need for caution on future ascents, but many individuals have made subsequent ascents without trouble. The prophylactic use of acetazolamide should be discussed and nifedipine should be included in the first aid kit.

28.5 BLOOD DISORDERS

28.5.1 Anaemia

Anaemia, when oxygen carrying capacity is reduced, should be treated prior to ascent. Premenopausal women may have inadequate iron stores (Richalet *et al.*, 1993) and might benefit from iron therapy before or during an excursion to altitude.

28.5.2 Patients on anticoagulants

Patients with recurrent clotting or bleeding problems may be taking unnecessary risks, whilst for those on anticoagulants, if well controlled, there is no increased risk from altitude *per se*, but their being remote from medical help will be a risk.

28.5.3 Sickle cell trait

Individuals with sickle cell trait may not be aware of the problem. Reports in the literature indicate that there is a 20–30% risk that altitude travel over 2000 m may precipitate a crisis in patients with either homozygous sickle cell disease (Hb SS), sickle cell/haemoglobin C disease (Hb SC) or sickle cell trait (Hb AS) (Adzaku *et al.*, 1993). These crises are either vaso-occlusive (mainly in Hb SS patients) or abdominal or splenic infarcts (mainly in Hb SC patients).

28.6 DIABETES MELLITUS

Glucose tolerance is normal at altitude when energy expenditure and food intake balance one another. Exercise at altitude may improve sugar uptake and for well controlled diabetics there appears to be no contra-indication to mountaineering.

Those taking insulin should appreciate, not only the considerable energy output that may be demanded over a few days (up to 6000 kcal day^{-1} or more, but also the variation from day to day and within the day. During severe exercise they may need less insulin than at sea-level because of increased glucose uptake by muscle metabolism. During rest days at altitude, insulin requirement will be similar to that at sea-level. Because of these great variations, diabetics should be encouraged to use quick acting insulin, having three or four injections each day and monitoring blood sugar.

Ready access to glucose in the form of sugar or chocolate is necessary; for emergencies intravenous glucose should be available, as hypoglycaemia can be produced very rapidly by severe activity.

As insulin freezes at 0°C it should be kept warm by carrying close to the body. Frozen insulin may be thawed out without loss of potency, but care should be taken to prevent breadage and spare ampoules carried. Accidents to diabetics may be complicated by diabetic coma.

The companions of diabetic trekkers or mountaineers should be carefully instructed in the rudimentary problems that diabetics face, should be able to recognize hypoglycaemia and diabetic coma and know what to do in emergencies. Hypothermia can produce hypoglycaemia and exhausted diabetic mountaineers are at considerable risk. Extra easily assimilated carbohydrates must be taken for bivouacs.

28.7 GASTROINTESTINAL DISORDERS

Intestinal colic and diarrhoea are frequently encountered in mountainous areas but altitude *per se* is not a factor. Simple traveller's diarrhoea can be treated by Lomotil or Imodium unless there is evidence of parasitic infection when specific medication should be given.

The incidence of peptic ulcer appears to be less at altitude (Singh *et al.*, 1977). However, patients with known peptic ulceration should be well controlled prior to the expedition as complications in the field can be fatal. Drugs taken because of joint problems (non-steroidal anti-inflammatory agents) or for headache (aspirin), may cause gastric haemorrhage which should be considered as a cause of unexpected weakness. These drugs should not be taken on an empty stomach.

Those with inflammatory disorders of the bowel, such as Crohn's disease or ulcerative colitis in an active phase, should not go on expeditions. An expedition which lasts weeks or months should be considered very carefully for an individual in the quiescent phase and medication and diet planned to ensure that the condition gets no worse. Adequate treatment for an acute exacerbation must be available and evacuation arrangements must be easy.

Haemorrhoids, perianal haematoma and fissure-in-ano are often considered trivial conditions except by sufferers. They are not, and pre-expedition treatment must be undertaken. On an expedition a prolapsed pile should be replaced as soon as possible. Perianal haematoma is classically a self limiting condition lasting 5 days before resolution, the clot however may be evacuated under local anaesthetic. Acute fissure-in-ano may be exquisitely painful; anaesthetic ointment should always be available, and a fissurotomy may be carried out if necessary, under local anaesthetic. Any recurrent perineal or ischio-rectal abscess must be dealt with prior to an expedition, as must fistulae and pruritus ani. Abscesses can be drained in the field, but even when an adequate anaesthetic is available this is painful postoperatively.

Patients with hernias must have these repaired prior to an expedition. Any hernia occurring in the field should be reduced and kept reduced by a home-made truss. Irreducible and strangulated hernias can and have been operated on under local anaesthetic and the simplest operation consistent with the operator's skill and the patient's condition should be carried out.

Patients with recurrent appendicitis should consider an interval appendicectomy prior to an expedition. In the past, prophylactic appendicectomy has been advised before very long periods away from good medical cover but this is not necessary. If appendicitis occurs during an expedition it should be treated conservatively with antibiotics, intravenous fluids and nothing by mouth. Often it resolves but if an abscess or appendicular mass forms this may resolve, or it will point on the abdominal wall or rectum and can be drained. Ruptured appendicitis and peritonitis should be drained under local anaesthetic. Successful appendicectomy has been carried out by an experienced abdominal surgeon at 5500 m (Franco, 1957) under combined general and local anaesthetic but this procedure is not recommended.

28.8 ORTHOPAEDIC CONDITIONS

Those with arthritis, particularly of the joints of the lower limb, should carefully consider the degree and amount of exercise that has to be taken on a mountain trek. Non-steroidal anti-inflammatory drugs can be very beneficial and should be started early rather than be heroic about the pain. Treatment of painful joints, particularly of the hip, whether by replacement prosthesis, arthrodesis or some other method, may make a short trek possible. One member of the successful Everest 1953 expedition who climbed to 8500 m had a fixed, flexed elbow, the result of an accident as a child.

28.9 ENT CONDITIONS AND DENTAL PROBLEMS

Nasal polyps or a deflected nasal septum which interferes with breathing should be treated prior to ascent. Patients with perennial rhinitis and sinusitis should ensure supplies of their usual medication.

Dental problems are not made worse by altitude, but any one planning a holiday or expedition out of range of dental help on the mountains or anywhere else, is well advised to have a thorough dental check-up, with any suspect teeth dealt with before setting out.

28.10 PREGNANCY AND ORAL CONTRACEPTION

The risk to a pregnancy of going to altitude is not known with confidence but it would seem wise to advise pregnant women against ascent to more than a modest altitude.

There are no data on the risk of using oral contraceptives at altitude, but it is well known that they increases the risk of thrombosis at sea-level (though the risk is small in non-smokers). The increased haematocrit at altitude and dehydration, should it occur, probably increases this risk. After some weeks at altitude, vascular episodes, some thrombotic in nature, which have a high mortality, have been reported, though not in women (Chapter 21). Thromboses may also play a part in the mechanism of high-altitude pulmonary oedema; cold stress also is associated with changes in blood viscosity. Therefore, although there is as yet no hard evidence of increased thrombosis among women taking 'the pill' at altitude, it would seem wise not to do so.

28.11 OBESITY

Obesity has been reported as being a risk factor for acute mountain sickness (Chapter 17) and those who are overweight will have an increased oxygen uptake for a given task. At night, obese individuals may suffer from a greater fall in arterial P_{O_2}, as the weight of the abdomen interferes with normal lung expansion. The repeated episodes of hypoxaemia lead to increased pulmonary hypertension. In addition, they are more likely to have sleep disorders with, in particular, obstructive sleep apnoea, during which the arterial P_{O_2} can fall precipitously. In residents at altitude this may cause an undue increase in red blood cells and may be implicated as a cause of Monge's disease (chronic mountain sickness).

28.12 NEUROLOGICAL PROBLEMS

Headaches are common on ascent to altitude, possibly because of cerebral vasodilatation and mild cerebral edema. These are features of acute mountain sickness and resolve spontaneously in a few days. There is anecdotal evidence that altitude tends to trigger migraine attacks which can be severe. One sufferer had an attack of transient nominal aphasia at 5500 m. A history of migraine is a risk factor for acute mountain sickness (Chapter 17).

There is no evidence that epileptics are affected or that fits are more frequent at altitude, however the consequences of an epileptic attack need to be considered, both on the affected individual and his companions. Understanding this, it is probably reasonable for patients with well controlled epilepsy, who have not had a fit for six months, to go on a trek but not to rock or ice climb. Some anti-epileptic preparations may affect adversely breathing during sleep, whilst others in high doses may affect co-ordination.

Nightmares and vivid dreams are not unusual at altitude and sleep may be very disturbed. Those who take drugs at sea-level to induce sleep should remember that these often depress respiration and can lead to severe transient hypoxia. In any event, sleep at altitude is usually lighter and often less refreshing than at sea-level (Chapter 12).

28.13 MENTAL OUTLOOK

Mountaineering is a potentially dangerous sport with an appreciable mortality. It requires time and patience to master all the skills necessary to move safely in mountain country, which is no place for the danger-mystic, with or without religious overtones.

Mental agility and emotional stability are important and the gregarious extrovert who can only be effective with constant activity and an impressionable audience is not so likely to function effectively as the more self-sufficient. Those who are obliged to live harmoniously in close proximity for long periods should be stable, loyal and have both a social and intellectual tolerance for their companions. Above all, a sense of humour and the ability to control and sublimate hostile and aggressive impulses is of great importance.

Considerable attention has been paid to the possible effects of emotional deprivation, with reference to sexual abstinence in isolated male communities. Most agree that sexual deprivation is usually of minor significance and, as a subject of conversation, ranks rather lower than food, drink or the task in hand. At high altitude, reduction in libido has been reported in some lowlanders. High-altitude residents do not appear to be affected. Instructions on the frequency of sexual intercourse are included in a work on traditional Tibetan medicine.

> During winter one can indulge in intercourse twice or thrice daily, since sperm increases in winter. In the autumn and spring there must be an interval of two days, and during the summer an interval of 15 days. Excessive intercourse affects the five sense organs.
>
> *(Rinpoche, 1973)*

Elderly, enfeebled Tibetans drank the urine of young boys to increase their sexual vigour (MacDonald, 1929).

28.14 COMMERCIAL ACTIVITIES AT ALTITUDE

Recently there has been a substantial increase in commercial activities at altitudes of 3500–6000 m. For example, new mines are being develop in northern Chile at altitudes of about 4500 m. Because most of the workers come from sea-level, intolerance of the high altitude is a major problem. As discussed elsewhere in this book, the degree of hypoxia encountered reduces work capacity, mental efficiency and sleep quality.

Three issues arise in connection with these new commercial activities. The first is whether anything can be done in the initial selection process better to predict which workers will tolerate altitude. There is little information on this point. The best predictor is probably previous work experience at a similar altitude. Of course it is assumed that potential workers will have a full clinical examination for evidence of lung and heart disease. Another possible predictor is hypoxic ventilatory response because there is some evidence that people with a low response are particularly likely to develop acute mountain sickness and high-altitude pulmonary edema. There is also some evidence that tolerance to extreme altitude is loosely related to hypoxic ventilatory response, although there are clearly exceptions. This measurement is relatively easily made at sea-level.

It might also be possible to obtain some information by looking at the responses to work on a treadmill or bicycle ergometer during acute hypoxia at sea-level. Again it is not clear that this would be a useful test. The responses to acute and chronic hypoxia are very different because the latter depends so much on the process of acclimatization. Nevertheless, this might be worth investigating.

Finally, it might be useful to look at the increase in pulmonary artery pressure which occurs in response to acute hypoxia at sea-level. This can be done non-invasively by echocardiography in most, but not all, subjects. The rationale for this is that there is a relationship between the risk of high-altitude pulmonary edema and pulmonary hypertension at high altitude.

In order to determine whether these tests are of value, it would be important to do a prospective study. This would involve careful measurement of tolerance to high altitude including a questionnaire on acute mountain sickness. One problem may be the unreliability of a questionnaire in this setting. Workers may anticipate that their answers would determine whether they could remain in employment, and in this case the results are likely to be unreliable. In addition to a questionnaire, an assessment of altitude tolerance might include simple clinical measurements such as heart rate, respiration rate, presence or absence of râles in the chest, and simple neurological measurements such as Romberg's test.

A second issue is the schedule of work at high altitude. In the new mines of northern Chile, the families remain at sea-level and the worker spends a period at high altitude followed by a period at sea-level. The optimal arrangement of these times in unclear. Schedules that have been employed so far include one, two or three weeks at high altitude, followed by a few days to a week or more at sea-level. Clearly it is advantageous to spend enough time at high altitude to benefit from acclimatization. The ventilatory response takes perhaps seven days to reach a steady state, so it would not be reasonable to spend less time than that at altitude. Other changes, for example polycythaemia, take several weeks, but how important this response is in acclimatization is unclear, and in any event workers would likely be unwilling to leave their families for more than two or three weeks.

Little is known about the rate of de-acclimatization, and more work should be done on this. There is some anecdotal evidence that some acclimatization lasts for at least seven days, so that workers returning to high altitude after a week at sea-level could be expected to have some residual high-altitude acclimatization. Another important factor in scheduling is the social interaction between workers and their families.

A final issue is the possibility of oxygen enrichment of room air to relieve the hypoxia of high altitude. This has become feasible because of the introduction of oxygen concentrators which only need electrical power to produce high concentrations of oxygen from the air. Oxygen enrichment is remarkably effective. For example at altitude of 4000–5000 m, increasing the oxygen concentration by 1% (e.g. from 21% to 22%) reduces the equivalent altitude by about 300 m (West, 1994). Thus if we have a mine at an altitude of 4500 m, increasing the oxygen concentration of the air by 5% reduces the equivalent altutide to 3000 m which is easily tolerated. The initial and running costs of the oxygen concentrator are both relatively small. The fire hazard is less than in air at sea-level. Initially, oxygen enrichment might be used in a small conference room or a laboratory; a more extensive facility could be developed for a dormitory to improve the quality of sleep. Some critics have argued that oxygen enrichment will interfere with acclimatization. However, the net result is no different from descending to a lower altitude for sleeping. Everybody now expects that the ventilation of a room will provide a comfortable temperature and humidity environment. Control of the oxygen concentration can therefore be regarded as a further logical step in man's control of his environment.

REFERENCES

Adzaku, F., Mohammed, S., Annobil, S. and Addae, S. (1993) Relevant laboratory findings in patients with sickle cell disease living at high altitude. *J. Wild. Med.*, **4**, 374–83.

Alpine Club Newsletter, 4. (1992) *Stok Kangri (6121 m)* (members activities), Alpine Club, London, p. 11.

Dill, D.B., Robinson, S., Balke, B. and Newton, J.L. (1964) Work tolerance: Age and altitude. *J. Appl. Physiol.*, **19**, 483–8.

Franco, J. (1957) *Makalu*, Cape, London, pp. 243–6.

Gillman, P. (1993) *Everest*, Little Brown, Boston MA.

Halhuber, M.J., Humpeler, E., Inama, A.K. and Jungmann, H. (1985) Does altitude cause exhaustion of the heart and circulatory system? Indications and contra-indications for cardiac patients in altitudes, in *High Altitude Deterioration*, (eds R.J. Rivolier, P. Cerretelli, J. Foray and P. Segantini), Karger, Basel, pp. 192–202.

Hultgren, H.N. (1992) Effect of altitude on cardiovascular diseases. *J. Wild. Med.*, **3**, 301–8.

MacDonald, D. (1929) *The Land of the Lama*, Seeley, Service, London, p. 184.

Mirrakhimov, M., Brimkulov, N., Cieslick, J., *et al.* (1993) Effect of acetazolamide on overnight oxygenation and acute mountain sickness in patients with asthma. *Eur. Respir. J.*, **6**, 536–40.

Oades, P.J., Buchdahl, R.M. and Bush, A. (1994) Prediction of hypoxaemia at high altitude in children with cystic fibrosis. *Br. Med. J.*, **308**, 15–18.

Pugh, L.G.C.E., Gill, M.B., Lahiri, S., *et al.* (1964) Muscular exercise at great altitudes. *J. Appl. Physiol.*, **19**, 431–40.

Rennie, D. (1989) Will mountain trekkers have heart attacks? *J. Am. Med. Assoc.*, **261**, 1045–6.

Rennie, D. and Wilson, R. (1982) Who should not go high? in *Hypoxia: Man at Altitude*, (eds J.R. Sutton, N.L. Jones and C.S. Houston), Thieme-Stratton, New York, pp. 186–90.

Richalet, J.-P., Souberbielle, J.-C., Antezana, A.-M., *et al.* (1993) Control of erythropoiesis in humans during prolonged exposure to the altitude of 6542 m. *Am. J. Physiol.*, **266**, R756–64.

Rinpoche, R. (1973) *Tibetan Medicine*, Wellcome Institute of the History of Medicine, London, pp. 54–5.

Savonitto, S., Cardellino, G., Doveri, G., *et al.* (1992) Effects of acute exposure to altitude (3460 m) on blood pressure response to dynamic and isometric exercise in men with systemic hypertension. *Am. J. Cardiol.*, **70**, 1493–7.

Shlim, D.R. and Houston, R. (1989) Helicopter rescues and deaths among trekkers in Nepal. *J. Am. Med. Assoc.*, **261**, 1017–19.

Singh, I., Chohan, I.S., Lal, M., *et al.* (1977) Effects of high altitude stay on the incidence of common diseases in man. *Int. J. Biometeorol*, **21**, 92–122.

Speechley-Dick, M.E., Rimmer, S.J. and Hodson, M.E. (1992) Exacerbations of cystic fibrosis after holidays at high altitude – a cautionary tale. *Respir. Med.*, **86**, 55–6.

West, J.B. (1994) Oxygen enrichment of room air to relieve the hypoxia of high altitude *J. Appl. Physiol., FASEB J.*, **8**, A298.

West, J.B., Boyer, S.J., Graber, D.J., *et al.* (1983) Maximal exercise at extreme altitudes on Mount Everest. *J. Appl. Physiol.*, **55**, 688–9.

29

Fitness and performance in the mountains

29.1 INTRODUCTION

In mountaineering and hill walking performance depends on fitness, which is the ability to perform successfully a particular task and to cope with the demands of that task. This depends on mental and physical ability and endurance. The psychological aspects of fitness are based on the confidence that the individual possesses the necessary skills, strength, endurance and experience, whilst physcially it means that the pulmonary and cardiovascular systems are effective in transporting enough oxygen to an adequate tissue substrate.

Fatigue is the inability to perform a task or exercise to the expected standard and is influenced by external stimuli such as hypoxia, cold or fear. Fatigue occurs during prolonged exercise when the individual can no longer sustain the initial energy output, which it may be possible, with great effort, to regain for a brief period.

Exhaustion occurs as a result of prolonged fatigue, when physiological mechanisms break down and the individual cannot cope mentally or physically with the demands of the situation. If allowed to continue there is a danger of death. In mountaineering, particularly at high altitude, exhaustion is likely because of excessive demands made on the body by the mind, itself influenced by hypoxia and cold.

However the other side of the coin is amusingly told by Tilman.

> I would not wish anyone to believe that because such arduous day-to-day exertions are passed over in silence the Himalayan climber is therefore a man of ape-like strength and agility, with an immense capacity for breathing rarefied air, drinking melted snow or raw spirit and eating fungi and bamboo shoots. True, on occasions he must live hard or exert himself to the point of exhaustion, necessarily when at grips with a big peak; but for the most part his condition is one of ease bordering upon comfort; he suffers from

heat rather than from cold, from muscular atrophy rather than nervous exhaustion, and for a variety of reasons – the weather, the worsening snow, the porters fatigue – his days are usually short. Thus he spends more time on his back than on his feet. His occupational disease is bed sores, and a box of books his most cherished load. *(Tilman, 1952)*

29.2 FITNESS

29.2.1 Fitness and feats of endurance

With training, outstanding feats are possible. For instance a man in his 50th year ran 391 miles in 7 days 1 h 25 min over lakeland fells in the UK. This involved a total ascent of 37 000 m, an average of over 5000 m day^{-1} (Brasher, 1986). In June 1988, 76 summits in the same region were reached in 24 h, involving an ascent and descent of 12 000 m (Brasher, 1988). At intermediate altitude, all 54 of the peaks over 4300 m in Colorado, USA were climbed in 21 days (Boyer, 1978) and the ascent of Mt Blanc (4807 m) from Chamonix, with return to Chamonix, was made in 5.5 h (Smyth, 1988). At high altitude, one ascent was made from 3000 m to 6000 m in 19 h (Rowell, 1982) and another climb was from 4900 m to 8047 m with return to 4900 m in 22 h (Wielicki, 1985). In 1986 an ascent and descent of Everest (8848 m) in 2 days by a new route on the north face was completed from the head of the West Rongbuk Glacier at 5800 m. Supplementary oxygen was not used (Everest, 1987). In 1990, Marc Batard ascended from base camp to summit in 22.5 h, also without the use of supplementary oxygen (Gillman, 1993).

As the main endurance muscles are the large limb muscles, increasing fitness should result in an increased ability to generate heat over a long period and, in conditions of cold stress, the fit person will be able to continue for longer periods, enabling them to reach safety before exhaustion occurs (Brotherhood, 1975; Edwards, 1975). The unfit will not be able to produce sufficient heat and the rate of heat loss will be maximal.

29.2.2 Fitness and cold

Increased fitness allows an increased oxygen intake to be sustained and hence increased heat production. Therefore the fit can work better in the cold than the unfit. Improved fitness also results in an improved ability to sleep in the cold and increases the peripheral temperature in cold conditions (Horvath, 1981).

Cold causes a sympathetic response, catecholamine release and increase in free fatty acids (FFA), some of which are used by the shivering muscles. Some FFA are converted by the liver into low density lipoprotein (LDLP) which is important as a source of thermogenesis (Hartung *et al.*, 1984). Fat utilization appears to be increased by exercise in a cold environment (Timmons *et al.*, 1985). The main sources of energy in endurance activities are FFA and LDLP, particularly after 2 h, and increasing fitness depends on the ability to use FFA and LDLP for energy requirements. At high altitude enhanced fat metabolism spares muscle glycogen (Costill *et al.*, 1977; Sutton, 1987).

29.3 FATIGUE

In an environment where the ambient temperature is at or below freezing, fatigue may be a factor in falling core temperature. Regular exercise improves performance and trained men can tolerate higher work rates. Hill walking may, in the unskilled, require 60% or more of the maximum oxygen uptake but only 40% for comparable performance in the skilled. Fatigue, therefore, occurs more rapidly in the unskilled and the level of performance will be lower. In cold conditions, this may not be enough to ensure adequate heat production and hypothermia occurs. Fatigue also occurs more rapidly if there is discomfort, and descent often causes more muscle soreness than ascent (Assmussen, 1956). Ascent requires five to six times as much energy expenditure as descent, whilst in isometric contraction the energy required depends on the force of contraction.

Dynamic exercise such as hill walking or mountaineering can be continued for several hours without fatigue, providing the work rate does not demand an oxygen uptake much greater than half the maximum. Mountaineers and hill walkers usually learn this rate by experience, but psychophysical tests may also be used to measure demand (Edwards *et al.*, 1972a). The pulse rate should not exceed 130 beats per minute if exercise over several hours is contemplated. At very high altitude the necessity to work near the maximum for ascent will force the mountaineer to work intermittently, though this may be more costly in physiological terms (Edwards *et al.*, 1973).

In isometric exercise, energy supplies are provided within the muscle and the time for such a contraction is short, a few seconds only. Great demands are placed on local energy stores, however fatigue is more likely to be due to reducing neural drive than insufficient energy supply. The energy cost of maintaining a contraction is less in the cold but the neural drive begins to fall if cooling is severe.

Cold muscles relax more slowly than normal and, as a result, the maximal rate of working is diminished and skilled movements are more difficult; thus the effects of fatigue are compounded (Edwards *et al.*, 1972b). Cold muscle fibres also contract less efficiently with resulting early onset of fatigue (Faulker *et al.*, 1987).

29.3.1 Terrain

Walking on a road demands 30–40% of maximum oxygen uptake and can be maintained for hours. The basic energy cost may be increased by 30% by protective clothing, heavy footgear and loads of 20–25 kg. Economy of walking is sensitive to any change in the normal swinging gait and terrain may do this either by requiring a greater lift of the feet or shortening of the stride. Surfaces found in mountain country may increase energy demand by 50%, whilst loose snow or sand can double the energy cost of walking. Horizontal speeds may have to be halved to keep energy demand tolerable. On gentle gradients the nature of the surface is important, as horizontal progress contributes greatly to total energy cost.

On slopes greater than 1 in 5, surface has less effect as energy demands depend on vertical ascent. However, on steep snow with a breakable crust both factors operate and extreme fatigue is common (Brotherhood, 1975).

For the average person, an ascent at 500–650 m^{-1} corresponds to 50% of maximal capacity. On descent, energy cost is about one-fifth of ascent, and leg strength and technique of descent rather than energy production are the limiting factors. Much potential energy is absorbed by muscles acting as brakes and appears as heat. Thus, despite low energy production, the individual becomes extremely warm.

29.3.2 Bad weather

The stresses imposed by bad weather arise as a result of increased energy demands from two sources, the direct effect of wind and the need to maintain body heat.

Wind

Strong head and cross-winds exert forces that have to be overcome to maintain progression. At normal walking pace, a fresh breeze increases oxygen uptake by about 30%, whilst a gale may double this. Speed will therefore suffer and head winds can halve the speed expected on a still day. Wind also increases skin cooling, the temperature of which is almost entirely dependent on the environment. By contrast, the core temperature is related more to energy production and increases during activity. Clothing insulation will modify skin temperature and the initial stages of hypothermia are often associated with loss of clothing insulation. Wind and movement may decrease insulation by 50% whilst wetting can further reduce this to a negligible amount so that, effectively, the individual may be almost naked (Chapter 22).

Cold

With incipient hypothermia the individual attempts to increase heat production by activity. If this is inadequate, the skin temperature falls and there is increase in muscle tone followed by shivering, the muscle acting as a heat engine but performing no mechanical work. Shivering may increase heat production by an amount equivalent to 20% of oxygen uptake. However, as shivering may occur whilst walking, this 20% must be added to the 50% incurred during continuous progression. The individual may, therefore, be working at 70% of the maximum oxygen uptake, even when dry, and be under considerable stress. Extremely fit individuals may be able to maintain such a high energy production but the less fit will become fatigued, and unable to maintain adequate heat production and become hypothermic.

In those individuals with poor insulation from subcutaneous fat, muscle cooling is more rapid and weakness and inco-ordination occurs with resulting rapid loss of voluntary and involuntary heat production. As a result of the failure to maintain heat production hypothermia is inevitable.

Low skin temperature is associated with extreme discomfort and has an appalling effect on morale and, with attendant cerebral dysfunction due to cold and hypoxia, plays an important part in the inability to take correct decisions in subjects with hypothermia. Below a central core temperature of about 34°C involuntary thermogenesis fails and the body cools, influenced only by environmental factors. Continuing to walk increases exposure and hastens collapse. The only way to reverse the situation is to prevent further heat loss. Shelter, reduction in movement, warm drinks, food, and prevention of evaporative heat loss (which increases the insulation of wet clothing) may prevent hypothermia even at very low temperatures (Pugh *et al.*, 1964; Pugh, 1966, 1967; Freeman and Pugh, 1969).

29.4 EXHAUSTION

Exhaustion may lead to reduced cardiac stroke volume, a falling peripheral resistance and shift in distribution of blood to the capacitance vessels (Ekelund, 1967). This failure of vasomotor regulation, with pooling of the peripheral venous blood, will, in cold conditions, cause maximum heat loss. Low blood pressure states have been described following ascent to extreme altitude (Pugh and Ward, 1956).

Continued exercise may result in complete collapse and increased heat loss and, unless the victim is very close to safety, shelter must be sought. Forcing a person to get up and go on may cause a drop in body temperature and death through loss of vasomotor tone (Hong and Nadel, 1979). A fall in skin blood flow has been observed in association with physical exhaustion. This might reduce nutritional blood flow sufficiently to render the fingers and toes more susceptible to hypoxia and cold injury (Wiles *et al.*, 1986).

Depleting the body's glycogen stores makes an individual more sensitive to fatigue, and, during a strenuous day's mountaineering, calorie intake may not equal work output (Guezennec and Pesquies, 1985). If the blood glucose can be kept above normal fasting levels, deterioration in performance and exhaustion may be prevented. An exhausted individual cannot increase his heat production in response to cold and his rate of heat loss is maximal.

29.4.1 Exhaustion at altitude

An altitude of 5950 m seems to represent the limit of permanent human habitation (West, 1986). Individual tolerance to altitude becomes more marked and there is a wide difference in performance and well-being from day to day and even within a day. Although at this altitude exhaustion is common after physical exertion, recovery can occur, though taking longer than at lower levels. Some improvement in physical performance still occurs but the placing of camps nearer to each other indicates a reduction in work capacity.

Deterioration, both physical and mental becomes more marked above 7000 m. $\dot{V}_{O_2}$ max, and hence work rate, falls in line with barometric pressure. Undue fatigue may be clear to a subject's companions but not to themselves.

Above 7600 m the effects of oxygen lack become more marked and supplementary oxygen more beneficial. Fifty-one individuals have climbed to the summit of Everest (8848 m) without supplementary oxygen (one Sherpa on seven different occasions), but this represents the limits of their capacity and the mortality rate is appreciable (Gillman, 1993).

Climbing rate varies according to conditions but appears to fall dramatically above 8500 m. Climbing at these altitudes has been described by one mountaineer as like a 'sick man walking in a dream'.

Because individuals are working at their limits, work rate slows and becomes intermittent. At 7500 m a rate of work of 2 min followed by 30 sec–1 min rest has been observed. Above this altitude the work period shortens and the rest periods lengthen. In 1978, on the last 50 m to the summit of Everest, Messner (1979) comments, 'We can no longer keep on our feet while we rest . . . Every 10–15 steps we collapse into the snow then crawl again.'

At extreme altitude hyperventilation is one of the most important responses, and its chief value is that it allows the climber to maintain a high alveolar P_{O_2}, and thereby keeps the arterial P_{O_2} above danger level. Even so there is some evidence of impairment of the central nervous system after ascent to extreme altitude without supplementary oxygen, for above 7000 m the maximum oxygen uptake falls precipitately.

Above 8000 m the body deteriorates rapidly and tolerance to extreme altitude and climbing performance is critically dependent on barometric pressure, which is a measure of weather and season (West, 1993).

29.4.2 Oxygen uptake and thermal balance

Measurements of maximum oxygen uptake at 7440 m show a reduction to 30–40% of sea-level values (Pugh *et al.*, 1964), which, at 1.33–1.48 l min^{-1} (in two subjects), is equivalent to an oxygen uptake of a person walking on the level at 6 km h^{-1} (3.75 mph) with a heat production of 220 kcal h^{-1} (921 kJ h^{-1}). Chapter 11 gives further discussion of maximum oxygen uptake at extreme altitude. As climbers are unable to maintain average oxygen uptakes greater than 50–60% of their maximum over a long period, metabolic heat production may be only a little over 100–120 kcal h^{-1} (420–500 kJ h^{-1}) which would hardly be enough to balance thermal demand at extreme altitude were it not for the mitigating effect of solar radiation and low air density on the dissipation of heat from mountaineers' clothing.

It is not surprising, therefore, that cold injury, certainly frost-bite, and possibly hypothermia, may occur in fully clothed exhausted mountaineers. As the maximum oxygen uptake near the summit of Everest is about 1.0 l min^{-1} (West *et al.*, 1983) the sustained oxygen uptake cannot be much more than 0.6–0.7 l min^{-1}, which is the oxygen cost of walking at about 5.0 km h^{-1} (3 mph) at sea-level. This means that heat production is very limited and the climber at extreme altitude is never far from hypothermia (Ward, 1987). A temperature of −27°C was measured at 8600 m on Everest at 0.300 hours on 29 May 1953 (Ward, 1993).

Heat gain from solar radiation, both direct and indirect, plays an important part in maintaining thermal balance. The gain at 5800 m is estimated at 350 kcal m^{-2} h^{-1} by comparison with 125 kcal m^{-2} h^{-1} in desert conditions at sea-level. Heat gain from solar radiation at altitudes is equivalent to a gain of about 20°C in ambient temperature (Pugh, 1962). The differences between environmental day and night temperatures may be of the order of 60–70°C at 6000 m (Pugh and Ward, 1953) and above, and this change occurs within an hour or so.

Clothing worn at extreme altitude has an insulating value of around

3 CLO units, but may lose 30% or more of its value due to wetting (perspiration, melting snow etc.) (Chapter 22). Loss of subcutaneous fat due to poor appetite, decreased food intake and increased excretion of faecal fat can be crucial (Blume, 1984). Once active movement has ceased, clothing, which may be adequate when moving, may not be sufficient to maintain thermal balance at rest and extra insulation will be necessary.

29.4.3 Death from exhaustion

Death from exhaustion, even in a snow hole or tent, may be due to hypothermia, the body metabolism failing to produce enough heat despite the 'adequate' insulation of clothing, sleeping bag and subcutaneous fat. Contributory factors are deficient calorie intake and dehydration. During a 3–4 day summit ascent particularly, on lightweight expeditions, a large calorie deficit may occur.

Despite strenuous efforts, dehydration also seems almost inevitable at extreme altitude (Blume *et al.*, 1984). Fluid requirement is high because of greater water loss from the lungs associated with increased breathing, and heat stress due to the high intensity of direct and indirect solar radiation. The fluid requirement for maintaining a normal urine output of about 1.5 l day^{-1} is 2.8–4.0 l, which is seldom obtained. Extreme dehydration affects physical performance and may be an additional factor in the occurrence of vascular episodes and frost-bite. While taking the correct precautions, survival without cold injury has been recorded at 8800 m without supplementary oxygen at temperatures of −35°C (Clarke, 1976).

The use of supplementary oxygen brings an immediate feeling of warmth, greatly improves recovery from exhaustion, increases sound sleep, prevents physical and mental deterioration, and increases the chance of survival. Whilst climbing, though giving no obvious boost, it increases endurance, decreases fatigue, decreases respiration, and improves overall climbing rate, as the mountaineer does not have to stop to repay his oxygen debt. It also increases appetite and fluid intake, and on the first oxygen ascent of Everest in 1953, Hillary and Tensing drank about 4 l of fluid on the day of the assault and their rations contained 3500 kcal day^{-1} (14 657 kJ day^{-1}); it included 400 g of sugar, most of which was eaten. Analysis of the diaries of Noyce and Ward suggested that food consumption when using supplementary oxygen did not fall below 2500 kcal day^{-1} (10 470 kJ day^{-1}). Examination of Hillary and Tensing after their successful ascent showed little evidence of significant dehydration as judged by weight change and urine analysis (Pugh and Ward, 1956).

Turning off supplementary oxygen appears to have little effect as long as the climber is at rest. Sudden failure during exertion causes shortness of breath, dizziness and incontinence of urine, and also extreme fatigue and paraesthesiae in the limbs (Ward, 1968). Gradual failure of supply often passes unnoticed, the mountaineer being brought to a halt by increasing breathlessness and fatigue without realizing that his oxygen set was at fault; this increases his chances of falling or making the wrong, often life threatening, decisions.

29.4.4 Individual variation

Individual variation may explain the random incidence of hypothermia and exhaustion. This variation depends on a number of factors: physical fitness, degree of clothing insulation, physical type, thickness of subcutaneous fat and sensitivity to cold. With the increasing popularity of all forms of outdoor pursuits, particularly mountain walking and allied pastimes as a substitute for field games, the number of children and adolescents exposed to the risk of cold injury has greatly increased. About 40% of the victims of mountain accidents in the British Isles are under 21 years of age and a number suffer from hypothermia, apart from other injuries.

As a normal part of the 'character-building' process, children and adolescents are exhorted to exhaust themselves physically whilst playing games under controlled, though often atrocious, climatic conditions. In the mountain environment the 'excelsior' spirit can and does lead to exhaustion hypothermia and death, and should be avoided. Adolescents and young people are more at risk than the mature, as they are less willing to conserve energy and become more rapidly exhausted. Being less emotionally mature, they tend to panic and use up more energy and become fatigued with a consequent fall in heat production. As a result, they may forget to take adequate precautions against hypothermia. Some have little subcutaneous fat and are, therefore, less well insulated. A recent illness may also result in the unduly rapid onset of fatigue, and exhaustion.

29.5 LOAD CARRYING

Loads are carried by all who visit mountainous regions. In the valleys of the Himalayas much of the merchandise is carried by professional porters and the economy depends on them, together with yak and mule transport.

Observations by Pugh in 1952 and 1953 on the March–In to Everest (Pugh, 1955) suggest that loads of 40–50 kg, with an addition of 10 kg personal baggage, are carried routinely by porters for 10–12 h over 10–12 miles each day. Often ascents and descents of 1000–1200 m are made, with loads of tea or paper weighing over 60 kg occasionally being carried.

As the body weight of porters is usually between 45–60 kg, and the average height just over 150 cm, each porter carries their own weight in merchandise.

Where possible loads are carried in a conical, light but strong, wicker basket, 22 cm × 30 cm at the base and 50 cm × 70 cm at the top, with a height of 60 cm. Larger sizes are available for carrying bulky loads such as leaf mould. Loads are supported by a strap passing over the forehead and under the lower end of the basket. When in position the upper end of the basket is level with the top of the porters head. The centre of gravity therefore is as close as possible to a vertical line passing through the centre of the pelvis, thus reducing the angular momentum. The advantage of the head band is that it allows direct transmission of the load to the vertebral column, with muscles being used for balancing rather than support, as when shoulder straps are used. This method of carrying has to be learnt as a child and the neck muscles in all such Himalayan porters are extremely well developed.

Marching technique depends on the weight of the load. With loads of 50 kg, stops are made every 2–3 min, with rests lasting 0.5–1.0 min after a distance of 70–250 m has been covered, depending on the gradient. With lighter loads, rests for 2–3 min every 10 min are normal. Longer pauses are made every hour.

During rests, the loads are supported on a T-stick about 1 m long, and the porter does not sit down. When longer rests are taken, loads are placed on the top of stone walls conveniently placed beside the track, usually in the shade of a large tree.

Heart rate in ascending porters varies between 140 and 160 beats per minute: on the level between 100 and 124 and downhill between 80 and 104 beats per minute.

At about 3700 m, porter loads are reduced to 25 kg (gross weight 35 kg) which are carried to 5700 m. Exhaustion, when it occurs is due to overwork, that is not enough rest days. Few porters have any interest in climbing mountains and so tend to give up when the effects of hypoxia appear.

With high altitude Sherpas, load carrying ability is considerable. Without supplementary oxygen on Everest in 1933 eight porters carried loads weighing 10–15 kg to an altitude of 8300 m, as they did on the Swiss Everest Expedition in 1952.

Low altitude porters carry their own food, eating tsampa or ata, which is made into a paste or dough, three times a day. Four seers (4 kg) of tsampa is the standard ration for each man for 3.5 days, equivalent to 3500 kcal per man per day.

Mountaineers also carry considerable loads to high altitude but use shoulder straps, climb more slowly and stop less frequently.

29.6 ATHLETES AND ALTITUDE

Pugh (1965) suggested that performance at altitude would result in lower times in the sprint events due to decreased wind resistance. In distance events, times would be increased because the maximum oxygen uptake falls with altitude.

Comparing the times of athletes in the 1965 Pan-American games held in Mexico (2250 m) with those of the Melbourne Olympics of 1956 at sea-level, he showed that there was an increase in time of 2.6% in the 800 m, and 14.9% in the 10 000 m events. In 100 m and 400 m, but not the 200 m races, times at altitude were better than at sea-level.

When the Olympic Games were held in Mexico City (2250 m) in 1968, several world records in short sprint events were broken, presumably due to decreased wind resistance at altitude. In the longer endurance events times were slower than at sea-level but not as slow as had been forecast.

The Kenyan team, who lived at 1675 m, an altitude similar to that at which the games were held, were remarkably successful. However, in the sea-level competitions that immediately followed the Olympic Games, no records were set in endurance events and this raised the question of whether altitude training conferred any special advantage.

29.6.1 Altitude training for sea-level performance

One of the first studies was carried out by Balke (1964), who described an increase in maximal aerobic power of 11% in three men who trained for a month at 600 m and a month at 3000 m.

By 1970, several conclusions had been made concerning altitude training, though some would be challenged. These were that maximum work capacity decreased by approximately 1% for every 100 m above 1500 m, but returned to sea-level values after prolonged stay at altitude, and that long residence at altitude did not enhance sea-level performance. In endurance events at intermediate altitude, athletes who have spent a life time at altitude appear to have an advantage over those born and bred at sea-level. However, in short explosive events, prior altitude acclimatization made little or no difference.

At present the effect of altitude training on sea-level performance is becoming clearer, though the question is by no means settled. Both acclimatization to altitude and exercise under hypoxic conditions play an important role in improving the oxygen carrying capacity of the blood and both are necessary to improve performance at altitude. For the untrained individual, endurance and work capacity are improved by altitude training. For elite athletes, training above 3000 m probably precludes great intensity of work and thus decreases any favourable impact of altitude acclimatization.

The most effective technique may be to live at altitude and train at sea-level but travel difficulties may well limit this approach (Levine *et al.*, 1992).

29.6.2 Training to improve performance at altitude

The two key factors are maximum oxygen intake ($\dot{V}_{O_2}$ max) and acclimatization.

The $\dot{V}_{O_2}$ max is a function of the uptake, delivery and extraction of oxygen and is limited by cardiac output and lung diffusion. Some individuals have a high $\dot{V}_{O_2}$ max for genetic reasons but all can improve their $\dot{V}_{O_2}$ max by training.

Individuals only work at their maximum for a short period, but the majority are able to work for long periods at 40–50% of maximum. The percentage of $\dot{V}_{O_2}$ max that can be sustained can be increased by training. Endurance also depends on muscle strength and substrate activity.

Acclimatization to altitude is the other key factor, and thus improves the ability to perform work. Gradual acclimatization reduces the incidence of mountain sickness. Endurance training can improve both $\dot{V}_{O_2}$ max and submaximal work capacity, but training must be specific.

There is evidence that endurance training at sea-level can increase both maximal aerobic power and endurance for altitude activity. A high level of fitness, however, does not protect against mountain sickness and, indeed, the ability to ascend rapidly may increase this likelihood, especially if the individual remains at the altitude which he has attained (Levine, 1991; Levine *et al.*, 1992).

If it is not possible to train at intermediate altitude before going higher, training in a decompression chamber may improve performance at altitude (Richalet *et al.*, 1992; Asano *et al.*, 1992; Kikuchi *et al.*, 1992).

REFERENCES

Asano, K., Kumazaki, Y., Suganuma, I., *et al.* (1992) Effects of simulated altitude training and climbing on aerobic work capacity, in *High-Altitude Medicine*, (eds Y. Ueda, J.T. Reeves and M. Sekiguchi), Shinshu University, Japan, pp. 428–34.

Assmusen, E. (1956) Observations on experimental muscle soreness. *Acta Rheumatal. Scand.*, **2**, 109–16.

Balke, B. (1964) Work capacity and its limiting factors at high altitude, in *Physiological Effects at High Altitude*, (ed. W.H. Weihe), MacMillan, New York, pp. 233–40.

Blume, F.D. (1984) Metabolic and endocrine changes at altitude, in *High Altitude and Man* (eds J.B. West and S. Lahiri), American Physiological Society, Bethesda, Maryland, pp. 37–45.

Blume, F.D., Boyer, S.J., Braverman, L.E., *et al.* (1984) Impaired osmoregulation at high altitude. *J. Am. Med. Assoc.*, **252**, 524–6.

Boyer, S.J. (1978) Endurance test on Colorado's 14 000 ft peaks. *Summit*, **24**, 30–5.

Brasher, C. (1986) Wizard of the peaks. *Observer*, 29 June.

Brasher, C. (1988) Ascent of Superman. *Observer*, 26 June.

Brotherhood, J.R. (1975) Fitness and the relation of terrain and weather to fatigue and accidental hypothermia in hill walkers, in *Mountain Medicine and Physiology*, (eds C. Clarke, M. Ward and E. Williams), Alpine Club, London, pp. 111–17.

Clarke, C. (1976) On surviving a bivouac at high altitude. *Br. Med. J.*, **1**, 92–3.

Costill, D.L., Coyle, E., Dalsky, G., *et al.* (1977) Effect of elevated plasma FFA and insulin on muscle glycogen usage during exercise. *J. Appl. Physiol.*, **43**, 695–99.

Edwards, R.H.T. (1975) Physiology of fitness and fatigue, in *Mountain Medicine and Physiology*, (eds C. Clarke, M. Ward and E. Williams), Alpine Club, London, pp. 107–10.

Edwards, R.H.T., Melcher, A., Hesser, C.M., *et al.* (1972a) Physiological correlates of perceived exertion in continuous and intermittent exercise with the same average power output. *Eur. J. Clin. Invest.*, **2**, 108–14.

Edwards, R.H.T., Harris, R.C., Hultman, E., *et al.* (1972b) Effect of temperature on muscle energy metabolism and endurance during successive isometric contractions, sustained to fatigue of the quadriceps muscle in man. *J. Physiol.*, **229**, 335–52.

Edwards, R.H.T., Ekelund, L.-G., Harris, R.C., *et al.* (1973) Cardio-respiratory and metabolic costs of continuous and intermittent exercise in man. *J. Physiol.*, **234**, 481–97.

Ekelund, L.-G. (1967) Circulatory and respiratory adaptation during prolonged exercise. *Acta Physiol. Scand.*, **70(suppl)**, 292.

Everest: The Hornbein Couloir direct from Tibet. (1987) *Am. Alpine J.*, **29**, 302–4.

Faulkner, J.A., Claflin, D.R. and McCully, K.K. (1987) Muscle function in the cold, in *Hypoxia and Cold*, (eds J.R. Sutton, C.S. Houston and G. Coates), Praeger, New York, pp. 429–37.

Freeman, J. and Pugh, L.G.C.E. (1969) Hypothermia in mountain accidents. *Int. Anesthesiol. Clin.*, **7**, 997–1007.

Gillman, P. (1993) *Everest*, Little Brown, Boston MA, p. 200.

Guezennec, C.Y. and Pesquies, P.C. (1985) Biochemical basis for physical exercise fatigue, in *High Altitude Deterioration*, (eds J. Rivolier, P. Cerretelli, J. Foray and P. Segantini), Karger, Basel, pp. 79–89.

Hartung, G.H., Myhre, L.G., Nunnely, S.A. and Tucker, D.M. (1984) Plasma substrate response in men and women during marathon running. *Aviat. Space Environ. Med.*, **55**, 128–31.

Hong, S.I. and Nadel, E.R. (1979) Thermogenic control during exercise in a cold environment. *J. Appl. Physiol.*, **47**, 1084–9.

Horvath, S.M. (1981) Exercise in a cold environment. *Exercise Sport Sci. Rev.*, **9**, 221–63.

Kikuchi K., Sato M. and Fujiwara M. (1992) Simulated training for the members of the Fukuoka Muztag Ata Expedition 1991. *Jpn. J. Mount. Med.*, **12**, 59–66.

Levine, B.D. (1991) Enhancing capacity for performance at altitude. *Proceedings of the 1st World Congress of Wilderness Medicine*, Wilderness Medical Society, Point Reyes Station CA, pp. 101–3.

Levine, B.D., Roach, R.C. and Houston, C.S. (1992) Work and training at altitude, in *Hypoxia and Mountain Medicine*, (eds J.R. Sutton, G. Coates and C.S. Houston), Queen City Printers, Burlington, VT, pp. 192–202.

Messner, R. (1979) *Everest: Expedition to the Ultimate*, Kaye and Ward, pp. 178–92.

Pugh, L.G.C.E. (1955) *Report on Cho Oyu 1952, and Everest 1953 Expeditions* (unpublished archival material).

Pugh, L.G.C.E. (1962) Solar heat gain by man in the high Himalayas. UNESCO *Symposium on Environmental Physiology and Psychology*, Lucknow, India, pp. 325–9.

Pugh, L.G.C.E. (1965) Altitude and athletic performance. *Nature*, **207**, 1397–8.

Pugh, L.G.C.E. (1966) Clothing insulation and accidental hypothermia in youth. *Nature*, **299**, 1281–6.

Pugh, L.G.C.E. (1967) Cold stress and muscular exercise with special reference to accidental hypothermia. *Br. Med. J.*, **2**, 333–7.

Pugh, L.G.C.E. and Ward, M.P. (1953) Physiology and medicine (appendix), in *The Ascent of Everest*, (ed. J. Hunt), Hodder and Stoughton, London, p. 275.

Pugh, L.G.C.E. and Ward, M.P. (1956) Some effects of high altitude on man. *Lancet*, **2**, 1115–21.

Pugh, L.G.C.E., Gill, M.B., Lahiri, S., *et al.* (1964) Muscular exercise at great altitude. *J. Appl. Physiol.*, **19**, 431–40.

Richalet, J.P., Bittel, J., Herry, J.P., *et al.* (1992) Pre-acclimatization to high altitude in a hypobaric chamber: Everest turbo, in *Hypoxia and Mountain Medicine*, (eds J.R. Sutton, G. Coates and C.S. Houston), Queen City Printers, Burlington, VT, pp. 202–12.

Rowell, G. (1982) High altitude pulmonary oedema during rapid ascent, in *Hypoxia, Man at Altitude*, (eds J.R. Sutton, N.L. Jones and C.S. Houston), Thieme-Stratton, New York, pp. 168–71.

Smyth, R. (1988) Alpine runners racing danger. *Observer*, 7 August.

Sutton, J.R. (1987) Energy substrates and hypoglycaemia, in *Hypoxia and Cold*, (eds J.R. Sutton, C.S. Houston and G. Coates), Praeger, New York, pp. 487–92.

Tilman, H.W. (1952) *Nepal Himalayas*, Cambridge University Press, Cambridge, p. 79.

Timmons, B.A., Ararujo, J. and Thomas, T.R. (1985) Fat utilisation enhanced by exercise in a cold environment. *Med. Sci. Sports Exercise*, **17**, 673–8.

Ward, M.P. (1968) Diseases occurring at altitudes exceeding 17 500 ft (thesis). University of Cambridge, Cambridge, p. 44.

Ward, M.P. (1987) Cold, hypoxia and dehydration, in *Hypoxia and Cold*, (eds J.R. Sutton, C.S. Houston and G. Coates), Praeger, New York, pp. 475–86.

Ward, M.P. (1993) The first ascent of Mount Everest 1953. The solution of the problem of the 'last thousand feet'. *J. Wild. Med.*, **4**, 312–18.

West, J.B. (1986) Highest inhabitants in the world. *Nature*, **324**, 517.

West, J.B. (1993) Acclimatization and tolerance to extreme altitude. *J. Wild. Med.*, **4**, 17–26.

West, J.B., Boyer, S.J., Graber, D.J., *et al.* (1983) Maximal exercise at extreme

altitude on Mount Everest. *J. Appl. Physiol.*, **55**, 688–98.
Wielicki, K. (1985) Broad Peak climbed in one day. *Alpine J.*, **90**, 61–3.
Wiles, P.G., Grant, P.J., Jones, R.G., *et al.* (1986) Lowered skin blood flow at exhaustion. *Lancet*, **2**, 295.

30

Clinical lessons from high altitude

30.1 INTRODUCTION

High-altitude medicine and physiology constitute a legitimate subject for study in their own right and if, like any branch of science, such study casts light on other fields of science including clinical medicine, that is a bonus.

However, it is often argued that a justification for human studies at high altitude is that the knowledge so gained may be applied in clinical medicine. Patients hypoxic because of pulmonary or cardiovascular disease present a complex picture in which hypoxia is only one of their many problems. In the study of humans at high altitude one can study the effects of hypoxia alone in otherwise healthy subjects. The stimulus, hypoxia, can be applied in a measurable controlled way at a time to suit the scientist, so that controlled measurements can be made before and after hypoxia.

The insight so gained can be applied to the more complicated uncontrolled situation of the hypoxic patient. This chapter discusses how good a model human subjects at high altitude are for the hypoxic patient, and the similarities and the differences between these two situations. It also reviews the extent to which high-altitude physiology has illuminated clinical medicine.

30.2 CHRONIC OBSTRUCTIVE LUNG DISEASE

Probably the commonest cause of hypoxia in medicine is chronic obstructive lung disease (COLD). Within this category are included patients with chronic obstructive bronchitis, emphysema and chronic fixed asthma. Patients with long standing severe deformity, such as kyphoscoliosis, also develop hypoxia in the latter stages of their disease. Table 30.1 lists the similarities and differences between a patient with COLD and subject at high altitude.

Table 30.1 Comparison of clinical aspects of chronic obstructive lung disease with people at high altitude

Symptom/finding	*At high altitude*	*Chronic obstructive lung disease*
Dyspnoea on exertion	Yes	Yes
Limited work capacity	Yes	Yes
Peripheral oedema	Seen in AMS	Frequent
Polycythaemia	Yes	Yes
Red cell mass	Increased	Increased
Arterial P_{O_2}	Reduced	Reduced
Arterial P_{CO_2}	Reduced	Normal or raised
Arterial pH	Raised	Normal or reduced
$[HCO_3^-]$ blood, CSF	Reduced	Raised
Work of breathing l^{-1}	Reduced	Increased
Work of breathing, total	Increased	Increased
CO_2 ventilatory response	Shift to left and steepened	Shift to right and flattened
Cerebral blood flow	Increased/normal	Increased
Pulmonary arterial pressure	Raised	Raised

30.2.1 Symptoms

The similarities include the symptoms of dyspnoea, especially on exertion, and the limitation of work capacity. Dyspnoea is a difficult sensation to describe and probably the term includes more than one sort of sensation. Patients with asthma, for instance, say that the sensation during an attack is quite different from the breathlessness felt by them at the end of a run when free of asthma. The dyspnoea of an individual at high altitude is probably more like the latter; the sensation is of needing to hyperventilate and being quite free to do so, whereas patients with COLD probably suffer a rather different sensation akin to that of the asthmatic patient in an attack, which is described as a difficulty in 'getting the breath' or of suffocation.

The reduction in work or exercise capacity is very similar in both patients and high-altitude subjects. In both, the dyspnoea is felt to play a part but both also complain that work is limited by a sensation of the legs 'giving out' or 'feeling like lead'. This is for large muscle mass dynamic work such as walking, cycling, climbing stairs. If the strength of a small muscle mass is tested (e.g. hand grip), it is found to be largely unimpaired in both cases.

In the patient with COLD the work of breathing (per litre) is increased because of airways obstruction. The total ventilation may be increased as well, even if there is alveolar hypoventilation, because of the increased dead space; thus the total work of breathing is further increased. At high altitude, the work of breathing per litre is modestly decreased because of the reduction in air density at reduced barometric pressure; however, the total work of breathing is increased due to the marked hyperventilation especially on exercise (Chapter 10).

30.2.2 Blood gases and acid-base balance

Subjects at high altitude and patients with COLD both have reduced Pa_{O_2}. At high altitude this is due to low inspired P_{O_2}, whereas in COLD patients it is due to a combination of alveolar hypoventilation (secondary to airways obstruction and possibly reduced respiratory drive) and gas transfer problems due to ventilation/perfusion ratio inequalities. In both cases, the hypoxaemia is made worse by exertion.

The CO_2 response, however, is different. In patients with COLD the Pa_{CO_2} is either normal or, in more severe cases, raised. The pH is consequently lowered; respiratory acidosis and secondary renal compensation results in elevated blood [HCO_3^-]. The CSF [HCO_3^-] is also elevated and there follows a shift to the right of the ventilatory CO_2 response line and the response becomes flattened (i.e. blunted). In contrast, at high altitude the Pa_{CO_2} is reduced, pH elevated, blood and CSF [HCO_3^-] reduced, and the CO_2 response shifts to the left and becomes more brisk (Chapter 4).

30.2.3 Haematological changes

At high altitude and in COLD patients there is an increase in red cell mass. This invariably results in polycythaemia at high altitude where it is accompanied at first by a reduced plasma volume (Chapter 7). In COLD the plasma volume is usually also increased, for reasons which are unclear, so that polycythaemia is often not seen until red cell mass is considerably increased by a more extreme hypoxia. In both cases the increase is due to more erythropoiesis, stimulated, it is believed, by higher levels of erythropoietin. After the first few days at a given high altitude, levels of erythropoietin fall to within the normal or control range (Chapter 7) and similarly, in over half the patients with polycythaemia due to hypoxic lung disease, erythropoietin levels are within the normal range (Wedzicha *et al.*, 1985).

Plasma volume, as already mentioned, is increased in COLD. Plasma volume is decreased on first going to altitude but returns towards normal after about three months (Chapter 7). In high-altitude residents plasma volume is decreased by about 27% compared with sea-level residents (Sanchez *et al.*, 1970).

30.2.4 Fluid balance and peripheral edema

Patients with COLD are at risk of developing peripheral edema, mainly dependent edema, and raised venous pressure. They have been shown to have a defect of sodium and water handling; they fail to excrete a water load at the normal rate if they have a high P_{CO_2} (Farber *et al.*, 1975; Stewart *et al.*, 1991). They have a reduced effective renal plasma flow and urinary sodium excretion. They may have raised plasma renin activity and aldosterone levels. The development of peripheral edema may take place without increase in body weight (Campbell *et al.*, 1975), suggesting a transfer of fluid from intra- to extracellular compartments. This is in contrast to edema formation in cardiac failure when, as expected, it is associated with weight gain. How these findings can be fitted into a coherent account of the mechanism of this condition is not clear at present.

The fluid balance in people at high altitude is also far from clear. It seems likely that the development of acute mountain sickness (AMS) is associated with fluid retention, whereas the healthy response on going to high altitude is a diuresis. Peripheral edema frequently occurs in AMS, often affecting the periorbital regions and hands as well as the ankles, whilst pulmonary and cerebral edema are the malignant forms of AMS (Chapters 17, 18, 19). In the acclimatized there is no evidence of any problem in fluid handling.

Whether there are analogies between the mechanism of AMS and cor pulmonale are questions for future research in both fields. For instance, it is the COLD patients with high Pa_{CO_2} that are likely to develop cor pulmonale, and in subjects at altitude higher Pa_{CO_2} is associated with AMS.

30.2.5 The circulation

The systemic circulation is not importantly affected by either COLD or altitude. There is often mild elevation of the blood pressure in both cases, but there are important changes in the pulmonary circulation. In both patients with COLD and those at high altitude there is increased pulmonary resistance, resulting in raised pulmonary artery and right ventricular pressures and similar ECG changes (i.e. right axis deviation) (Chapter 6).

30.2.6 Cerebral blood flow (CBF)

In patients with COLD the CBF is increased due to the cerebral vasodilatory effects of both hypoxia and hypercarbia. On going to altitude the CBF is normally modestly increased at first, then tends to fall towards sea-level values (Severinghaus *et al.*, 1966). This is due to the low Pa_{CO_2}, which tends to reduce CBF, opposing the effect of hypoxia. Polycythaemia, as it develops in both COLD patients and those at high altitude, will tend to reduce CBF. Very low CBF values have been inferred from the large (a–v) cerebral oxygen difference in Andean altitude residents with marked polycythaemia (Milledge and Sorensen, 1972) whereas patients with COLD are to a degree protected from cerebral hypoxia by their hypercapnia which causes increased CBF.

30.2.7 Alimentary system

There has been little work on the effect of hypoxia on bowel function in either patients or individuals at high altitude. Milledge (1972) showed that small bowel absorption, as measured by the xylose absorption test, was reduced in patients with either hypoxic lung disease or cyanotic heart disease, when the saturation fell below about 70%. It was suggested that this finding might explain the loss of weight which often characterizes patients with severe emphysema towards the end of the course of their disease.

Subjects at high altitude tend to lose weight and, although much of this weight reduction may be due to reduced calorific intake, there has been uncontrolled evidence that at altitudes above about 5500 m there is continued weight loss even with adequate calorific intake (Pugh, 1962). During the American Medical Research Expedition to Everest, 1981, there was a significant reduction in both fat and xylose absorption in subjects at 6300 m (Blume, 1984) (Chapter 13).

30.2.8 Mental effects

Patients with hypoxia due to COLD frequently have disturbance of mental function, especially during exacerbations, when their P_{O_2} falls to very low levels. In the milder stages these disturbances may be quite subtle but, as hypoxia becomes severe, patients become irritable, restless and confused. Motor function may become impaired with ataxia. These changes are very similar to those observed in healthy subjects exposed to acute hypoxia in decompression chambers. However, in acclimatized subjects, very low saturations may be seen, especially on exercise, with very little mental disturbance, though at extreme altitude and with AMS these mental problems may be seen (Chapter 15).

30.2.9 Summary

Table 30.1 summarizes the similarities and differences between patients with COLD and those at high altitude. Healthy people at altitude differ in a number of important respects from the patient with hypoxia due to COLD. Most of these differences are attributable to the one being hypocapnic and the other hypercapnic. However, the hypoxia is, of course, similar and results in similar effects on a number of bodily systems, including erythropoiesis, muscles, the alimentary system and mental function. Providing the CO_2 effect is borne in mind, persons at high altitude can be considered as a model for the hypoxia of COLD.

30.3 INTERSTITIAL LUNG DISEASE

Within this category are included such conditions as sarcoidosis, fibrosing alveolitis, allergic alveolitis (farmer's lung etc.), pneumoconiosis (including silicosis) and other causes of diffuse pulmonary fibrosis. Some types of pneumonia, for instance that due to *Pneumocystis pneumoniae*, which are diffuse rather than lobar, present similar pathophysiology. In all these conditions the main problem is an impairment of gas exchange. There usually develops some restriction of lung volumes as well but, unlike COLD, there is little or no airways obstruction. The result is that hypoxia develops without any rise in P_{CO_2}. Indeed, the Pa_{CO_2} is characteristically decreased as it is in subjects at high altitude.

The dominant symptom in these patients is breathlessness on exertion and, later, even at rest. The arterial desaturation becomes worse on exertion just as it does in those at extreme altitudes (Chapter 11). The cause of the hypoxaemia in these patients is a defect of gas transfer. This is due to ventilation/perfusion ratio inhomogeneity and an increase in the diffusion path length, that is, a thickening of the alveolar capillary membrane by cellular infiltrate or fibrosis. In most cases the ventilation/perfusion mismatch problem is the more important. These conditions usually develop over a period of months and those who are well acclimatized to high altitude are very good models for the hypoxia of patients with interstitial lung disease.

30.4 CYANOTIC HEART DISEASE

Most patients in this group have congenital cardiac defects which result in right to left shunts and therefore in cyanosis. Diagnoses include tetralogy of Fallot, ventricular and atrial septal defects with reversed shunts, patent ductus arteriosus with reversed shunt, and most forms of anomalous venous drainage.

These patients, often hypoxic from birth, sometimes have most extreme cyanosis with severe polycythaemia. Pa_{CO_2} is usually in the normal range but may be low as is found at high altitude. Those with extreme polycythaemia, in whom the PCV can be up to 70%, resemble cases of chronic mountain sickness and may suffer the same symptoms of lethargy, poor concentration, being easily fatigued etc. (Chapter 20). Though they do get out of breath on exertion, dyspnoea is not a prominent symptom, perhaps because the condition has been present since birth. Again, like chronic mountain sickness and the 'blue bloater' type of COLD patient, it may be due to a blunted respiratory drive. The histopathology of the pulmonary circulation of these children is comparable to that of high altitude residents (Heath and Williams, 1981). The normal demuscularization of pulmonary arteries after birth is retarded so that the wall thickness, especially of the resistance arterioles, is increased compared with the normal pulmonary arterial tree (Chapter 16).

These children have retarded growth, as do children at altitude (Chapter 16). If their defect can be corrected by surgery, growth accelerates and they catch up with their peers. If their arterial saturation is below about 70% they will have impaired small bowel absorption which may contribute to their growth retardation. Surgical repair of the defect relieves the cyanosis and the small bowel absorption improves (Milledge, 1972). In this respect they resemble those at high altitude (Chapter 13).

30.5 LOW OUTPUT CARDIAC CONDITIONS

Ischaemic heart disease and cardiomyopathy can result in low cardiac output. In milder forms of this condition the output at rest is normal but there is failure of the normal response to exercise of an increase in cardiac output. Patients are symptom free at rest but find that their exercise tolerance is markedly diminished; they can only walk slowly and the slightest uphill slope causes them to stop and rest. They are not limited by dyspnoea but by fatigue in the leg muscles. In these patients the Pa_{O_2} is normal, but blood flow is limited, which reduces oxygen delivery and results in tissue hypoxia. The tissues most affected are those which have a high extraction of oxygen and which increase their oxygen demand on exercise, that is, the working muscles. The mixed venous P_{O_2} is very low but Pa_{CO_2} is normal.

The subject at high altitude is obviously not such a good model for this type of patient, but, especially at extreme altitude, there are physiological similarities. The maximum cardiac rate and output is limited to some degree (Chapter 11), so that, during large muscle mass dynamic exercise, oxygen delivery to the working muscles is limited. There is certainly tissue hypoxia, especially of these muscles, due to a reduction in delivery of oxygen and possibly also to limitation of oxygen diffusion at the tissue level (Chapter 11). As mentioned in section 30.2.1, the sensation of work being limited by 'the legs giving out' rather than dyspnoea alone is common to both individuals at high altitude and to these patients.

30.6 CHRONIC ANAEMIA

Patients with chronic anaemia have a very similar pathophysiology to patients with low cardiac output. The oxygen delivery to the tissues is reduced in their case by the reduced oxygen capacity of the blood. Cardiac output increases partly due to a decreased viscosity of the blood, and this partially compensates for the loss of oxygen carrying capacity. Nevertheless, oxygen delivery is reduced, especially to the working muscles, during exercise. The resulting symptoms are similar to those of low cardiac output and have their analogy in those at extreme altitude.

30.7 HAEMOGLOBINOPATHIES WITH ALTERED OXYGEN AFFINITY

These are a rare, but interesting, group of conditions in which patients have a genetic defect resulting in minor changes to their haemoglobin. These changes result in their haemoglobin having either a greater or a reduced affinity for oxygen compared with normal haemoglobin. The oxygen dissociation curve is shifted either to the left (increased affinity) or to the right (decreased affinity).

Patients with **increased** affinity haemoglobin experience a degree of tissue hypoxia because oxygen is not readily unloaded in the tissues. This evidently stimulates erythropoietin production since these patients are typically polycythaemic.

Conversely, patients with **decreased** affinity haemoglobins are anaemic, presumably because their tissue P_{O_2} is higher than normal, as evidenced by the ease with which oxygen is unloaded there. At moderate altitude this may confer some advantage, though this has not been demonstrated, and on exercise the difficulty of oxygen loading in the lungs would probably outweigh any advantage in the tissues. At higher altitude the difficulty in loading oxygen into the blood in the lungs would certainly be a disadvantage.

Indeed, **increased** oxygen affinity is probably beneficial, since, at high altitude, the advantage in the lungs more than outweighs the disadvantage in the tissues. A study by Hebbel *et al.* (1978) of two subjects with Hb Andrews-Minneapolis, a high affinity Hb (P_{50} =

17 mmHg), found that they had less reduction in exercise capacity on going to altitude than their siblings with normal Hb.

Normal subjects at high altitude, especially at extreme altitudes above 8000 m, have their oxygen dissociation curves shifted to the left by respiratory alkalosis; this is probably advantageous for the above reason (Chapters 8 and 10). Thus, those at high altitude can be a model for some aspects of haemoglobinopathies.

30.8 CONTRIBUTION OF HIGH-ALTITUDE PHYSIOLOGY TO CLINICAL MEDICINE

30.8.1 Partial pressure of gases

It is not easy to overestimate the importance to clinical medicine of Paul Bert's work published in his landmark 'La Pression Barométrique' in 1878. This work clearly showed that it is the partial pressure of oxygen, rather than the barometric pressure or oxygen percentage, that determines the effect of hypoxia in causing mountain sickness and death. Although he did not work at altitude himself he corresponded with and encouraged people who did, and he used chambers to reduce the ambient pressure for both human and animal subjects. He can be truly claimed as a father figure by both altitude physiology and aviation medicine. Of course, other physiologists and clinicians after Paul Bert have developed the idea of the partial pressure of gases and its importance, including such workers as Haldane, Douglas, Fitzgerald, Henderson, Schneider, Bohr, Krogh and Barcroft, all of whose work has been stimulated by the problems of altitude physiology.

The concept of the effect of gases on the body being due to their partial pressures is fundamental to respiratory medicine and physiology, anaesthesia, and aviation and underwater medicine.

30.8.2 Haematology

The polycythaemia of high altitude was first documented by Viault (1890) and has been extensively studied ever since. As a tool in haematological research, this stimulus to erythropoiesis has been invaluable. Much of the early work on the oxygen dissociation curve, by Haldane, Barcroft and others, owes its stimulus to the question of human survival and acclimatization to high altitude. These 'lessons from high altitude' are amongst the foundation stones of modern haematology, open heart surgery, respiratory medicine, cardiology and anaesthetics. More recently, research on 2,3-diphosphoglycerate and its influence on the position of the oxygen dissociation curve has been studied at altitude (Chapter 8) and the results incorporated into the body of haematological knowledge.

30.8.3 Respiratory medicine

Work on the effect of altitude acclimatization on the control of breathing (Chapter 4) has helped in the understanding of the changes in control of breathing in patients with COLD with hypercapnia. These patients 'acclimatize' to a high P_{CO_2} and their CO_2 ventilatory response becomes blunted, the opposite of altitude acclimatization. They are then dependent on hypoxia as a drive to ventilation and may have their breathing depressed if given high inspired oxygen mixtures to breathe.

In patients with asthma, as the condition worsens, their Pa_{O_2} falls. At first the Pa_{CO_2} is reduced because of the hypoxic drive to ventilation; then, with increasing airways resistance, Pa_{CO_2} rises to 'normal' and finally rises above normal. Cochrane *et al.* (1980) have pointed out that the Pa_{CO_2} in the middle of these three stages should be below 'normal', depending on the degree of hypoxia. Drawing on altitude data, Wolff (1980) gives a predicted value for Pa_{CO_2} dependent upon Pa_{O_2}. The patient should be considered to be in respiratory failure if the P_{CO_2} is above this value. For instance a patient with a Pa_{O_2} of 60 mmHg has a predicted Pa_{CO_2} of 30 mmHg, assuming full acclimatization to this degree of hypoxia.

Study of the increasing arterial desaturation due to diffusion limitations found in climbers on exercise at altitude (Chapter 5) helps in the understanding of the similar problems in patients at sea-level with interstitial lung disease and limited diffusing capacity.

30.8.4 Cardiology

The phenomenon of the hypoxic pulmonary pressor response has been studied at sea-level and altitude in humans and animals, with results from altitude stimulating work at sea-level and vice versa. The insights gained have helped in the understanding of patients with pulmonary hypertension due to hypoxia secondary to heart or lung disease.

30.8.5 Other areas of clinical medicine

High-altitude physiology and medicine have lessons for other branches of clinical medicine including: small bowel function, which is impaired at altitude as well as in hypoxic patients (Chapter 13); metabolism, in the slower growth of children at altitude, and patients hypoxic due to congenital heart disease; reproductive medicine, in the problem of fertility at altitude; and endocrinology, in the effect of hypoxia on various endocrine systems (Chapter 14), and their counterparts in patients with similar conditions. However these fields have been less thoroughly explored both by high-altitude and clinical scientists. No doubt high altitude has yet more lessons to teach clinical medicine in the future.

REFERENCES

Blume, F.D. (1984) Metabolic and endocrine changes at altitude, in *High Altitude and Man*, (eds J.B. West and S Lahiri), American Physiological Society, Bethesda, Maryland, pp. 37–45.

Campbell, R.H.A., Brand, H.L., Cox, J.R. and Howard, P. (1975) Body weight and body water in chronic cor pulmonale. *Clin. Sci. Mol. Med.*, **49**, 323–35.

Cochrane, G.M., Prior, J.G. and Wolff, C.B. (1980) Chronic stable asthma and the normal arterial pressure of carbon dioxide in hypoxia. *Br. Med. J.*, **301**, 705–7.

Farber, M.O., Bright, T.P., Strawbridge, R.A., *et al.* (1975) Impaired water handling in chronic obstructive lung disease. *J. Lab. Clin. Med.*, **85**, 41–9.

Heath, D. and Williams, D.R. (1981) The pulmonary trunk, in *Man at High Altitude*, Churchill Livingstone, London, pp. 119–27.

Hebbel, R.P., Eaton, J.W., Kronenberg, R.S., *et al.* (1978) Human llamas. Adaptation to altitude in subjects with high haemoglobin oxygen affinity. *J. Clin. Invest.*, **62**, 593–600.

Milledge, J.S. (1972) Arterial oxygen desaturation and intestinal absorption of xylose. *Br. Med. J.*, **2**, 557–8.

Milledge, J.S. and Sorensen, S.C. (1972) Cerebral arteriovenous oxygen difference in man native to high altitude. *J. Appl. Physiol.*, **32**, 687–9.

Pugh, L.G.C.E. (1962) Physiological and medical aspects of the Himalayan Scientific and Mountaineering Expedition, 1960–61. *Br. Med. J.*, **2**, 621–634.

Sanchez, C., Merino, C. and Figallo, M. (1970) Simultaneous measurement of plasma volume and cell mass in polycythemia of high altitude. *J. Appl. Physiol.*, **30**, 775–8.

Severinghaus, J.W., Chiodi, H., Eger, E.I., *et al.* (1966) Cerebral blood flow in man at high altitude. *Circ. Res.*, **19**, 274–302.

Stewart, A.G., Bardsley, P.A., Baudouin, S.V., *et al.* (1991) Changes in atrial natriuretic peptide concentrations during intravenous saline infusion in hypoxic cor pulmonale. *Thorax*, **46**, 829–34.

Viault, F. (1890) Sur l'augmentation considerable du nombre des globules rouges dans le sang chez les habitants des hauts plateaux de l'Amerique du Sud. *Comptes Rendus*, **111**, 917–18.

Wedzicha, J.A., Cotes, P.M., Empey, D.W., *et al.* (1985) Serum immunoreactive erythropoeitin in hypoxic lung disease with and without polycythaemia. *Clin. Sci.*, **69**, 413–22.

Wolff, C.B. (1980) Normal ventilation in chronic hypoxia. *J. Physiol.*, **308**, 118–19P.

31

Practicalities of field studies

31.1 INTRODUCTION

31.1.1 Planning, testing and practice

Much of the data referred to in this book has been collected on expeditions to the major mountain regions of the world. Good scientific work under these conditions can be difficult but is perfectly possible, providing adequate time, thought and effort is given to planning and preparation. The preparation time will be at least three to six months for a small expedition and two years or more for a major scientific expedition.

The techniques and apparatus to be used must be tested adequately beforehand. Many studies require control measurements as sea-level and these are best carried out using the same equipment as will be used in the field. Not only are results more reliable if the same equipment is used, but problems and deficiencies are identified before leaving for the mountains. Practice with the equipment in the comfort of a standard laboratory is also highly desirable, though not absolutely essential. One of the authors of this book taught one of the others the technique of gas analysis using the Lloyd–Haldane apparatus during the course of their first Himalayan expedition at 5800 m. Even if study protocols do not demand control measurements before leaving, it is advisable to carry out a complete dummy run of the observations to be made, listing all the equipment needed, down to the last rubber band and needle.

31.1.2 Field versus chamber studies

Although this chapter is concerned with field studies at altitude, much valuable work has been done in decompression chambers and the advantages and disadvantages of these two ways of studying altitude will be discussed. The advantages of chamber studies over field studies are as follows.

- Rate of ascent, descent, and altitude can be controlled to suit the problem under study.
- Other factors such as temperature, and humidity can be controlled.
- More invasive procedures can be justified since, in the event of some complication, help is more readily available.

The disadvantages are perhaps not so obvious, especially to people who have not been involved with such work. Living for more than a few hours in a decompression chamber is not pleasant. The environment is usually noisy, confined and often smelly – though this is less true of large modern facilities such as the chamber at Natick, MA, operated by the US Army Insitute of Environmental Medicine. However even the largest chamber is cramped compared with the mountains and it is difficult and very boring to take much exercise. Although proof is lacking, most authorities believe that acclimatization is slower and less complete in the absence of exercise (Rahn and Otis, 1949; West, 1988). In studies lasting more than a few hours, boredom, and hence morale, is a problem. A limiting factor for chamber studies is the number of subjects that can be accommodated. This will not be a drawback for most physiological studies but it will be in studies of acute mountain sickness where a large number of subjects is needed to ensure that some have symptoms and others are unaffected. Finally, chambers are built with specific tasks in mind; usually their use is geared to short term experiments on acute hypoxia and so they may not be available to altitude scientists for prolonged experiments.

In comparing the results of studies carried out in the field, with those done in low-pressure chambers, it is useful to look at the results obtained from the Silver Hut Expedition and the American Medical Research Expedition to Everest (AMREE), and compare these with the two major simulation studies to date, Operation Everest I and II. In many areas, the results of the two types of studies have been very similar. For example, the measurements of maximal oxygen consumption for the inspired P_{O_2} on the summit of Mt Everest were almost identical in AMREE and Operation Everest II. However, the two types of studies have yielded quantitatively different information in some areas presumably because of the different periods of acclimatization. The main differences are seen in three areas.

Alveolar gas composition

The shorter period of acclimatization in the two low-pressure chamber studies to date resulted in very different alveolar P_{O_2} and P_{CO_2} values at extreme altitudes compared with the results from the field studies (Figure 11.4). The differences are particularly marked for Operation Everest I and are discussed in section 11.3.3.

Blood lactate concentration

Blood lactate concentrations after maximal exercise were appreciably higher on Operation Everest II than on the AMREE and extensive field measurements made by Cerretelli (1982). These are shown in Figure 11.5 and discussed in section 11.3.4. Again the differences are presumably due to the shorter period of acclimatization on Operation Everest II. This topic is discussed fully by West (1993).

Exercise ventilation at extreme altitude

As was pointed out in section 10.3, both the Silver Hut and AMREE expeditions found a decrease in ventilation at maximal exercise at extreme altitude (Figure 10.3). By contrast, maximal exercise ventilation on Operation Everest 11 continued to increase with greater altitude. The reason for the differences is not clear; it is presumably related to the different degrees of acclimatization.

31.1.3 Cost

It is often assumed that chamber studies must be cheaper than field studies. This is not necessarily the case. Accounting in both cases is a very inexact science. The cost of a mountaineering expedition is clear but in many cases the climbers are going to the mountains anyway and the scientific work can be carried out at very little extra cost. Chambers represent a huge capital cost but usually the altitude scientist is not called upon to contribute to this. However even the running costs of a chamber are not inconsiderable if they are all charged realistically to the study.

In summary, chambers are very useful in studies of acute and subacute hypoxia lasting a few hours. Their advantage over field studies becomes less as the duration of the study and the number of subjects increase. Thus the two modes of research are complementary.

31.1.4 Personnel management

The psychodynamics of a mountaineering expedition are fascinating and of vital importance in achieving both climbing and scientific goals, but too great an emphasis on psychological factors may well be self-defeating. The essential aspect of leadership of a scientific expedition is to ensure that the whole team is as fully aware of the scientific programme as possible and in sympathy with it. Climbers may be suspicious of scientists but can understand quite abstruse scientific argument providing terms and concepts are explained in everyday language. They are naturally interested in topics such as acute mountain sickness, work performance at altitude and the effect of altitude on various biological systems and can become enthusiastic participants, providing the issues are clearly explained.

Time spent in presenting the scientific programme to the whole team is well spent, as was evident from experience on the AMREE, where climbers as well as climbing scientists were enthusiastic in working on the scientific programme as well as climbing the mountain. In a large party with a number of scientists it is equally important that the various scientific members understand the importance of each other's projects and are in sympathy with them.

After presenting the programme, the next essential is to delegate responsibility as widely as possible. It is highly desirable that every member of the expedition has a job to do in relation to the scientific programme, for two reasons.

- The programmes are usually over ambitious in terms of what can be achieved in the time available and, by sharing the work out, the load on the main scientists is reduced.
- By having a designated job, each member more readily feels that they are personally committed to the scientific programme, with consequent improvement in morale. This is particularly important if non-scientific members are expected to act as subjects. By having a job to do as well as being a subject avoids the feeling, 'they only want me as a guinea pig'. There are many jobs which can be carried out perfectly well by non-scientifically trained members, such as measurement of urine volume, body weights, clerking results as they are read off by another member. Even the spinning and pipetting of blood samples can be quickly taught to an intelligent lay member. A further important aspect of delegating work as widely as possible is that it helps to keep the work going should any of the scientific members be unable to function due to illness or accident.

31.2 LABORATORY WORK IN THE FIELD

31.2.1 Laboratory accommodation

However small the expedition, some form of designated laboratory accommodation is recommended. For small expeditions this will be a tent; if at all possible it should be of the type high enough to stand up in, and have a folding table and chairs. Cold is a major problem in the mountains. Most types of scientific work cannot be carried out in temperatures below 5–10°C, and certainly not below freezing. Battery operated instruments work poorly below freezing, plastic bags crack easily and venepuncture is difficult because of vasoconstriction. Under severe freezing conditions blood samples will freeze and haemolyse. If there is no space heating available, the time for scientific work will be limited to the warmest hours of the day. However, it must also be said that at high altitude the sun is strong and when it is shining on a tent the temperature rises rapidly inside, even though the outside shade temperature remains well below zero.

On a large expedition, almost ideal laboratory conditions can be achieved by using a modern 'tent', such as a 'Weatherport' (Hansen Weatherport, Gunniston, Colorado). This is a tubular aluminium frame with padded plastic cover made in various sizes which proved very satisfactory in the Western Cwm in 1981 (West, 1985). Heating was provided from a propane stove of the type designed for mobile homes in which a heat exchanger heats the air, which is blown into the tent. In this way there is no possibility of carbon monoxide from the burning propane getting into the tent. Carbon monoxide poisoning is a real danger from less sophisticated forms of heating.

The Silver Hut similarly provided almost ideal conditions in 1960–1961, though at far greater expense. It was a prefabricated hut made from boxed-up marine plywood members with foam insulation within the box sections. A similar hut but using fibreglass sections was used at base camp on the AMREE and was also successful. Work surfaces, seating and lighting should also be provided. In such conditions, the working day can be prolonged into the night if necessary and allow much more work to be carried out than in an unheated laboratory, as well as avoiding the problem of cold as an interfering factor if one is examining the effects of chronic hypoxia.

31.2.2 Electrical supply

Early in the planning of an expedition the decision will have to be made about whether to use mains voltage apparatus or to restrict work to battery operated and non-electrical equipment.

The advantages of mains voltage equipment are obvious and certain types of equipment are only available as mains operated versions. It is possible to get petrol-powered generators that weigh not more than one porter load, and on a large expedition this is the option that will be chosen. The disadvantages are not inconsiderable. In order to try and ensure that one generator is working, at least two must be taken; even then it is quite likely that both will break down. Extra spare parts must be taken and at least one expedition member should be a mechanic and have knowledge of that particular generator. Altitude affects petrol engines as it does the animal organism and adjustments must be made to the fuel mix, usually by changing the jets in the carburettor. Some generators are available with variable jets, in which case the settings required for various altitudes should be ascertained before the expedition. The power output declines with altitude, as it does in humans, so a more powerful generator must be taken than would be needed for the same equipment at sea-level. Petrol and oil must also be carried.

Alternative sources of electrical power have been used. In the Silver Hut expedition much of the electricity used over the winter was derived from a wind generator and on the AMREE a battery of solar cells gave up to almost 30 A at 15 V. In both cases this power was fed into 12 V storage batteries and mains voltage was obtained by using convertors, which introduced their own degree of inefficiency, as well as further expense and transport penalties. These alternative sources cannot be relied upon and petrol generators are needed for back up.

31.2.3 Water, reagents etc.

Water at altitude is derived either from melting snow or ice, or from mountain streams. In either case it has a fairly high degree of purity so that for most chemical uses it will be adequate if water is passed through a de-ionizing column which will include a filter. If distilled water is essential it will have to be carried out from home.

Analytical balances are impractical in the field. Reagents should be weighed at the home institution into capped tubes. These can then be made up in the field as needed by dissolving in de-ionized water.

31.3 RESPIRATORY MEASUREMENTS

31.3.1 Classical methods

Classical measurements of ventilation and oxygen consumption using Douglas bags, taps and valves are as easy to carry out in the field as in the laboratory (providing all the bits are remembered, including the nose clip). The gas meter will be of the dry type or a Wright's respirometer (anemometer) can be used if care is taken not to empty the Douglas bag too fast through it (accuracy ±2%). The gas analysis is more of a problem for the physiologist used to using a mass spectrometer. If mains voltage is available (section 31.2.2) an infra-red CO_2 meter and paramagnetic oxygen meter can be used, though calibrating gases will have to be carried. Paramagnetic oxygen analysers are available as battery operated instruments but CO_2 meters are not. Alternatively, one can be really classical and use the Lloyd–Haldane or Scholander apparatus and analyse samples chemically.

Care should be taken with modern Douglas bags. The plastic that is used now for these bags becomes hard and brittle in the cold. If the bag is unfolded in temperatures below zero it will crack and the bag will leak. A repair kit should be taken. An alternative is to use meteorological balloons which, being made of latex rubber, are free of this problem; it must be remembered that they are permeable to CO_2, so that if used for expired gas collection, samples for analysis should be taken rapidly or even during collection from a fixed point beyond a gas mixing box.

31.3.2 Alveolar gas sampling

Alveolar or end tidal gas samples have been taken from subjects at altitude on a number of expeditions; in 1981 from the summit of Everest itself.

Glass ampoules were successfully used on a number of expeditions, including the Silver Hut expedition, when samples were brought back from 7830 m. These were of 50 ml capacity and had a stem with two necks in it. The ampoules were pre-evacuated before leaving. In the field, a Haldane–Priestley sample was delivered down a tube with the ampoule attached to a side arm by a short length of pressure tubing. Surgical forceps were then used to break the glass within the pressure tube and the sample entered the ampoule. With the rubber tube clamped the ampoule was brought back to base where, with a suitable gas flame, the ampoule was sealed at the lower neck and transported back for analysis.

More recently, 20 ml aerosol cans of the type used in asthma inhalers have been successfully used. These cans, supplied by the pharmaceutical industry, had the metering device removed and were then pre-evacuated. They were shown to hold their vacuum for at least six months. In the field, the simplest apparatus involved merely a T-shaped piece of tubing into the stem of which the can was fitted with its nozzle resting on a shoulder. The subject delivered a Haldane–Priestley alveolar sample across the T to which was added a soft, wide-bored tube; the can was then depressed, which opened its valve and the sample entered the can. Releasing the can sealed it again and it was then transported back for analysis.

The actual device used on the summit of Everest was rather more complicated (West, 1985); it held six pre-evacuated cans in a rotating cylinder to which two handles were attached. The subject blew across the top of the cylinder through two one-way valves and the end tidal gas was caught between them. On squeezing the handles, one can was opened and a sample taken. On releasing the handles the can was closed; the cylinder rotated to present the next can for a second sample (Maret *et al.*, 1984).

Analysis at the home institute was by mass spectrometry using a special inlet device which would accept the aerosol can. The sample volume at sea-level pressure would be only 5–7 ml.

31.3.3 The Oxylog and electronic spirometers

The Oxylog is a portable electronic instrument giving a continuous read-out of minute ventilation and oxygen consumption (updated each minute), and the total ventilation and oxygen consumption since it was last re-set. The subject wears a mask, into the inspiratory port of which is fitted an electronic spirometer or anemometer. It is normally supplied with rechargeable batteries but can be modified to take non-rechargeable batteries. The output ($\dot{V}$ and $\dot{V}_{O_2}$) can be recorded for hours on a portable tape recorder. It is accurate for submaximal work rates (Milledge *et al.*, 1983) but is not suitable for $\dot{V}_{O_2}$ max measurements.

Ventilation alone can be recorded using one of a number of electronic spirometers such as that used in the Oxylog, though the resistance of most commercially available models is not well tolerated at the very high ventilation found in climbers exercising at altitude. Such an electronic spirometer was successfully used by Pizzo near the summit of Everest (West *et al.*, 1983).

31.3.4 Pulse oxymetry

The pulse oxymeter is a considerable advance over older oxymeters and allows measurement of arterial oxygen saturation with a reasonably light instrument. Most models are mains voltage but one using rechargeable batteries is available and presumably could be converted to use non-rechargeable batteries. These models also give a reading for heart rate and both saturation and heart rate can be recorded over prolonged periods, such as in sleep studies. At present they are not suitable for ambulatory measurements, though they can be used during exercise on a cycle ergometer. The sensors are made for use either on the finger or ear lobe, the former being usually preferred. It is essential for the finger to be warm in order to get a good signal.

31.4 CARDIOLOGICAL MEASUREMENTS

The ECG is easy to record at altitude, either the classical 12-lead ECG at rest, or ambulatory recording over many hours. Such recordings have been made on Everest climbers (West *et al.*, 1983). The pulse rate can be obtained from such recordings. Computer analysis can be carried out looking for arrhythmias and patterns of R–R intervals etc. Care is needed in the electrode placement and attachment (as at sea-level). More invasive cardiac techniques, such as right heart and pulmonary artery catheterization, have been discussed and, though possible under field conditions with mains voltage electricity available, are probably not justified, though this is debatable. Catheterization has been carried out in chamber studies, most extensively in Operation Everest II (Houston *et al.*, 1987); in skilled hands it carries very little risk.

31.5 SLEEP STUDIES

Sleep studies have been carried out on a number of expeditions where mains voltage was provided (Chapter 12). ECGs, EEGs, electro-oculograms, ear oxymetry and respiratory movements have all been monitored simultaneously and recorded on tape and paper while the subject was asleep. Most of this monitoring can be carried out with battery operated instruments but it is important that some way of monitoring the signals during the recording is provided, even if the analysis from tape is left until after the expedition.

31.6 BLOOD SAMPLING AND STORAGE

31.6.1 Venepuncture

There is little problem in performing venepuncture in the field. Two physician climbers took samples from each other on the South Col of Everest the morning after climbing to the summit (Winslow *et al.*, 1984). 'Vacutainer' systems using pre-evacuated tubes and double ended needles are particularly convenient, as the sampling tubes are used for centrifuging. They fill (from the vein) perfectly well at altitude.

31.6.2 Centrifuging blood samples

If mains voltage is available, a small electrical centrifuge can be used and this presents no problem. Hand centrifuges can be used but require quite a lot of muscle power. They need to be spun very vigorously for 15–20 min; even then the cells are not packed as tightly as by even the lowest powered electrical centrifuge. This means that the yield of plasma is less, typically a maximum of 5 ml from 10 ml of blood. When subjects become polycythaemic the problem becomes worse.

These hand centrifuges usually take four 10 ml tubes compared with six or eight in the small electrical centrifuges; they are not really designed for such vigorous spinning. Older designs with brass gears and cast metal casings stand up better than do modern models with nylon gears and plastic cases. A firm bench is essential on which to clamp the centrifuge. However, with all these drawbacks, hand centrifuging of blood is possible if mains voltage is unavailable. A dry battery centrifuge is not a viable possibility.

31.6.3 Arterial blood sampling and analysis

If the usual precautions are taken and if the doctor is experienced in the procedure, there should be no problem in arterial puncture. Arterial cannulation is more hazardous and probably not justified in the field. The measurement of arterial pH, P_{CO_2} and P_{O_2} is really not possible without mains voltage for the various meters and thermostatting. Although there is no inherent reason why these electrodes could not be run from battery operated electronics, the market is not big enough for manufacturers to develop them commercially.

31.6.4 Sample storage

Plasma, serum and urine samples can be deep frozen, stored and transported back to the home laboratory by using a cryostat or Dewar flask. These are the standard containers used for liquid nitrogen, being flask shaped with a narrow neck. Their characteristics vary depending upon their capacity and insulative properties. If filled with liquid nitrogen, they typically lose the nitrogen by evolution in about three weeks.

E.S. Williams (personal communication) realized that if some heat sinks were added with the liquid nitrogen the time of low temperature would be prolonged. He considered water ice at first but decided to use dry ice (solid CO_2). He first filled the 28-litre flask with dry ice using small lumps or pellets, then added liquid nitrogen. This has to be done carefully because the first few litres of liquid nitrogen evolve at once, cooling the dry ice down to the temperature of liquid nitrogen (−195°C). Liquid nitrogen added later remains as liquid.

Figure 31.1 shows Williams' first trial. It will be seen that the weight of the filled cryostat decreases with time but that there are three distinct phases. Over the first 12 days liquid nitrogen is evolved and the cryostat loses weight. Over the next 15 days the dry ice warms up slowly from −195°C to −80°C, when it begins to evolve. Over this phase there is no weight change. As the dry ice evolves, the weight falls steadily again until reaching the weight of the empty cryostat after a further 42 days.

In later trials, Williams was able to extend to life of the 'deep freeze'

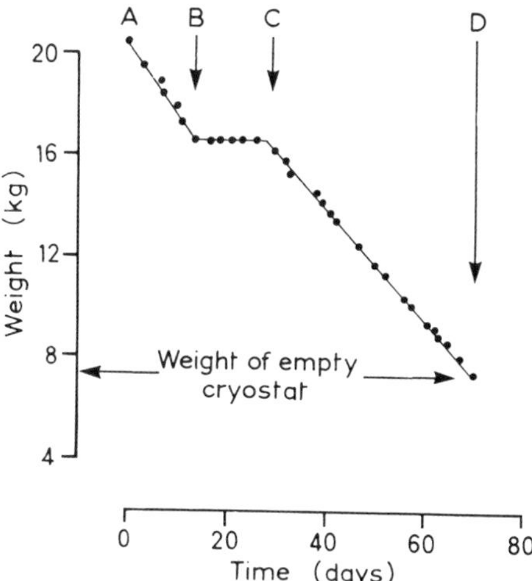

Figure 31.1 The loss of weight of a cryostat (Dewar flask) filled with liquid nitrogen and dry ice (solid CO_2). From A to B, liquid nitrogen is evolving; from B to C, the dry ice is warming from −198°C to −80°C; and from C to D the dry ice is evolving, giving a total of 70 days of portable deep freeze. In later trials, up to 137 days were achieved with more careful packing.

by packing the dry ice more carefully and adding liquid nitrogen more slowly, to achieve greater weight. He eventually managed to make the deep freeze last 137 days. The addition of samples in the field will shorten the time available at low temperature but, since the weight of the samples is small compared with the weight of dry ice, the effect is not large. In filling the cryostat it is important to use dry ice and not CO_2 snow and to fill the flask as completely as possible.

This method was used by S.P.L. Travis (personal communication, 1993) on the 1992 winter Everest Expedition. Two flasks were used, one with liquid nitrogen only, which was used to top up the other which was filled with liquid nitrogen and 5 kg of dry ice. The latter was used as the sample store. Over 150 2 ml samples were stored and remained frozen until return to the UK after three months.

Samples should be taken into PTFE tubes with good screw caps. Tubes should have a matt surface for labelling, which should be done in pencil; they should then be covered in low temperature Sellotape. During transportation, these tubes are constantly chafed together by the dry ice, and unless the labels are firm they will come off or run and all will be lost. It was found that pencil under low temperature Sellotape is safe.

For shorter periods of up to two to three weeks, it may be adequate to use polystyrene boxes of dry ice. It should be noted that airline regulations require that dry ice (or liquid nitrogen) conforms to regulations for dangerous goods. The cryostat has to be crated and sent as cargo. Airlines are usually familiar with handling 'medical samples' in this way but expect to deal with recognized shippers. The bureaucracy and expense of such a shipment is not inconsiderable and delays of a few days at each end can be anticipated.

31.7 HAEMATOLOGY

Much haematology can be done with quite simple equipment in the field. Battery operated microcentrifuges for packed cell volume are available commercially. Haemoglobin can be measured by the cyanmethaemoglobin method and a battery operated spectrometer. Cell count can be carried out by classical microscopy techniques. With mains voltage electricity and P_{O_2} electrodes the oxygen dissociation curve and P_{50} can be measured (Winslow *et al.*, 1984).

REFERENCES

Cerretelli, P. (1982) Gas exchange at high altitudes, in *Pulmonary Gas Exchange*, Vol. II, (ed. J.B. West), Academic Press, New York, pp. 97–147.

Houston, C.S., Sutton, J.R., Cymerman, A. and Reeves, J.T. (1987) Operation Everest II: man at extreme altitude. *J. Appl. Physiol.*, **63**, 877–82.

Maret, K.H., Billups, J.O., Peters, R.M. and West, J.B. (1984) Automatic mechanical alveolar gas sampler for multiple sample collection in the field. *J. Appl. Physiol.*, **56**, 1435–8.

Milledge, J.S., Ward, M.P., Williams, E.S. and Clarke, C.R.A. (1983) Cardiorespiratory response to exercise in men repeatedly exposed to extreme altitude. *J. Appl. Physiol.*, **55**, 1379–85.

Rahn, H. and Otis, A.B. (1949) Man's respiratory response during and after acclimatization to high altitude. *Am. J. Physiol.*, **157**, 445–9.

West, J.B. (1985) *Everest, the Testing Place*, McGraw-Hill, New York.

West, J.B. (1988) Tolerable limits to hypoxia – on high mountains, in *Hypoxia: the Tolerable Limits*, (eds J.R. Sutton and C.S. Houston), Benchmark Press, Indianapolis, pp. 353–62.

West, J.B. (1993) The Silver Hut expedition, high-altitude field expeditions and low-pressure clamber simulations, in *Hypoxia and Molecular Medicine*, (eds J.R. Sutton, C.S. Houston and G. Coates), Queen City Printers, Burlington VT, pp. 190–202.

West, J.B., Boyer, S.J., Graber, D.J., *et al.* (1983) Maximal exercise at extreme altitudes on Mount Everest. *J. Appl. Physiol.*, **55**, 688–98.

Winslow, R.M., Samaja, M. and West, J.B. (1984) Red cell function at extreme altitude on Mount Everest. *J. Appl. Physiol.*, **56**, 109–16.

Index

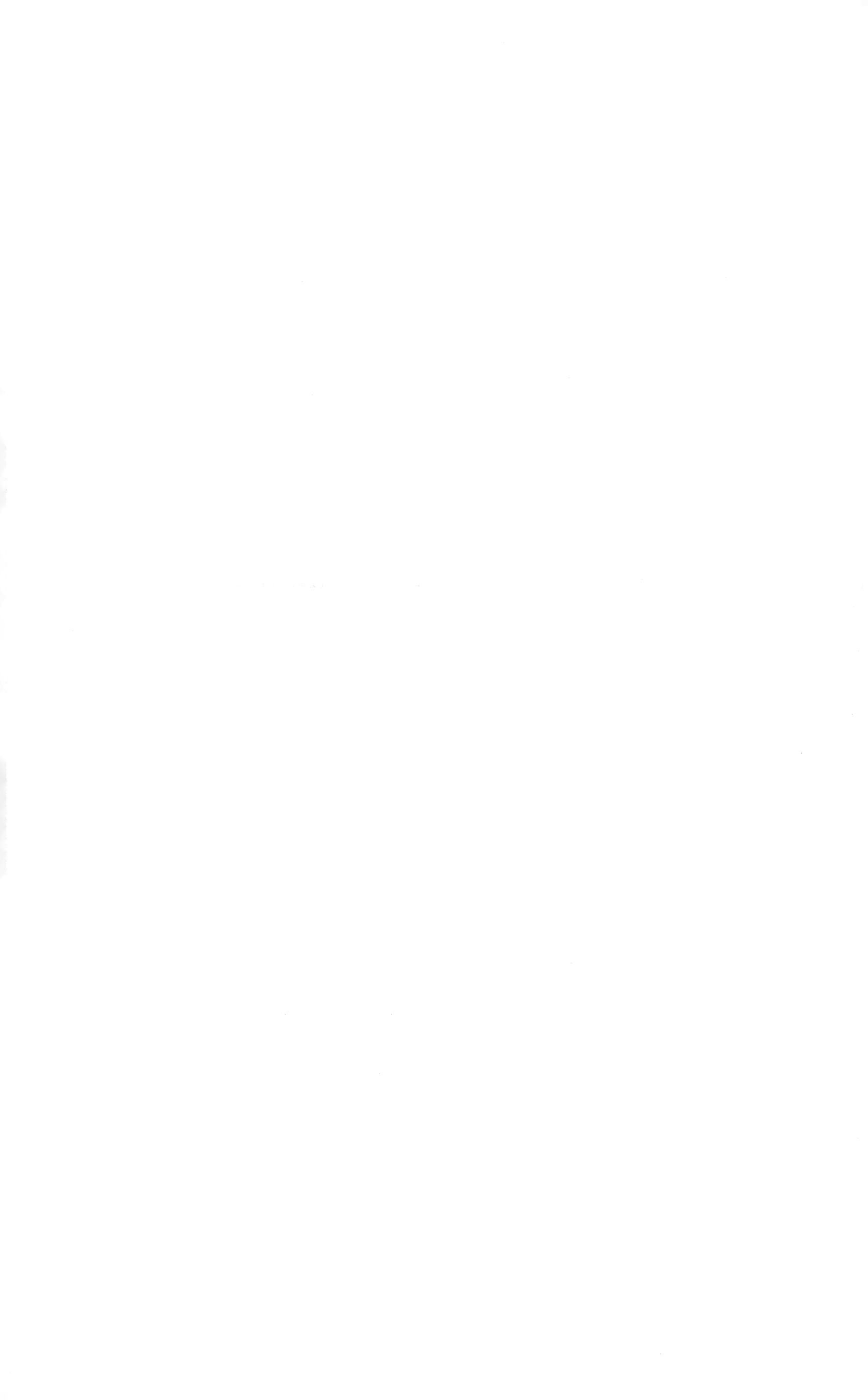

P9-APM-562

Donated by
James M. Buchanan
BUCHANAN LIBRARY
George Mason University

Economic Behavior

of the Affluent

Studies of Government Finance

TITLES PUBLISHED

Federal Fiscal Policy in the Postwar Recessions, by Wilfred Lewis, Jr.

Federal Tax Treatment of State and Local Securities, by David J. Ott and Allan H. Meltzer.

Federal Tax Treatment of Income from Oil and Gas, by Stephen L. McDonald.

Federal Tax Treatment of the Family, by Harold M. Groves.

The Role of Direct and Indirect Taxes in the Federal Revenue System, John F. Due, Editor. A Report of the National Bureau of Economic Research and the Brookings Institution (Princeton University Press).

The Individual Income Tax, by Richard Goode.

Federal Tax Treatment of Foreign Income, by Lawrence B. Krause and Kenneth W. Dam.

Measuring Benefits of Government Investments, Robert Dorfman, Editor.

Federal Budget Policy, by David J. Ott and Attiat F. Ott.

Financing State and Local Governments, by James A. Maxwell.

Essays in Fiscal Federalism, Richard A. Musgrave, Editor.

Economics of the Property Tax, by Dick Netzer.

A Capital Budget Statement for the U.S. Government, by Maynard S. Comiez.

Foreign Tax Policies and Economic Growth, E. Gordon Keith, Editor. A Report of the National Bureau of Economic Research and the Brookings Institution (Columbia University Press).

Defense Purchases and Regional Growth, by Roger E. Bolton.

Federal Budget Projections, by Gerhard Colm and Peter Wagner. A Report of the National Planning Association and the Brookings Institution.

Corporate Dividend Policy, by John A. Brittain.

Federal Estate and Gift Taxes, by Carl S. Shoup.

Federal Tax Policy, by Joseph A. Pechman.

Economic Behavior of the Affluent, by Robin Barlow, Harvey E. Brazer, and James N. Morgan.

Economic Behavior of the Affluent

ROBIN BARLOW

HARVEY E. BRAZER

JAMES N. MORGAN

Studies of Government Finance

THE BROOKINGS INSTITUTION

WASHINGTON, D.C.

© 1966 by

THE BROOKINGS INSTITUTION
1775 Massachusetts Avenue, N. W., Washington, D. C.

Published November 1966

Library of Congress Catalogue Card Number 66-28715

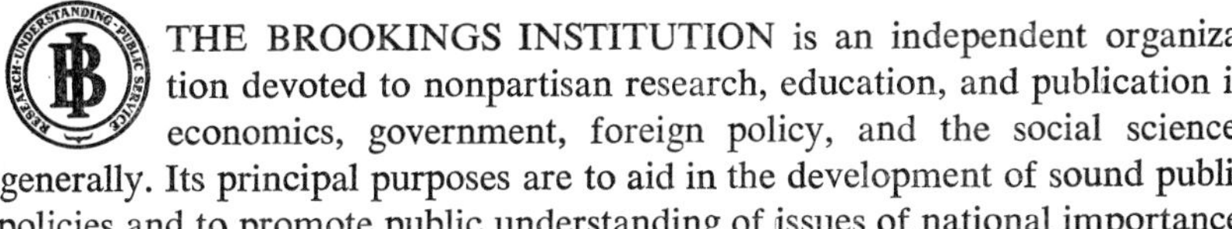

THE BROOKINGS INSTITUTION is an independent organization devoted to nonpartisan research, education, and publication in economics, government, foreign policy, and the social sciences generally. Its principal purposes are to aid in the development of sound public policies and to promote public understanding of issues of national importance.

The Institution was founded December 8, 1927, to merge the activities of the Institute for Government Research, founded in 1916, the Institute of Economics, founded in 1922, and the Robert Brookings Graduate School of Economics and Government, founded in 1924.

The general administration of the Institution is the responsibility of a self-perpetuating Board of Trustees. The trustees are likewise charged with maintaining the independence of the staff and fostering the most favorable conditions for creative research and education. The immediate direction of the policies, program, and staff of the Institution is vested in the President, assisted by the division directors and an advisory council, chosen from the professional staff of the Institution.

In publishing a study, the Institution presents it as a competent treatment of a subject worthy of public consideration. The interpretations and conclusions in such publications are those of the author or authors and do not purport to represent the views of the other staff members, officers, or trustees of the Brookings Institution.

BOARD OF TRUSTEES

EUGENE R. BLACK, *Chairman*
ROBERT BROOKINGS SMITH, *Vice Chairman*
WILLIAM R. BIGGS, *Chairman, Executive Committee*

Dillon Anderson
Elliott V. Bell
Louis W. Cabot
Robert D. Calkins
Leonard Carmichael
Edward W. Carter
Colgate W. Darden, Jr.
Douglas Dillon
Gordon Gray
Huntington Harris
Luther G. Holbrook
David M. Kennedy
John E. Lockwood
Arjay Miller
Herbert P. Patterson
J. Woodward Redmond
H. Chapman Rose
Sydney Stein, Jr.
Donald B. Woodward

Honorary Trustees

Arthur Stanton Adams
Daniel W. Bell
Marion B. Folsom
Raymond B. Fosdick
Huntington Gilchrist
John Lee Pratt

Foreword

PUBLIC POLICY—in particular fiscal and tax policy—can benefit from a better understanding of how people make decisions about their work and their investments. Do high marginal tax rates keep people from working as hard or as long as they might? Are people "locked in" with their present assets because they do not wish to pay the capital gains tax? Are investors familiar with special tax provisions? How do these provisions affect investment decisions?

The objective of this study is to help answer such questions by presenting the results of a field survey, conducted in 1964, of the investment and working behavior of a nationwide sample of 957 individuals with yearly incomes of $10,000 or more. The interviews also included questions on estate planning, charitable donations, the information sources used by investors, motives for saving, and other matters.

The authors are members of the Economics Faculty of The University of Michigan. The study was made as part of the program of The University of Michigan Survey Research Center.

The field work for the study was financed by the National Science Foundation, and the policy-oriented aspects were financed by the National Committee on Government Finance of the Brookings Institution.

The authors had the benefit of the advice and guidance of an advisory committee consisting of Richard Goode, Richard A. Musgrave, Richard Ruggles, Richard E. Slitor, Lawrence E. Thompson, James Tobin, and Norman B. Ture. George Katona, Eva Mueller, John B. Lansing, Charles Cannell, and several other members of the staff of the Survey Research Center made contributions to the design and execution of the study. New and complex sampling problems requiring some important innovations were expertly handled by Irene Hess, head of the sampling section. And the ultimate quality of the data is due to the work of the Center's excellent, intrepid, and persistent staff of interviewers across the country. Contributions to the early design were also made by Richard Kosobud, Warren L. Smith, and Ronald L. Teigen. Nancy Baerwaldt had a major part in the conduct of the study from the beginning and is directly responsible for two appendixes. The authors are also grateful for the many constructive suggestions and comments on the manuscript by George F. Break, Richard Goode, Daniel M. Holland, George Katona, Richard A. Musgrave, Guy Orcutt, Joseph A. Pechman, Lawrence E. Thompson, and Carl S. Shoup. Virginia Haaga edited the manuscript and prepared the index. The coding of the responses to the questions was supervised by Joan Scheffler. Carl Bixby and David Schupp handled the computer operations.

The National Committee on Government Finance was established in 1960 by the trustees of the Brookings Institution to supervise a comprehensive program of studies on taxation and government expenditure. The program, sponsored by the National Committee, is supported with funds provided by the Ford Foundation.

The views expressed in this study are those of the authors and are not presented as the views of the National Committee on Government Finance or its Advisory Committee, or the staff members, officers, or trustees of the Brookings Institution, the Ford Foundation, or the National Science Foundation.

Robert D. Calkins
President

August 1966
Washington, D.C.

Studies of Government Finance

Studies of Government Finance is a special program of research and education in taxation and government expenditures at the federal, state, and local levels. These studies are under the supervision of the National Committee on Government Finance appointed by the trustees of the Brookings Institution, and are supported by a special grant from the Ford Foundation.

MEMBERS OF THE NATIONAL COMMITTEE ON GOVERNMENT FINANCE

HOWARD R. BOWEN
President, University of Iowa

ROBERT D. CALKINS (Chairman)
President, The Brookings Institution

MARION B. FOLSOM
Director and Management Advisor, Eastman Kodak Company

ERWIN NATHANIEL GRISWOLD
Dean, Law School of Harvard University

ALVIN H. HANSEN
Emeritus Professor of Political Economy, Harvard University

GEORGE W. MITCHELL
Board of Governors, Federal Reserve System

DON K. PRICE
Dean, Graduate School of Public Administration, Harvard University

JACOB VINER
Emeritus Professor of Economics, Princeton University

WILLIAM C. WARREN
Dean, Columbia University Law School

HERMAN B WELLS
Chancellor, Indiana University

JOSEPH A. PECHMAN, Executive Director

MEMBERS OF THE ADVISORY COMMITTEE

ROBERT ANTHOINE
Attorney, Winthrop, Stimson, Putnam and Roberts

WALTER J. BLUM
Professor of Law, University of Chicago Law School

E. CARY BROWN
Professor of Economics, Massachusetts Institute of Technology

JAMES M. BUCHANAN
Professor of Economics, University of Virginia

JESSE BURKHEAD
Professor of Economics, Maxwell School, Syracuse University

GERHARD COLM
Chief Economist, National Planning Association

L. LASZLO ECKER-RACZ
Assistant Director, Advisory Commission on Intergovernmental Relations

OTTO ECKSTEIN
Professor of Economics, Harvard University

LYLE C. FITCH
President, Institute of Public Administration

RICHARD GOODE
Director, Fiscal Affairs Department, International Monetary Fund

HAROLD M. GROVES
Professor of Economics, University of Wisconsin

WALTER W. HELLER
Professor of Economics, University of Minnesota

NEIL H. JACOBY
Dean, School of Business, University of California at Los Angeles

RICHARD A. MUSGRAVE
Professor of Economics, Harvard University

RICHARD RUGGLES
Professor of Economics, Yale University

LOUIS SHERE
Professor of Economics, Indiana University

CARL S. SHOUP
Professor of Economics, Columbia University

DAN THROOP SMITH
Professor of Finance, Harvard Graduate School of Business Administration

STANLEY S. SURREY
Assistant Secretary, U. S. Treasury Department

GEORGE TERBORGH
Director of Research, Machinery and Allied Products Institute

NORMAN B. TURE
Director of Tax Research, National Bureau of Economic Research

Contents

Text Tables

Charts

Appendix Tables

CHAPTER I

Introduction and Summary

THIS STUDY IS CONCERNED with high-income individuals in their roles as investors and workers. How do they invest what they save? How hard do they work? What influences them in their choices? To find out the answers to these and other questions, a representative sample of high-income individuals—those whose decisions in these areas have such an important impact on the American economy—was asked about their asset holdings, their motives for saving, and their investment decisions. They were asked how much they worked, whether their wives were employed, and whether the progressive income tax influenced their decisions on these matters. These and other questions brought some surprising answers and showed a few long-held beliefs to be myths.

The Sample

An unbiased sample was drawn representing income in 1961 of residents of the continental United States, clustered geographically to reduce the cost of interviewing. Personal interviews were held in the spring of 1964 with 957 individuals whose incomes in 1961 were $10,000 or higher, hereinafter referred to as the "high-income group." A disproportionately large number of interviews was purposely secured from individuals with very high incomes. Indeed the chance of selection was roughly proportional to income.

In presenting the statistical results it was felt that each individual should be weighted in accordance with the number of income-dollars he represented. This was because the economic significance of the attitudes and behavior under analysis depends not so much on the number of individuals involved as on the number of dollars they represent. One could perhaps ignore the harmful effects of taxation if it were found, for example, that only 1 percent of all individuals are "locked-in" by capital gains taxes and only 1 percent work less because of progressive income taxes. But if it were revealed that these small groups account for, say, 25 percent of aggregate stockholdings and receive 10 percent of aggregate earnings, one might take a different view of the effects of taxation. Thus each individual was weighted according to his "economic importance," and income was taken to be the best available measure of such importance. Other relevant measures (such as the value of asset holdings, the value of work earnings, etc.) might provide more appropriate weights for some types of behavior, but they are highly correlated with income in any case. *Consequently the percentages and proportions cited in this book refer not to numbers of people but to shares of the aggregate income of those with incomes over $10,000.* The aggregate income of this group was about two-fifths of total personal income in the United States in 1961 and was received by about one-fifth of all families.

The Findings

The picture of the high-income individual emerging from our study is that of a hard-working executive or professional, whose decisions about how much to work are dictated by the demands of his job and by his health, rather than by taxes or other purely pecuniary considerations. These people reported that on the average they work 48 hours a week and 50 weeks a year. They usually manage their own investments, and even those who have delegated this task to someone else still retain considerable control over the final decisions. Although they are aware of many opportunities for reducing their taxes, most of these opportunities are regarded as involving more trouble than they are worth, and the only ones of which they frequently take advantage are those associated with capital gains, tax-exempt securities, and the making of gifts.

Only one-eighth of the sample said that they have actually curtailed their work effort because of the progressive income tax, and many members of this group in fact continue to work 60 or more hours a week. Those facing the highest marginal tax rates reported work disincentives only a little more frequently than did those facing the lowest rates. Curiously enough, those whose rates were in the middle of the tax rate schedule—around 50 percent—were more likely to say that their work effort was deterred. Very few reported that their wives' participation in the labor force or the timing of retirement was affected by taxes. The implication of these findings is that the loss of annual output due to work disincentives caused by the progressive income tax is of negligible proportions.

Decisions about the investment of family assets can be influenced by the purposes for which people accumulate or hold them. The reasons given for saving varied with age and income. The young mentioned most frequently the education of their children, the middle-aged save mainly for their own retirement, and the elderly (and those with the highest incomes) often mentioned a desire to make bequests. But a substantial minority of all high-income respondents mentioned the desire for security as a motive for saving. In an ordinary representative sample of people, retirement is usually the reason most commonly given for saving, followed by the education of children and provision for emergencies.

Gifts and inheritances received in the past account for one-fifth of total current wealth holdings of the entire high-income sample, even after allowance is made for appreciation in their value. Omitting the rare cases where some restrictions had been placed on the disposition of inheritances or gifts, a majority had divested themselves of all or part of the assets received. Most of the proceeds had been reinvested in other earning assets, generally common stock or other variable-return investments.

Most people had full control over the management of the assets they had received as gifts and inheritances. Even those who did have some beneficial interest in a trust frequently reported that they had some control over how the assets were invested.

Most of the high-income individuals are fairly active in the management of their portfolios. They seek information from investment advisory publications, stockbrokers, bank officials, and other qualified professionals, but they ordinarily make their own investment decisions. And even when they delegate some authority over day-to-day transactions, they usually give fairly specific instructions about the handling of their portfolios. Only among female rentiers is there often a substantial separation between the ownership and the control of financial assets.

Capital gains are preferred to current yield by most high-income individuals as an investment objective. Safety and liquidity are also considered important, even at the higher levels of income. Only a few consider current yield to be more important than capital gains, and these individuals are generally the less well informed. Those who are employed in the financial sector (banking, insurance, accountancy, etc.) are the most likely to belittle the importance of current yield. They are also the most informed and sophisticated about investment management and are the most interested in liquidity.

To interpret the investment goals expressed by the respondents it is necessary to look at their actual portfolios, recent transactions, and plans for future changes in their portfolios. Almost all have some of their wealth in the form of common stock, and common stock comprises the largest component of the portfolio for half of the entire high-income sample. The attractiveness of common stock is shown, too, by the fact that past and expected future changes in portfolio composition consist largely of the substitution of common stock for fixed-yield assets. A major exception to this attitude toward stock is evident among those individuals with the very highest incomes, who tend instead to favor tax-exempt municipal bonds and certain other fixed-yield securities when making adjustments in the composition of their portfolios. Many of the high-income individuals have invested in their own businesses; one-third have an ownership interest in a corporation that they manage; and one-fourth have an interest in an unincorporated enterprise.

Investment activity is fairly concentrated. A third of the high-income sample had neither purchased nor sold stock, bonds, real estate, or unincorporated business interests during the 15 months prior to the survey. The active investors tend to be better informed about investment opportunities generally, less satisfied with their present portfolios, and more conscious of taxes than those who are inactive. Investment activity increases with income up to a point, but quickly reaches a ceiling. For those with incomes above $150,000, activity is unrelated to income level—the very affluent may have more assets to manage, but they are no more active in managing them than are those with somewhat lower incomes.

The sale of assets usually involves the realization of a capital gain or loss, and most of the high-income sample had experienced such a gain or loss within the recent past. Irrespective of whether the sale had produced a gain or a loss, most of the sellers expressed satisfaction with the transaction, primarily because of the market's subsequent behavior.

An asset is often sold at a loss for tax reasons, the loss being used as an offset against realized gains and thus reducing tax liabilities. Many of the realized losses reported by respondents appear to be related to tax considerations. By contrast, tax considerations may be a deterrent to the sale of an asset for a gain. About one-fifth of the investors owning appreciated assets gave evidence of being locked-in to some extent by taxation. The distinction made in the tax law between "short-term" and "long-term" gains, the former being more heavily taxed than the latter, may affect the timing of sales for gains. Only a small fraction of the high-income population, however, appears to be affected by this provision.

The discussion of investment purposes, policies, activities, and plans proceeded without the question of taxes being explicitly introduced. In this way we could see how often taxes were mentioned voluntarily.[1] Although there were thirty-nine questions that could have led to a voluntary mention of taxes as a reason for some action, more than half of the sample failed to mention taxes even once. Of those who did mention taxes, over two-thirds mentioned them only once or twice. The most frequent references to taxes were the following: 17 percent of the entire sample said they preferred growth stocks to income stocks because of tax considerations

[1] The interviewing period included the date when the Revenue Act of 1964 was passed and the annual filing date for federal income taxes, and so the respondents' awareness of the tax structure should have been unusually high.

(presumably favorable treatment of capital gains); 13 percent said that taxes kept them from selling appreciated assets; 10 percent said that their most recent sale at a loss had been advantageous for tax reasons; 8 percent had made large gifts to relatives because of tax considerations; 7 percent had made estate arrangements with taxes in mind; and 7 percent mentioned tax considerations in explaining a recent sale of common stock. The frequency with which taxes were mentioned increased markedly with income and with total assets. Except for questions of capital gains and losses, then, only the transfer of assets to children and other relatives seems to involve appreciable concern with tax avoidance.

Indeed, the timing of large gifts to children and other relatives appears to be dominated by tax considerations. Concern for the welfare of the recipients may also be assumed to be a common motive for making gifts, though this motive was less frequently expressed. The making of large gifts *inter vivos* was one aspect of estate planning that some of the high-income individuals had undertaken. Also involved was the establishment of trusts and insurance arrangements. Most of the high-income individuals had given some thought to how their estates would be handled at their death, but only a few had actually done anything about it.

Respondents were asked whether they had ever given an appreciated asset to charity. Only a small fraction had, yet most individuals in the sample did own appreciated assets, and most had made some donations. Making the donations in the form of appreciated assets gives the donor an important tax advantage since the full value of the asset is deductible as a contribution, while the capital gain on it is not taxed. At higher income levels, there was a substantial increase in the proportion who had donated appreciated assets.

An even more direct question was asked about the special tax advantage of investing in real estate. Only half had even heard of the possibilities, and only one-fifth had actually made or thought of making such investments. And a final question about any other features of the tax law that affected investment decisions elicited nothing but a reiteration of the favorable treatment of capital gains, except for the few who mentioned tax-exempt municipal bonds and percentage depletion allowances.

Conclusions

It is clear that there are many more powerful motives affecting the working behavior of high-income people than the marginal income tax rates. People are aware of taxes and do not enjoy paying them, but other considerations are far more important to them in deciding how long to work.

As for investment decisions, it appears that high-income people tend to make their own decisions, often without seeking detailed information and understanding. Sensitivity to taxes appears in only two places: where income can be received in the form of capital gains, and where it is possible to transfer assets to relatives and reduce one's tax liabilities by so doing.

Only a very small fraction of the high-income population is making use of the other special provisions in the tax law. This means that these provisions are inequitable not only as between high-income and low-income people but also within the high-income group. Their modification would adversely affect fewer people than some have thought.

CHAPTER II

Methods and Definitions

PREVIOUS STUDIES ON a local and restricted basis have shown that the financial decisions of high-income people are qualitatively as well as quantitatively different from those of middle-income and low-income people.[1] It can be estimated from a study conducted recently by the Federal Reserve Board and from Internal Revenue Service statistics that families with incomes over $10,000 accounted for only one-fifth of the families in the United States in 1961 but received two-fifths of the aggregate income and owned more than three-fifths of the aggregate personal net wealth.[2] Since people with high incomes control income and assets far more than in proportion to their numbers, a special study of their investment and working behavior seemed desirable.

Before such a study was possible, however, a national sample properly representing high-income people was required. Since sam-

[1] George Katona and John B. Lansing, "The Wealth of the Wealthy," *Review of Economics and Statistics* (February 1964), pp. 1-13; J. Keith Butters, Lawrence E. Thompson, and Lynn L. Bollinger, *Effects of Taxation, Investments by Individuals* (Harvard University, Graduate School of Business Administration, 1953).

[2] "Survey of Financial Characteristics of Consumers," *Federal Reserve Bulletin* (March 1964), pp. 285-93. For estimating the percentage of tax returns in the highest brackets and shares of income, see U.S. Treasury Department, Internal Revenue Service, *Statistics of Income, 1961,* p. 32.

pling such people by particular geographic locations or locating them by a screening interview would have been cumbersome and expensive, the Survey Research Center had to develop a technique whereby a sample could be drawn with the chance of selection specified according to income. Fortunately, with the help of other organizations, it was possible to secure a list of names containing a known and disproportionate number of people with incomes higher than the average. A sample was drawn from this list and interviewing took place in the spring of 1964. Interviews were obtained with 1,051 individuals, 957 of whom had 1961 incomes of $10,000 and over. The 94 cases with incomes of less than $10,000 were omitted from the analysis.

Sampling

The list of names used by the Survey Research Center to draw its representative national sample was unlike a random list of individuals since it contained a disproportionate number of people with incomes higher than the average. It did, however, contain a few people with low incomes, so that we could if necessary assure our respondents and others that the mere fact of inclusion in the list revealed nothing about any individual's income. This, of course, involved some cost and inefficiency. One interviewer actually had to hire two horses and an interpreter and ride many miles into the desert to interview an Indian, who proved to have a very low income!

Even at incomes of over $10,000, varying rates of selection for inclusion in the sample had to be applied because those with incomes slightly over $10,000 are numerous relative to their aggregate income and wealth. For instance, those with incomes between $10,000 and $15,000 account for about two-thirds of the total number of individuals with incomes over $10,000, but receive less than half the aggregate income of those with incomes over $10,000.[3]

Hence, selecting all individuals with incomes of over $10,000 at the same rate would have produced a sample in which two-thirds of the interviews accounted for less than half of the aggregate income. Instead, each income class was sampled at a different rate,

[3] *Statistics of Income, 1961.*

calculated so that the probability of selection increased with the level of income. (See Appendix A.) We were interested in sampling dollars of income, not numbers of people.

Response Rates

A sample may begin by being representative and end by being biased if some people are harder to find and interview than others. Some of the names selected for this sample could not be used because the addresses listed were either obsolete or were those of financial institutions or lawyers acting as financial agents for the individuals in question. Also not everyone was willing or even able to be interviewed personally.

Response rates were lower than those achieved in more evenly representative national samples of households. Thirteen percent of the names selected for interviewing were unusable because of inadequate addresses, and another 25 percent were unable or unwilling to give an interview. Thus, of the original sample of individuals selected, 62 percent were actually interviewed. Further information on the response rates and potential nonresponse biases is given in Appendix C.

Weights

The variations in sampling fractions from a perfect representation of dollars of income and the variations in response rates required that each response be weighted according to the proportion of aggregate income it represented. In a particular income group where there was more nonresponse than in another income group, those who were successfully interviewed were given higher weights. In a group where the selection rate was higher per dollar of aggregate income, those interviewed received lower weights.

The grouping by income for weighting purposes was based on the respondent's own report of his 1961 income since we knew only the total distribution of aggregate income within the sample—not any one individual's income. Thus errors in reporting income could cause errors in the weights. However, the adjustments for the different sampling and response rates did not vary a great deal from one income class to the next, so errors that moved an individual to a neighboring income class did not create serious problems.

The principal set of weights, then, valued each response according to the share of the aggregate income of individuals with incomes over $10,000 that it represented.

These weights are used throughout the analysis except where noted, so that the proportions given are always the proportions of income represented by those giving particular replies. For example, when we report that "three-fourths of the high-income respondents own common stock," what is actually meant is that among individuals with incomes of $10,000 or higher, those who own stock receive three-fourths of the group's total income.

A second set of weights, far more varied from one income class to another, was calculated in such a way that each respondent is weighted according to the number of people with incomes over $10,000 whom he represents. In this case, the respondents with the highest incomes represent so few individuals that their weights round to zero. They represent a substantial fraction of the aggregate income but practically no individuals at all! Appendix E gives the distribution of answers to each question using each of these two sets of weights—one giving the distribution of aggregate income and the other the distribution of individuals, eliminating in both cases respondents with incomes under $10,000.

A third set of weights could have been calculated according to the wealth owned by each individual; and for assessing the importance of certain investment decisions this might have been preferable. However, the information on which such weights would be based was tenuous, and the variation in weights would have been so great as to make the weighted estimates somewhat unstable. Also the importance of work decisions and perhaps even the importance of investment decisions may be measured better by income than by total assets.

Precision of Data from a Sample

A percentage estimated from a sample may be different from the true percentage based on the whole population. The variation of possible sample estimates around the true population figure is generally misnamed the "sampling error." The extent of this variation depends both on the size of the sample and on its design. The whole purpose of oversampling individuals in the higher income classes in this study was to reduce the sampling errors in estimates of the aggregate income represented by a given answer, where most of the variability can be attributed to the higher incomes. Estimates of sampling errors for some of the more important percentages are given in Appendix A.

The precision of survey data depends not only on the extent to which the sample size and design reduce the sampling errors, and on the extent to which the failure to interview some people introduces a bias, but also on the reliability of the replies given in the interviews, to which we now turn.

Interviewing

The accuracy with which respondents report the desired information to an interviewer depends on the respondent, the interviewer, the questionnaire, and the kind of information sought. The questionnaire in this case focused on people's concerns, motives, attitudes, levels of information, insights, and understanding, rather than on the dollar details of financial assets and transactions. Questions about the value of assets were asked only to get rough approximations. Broad questions were asked about the composition of the investment portfolio, past trends therein, recent capital gains and losses realized, charitable contributions, gifts and inheritances, and income. Even if respondents had been willing and able to provide detailed financial information, it was felt that trying to infer motives and purposes from such information would be less fruitful than using a combination of reported behavior, plans, financial situation, attitudes, and expressed reasons.

Efforts were also made to keep the interviews short. Those respondents who were pressed for time were able to answer all the questions in less than an hour. In the later stages of the study, interviewers found it helpful to be able to assure respondents of this.

Quantification of attitudes and reasons requires that there be reasonable consistency from one respondent to the next in what is asked and how the replies are treated. The fixed-question, open-answer technique was used. This means that interviewers asked questions exactly as they were worded for the interviews and used only a limited set of specified nondirective probes, such as "Why is that?" or a repetition of the question. They wrote down the respondent's answer as fully as possible. The interpretation and analysis of the replies were then made systematically by the coding staff in the Ann Arbor office, under the close supervision of trained economists.

With such a procedure, the interviewers had to have some general familiarity with the terms used in finance and investment, but they did not have to know enough to phrase their own questions or to interpret the responses. The experience of the Survey Research Center in earlier studies of business executives and of congressmen had shown that with a fixed questionnaire, trained interviewers were more successful in securing interviews with interpretable responses than were professional experts, such as economists or political scientists.

Response Errors

Even with the fixed-question technique of interviewing, there may still have been misinterpretation of some questions, or memory errors in recalling past actions or dates. Most respondents provided a consistent and credible picture, but people can develop self-images that are consistent yet erroneous.

One type of possible response error was particularly crucial in this study because the weighting for nonresponse depended on it, namely the possible errors in reporting 1961 income. The procedure for asking about this income was necessarily cumbersome. Questions were first asked about 1963 income in such a way as to approximate income as defined in our sample, that is, to exclude tax-exempt interest, social security benefits, and half of all long-term capital gains. Respondents were then asked what that figure, which approximates "adjusted gross income" as defined for tax purposes, had been two years earlier in 1961. No additional questions about types of income or other earners in the family seemed feasible in this situation.

Appendix D shows that there was evidence of frequent understating of income. Because we knew only the distribution of income for the entire sample and no one individual's 1961 income, there was no way to match what the individual had reported with any other record. Such matching would have revealed whether the understatement resulted from numerous small understatements, moving many people down by one income class, or from a smaller group of very great understatements. However, from the observed consistency within the interviews, there is some reason to believe that the former interpretation is the right one. If so, the errors in weighting are quite small since the weights do not vary substantially from any one income class to the adjacent one. In any case, the weights would have to be very substantially in error before much bias would be produced in the resulting estimates of the percentage who gave any particular answer. Precision in weighting would have been far more crucial if our purpose had been to estimate mean and aggregate dollar amounts of assets where the distribution is highly skewed. In that case the weights of the few extreme cases would have been very influential.

Given the understating of income, however, the use of the original income-bracket boundaries as reported by respondents would have given a biased impression in discussing our findings about differences among income groups. Consequently, the income brackets were adjusted so as to give a more accurate impression of the income levels being discussed. (See Appendix D.)

As for the many other items of information, concerning both fact and attitude, it would be a major undertaking to provide a thorough check of the validity of any one of them. Imperfect checks can be made by looking for meaningfulness and consistency. Some investigating was done to determine whether respondents' reports of their own marginal tax rates were reasonable, given their incomes and family situations. But this was only a loose check because the marginal tax rate can vary widely even at the same income level. In general the only check on the reliability of the remaining responses must be based on our statement that the replies were generally consistent and meaningful and the reader's own intuitive reaction to the clarity of the questions actually asked.

In addition to possible biases from sampling variability, selective nonresponse, and response errors, there is always the possibility of conceptual errors or discrepancies between what is important and what is measured.

Concepts and Definitions

Both for selecting high-income people, and for categorizing people according to income, the 1961 income concept used is an imperfect measure. The concept was defined to conform with the income definition used in deriving the original list of names from which the sample was selected. The concept excludes tax-exempt interest, social security benefits, half of long-term capital gains, nonmoney income such as employer-paid insurance or retirement contributions, stock options, and unrealized capital gains in general. Insofar as some of these types of income are more important for female rentiers (tax-exempt interest), self-employed (capital gains), or business executives (retirement plans, stock options, group term life insurance), these groups are under-represented and their income level understated.

To minimize our requests for detailed financial information, we asked only broad ranges of asset values and only for each of three broad types of assets. We were thus able to characterize the size of the total portfolio only as being "large," "medium," or "small." The estimated size of the total portfolio also omitted the value of any personal residences owned, pension rights, life insurance, and expected inheritances.

For those who owned stock in corporations in which they were also officers or executives, it was not always clear whether they were really owner-managers who decided on such things as dividend policy, or merely executives who happened to own stock in the company for which they worked.

Finally, there may have been some minor misunderstanding as to our concepts of "investments that pay a fixed amount each year" or our distinction between "direct business investments" and common stock ownership, or how large a "large gift" or inheritance had to be before it was to be reported. In general, however, the respondents seemed to understand the questions and answered them easily and rapidly.

Social Characteristics of the Sample[4]

Apart from the fact that those included in the analysis had 1961 incomes of $10,000 or more and hence were wealthier than a representative national sample, the sample had a few other distinguishing features.

Most respondents were middle-aged, the median age being fifty-one. One-third (weighted by dollars of income) were between forty-five and fifty-four years old, compared with one-fifth for a representative (unweighted) national sample of heads of spending units. About the same proportion were sixty-five or older as in a representative sample of spending-unit heads. Most of the respondents were men. They were less likely to be retired than those in a representative national sample. Fewer than a tenth were retirees, compared with one-sixth for a representative sample of heads of families. One-third of our sample were business owners, compared with 8 percent in a representative national sample, and one-fourth were professionals as against 12 percent in a representative national sample.

There were somewhat more Jews and somewhat fewer Catholics than in a representative national sample of family heads. The most noticeable relationship between religion and occupation was the almost complete absence of Catholics in the financial sector. There were more than three times as many Episcopalians in the high-income group as in a representative national sample, and Presbyterians were also "over-represented." By contrast, there were relatively few Baptists and other fundamentalist Protestants in the high-income group. However, the proportion attending church more than once a month was exactly the same as in a representative national sample of family heads!

Nine-tenths owned their own homes, half again as many as in a representative national sample of families. Nearly six-tenths said that they were covered by a retirement program other than social security. About a third reported that their wives had had a job sometime in the last ten years and a fourth said their wives had

[4] All the data in this section refer to proportions of the aggregate income of those with 1961 incomes over $10,000.

earned money in the last year, substantially fewer than the 46 percent making this report in a representative sample. But one-fifth said that their wives worked full time, not many fewer than in a representative sample of families.

Less than two-fifths had lived in only one state, compared with nearly two-thirds of a representative sample of family heads, indicating that upper-income people are more mobile. They had also received more education, with nearly half reporting a college degree and 17 percent reporting an advanced or professional degree. Finally, there were more Republicans than Democrats. Most of these differences were as expected.

Summary

• A sample of high-income individuals was selected by probability methods and weighted to represent dollars of income.

• It proved possible to interview personally 62 percent of the sample originally selected for interviewing.

• Each completed interview was given a weight to adjust for remaining variations in the probability of a dollar of income being selected, and to adjust for variations in response rates among subgroups.

• A fixed-question, open-answer technique of interviewing was used. The analysis of responses was supervised in the Ann Arbor office to assure uniformity and proper quantification.

• There was widespread understating of income, requiring adjustment of the brackets used in describing the income groups.

• This sample of people with incomes over $10,000, who were weighted for dollars of income, differs from a representative national sample in a number of expected ways. Their average age and average education were higher than those of a representative national sample of adults. A relatively high proportion of them were Presbyterians, Episcopalians, or Jews, and a relatively low proportion were Catholics and fundamentalist Protestants.

CHAPTER III

Separation of Ownership from Control

THIS CHAPTER REPORTS our findings on the separation of the ownership of wealth from its control through such devices as the use of trusts, joint ownership of assets, or the delegation of investment decisions.[1] In studying the factors affecting the investment of personal wealth, it would have been quite inappropriate to interview the wealth-owners themselves if control over the investment of their wealth actually rested with trust officers, investment counselors, and other financial experts. But, as it turned out, the separation of ownership from control appeared to be not at all widespread.

Assets in Trust

The relative importance of trusts in the economy can be assessed from aggregate data available from the Internal Revenue Service. Out of an aggregate adjusted gross income of $329.9 billion in 1961, only 0.2 percent was taxable individual income from

[1] All the data in this chapter refer to proportions of the aggregate income of those with 1961 incomes over $10,000.

estates and trusts. Excluding those returns with adjusted gross incomes under $10,000 leaves an aggregate adjusted gross income of $101.7 billion, and of this amount 0.4 percent was from estates or trusts (not counting $15 million in trust losses).[2] These percentages underestimate the importance of assets that are outside the control of the beneficial owner. The delegation of investment decisions is not accounted for nor is undistributed trust income, which does not need to be declared on individual income tax returns.

A further indication of the importance of assets tied up in trusts or estates not yet distributed can be gained from a sample of fiduciary income tax returns for 1960.[3] These trusts and estates had a total income of $5.3 billion, of which $2.4 billion was distributed and presumably became the income of individuals. Various deductions reduced this latter figure to a taxable amount of $1.0 billion, nearly 80 percent of which went to trusts with total incomes of more than $10,000 each.[4]

At any rate, statistics from all sources indicate that income from estates and trusts accounts for only a very small fraction of the aggregate income of individuals.

Beneficial Interest in Trusts

Trusts may vary from small tax-avoidance plans, where assets are placed in trust for the benefit of minor children (with parents or bank officers as trustees), to major asset accumulations that are professionally managed for the benefit of several generations of a

[2] U.S. Treasury Department, Internal Revenue Service, *Statistics of Income, 1961.*

[3] *Statistics of Income, 1960, Fiduciary, Gift, and Estate Tax Returns.*

[4] The Internal Revenue Service statistics on individual income indicate that income from estates and trusts was $669 million in 1961, while the fiduciary return data show that distributions of income to beneficiaries totaled $2,398 million. These two amounts are different because those who received income from trusts which was originally in the form of dividends or capital gains were allowed to report it as dividend or capital gain income rather than as income from a trust. They benefited from doing so because they could then take advantage of the dividend credit and exclusion and the special treatment of long-term capital gains. In addition, some of the distributions of estates and trusts went to individuals with low incomes who did not file tax returns. Finally, the reported distributions of $2,398 million were really deductions for distributions, not the precise amount of the distributions themselves. (Letters from J. A. Stockfisch, Deputy Assistant Secretary of the Treasury, March 16, 1965, and from Vito Natrella, Director, Statistics Division, U.S. Internal Revenue Service, March 22, 1965.)

single family. In the case of assets held in the name of children, someone else in the family (usually one or both parents) has some control over the investment of the assets in trust.[5]

The following question was asked:

> Do you have any control over how it [the trust] is invested?

Some illustrative replies from three different respondents were:

> I have control of trusts for my three grandchildren for their education. Of course the bank is the executor, but only in an advisory capacity.
>
> No. These are short-term trusts over which the bank has control. They are revocable, and the trustee has to be able to control them. Under the Keogh Bill I do make some of the decisions in keeping with the law.
>
> Yes, I have control over one (mine) but not over those of the other members of my family. If I did have, it would have been silly for me to have created the trusts because they would all have been taxable to me. [The respondent said later that he spends full time managing these family trusts. There is a general policy that he and the legal trustees follow, but he makes the decisions and tells the trustees what to do. The trustees are all relatives—though somewhat remote. He and the trustees review the investments quarterly.]

Nearly one-fourth of our respondents said that they or someone else in their immediate families held a beneficial interest in a trust fund. At incomes over $150,000 the proportion rose to more than half. Six in ten of those reporting a beneficial interest in a trust said that they had some control over the investment policy of the trust, and the higher the income the larger that proportion. At very high income levels, three-fourths of those with beneficial interests in trusts said they had some control over the investment of these assets.

[5] Since a trust involves some separation of ownership from control, with control often vested in a trustee who specializes in this kind of work, it can be assumed both that there is less flexibility in the investment of such assets and that there is little point in asking the beneficiaries about the management of the investments. A special study of trustees would be required to analyze the decisions about the investment of assets held in trust. Hence the present study did not ask whether the respondent or anyone in his family was acting as a trustee, but only whether anyone had a beneficial interest in a trust.

The wealthiest respondents were more likely to report that someone in their immediate family was the beneficiary of a trust, and also more likely to report having some control over the trust's investment policies. Therefore, especially at the highest income levels, many trusts have both the trustee and the beneficiary in the same immediate family. Most of the trusts reported by the high-income sample were set up by the respondents for their children rather than by others for the respondents, since very few reported elsewhere in the interview that they had ever received either inheritances or large gifts in trust form.

Receipt of Gifts or Inheritances in Trust

Of the 40 percent who reported inheriting assets at some time in the past, fewer than one-tenth reported any trust or other restrictions on them. And of the 18 percent who reported receiving large gifts, only one-tenth reported any restrictions on their disposition. It is possible that some beneficiaries with an interest in trusts that do not pay current income may have failed to report them, and may even have failed to think of them as a gift or inheritance. (But the general picture, consonant with published data, is *not* one in which private trustees administer any substantial part of personal wealth.) There are, of course, substantial investments managed by pension fund trustees, insurance companies, and nonprofit institutions.

Gifts in Trust Form

To investigate the setting up of trusts from the donor's side, we asked:

> Within the last couple of years, have you transferred any money or property to your children or other relatives?
>
> To whom have you given these gifts (and transfers)?
>
> Now, about these gifts (and transfers)—were they outright gifts or in the form of a trust, or what?

Here trusts seemed to be of somewhat more importance. Even within the limited time period of "a couple of years," nearly one-fifth of our sample had made such large gifts, and more than one-third of these gifts were in the form of trusts. The proportion making gifts rose from 5 percent in the \$10,000-\$15,000 income group to 71 percent of those with incomes over $300,000. The recipients of many of these gifts in trust form may well have been low-income people or minors, who are not represented in our sample at all. There may also be a tendency to forget gifts received more than gifts given. Among the group who had given large gifts, 42 percent of those with dependent children reported having made their gifts in the form of trusts, as against 28 percent of those without dependent children. Those with higher incomes were more likely to have made their gifts to relatives in the form of trusts. Among those with incomes of over $300,000 nearly half of the donors had used trust arrangements. Combining this with the fact that 71 percent of those with incomes over $300,000 had made gifts to relatives or children, we see that one-third of those with incomes over $300,000 had put assets in trust for their children or other relatives within the last few years. This might seem to belie the other evidence that separation of ownership from control through trusts is not very important. But many of these trusts were for minor children who were part of the respondent's immediate family, probably with the parents as trustees. In any case these assets in trust frequently become the outright property of the children when they come of age.

Those who were tax conscious (that is, those who mentioned taxes voluntarily in the interview as a reason for certain attitudes or behavior) were more likely to have made gifts and more likely to have used the trust device than were those in the high-income sample as a whole. Similarly, those with large total portfolios and those with accumulations of unrealized capital gains were more likely to have made gifts to relatives and more likely to have made them in the form of a trust. Since income, the value of assets, and the possession of appreciated assets are all highly correlated with one another, we cannot determine which of these characteristics made the difference, but certainly their combined influence was powerful.

Joint Ownership of Assets

Another way in which authority over investment decisions is restricted, delegated, diffused, or even confused, is through some form of joint ownership of assets. Several legal forms are possible. "Joint tenancy" usually means that either party can legally sell the asset and reinvest the proceeds elsewhere. "Tenancy in common" usually means that both must sign for any transaction. Interpretations vary from state to state depending on state laws and court decisions. But the legal form of joint ownership does not determine who actually feels responsible for the decisions.

If assets are jointly owned within the immediate family, there seems little need to be concerned about who makes the decisions. Hence, we asked only about assets owned jointly with someone not in the immediate family:

> Do you have some things that are jointly owned with friends or with relatives who do not live with you?
>
> What kinds of investments are these? Anything else?
>
> With whom are they owned—your parents, your children, a friend, or whom?
>
> What are the reasons why these investments are jointly owned?
>
> Who would be responsible for deciding what to do with these things—whether to sell them and invest the money somewhere else, for instance?

Twenty-nine percent of the high-income sample reported joint ownership of assets with someone outside the immediate family. The proportion did not increase with income. The most common type of joint ownership involved unincorporated businesses or real estate (19 percent of the entire high-income group), with common stock in second place (11 percent). Only 3 percent reported joint ownership of fixed-yield assets, and this was virtually nonexistent at the highest incomes. Who were these other owners? They were parents or brothers and sisters (18 percent), business associates (12 percent), and the respondent's children living outside the immediate family (3 percent). (These percentages add to more than 29 percent because some people owned assets jointly with more than one category of individuals.)

However, joint ownership of assets with one's own children living outside the immediate family became more common at higher incomes, having been reported by 14 percent of those with incomes over $300,000. The people with the higher incomes were also older, of course. Interestingly enough, the type of asset jointly owned bore no relation to who the other owners were.

Most assets were jointly owned because they had been inherited or otherwise received in that particular form, or because of a business partnership, as is shown by the following responses:

> Well, they helped finance it at the start, and it's difficult to eliminate them [the other owners] if you make money.
>
> That was a cold turkey business deal.
>
> It means I have a larger investment than I could have alone.
>
> In the first place to hold the assets together during the depression. [Has that reason changed?] Now it's a profitable arrangement, so we do not plan to change it.

Tax considerations as a reason for joint ownership were mentioned by only 4 percent of those with joint ownership, or by 1 percent of the entire high-income group.

It must be kept in mind that joint ownership within the immediate family, not investigated here, may well be more common, and more influenced by tax considerations than is joint ownership outside the immediate family. It is interesting, however, that there was relatively little joint ownership of passive investments with people outside the immediate family. (Some of the jointly owned stock was undoubtedly in small incorporated business ventures.)

The extent of joint ownership did not vary with the presence or absence of children, dependent or not. Neither did joint ownership vary systematically with the reported marginal tax rate, nor with stated investment policies,[6] nor according to whether large gifts had recently been made to individuals or charities. Since so many jointly owned assets were business ventures, it is not surprising that the occupational group most likely to own assets jointly with others were the business owners. Virtually none of the rentiers held any jointly owned assets. Of course, owning some assets jointly was more common among those with more total assets. As the size of the total portfolio increased, there was an increase in the likelihood of joint ownership of direct business investments, but not of common stock nor of fixed-yield assets.

The final question in this series asked who would be responsible for deciding what to do with the assets. The most common answer was that the decisions would be jointly made. One in four said he

[6] That is, whether the respondent preferred current yield or capital gains.

could decide by himself, and one in ten said that the other owner would make the decisions. This asymmetry could mean that the existence of such assets may or may not be completely reported, depending on the extent of control and responsibility on the part of the individual reporting. It may also reflect an egoistic bias, similar to that found when husbands and wives are asked which of them makes the decision in a particular situation.[7]

As might be expected, responses indicating that the respondent himself was solely responsible for managing jointly owned assets were most common when the other owners were grown children, rather than when the other owners were parents, siblings, or business associates. But even when the other owners were grown children, the respondent claimed sole responsibility in only about one-half the cases. Typical responses regarding control over jointly owned assets were:

> In the hotel business, I make the decisions; as to the unimproved property, its a fifty-fifty proposition.
>
> All of us. We'd have to agree about selling it. Then we'd handle any reinvestment individually—no more co-ownership as far as I'm concerned.

Delegation of Investment Decisions

Even if wealth is not under the control of a trustee or a joint owner, decisions regarding its management can be delegated to someone else. Respondents were asked:

> Do you (and your immediate family) handle the job of managing your investments, or have you turned over some of your investment decisions to someone else?
>
> What kind of investments are managed by someone else?
>
> Is the person who manages them a stockbroker, a bank officer, or what?
>
> What kind of policy or instructions is he following in handling your investments?

[7] *Male vs. Female Influence in Buying and Brand Selection* (Fawcett Publications, 1958).

How frequently does he check with you about your investments—once a month, once a year, or what?

Only one-tenth reported delegating some or all authority over their investments, and this proportion reached one-fourth only for those with incomes over $300,000. Only 2 percent of the entire high-income group said that they delegated "all" authority.[8]

When delegation was reported, in three-fourths of the cases it was delegation of the management of a common stock portfolio. Usually the portfolio had been entrusted to a stockbroker or a professional investment manager.

Only a minority of those delegating reported that they had given specific instructions to their managers. A few, mostly those with the highest incomes, had specified that they wanted capital gains; still fewer had mentioned safety; and almost no one reported that he had explicitly instructed his investment manager to secure tax advantages.[9] On the other hand, many of the delegators checked with their investment managers "every few months" or "a few times a year," so that the lack of even general instructions does not mean that the respondents were not taking some part in setting their own investment policy.

Delegation was most common among female rentiers, one-third of whom said that they delegated "all" authority. The more tax conscious were also more likely to have delegated some authority over their investments, and if they did so, they were also more likely to have given specific instructions to their investment managers. Nine-tenths of them had given some instructions to their investment managers.

Older people were also more likely to have delegated, in spite of the fact that they presumably had more time to manage their own assets. Eighteen percent of those sixty-five or older had delegated some or all authority, compared with only 8 percent of those aged under sixty-five. However, the aged were *more* likely to give instructions from time to time, 62 percent as against only 23 percent of the younger delegators.

[8] This fraction might well be an underestimate, however, because several of the female rentiers could not be located or interviewed. See Appendix C.

[9] The search for capital gains involves tax advantages, but it brings other advantages as well.

Those with more formal education also were more likely to have delegated some decision-making, but also more likely to check with their asset managers frequently. College graduates were twice as likely to have delegated some or all authority (14 percent versus 7 percent for those not graduating from college), but among the few who had delegated, the college graduates were twice as likely to consult with their managers every few weeks or more frequently (34 percent versus 17 percent). The self-employed also had delegated more than the average, and consulted more. Two other factors associated with delegation of investment decisions were (1) having inherited a large fraction of one's total assets and (2) living in one of the twelve largest metropolitan areas. But whether the respondent preferred high current yield to capital gains was not related to whether or not decision-making authority had been delegated.

It appears then that delegation of "all" decisions concerning the investment of one's assets, without rechecking at frequent intervals, is relatively rare. This finding is not surprising. Certainly an individual wants to be sure through personal verification that his assets are being handled properly, and the "expert" to whom some decisions are delegated feels safer if he has received specific confirmation of his decisions at relatively frequent intervals, as is shown by the following responses:

> He [my investment counselor] has the authority to buy and sell the securities but not to withdraw funds. He deals with a broker. The securities are held in my name. He can call the broker and tell him to buy and sell, but he can't withdraw any cash. In practice he's so conservative that he usually talks to me before he does anything.
>
> He reports to me every three months but if he does something in between, he talks to me first most of the time.

A similar finding that few investors delegate authority was found in a previous study of high-income people in one midwestern city conducted in 1959-60 by the Survey Research Center.[10]

This general absence of total delegation does not imply that all individuals who make their own investment decisions are well in-

[10] See George Katona and John B. Lansing, "The Wealth of the Wealthy," *Review of Economics and Statistics* (February 1964), pp. 1-13.

formed. The extent and sources of the information used by investors are reported in Chapter VI.

Summary

- The use of trusts—in which the beneficial interests in the assets are legally owned by one person but the assets are managed by another—was relatively infrequent; and many of those who reported some beneficial interest in a trust also reported some control over how its assets were invested.
- Of those who received large gifts, only one in ten reported any trust or other restrictions on their use or reinvestment. Only one in five reported receiving such large gifts, so only 2 percent of the entire high-income group had beneficial interests in trusts as a result of gifts received.
- A similarly small fraction of inheritances was reported as being restricted. Since only two-fifths of the entire high-income sample reported having received inheritances, no more than 4 percent of the entire high-income group reported holding trusts or other restricted assets as a result of inheritances.
- Three-tenths of the high-income sample reported that they owned an asset jointly with someone not living in their immediate household. These assets tended to be unincorporated businesses, real estate, or common stock. Joint ownership of fixed-yield assets was rare. The other owners were mostly parents or siblings.
- Delegation of portfolio management was relatively rare, the proportion who delegated increasing from 5 percent for those with incomes around \$12,000 to 25 percent for those with incomes over \$300,000. Among asset types, delegation of management was most frequent in the case of common stock. The owner who had delegated management usually checked on the manager several times a year. Female rentiers most frequently delegated their investment decisions.
- There was probably a great deal of joint ownership *within* families; and the practice of placing assets in trust for minor children may be widespread, but in such cases the management decisions are still made within the immediate family owning the assets.

CHAPTER IV

Saving Objectives and Investment Policies

IN THIS CHAPTER "saving objectives" are defined as the ultimate purposes for which saving out of income is undertaken—for example, the individual's own future consumption. "Investment policies" are defined as the principles that guide the individual in choosing between alternative investments—for example, an aversion to a high degree of risk.[1]

Economic Significance of Saving Objectives and Investment Policies

The nature of saving objectives in the population affects the structure of the economy in a number of ways. If individuals saved in part in order to make bequests to their heirs, then in the long run aggregate saving and hence the rate of economic growth would probably be higher than it would if all individuals saved wholly for their own future consumption. In representative cross-section sam-

[1] All the data in this chapter refer to proportions of the aggregate income of those with 1961 incomes over $10,000.

ples, the Survey Research Center has never found that more than a small minority had a desire to bequeath wealth.[2] Advocates of the "life cycle hypothesis of saving" have built their models on the assumption that the bequest motive is in fact a rarity.[3]

The prevalence of the bequest motive also affects the distribution of income in the economy. The greater the volume of saving in order to make bequests, the more unequal the distribution of income becomes. In the sphere of tax policy too the effects of various tax changes on the aggregate amount of saving depend in part on the nature of saving objectives.[4]

Given the volume of personal saving, the policies pursued by individuals in investing those savings have an important influence on the rate and direction of economic growth. For example, the willingness of individuals to invest in venturesome, risky enterprises will affect the rate of economic growth, in some respects positively and in other respects negatively. It is of interest to policymakers to know how investment policies can themselves be influenced by other forces, in particular by the tax environment. Much has been written about how taxation has distorted investment decisions or has discouraged risk-taking, while others have seen taxation as a potent instrument for deliberately influencing investment decisions to further national economic goals. But there is little empirical evidence on how influential taxation has been in this sphere.

These issues must be explored most intensively among the high-income population since this group is responsible for a disproportionately large share of annual saving and also includes the individuals who are most active in transferring funds among alternative investments. The high-income group, while containing only one-

[2] Eva Mueller and Harlow Osborne, "Consumer Time and Savings Balances: Their Role in Family Liquidity," *American Economic Review* (May 1965), pp. 265-75, 286; George Katona, *The Mass Consumption Society* (McGraw-Hill, 1964), p. 176.

[3] See, for example, Franco Modigliani and Richard Brumberg, "Utility Analysis and the Consumption Function: An Interpretation of Cross-Section Data," K. K. Kurihara (ed.), *Post-Keynesian Economics* (Rutgers University Press, 1954); and Franco Modigliani and Albert Ando, "Tests of the Life Cycle Hypothesis of Savings," *Bulletin of the Oxford University Institute of Statistics* (1957), pp. 99-124.

[4] For a full discussion of this point, see Richard A. Musgrave, *The Theory of Public Finance* (McGraw-Hill, 1959), pp. 257-72.

fifth of all families in the United States, is responsible for well over two-thirds of aggregate personal saving.[5]

Saving Objectives

Questions about saving objectives were asked as follows:

Different people have different reasons for saving. In your case what are the purposes for saving?

Anything else?

The most common objective—mentioned by half of the respondents—was to accumulate funds for the retirement years. Several persons giving this reply expressed a strong determination to avoid being dependent on the government in their old age, like the respondent who said:

Being an American citizen of the old school, not the present generation, I'm not going to rely on Uncle Sam to do it all. I came up the hard way and believe in that purpose even though you stray from American history. We have lost the individual incentive our forefathers gave us, which was a drive to create something of your own financially and in old age to prove your independence in what you had accomplished. . . .

One-third of the respondents said that they saved "for a rainy day," that is, to provide themselves with security against future emergencies. Another third said that they were saving for their children's education. One in four mentioned the bequest motive:

I think it's to build up an estate basically, and the second reason would be to have support in case of emergency. The building up of the estate is to help the posterity somewhat.

Some respondents appeared to save not with any ultimate purpose in mind but because of past conditioning or simple inertia:

[5] U.S. Bureau of Labor Statistics, *Consumer Expenditures and Income, Total United States, Urban and Rural, 1961,* Bureau of Labor Statistics Report No. 237-93 (February 1965), p. 11. This estimate does not include unrealized capital gains or equity in retirement programs or in life insurance policies. See also Charles Lininger, "Estimates of Rates of Saving," *Journal of Political Economy* (June 1964), pp. 306-11.

Because I was taught by my parents that thrift is a good thing. I always want a backlog, always abhor debt.

This is a strong question. I haven't thought of anything like this for a long time. You usually think of saving in terms of buying a home for your family, or education for your children, or for your old age. But I'm already too old to think of saving for these purposes. The question somehow doesn't apply to me. . . .

A few of the high-income respondents denied that they were able to save anything at all, like the respondent who declared that he saved

. . . to pay taxes. I'm really not able to save anything. I want to save for my grandchildren's education, but each year I sell securities to have cash in the bank with which to pay the estimated income tax. My grandchildren are being deprived.

The relative importance of the main saving objectives differed markedly among income levels, as is illustrated in Chart 4.1. As income increased, there was a steady decline in the proportions saving for retirement or for their children's education. Presumably at the highest income levels most individuals felt confident of meeting these particular needs out of the current income provided by the capital they had already accumulated. One might have expected similar responses on the objective of saving to meet future emergencies, but this objective maintained roughly the same importance at all income levels.

As income rose, the bequest motive, however, became more prominent, being mentioned by about half of those with incomes over $300,000. Unlike the other saving objectives described in Chart 4.1, the bequest motive appears almost exclusively among the high-income group as defined. Other studies have shown that among families with incomes under $10,000, no more than 2 or 3 percent mention the bequest motive.[6]

[6] Representative national samples have been asked about the purposes of saving in a number of surveys conducted by the Survey Research Center. In general the most frequently mentioned purpose is that of saving for emergencies, illness, or unemployment. Next comes saving for retirement, old age, or burial expenses, and then saving for the education of children. See, for example, George Katona, Charles Lininger, and Eva Mueller, *1964 Survey of Consumer Finances* (Survey Research Center, Institute for Social Research, The University of Michigan, 1965), pp. 111-12.

CHART 4.1. Saving Objectives and Income

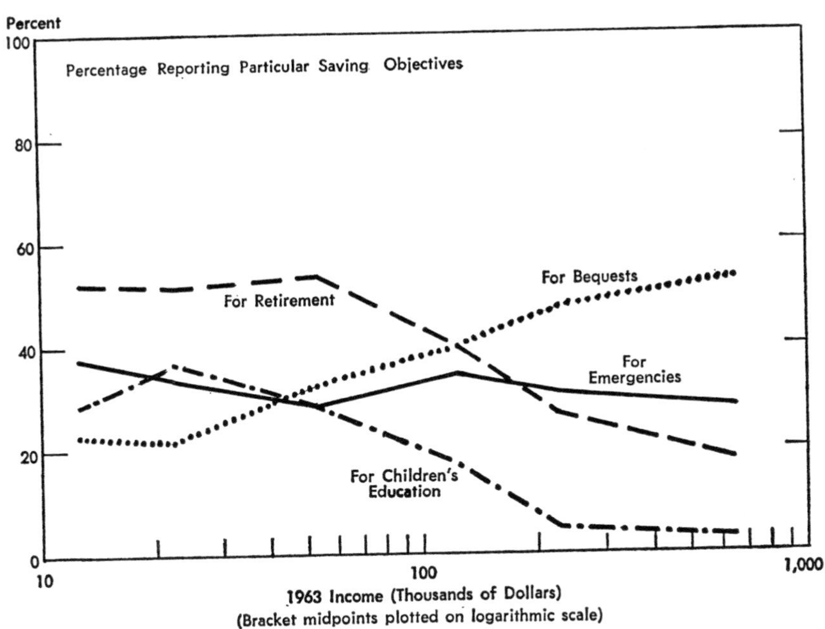

Saving objectives varied with age. The young tended to save for their children's education, the middle-aged for retirement, and the elderly in order to make bequests. Whether or not there were children in the family also made a big difference. The objective of saving for the education of children was, of course, confined to families with dependent children. And respondents without children were less likely to talk of saving to leave an estate. These respondents often mentioned the alternative objective of saving for future vacations or their own consumption in general. One in five of the latter group gave this reason for saving, compared with only one in ten of those with children.

Investment Policies in General

Our investigation of investment policies proceeded in two stages. We first asked the respondent to state how important each of the following investment characteristics was to him: (1) a high current yield (rent, interest, and dividends), (2) safety, (3) liquidity,

CHART 4.2. Factors Associated With a Preference for Current Yield Over Capital Gains

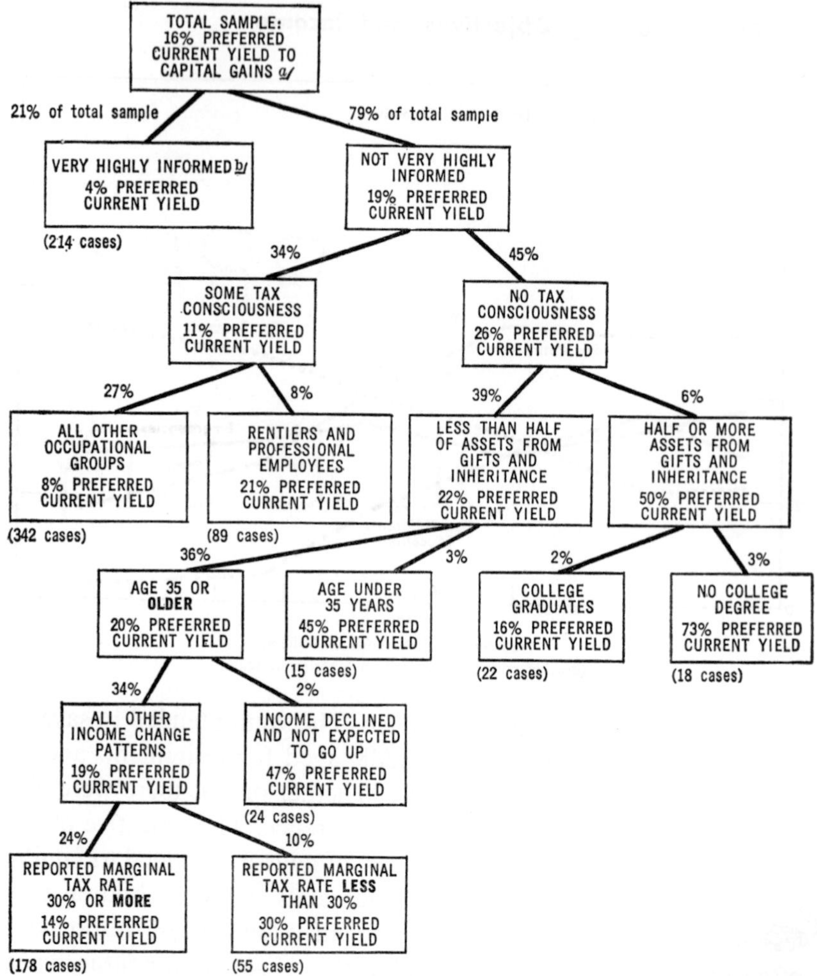

[a] A respondent who ranked current yield as "very important," "important," or "somewhat important" and who also attached less importance to capital gains than he did to current yield was classified as preferring current yield to capital gains.

[b] For technical reasons, this box includes respondents whose total "savings and investments" were worth less than $1,000.

NOTES: Starting with the whole sample in the box at the top of the chart, the program examines all the possible ways of using each of the predictors to split the sample into two subgroups. It selects the "best" split and then repeats the process with each of the two new subgroups. The "best" split is that which makes the biggest contribution toward predicting the dependent variable. The following predictors were used, listed in order of their explanatory power with a single split over the whole sample: (1) level of investment information (for definition, see Chap. VI); (2) tax consciousness (for definition, see Chap. XI); (3) reported marginal income tax rate; (4) whether any dependent children; (5) size of total portfolio; (6) percentage of assets from gifts and inheritances; (7) 1963 adjusted gross income; (8) past and future income changes (for definition, see Appendix E); (9) occupational group; (10) education; (11) age.

Figures on the lines joining the boxes are percentages of the sample in the next lower box.

Figures in the boxes are percentages of that subgroup preferring current yield to capital gains.

Figures below the final boxes in parentheses are the numbers of cases. In this and subsequent tables the number of cases is indicated only for the final groups, because it can be inferred for the others by simple addition. Stability of the estimates is always an inverse function of the number of cases on which they are based.

The nine final groups at the ends of the branches accounted for 17 percent of the total variance.

Details may not add to totals due to rounding.

For further information on this method of analysis, see Appendix F and references given therein.

and (4) capital gains. We then asked them to rate the characteristics as "very important," "important," "somewhat important," "not very important," or "not important at all."[7] Later in the interview the respondent was asked to explain some of his preferences or some specific investment transactions. In this way we were able to observe what investment policies were operative in particular situations.

One would expect that the high-income respondents, in answering the questions about the importance of the four investment characteristics, would seldom have regarded current yield as being more important than capital gains. For persons in the upper income brackets, the differences (in percentage points) between the tax rates applied to ordinary income and those applied to capital gains are too large to be ignored. Nevertheless about one-sixth of the respondents did express a preference for current yield. A multivariate analysis of the sample was performed in an attempt to identify the personal characteristics associated with this preference. Eleven explanatory variables were used in the analysis, the results of which are presented in Chart 4.2.

The analysis suggested that the preference for current yield over capital gains was associated with a general unawareness of investment possibilities rather than with any special financial circumstances that would have rendered such a preference rational. The variable that was most important in predisposing an individual to prefer current yield over capital gains was the adequacy of his investment information.[8] Almost none of those classed as "very highly informed" showed this preference. (This group incidentally included by definition all those employed in the financial sector.) The next most important variable was the level of tax consciousness.[9]

[7] A nearly identical question about the importance of each of the four investment characteristics was asked of a representative national sample in the 1964 Survey of Consumer Finances. Whether one uses only those saying an objective was "very important" or includes also those saying it was "important" or "somewhat important," safety was ranked first by the respondents in the representative sample, then capital gains, then a high current yield, with liquidity in last place. See Katona *et al., op. cit.*, pp. 118-19.

For the high-income sample, however, the ranking put safety and capital gains together in first place, with liquidity next, and a high current yield in last place.

[8] See Chap. VI for a full description of this variable.

[9] See Chap. XI for a full description of this variable.

Among the investors who were less well informed, those who showed no tax consciousness at all were most likely to express a preference for current yield.

Besides current yield and capital gains, we also asked investors about the importance they attached to safety and liquidity. As an investment characteristic, safety was regarded as important by a large majority at all income levels. Moreover, neither age nor the size of the investor's portfolio seemed to affect opinions on the importance of safety. Of the several variables inspected, only the individual's expectations about future income seemed to be strongly related to his views on safety. Those who expected their income to decline in the future were most likely to view safety as a "very important" investment characteristic.

About half of the investors regarded liquidity as being "important" or "very important," and this proportion tended to increase slightly as income rose. But the size of the investor's portfolio apparently did not affect his views on liquidity. Perhaps surprisingly, among the different age groups, the elderly (aged 75 and over) were the least concerned with liquidity. One might have expected that such persons above all others would have sought liquidity, in part to anticipate death tax liabilities and in part to render their estates more attractive to their heirs, but the reverse was true. Nearly half of the elderly said that liquidity was "not very important" or "not important at all," while among the younger respondents less than one-third gave this report.

Interestingly enough the experts in the field of investment management—those respondents who were employed in the financial sector—held a high opinion of liquidity. Only one in seven of this group believed that liquidity was "not very important" or "not important at all."

As an adjunct to the questions on the importance of current yield, capital gains, safety, and liquidity, we asked the following questions:

> Is there anything else important to you in managing your investments?
>
> What is it?

Only a third of the investors said that they took other things into consideration besides the four factors mentioned earlier. These investors most commonly said that they thought it was important to have some familiarity with the company in which they were investing and some acquaintance with its management. Typical of such replies were the following:

> I select securities on the basis of the caliber of management. . . .
>
> I might put money in a company that I'm with even though I could make more elsewhere. I want to be a factor in it.

Some respondents, many of them rentiers, stressed the importance of minimizing anxiety, a concern that was repeated many times in other contexts throughout the interviews:[10]

> What we are striving for is peace of mind. To accomplish this takes a beautifully planned and executed program. I am not sure if a person can ultimately accomplish this peace, but we are striving for it in the planning. . . .
>
> I don't like to turn over my investments. I'm afraid of a tumbling market. I did not want to be involved and so I decided many years ago to purchase land in suburban areas. In this way I don't have to spend too much time, don't have to be bothered thinking and worrying about my investments on a day-to-day basis.

A few respondents said that an important aim of their investment policy was to avoid taxes. These respondents tended to be those with the highest incomes and the largest portfolios:

> The whole area of taxation is a key item. I manage investments so as to legally minimize taxes, conserve as much as possible.
>
> Oh yeah, there is one other thing, and that is to minimize my tax burden in the process.
>
> I regard highly the fact that one can deduct depreciation on real estate when paying income tax. The amount permitted by the government as a deduction for depreciation on property compensates for the capital gains when the property is sold.[11]

[10] See Chap. IX, for example.

[11] For a further discussion of the tax loophole to which this respondent referred, see Chap. XI.

One is impressed by the acumen of such answers but should remember that they were representative of only 4 percent of the entire high-income sample. An awareness of tax considerations was, however, not confined solely to those few who explicitly mentioned taxes in this context. Many of those who regarded capital gains as important were doubtless thinking chiefly of tax considerations.

Preferences Between Growth Stocks and Income Stocks

Further information on investment policies was provided by some inquiries into the reasons behind specific preferences and transactions. For example, we asked stockholders these questions:

> Do you try to keep stocks with high current dividends, or ones that are likely to increase in price, or what?
>
> What are the reasons why you do that?

Of every twelve stockholders, eight expressed an interest in growth stocks exclusively, while only one claimed to have an exclusive interest in income stocks; two expressed an interest in both varieties. The explanations offered by the stockholders for these preferences followed expected patterns. Nearly half of those with an exclusive interest in income stocks said that they needed income at the present rather than in the future. For example, one said:

> I keep stocks with high current dividends for income purposes. That's what I live on.

About a third of the group believed that income stocks offered them a higher return on their investment; and about one in eight thought that such stocks offered the advantage of safety. Very few claimed that there were any tax advantages in income stocks.

Those with an exclusive interest in growth stocks appeared to be reasonably well aware of the tax advantages of such stocks. About a third of the group cited tax considerations, and this proportion tended to increase with income. Among the replies of this nature were the following:

I keep growth stocks—those which have a good future, both current and long-term growth, and a good past history. You lose too much in taxes on current dividends.

I'm interested in earnings, not yield, because of the tax reasons. Capital gains are better than dividends.

Another one-seventh said that growth stocks provided a higher return on their investment, and some of these may have had tax considerations in mind. A third of the group justified their preference by saying that they needed income in the future rather than currently:

I keep stocks that are likely to increase in price. I've no need to use my funds, so I can wait for the increase.

I have mostly growth stocks. I want to build an estate. I'm able to earn professionally, so I don't need the earnings.

One in six of those interested exclusively in growth stocks explained that safety was a major concern to them. However, safety was of more concern to those who were interested in both growth stocks and income stocks. It was mentioned by about one-third of the latter group.

It seems clear from these answers that many of the stockholders were concerned chiefly with avoiding the necessity of having to make frequent decisions in the management of their assets. Those who did not need current cash income from their stockholdings tended to prefer growth stocks because these securities provide a means of accumulating wealth without the necessity of making decisions. For such persons the cash dividends yielded by income stocks would have required continual decisions about reinvestment. Similarly those who did need current income from their stockholdings tended to prefer income stocks because they found it easier to be passive recipients of cash dividends than to make the periodic sales that a portfolio of growth stocks would have entailed. Such persons may have felt that the tax advantages of growth stocks were outweighed by their comparative inconvenience, or more probably, as was suggested by the multivariate analysis of investment policies described above, they may not have been fully aware of the tax situation. At any rate, given the widespread aversion to decision-making, the differential tax treatment of income stocks and growth stocks appears to discriminate among stockholders on the basis of the timing of their income needs. Few would argue that this constitutes a sensible basis for taxation.

As for the personal characteristics of the small group who preferred income stocks, a multivariate analysis probably would have produced results similar to those shown in Chart 4.2. By and large those who claimed to prefer income stocks to growth stocks had also stated earlier in the interview that they regarded a high current yield as more important than capital gains. Correlations with individual variables indicated that the preference for income stocks was most prevalent among those with the lower incomes, those with the smaller portfolios, and those in the older age groups.

Motives for Holding Real Estate

Like common stock, real estate may be held either for current cash income or for appreciation. To find out our respondents' motives for holding real estate we asked:

> Do you or your immediate family own any real estate, land, or a farm (excluding your home)?
>
> (If yes) Is this something you hold mainly for current income, or mainly for long-term increase in value, or what?

Nearly half of the high-income sample owned some real estate. Two-thirds of these owners said that they held the property mainly for appreciation. Most of the remainder held it mainly for current income. A few of the owners reported that they held the property for nonfinancial reasons—for example, out of sentiment because the property had been inherited.

The characteristics of the minority holding real estate for current income paralleled those of the minority who held common stock for the same purpose, with one interesting exception. Like the preference for income stocks, the holding of real estate for current income was most prevalent at the lower incomes and in the older age groups. But whereas the preference for income stocks was associated with smaller portfolios, the holding of real estate for current income was associated with larger portfolios. The explanation for this apparent paradox probably lies in the fact that "income property," such as an apartment building, is usually indivisible and exists only in large units. Hence an investor holding income property possesses *ipso facto* a fairly large portfolio; or conversely, those with small portfolios do not have the means to own income property, although they may have enough to own one or two small lots of vacant land, which they hold for future appreciation.

Past Changes in Portfolio Composition

Respondents were asked to view their portfolios as consisting of three components: fixed-yield assets, common stock, and interests in real estate and unincorporated businesses. We then asked:

> How does your present distribution among these categories differ from the distribution of five years ago?
>
> What are the main reasons for those changes?

The answers to these questions are discussed fully in the next chapter, but the investment policies revealed in the reasons that the respondents gave for the changes in their portfolios are noted here. The chief theme emerging is one of rich diversity of policies and motives. Most commonly the investors who had changed the composition of their portfolios said they had done so to secure more capital appreciation, but only one in eight gave this reply. An almost equal number said that they had been motivated by a desire for more safety in their portfolios, while a few explained that they were less concerned with safety than previously. Among the other leading reasons for changes in portfolio composition were a desire for more liquidity, a policy of expanding one's own business, a preference for investments whose management would involve less trouble and responsibility, and a desire to avoid taxes. But each of these reasons was mentioned by no more than 2 percent of the high-income respondents.

Planned Changes in Portfolio Composition

More information on investment policies was obtained when we asked respondents whether they planned to make some changes in the future in the distribution of their portfolios among the three types of assets mentioned above, and then:

> Why are you thinking of doing this?

About one-fourth of the high-income respondents said that they planned to make changes in the composition of their portfolios. Of every ten respondents in this group, five said that they were motivated by a desire for a higher net return on their investment: two out of the five expressed this motive by saying that they wanted more capital gains, another two simply said that they wanted a higher yield (not specifying whether in the form of appreciation or of cash income), and one mentioned tax considerations. Among the remaining respondents the most important motive was a desire for more safety or diversification.

The desire for more capital gains was most marked among those with the lower incomes and smaller portfolios. Among the wealthiest respondents, the chief concerns were with safety and tax matters. In talking of taxes these persons were not primarily expressing a desire for more capital gains; more often they had municipal bonds in mind. (This point is discussed further in Chapter V.) There is a suggestion in these results that those with the lower incomes felt that they had not yet taken full advantage of the primary means of expanding their wealth, of which the purchase of appreciating assets is one of the most obvious. On the other hand, those with the highest incomes were already using these opportunities to the full and were therefore anxious to consolidate their position through diversification. But it should be stressed that these considerations were of concern to only a minority of the total sample. Three-fourths claimed to be satisfied with the composition of their portfolios and were planning no changes.

Summary

• The objective of saving most frequently mentioned by the high-income group was to provide for retirement or old age. Next in importance was saving for future emergencies, then saving for the education of children, and then saving to bequeath an estate to heirs. Saving for retirement or for children's education became less important as income rose, while the bequest motive became more important.

• In investing their savings, most respondents thought capital gains more important than current cash income. The few who thought otherwise were found to be generally ill-informed about the management of their investments and generally unaware of the tax situation.

• The preference for capital gains was revealed both in general questioning about investment policies and in specific questioning about the holding of growth stocks and income stocks, the motives for owning real estate, and the changes that had been made and were going to be made in the structure of the investors' portfolios.

• Safety and liquidity were regarded as important characteristics of an investment by respondents at all income levels, especially by those employed in the financial sector.

CHAPTER V

Portfolio Composition

THE POLICIES THAT the high-income persons claimed to follow in their personal investment decisions were examined in Chapter IV. This chapter looks at the actual assets that they chose to hold in their portfolios.[1] The term "portfolio" as used here encompasses not only the financial securities owned by the investor but also some of his other assets, such as real estate and interests in unincorporated businesses. A wide variety of assets will be discussed, ranging from those, like unincorporated business interests, where the owner plays an active role in managing the enterprise, to those where the investor is a passive receiver of income, as in the case of government bonds.

Little attempt was made in the survey to get details on the dollar values of the assets owned. It was felt that, given the limited amount of cooperation that could be expected from each respondent, time would be better spent on exploring behavior and motives. Three recent studies that have paid major attention to financial measurement in this area are a Federal Reserve Board sample

[1] All the data in this chapter refer to proportions of the aggregate income of those with incomes over $10,000.

survey of high-income persons, a study of stock ownership, and a longitudinal income and asset study in Wisconsin.[2]

Specific Assets Held

In the survey we inquired about nineteen types of assets. These types are listed in Table 5.1, which shows also how the extent of ownership of the different assets varied with income. For nine of the nineteen types, ownership became more prevalent as income rose; for another six, the extent of ownership remained roughly the same in all income classes over $10,000; and for a small group of four—all of which were of the "fixed-yield" variety—ownership actually declined at the highest income levels. In particular, credit union deposits were rarely held by those with incomes over $30,000, while savings accounts were less popular among those with incomes over $300,000 than among those with incomes between $15,000 and $150,000.

Businesses Both Owned and Managed

Nearly half of the high-income respondents were occupied primarily in running businesses or professional enterprises in which they held ownership interests. (About one in four of this group was a self-employed professional, such as a doctor or lawyer.) For these owner-managers, their holdings in their own enterprises were usually a principal asset. Out of every six respondents in this group, three operated one or more corporations, two operated one or more unincorporated businesses, while one found time to operate businesses of both types, incorporated and unincorporated.

CORPORATIONS. It is often difficult to say who should be regarded as the "owner-manager" of a corporation. To discover whether the respondent was truly a "manager" or "entrepreneur" would have required detailed questioning about his role in the enterprise, the

[2] Dorothy Projector, "Consumer Asset Preferences," *American Economic Review* (May 1965), pp. 227-51; "Survey of Financial Characteristics of Consumers," *Federal Reserve Bulletin* (March 1964); and Jean Crockett and Irwin Friend, "Characteristics of Stock Ownership," *Proceedings of the Business and Economic Statistics Section* (American Statistical Association, 1963), pp. 146-68. The University of Wisconsin study is not yet published.

TABLE 5.1. Ownership of Selected Assets by Income Class

(Percentage in each income group owning asset indicated)[a]

Asset	1963 adjusted gross income						All cases with 1961 income
	$10,000–15,000	$15,000–30,000	$30,000–75,000	$75,000–150,000	$150,000–300,000	$300,000 and over	$10,000 or over
Group I. Assets more widely owned at upper income levels							
Common stock[b]	49	77	85	96	99	99	73
Real estate[c]	35	48	53	63	60	67	47
Own corporation[d]	12	26	43	61	75	64	31
Unincorporated business interests	21	21	30	32	32	36	25
Preferred stock	19	19	32	33	39	33	24
Corporate bonds	10	17	24	31	36	35	19
Municipal bonds	10	8	23	48	52	65	19
U. S. bonds paying currently	4	10	18	21	27	35	13
Treasury bills and notes	1	6	9	14	20	29	7
Group II. Assets owned to about same extent at all income levels							
Own home	88	91	95	92	95	99	91
Checking account	81	94	99	99	99	100	92
Cash-value life insurance	79	90	90	91	85	79	86
Private pension fund	62	61	51	51	57	54	58
Group term life insurance	49	56	58	61	70	50	55
Mutual fund shares	24	29	30	30	32	29	28
Group III. Assets less widely owned at upper income levels							
Savings accounts	67	79	84	78	74	70	76
U. S. savings bonds	46	53	50	51	46	45	50
Mortgages and land contracts	15	16	22	25	22	17	18
Credit union deposits	20	24	5	3	1	8	15
Respondents with total "savings, investments, or reserve funds" under $1,000	15	4	1	0	0	0	6

[a] Respondents with total "savings, investments, or reserve funds" under $1,000 were not asked whether they owned the specific assets listed above, except in the case of pension funds, life insurance, and housing. Therefore, with these exceptions, the percentages given above rest on the assumption that these respondents owned none of the assets in question.
[b] Including stock held in own corporation; excluding mutual fund shares.
[c] Including farms; excluding own home.
[d] Cases where the respondent held stock in a corporation of which he was an executive or director.

kinds of decisions for which he was responsible, etc. To discover whether he was truly a controlling owner would have involved asking what proportion he held of the shares of the enterprise—sometimes a matter of some delicacy. We decided to be content with a crude measure of which respondents were corporate owner-managers, and asked the following questions:

> Do you work for any company in which you own stock?
> Are you an executive or director of the company?

Those answering yes to both questions can be called "stockholder-managers." The individuals in this category, who numbered altogether about a third of the high-income sample, varied greatly in the ownership control and the management control that they exercised over their businesses. At one extreme were sole owners of small privately-held enterprises, while at the other extreme were junior executives holding a few shares in the large corporations for which they worked. The bulk of the group, however, fell into the class of "top management."

Within the total high-income population, the stockholder-managers tended to have the highest incomes and the largest portfolios. Among those respondents with incomes over $150,000, more than two-thirds had the status of stockholder-manager, but among those with incomes between $10,000 and $15,000, only one in eight did.

Stockholder-managers had some possible control over what happened to corporate earnings and also some personal financial interest in the outcome. To find out the usual practices on this, we asked the following questions:

> In those companies in which you are active, are most of the earnings reinvested, or most paid out in dividends, or what?
>
> Why is it done that way?

Nearly two-thirds of the stockholder-managers replied that "most" earnings were reinvested, while only one in eight said that "most" earnings were paid out in dividends. Those who claimed that their company reinvested most of its earnings usually explained that the growth of the business was a prime objective:

> Most of the earnings are reinvested so that the business will perpetuate and grow. This is the only sensible way.
>
> We need the money for growth and expansion.
>
> In our own company we don't aim to pay over half in dividends. We have no borrowed capital in this company. We have grown from within from a capitalization of $30,000 to $60,000,000. At one time we didn't pay any dividends; we believed in plowing money back in. After we became a public company, we set a policy of not paying more than a half. We used the earnings to generate improvements funds.

A few respondents seemed to say that the distribution of earnings was governed by tradition:

Manufacturing, retailing, and utilities historically pay 50 percent of profits out in dividends.

Only one in fourteen among the stockholder-managers explicitly said that tax considerations affected the disposition of corporate income. One respondent, for example, remarked as follows:

Most earnings are reinvested. The stockholders are primarily interested in capital gains and avoiding income subject to income tax.

Tax considerations usually dictate that corporate earnings be retained rather than paid out. However, one feature of the tax law has the effect of discouraging retention of earnings, namely the imposition of the penalty tax on "improper accumulations of surplus." Among our respondents, those who said that most corporate earnings were paid out were more likely to mention tax considerations in explaining their policy than were those who said that most earnings were reinvested. It should be stressed, however, that in neither case were taxes mentioned by more than a few of the respondents.

Were the differences in policy regarding earnings distribution associated with any differences in personal characteristics? Those saying that most earnings were paid out were remarkably similar in most respects to those saying that most earnings were reinvested. The two groups differed, neither in income, nor in portfolio size, nor in tax consciousness. There was not even any special tendency for those in "reinvestment" situations to have declared earlier in the interview that they preferred capital gains to current yield. Only one variable appeared to distinguish clearly between the two groups—the respondent's age. Almost none of the stockholder-managers under forty-five years of age said that most of their company's earnings were paid out; but this reply was relatively frequent among the older businessmen, such as the one who said, "At my age and income I'm not interested in expanding my business." Corporate growth, it seems, was pursued most enthusiastically by those businessmen who expected to live long enough to see the results of their efforts.

UNINCORPORATED BUSINESSES. One-fourth of the high-income group had money invested in an unincorporated business, and this proportion tended to increase as income rose. About two-thirds of these owners worked full time in the business, and another one in seven worked part time. About one-fifth of the owners—that is, 4 percent of the entire high-income sample—were "sleeping partners." They had retired from the business but retained a financial interest, or they had never been active in the management of the business. (One-fifth of the "sleeping partners" were male rentiers; almost all of the remainder were actively working elsewhere in the labor force.)

Like the corporate owner-managers, the owners of unincorporated businesses were asked about their policies regarding the disposition of earnings. Compared with the corporate sector, a higher rate of "pay-out" was observed. Fewer than half of the unincorporated business owners said that most earnings were usually reinvested (compared with nearly two-thirds of the corporate owner-managers), while one-third of the owners (compared with one-eighth of the corporate owner-managers) said that most earnings were usually paid out. This difference between the sectors in the disposition of earnings was not unexpected, since the unincorporated sector includes many enterprises, like those involving a professional practice, which require little in the way of physical plant.

Only one-twelfth of the unincorporated business owners explicitly said that tax considerations affected the distribution of their profits. This is not surprising, however, because in the case of unincorporated businesses the owner's current tax liability does not depend on whether the earnings are retained or distributed.

The owners of unincorporated businesses were asked how long they planned to stay in the business, and three-fourths replied that they would stay "indefinitely." Several of these expressed intentions —or predictions—about dying in harness, saying that they would continue working in the business "till I die" or "till I fall out of my chair." Only one in eleven owners planned to quit within the next five years.

The owners were then asked what would happen to their businesses after they had withdrawn from them. Out of every ten owners, two said that they would eventually pass on their interests to relatives (usually a son); one out of ten planned to transfer his interest to an unrelated partner who was already in the business; one out of ten planned to sell his interest to outsiders; and one out of ten planned to liquidate or wind up the business. Three out of ten, however, had no idea what would happen to their businesses when they no longer ran them.

Common Stock

Holdings of common stock account for a major part of the wealth of the wealthy. Three-fourths of the high-income respondents owned some common stock,[3] and ownership became almost universal at the highest incomes. Among the 150 individuals in the sample whose incomes exceeded $150,000, only two owned no stock. Stock ownership was most extensive among female rentiers and those working in the financial sector, both owner-managers and employees. In these groups about nine out of ten owned stock.

Out of every seven high-income stockholders, two owned holdings worth less than $10,000 and, on the average, held stock in only two companies.[4] Three out of seven had holdings worth between $10,000 and $100,000, in an average of six companies. One out of seven held common stock worth between $100,000 and $500,000, in an average of fourteen companies. Finally, one out of seven—or about one-tenth of the entire high-income sample—reported owning stock worth over half a million dollars, and these respondents on the average held stock in twenty-five companies.

Mutual Fund Shares

One-fourth of the high-income group held shares in a mutual fund, and this proportion remained roughly constant at all income levels. Moreover, the different occupational groups were remarkably similar in the extent of mutual fund ownership. Only the self-employed professionals, among whom two out of five held such assets, departed noticeably from the norm.

[3] The data in this section refer to "portfolio" holdings in companies where the stockholders held no management role and to holdings of stockholder-managers in their own businesses. Virtually all of the stockholder-managers owned "portfolio" stockholdings in addition to their interests in their own businesses. Among all stockholders in the sample, only 4 percent were in the position of owning some stock in the company which they helped to manage but no stock in any other enterprise.

[4] The dollar values cited here and in the following sentences include mutual fund shares as well as common stock owned directly, but all other information in this section excludes mutual fund shares. For more details on mutual fund ownership, see below. The "average" number of companies cited here and in the following sentences is a median figure.

Of the several explanatory variables tested, only the degree of tax consciousness appeared to be strongly associated with mutual fund ownership.[5] Among those respondents who showed no tax consciousness throughout the interview, only one in five held mutual fund shares, whereas among the others nearly two in five did. Many respondents were presumably attracted by the combination of advantages of mutual funds—the tax advantages inherent in the earning of capital gains, the convenience of having those gains provided regularly in the form of a cash flow, and the escape from the chores of decision making. About one-third of the mutual fund owners, it may be noted, said that they had invested in a "growth" fund.

Real Estate

Nearly half of the high-income group owned some real estate other than their own homes. This proportion increased steadily with income, but ownership was fairly widespread, even at the lower incomes. Of those with incomes between $10,000 and $15,000, slightly less than two-fifths owned this type of asset. In the sample as a whole, the popularity of real estate as an investment varied somewhat as between residents of large cities and those in smaller places. Among those respondents living in the twelve largest metropolitan areas in the United States, less than two-fifths owned real estate, but of those living in smaller communities, more than half did.

Fixed-Yield Assets

These are assets that pay a fixed amount of interest annually. Among the nine assets of this type that we investigated, savings accounts, held by three-fourths of the high-income respondents, and U.S. savings bonds, held by one-half, were the most widely owned. But both of these kinds of assets were somewhat less popular at the highest levels of income. Presumably many of those with the highest marginal tax rates found that whatever advantages these assets had in the way of liquidity and safety did not compensate for the meagerness of their after-tax yields. Nevertheless some high-income respondents continued to place great stress on the attributes of safety and liquidity. A few said that they regarded savings accounts as an

[5] The tax-consciousness variable is defined fully in Chap. XI.

attractive investment because of the insurance of deposits (to a maximum of $10,000 on each account) by the Federal Deposit Insurance Corporation, though no others had taken as full advantage of this insurance feature as the respondent who said:

> I really have overloaded on this. I have more than half a million in savings banks. I have it in $10,000 amounts in perhaps 55 banks in different cities throughout the country.

Two other types of fixed-yield assets—mortgages and land contracts, and credit union deposits—also were less popular at the highest levels of income. One feature worth noting about mortgages and land contracts is that, as between occupational groups, ownership was most extensive among realtors and contractors, for whom the acquisition of such investments was a natural part of their business. Two-thirds of these respondents owned mortgages or land contracts, compared with only one-sixth of the remainder.

By contrast, the other five types of fixed-yield assets—preferred stock, corporate bonds, U.S. bonds paying interest currently, Treasury bills and notes, and state and local government bonds ("municipals")—were all owned more extensively at the upper income levels. Not unexpectedly, the most dramatic increase in popularity (as income rose) was enjoyed by municipal bonds, the interest from which is tax-exempt. Among respondents with incomes over $300,000, each of the other four types of assets was owned by about a third of the group, but municipals were owned by two-thirds. We now turn to some further details concerning the ownership of municipals.

MUNICIPAL BONDS. One-fifth of the high-income group owned municipal bonds. In one-third of these cases, the interest yielded by the municipal bonds was more than one-tenth of total family income.[6]

[6] The estimate of aggregate interest payments obtainable from these survey data is remarkably close to independent estimates from other sources. Using the survey data, Okner has estimated that payments of municipal bond interest to individual investors in 1962 totaled $1,167 million. See Benjamin A. Okner, *Income Distribution and the Federal Income Tax* (Institute of Public Administration, The University of Michigan, 1966).

An independent estimate, based on *total* interest paid on state and local bonds and Federal Reserve Flow of Funds estimates of the proportion of recipients that were consumers and nonprofit institutions, is $1,046 million. See Federal

As was noted above, the extent of ownership increased rapidly with income, from about one-tenth among those with incomes between $10,000 and $30,000 to about two-thirds of those with incomes over $300,000. Indeed, it is surprising that those with the lower incomes owned any municipals at all. The tax-exempt status of municipals causes these bonds to carry an interest rate lower than that on taxable securities of comparable quality. Hence for those individuals with marginal tax rates below a critical level, taxable securities offer a more profitable investment than do municipals. (In addition, the high unit value of municipal bonds poses a formidable barrier for the small investor. Some but not all of the taxable investments available to him have this disadvantage.) As for those at the other end of the income scale, where high marginal tax rates increase the attractiveness of municipals relative to taxable securities, one might wonder why the ownership of municipals was not practically universal. The answer presumably is that many of these individuals exploited tax havens that were even more lucrative than the ownership of municipals or enjoyed business opportunities whose after-tax yield exceeded that on municipals. After all, an investment yielding capital gains needs only to yield one-third more than do municipals to be a better investment, even at the highest incomes.[7]

In order to throw more light on the personal characteristics of the respondents who owned municipal bonds, we performed a multivariate analysis. Eleven explanatory variables were used, and the results are presented in Chart 5.1.

Reserve System, *Flow of Funds Accounts, 1945-1962,* 1963 Supplement, p. 34, Table 24.

A third estimate made by the Treasury Department and the Joint Economic Committee is that consumers receive a total of $900 million in tax-exempt interest. See U.S. Congress, Joint Economic Committee, *The Federal Tax System: Facts and Problems,* 88 Cong. 2 sess. (1964), p. 19.

[7] Other views on this question have recently been expressed by Maxwell as follows: "The volume of exempts held by this group [of high-income persons] has always been less than an inspection of the tax advantages might suggest. The explanation is that many high-income persons prefer to be active rather than passive investors; they prefer an investment that may bring either appreciable capital gains, or, as with ownership of equities, involves participation in the operation of a business. To them the tax advantages of exempts are not decisive." See James A. Maxwell, *Financing State and Local Governments* (Brookings Institution, 1965), p. 193.

CHART 5.1. Factors Associated With the Ownership of Municipals

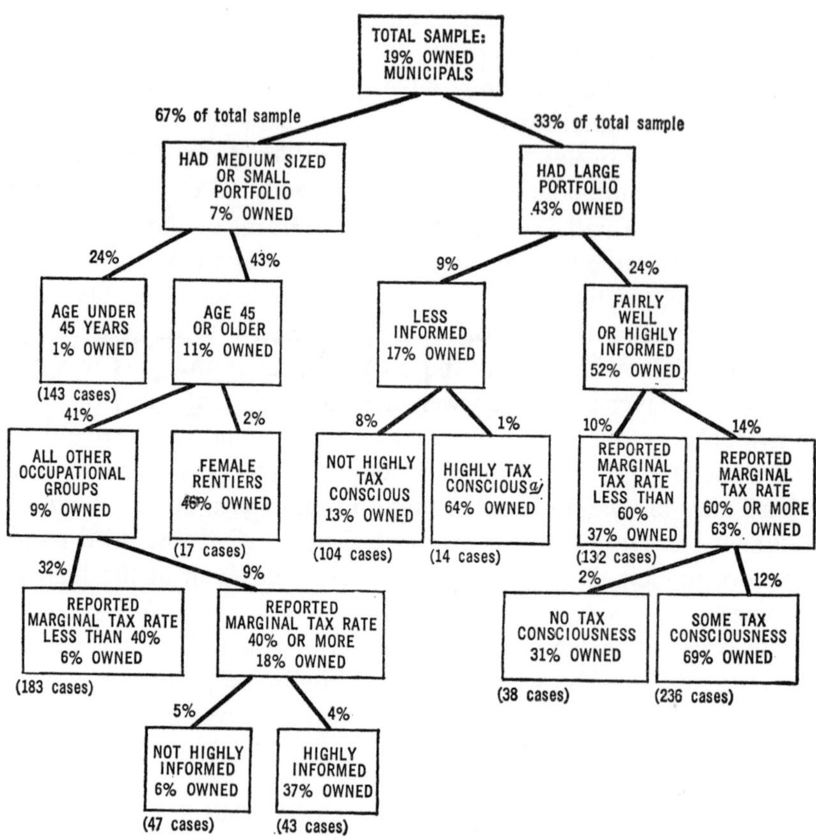

[a] Tax consciousness index of 4 or more.

NOTES: For explanation, see notes to Chart 4.2. In this chart the following predictors were used, listed in order of their explanatory power with a single split over the whole sample: (1) size of total portfolio (for definition, see Table 5.2); (2) 1963 adjusted gross income; (3) tax consciousness (for definition, see Chap. XI); (4) reported marginal tax rate; (5) level of investment information (for definition, see Chap. VI); (6) age; (7) occupational group; (8) preference between capital gains and current yield; (9) whether any dependent children; (10) education; (11) whether lived in a metropolitan area. The ten final groups at the ends of the branches accounted for 34 percent of the total variance.

The analysis showed that the variable most important in distinguishing between the owners of municipal bonds and the nonowners was the size of their total portfolios. That is, to some degree municipal bonds were a standard or customary component of large portfolios but were rarely held in small portfolios. Next, it appeared that ownership of municipals was a sign of a sophisticated investor. Among those with large portfolios, there was a wide gap between those classified as "fairly well or highly informed," half of whom held municipals, and those who were less well informed, only one-sixth of whom held these assets. Sophistication was also indicated by the respondent's degree of tax consciousness, and at two points in the analysis this variable emerged as differentiating sharply between owners and nonowners.

As expected, the analysis showed that ownership was fairly sensitive to the level of the investor's marginal tax rate. Finally, it appeared that, other things being equal, municipals were favored more by the old or retired than by the young. This may be because municipals do not offer much capital appreciation or growth, and long-run growth was often a major concern among the younger respondents.

THE TOTAL VALUE OF FIXED-YIELD ASSETS. Nine-tenths of the high-income group owned fixed-yield assets, and these respondents were asked to estimate the value of their total holdings of such assets. One-third said that the assets were worth under $10,000, one-half said they were worth between $10,000 and $100,000, while one-sixth said they were worth over $100,000. Among occupational groups it was the rentiers who had invested the most heavily in fixed-yield assets. In particular, nearly three-fifths of the female rentiers owned fixed-yield assets worth over $100,000. By contrast only one in eight among the self-employed professionals had invested that much in fixed-yield assets.

Life Insurance

Life insurance rights form a major asset for many high-income persons, and as an investment receive favorable tax treatment in several ways.[8] One popular form of insurance with important tax advantages is group term life insurance provided by a company to

[8] For a further discussion of the tax advantages of life insurance, see Chap. XI.

its executive employees as a fringe benefit. To find out how extensive such arrangements were, we asked:

> Do you have any group term life insurance that is paid for by a company?

More than half of the high-income respondents had such insurance, and this proportion remained roughly the same at all income levels. As would be expected, employees were covered more extensively than were the self-employed. Among non-professional employees, no less than four out of five held such insurance. For professional employees (those employed as physicians, lawyers, engineers, architects, or scientists), the proportion was two-thirds. By contrast, only one-fifth of the self-employed professionals held group term life insurance.

We then asked about non-term life insurance:

> Do you have any life insurance that has a cash value, or that you can borrow on if you want to?

Six out of seven in the high-income group held such life insurance. This proportion tended first to rise with income, and then ultimately to fall. Among those with incomes between $10,000 and $15,000, and also among those with incomes over $300,000, only eight out of ten held ordinary insurance; but among those with incomes between $15,000 and $300,000, nine out of ten did.

The older respondents were less likely to hold life insurance. Among those aged seventy-five or over, only 60 percent held such insurance, whereas among respondents who were under thirty-five, 95 percent did. The unmarried respondents were also less likely to hold insurance: only 60 percent did, compared with 89 percent of the married respondents.

Among occupational groups, the holding of non-term life insurance was extensive in all except that of female rentiers, of whom only one-fourth held such insurance. Finally, it was noted somewhat unexpectedly that there was no tendency for wealth to be substituted for insurance. Those with the largest portfolios were just as likely to hold insurance as were those with the smallest portfolios.

The purchase of non-term life insurance has at least two features to recommend it as a way of saving money. First are the tax advantages. Second, the regular payment of premiums imposes a sort of discipline which the would-be saver might otherwise find hard to sustain. Of course, these advantages are to some extent offset by the insurance company's loading charges and by the fact that the interest yield is generally a fixed return which does not increase with inflation.

To find out our respondents' opinions on this we asked:

What do you think of life insurance as a way of saving money?

Opinion was very evenly divided on this issue. One-third of the respondents thought that life insurance was a good way of saving money, one-third thought it was a bad way, and one-third was on the fence. Those who held a good opinion of life insurance in this context usually said that they liked being compelled to set money aside with regularity:

I think it's an excellent way, because you have to make monthly payments and the only way I can get something saved is when I get a monthly bill.

I think it is a very fine way. Anything that organizes savings on a regular basis is good even though it is not as good percentagewise as some other investments.

Those who held a poor opinion of life insurance as a method of saving usually referred to the low rate of return:

Well, of course, life insurance is necessary, but I think it is far from a good way to save. The return is too low. If I weren't married, I would have no insurance.

I'm rather disillusioned with life insurance. You only get back what you pay. It doesn't allow for changes in prices and money values.

I think of it only as a way of producing cash for the payment of inheritance taxes.

It is bunk. I buy stock in life insurance companies. I figure if anyone's going to be sap enough to spend his money that way, I'll take some of it.

The high-income respondents were generally unaware of the tax advantages of buying life insurance. Only 1 percent of the entire group mentioned tax considerations when talking about life insurance as a method of saving.[9]

What personal characteristics were associated with these varying opinions? Those with favorable opinions did not differ significantly from those with poor opinions in any of the following characteristics: income, portfolio size, degree of tax consciousness, or percentage of personal wealth derived from gifts and inheritances. It was found, however, that the respondent's age did make a difference. Among the respondents aged sixty-five or over, those who believed life insurance to be a good method of saving were twice as numerous as those who did not. But among the respondents aged under thirty-five, they were only half as numerous. This difference in views presumably reflects the preoccupation of the younger respondents with long-run capital appreciation, a characteristic which life insurance does not usually have.[10]

Finally, it appeared that the best-informed investors were somewhat inclined to hold unfavorable views about life insurance as a method of saving. Among those investors classified as "highly informed" or "very highly informed,"[11] those holding a low opinion of life insurance outnumbered by five to four those with a favorable view; but among the other investors, those with a high opinion were in the majority. This should not be taken as a fully authoritative assessment of life insurance as a method of saving since, as was

[9] When asked about life insurance in other studies of the Survey Research Center, lower-income people talked almost entirely about provision for dependents, and middle-income people somewhat more about insurance as a method of saving funds for emergency borrowing, children's education, or retirement. But interest in life insurance for saving purposes was no greater in high-income families than in middle-income ones. And the Center's Midwest City Study of high-income people also showed only moderate interest in insurance for saving purposes. See J. L. Miner, *Life Insurance Ownership Among American Families, 1957* (Survey Research Center, The University of Michigan, 1958); and George Katona and John Lansing, "The Wealth of the Wealthy," *Review of Economics and Statistics,* Vol. 46 (February 1964), pp. 1-13.

[10] The fact that the elderly respondents held a relatively favorable view of life insurance as a method of saving does not imply that they were more likely than other groups in the population to own this kind of asset. As is clear from results presented in the previous section, whatever the elderly may have thought of life insurance *qua* method of saving, they were relatively uninterested in life insurance *qua* insurance.

[11] For a full description of this variable, see Chap. VI.

noted above, one of the chief advantages of this form of investment —the tax-avoidance feature—was not adequately recognized, even by those investors who appeared in other ways to be well informed.

Pension Funds

Nine out of ten high-income respondents were covered by social security, but only three out of five were covered by a private pension plan. The latter proportion was fairly constant throughout all income groups and also throughout all age groups below sixty-five.[12] Among older respondents, only two out of five were covered by a private plan. To some extent, the possession of other assets acted as a substitute for a pension. Among those with small portfolios, four out of five were covered by a private plan, but among those with large portfolios, only two out of five were so covered.[13]

About one-fourth of the respondents who were covered by a private plan had been offered various choices as to the form of the plan, such as whether it should provide a lump-sum payment or an annuity, or whether the funds should be invested in low-risk or medium-risk securities. Asked about the factors governing their choices among these options, the respondents usually talked about the particular needs of their dependents (usually their wives) or the type of retirement income they wanted. Only rarely were tax considerations mentioned in this context.

The respondents were then asked specifically about the option of deciding how much money should be paid regularly into their retirement plans. Those who had some freedom in this matter usually said that their decisions rested on their need for income during retirement relative to their need for income at present. Virtually none said that the size of their pension contributions had been governed by tax considerations.

[12] In the working population as a whole only a little more than a third of the individuals and family heads were covered by private pension plans in 1962-63. See George Katona, *Private Pensions and Individual Saving,* Monograph 40 (Survey Research Center, The University of Michigan, 1965).

[13] For a detailed definition of the various portfolio sizes see Table 5.2. Pensions were *not* a substitute for asset accumulation for the whole working population studied in the pension study referred to in note 12 above. In that study those with a private pension were found to be saving more than those without one, even when the pension payments themselves were not counted as saving.

TABLE 5.2. The Size and Composition of Portfolios

(Percentages of the aggregate income received by those with 1961 adjusted gross income over $10,000)

Value of common stock[b] owned	Individuals owning fixed-yield assets[a] worth: Under $10,000			Between $10,000 and $100,000			More than $100,000			Total
	and interests in real estate and unincorporated businesses worth									
	Under $10,000	*Between $10,000 and $100,000*	*More than $100,000*	*Under $10,000*	*Between $10,000 and $100,000*	*More than $100,000*	*Under $10,000*	*Between $10,000 and $100,000*	*More than $100,000*	
Under $10,000	21[c]	6	2	6	7	1	0	1	1	45
Between $10,000 and $100,000	6	3	1	9	7	2	1	0	1	30
More than $100,000	2	1	1	3	2	2	4	2	5	22
Total	29	10	4	18	16	5	5	3	7	100[d]

Note: The information above was used to define portfolio sizes as follows:

Large portfolios (more than $100,000 in one or more asset-types) 30%
Medium-sized portfolios (where the largest asset-type had a value between $10,000 and $100,000) 40
Small portfolios (where the largest asset-type had a value below $10,000) 27

Details may not add to totals due to rounding.

[a] Savings accounts, credit union deposits, corporate bonds, preferred stock, U. S. savings bonds, U. S. bonds paying interest currently, Treasury bills and notes, state and local government bonds, mortgages and land contracts.

[b] Including mutual fund shares.

[c] Including those cases (numbering 6 percent of the entire sample) with total "savings, investments, and reserve funds" under $1,000.

[d] Including those cases (numbering 2 percent of the entire sample) where the value of any of the three asset-types was not ascertained.

The Size and Composition of Portfolios

In the case of three major asset types—common stock, fixed-yield assets, and interests in real estate and unincorporated businesses—the respondents were asked in which of three broad dollar brackets—under $10,000, $10,000 to $100,000, or over $100,000—the value of their total holdings fell. The results of these inquiries are presented in Table 5.2.

The principal pattern emerging from Table 5.2 is that most of the high-income individuals struck a fairly even balance in their portfolios among the three types of assets. For one-third of the group, the values of the three asset types fell in the same dollar bracket. For another one-fourth, the values of two of the types were in the same bracket, with the value of the third in the next lower bracket. Only 4 percent of the entire group were in the extreme situation of owning more than $100,000 of one asset type and less than $10,000 of each of the other two.

The respondents were also asked in which of the three types of assets they had the most money invested. Roughly speaking, one-half of the high-income group had most invested in common stock, one-fourth had most invested in fixed-yield assets, and one-fourth had most invested in interests in real estate and unincorporated businesses. The proportion having most invested in common stock rose steadily with income, reaching about three-fourths among those with incomes over $300,000. The proportion whose major asset type consisted of interests in real estate and unincorporated businesses remained roughly the same at all income levels below $300,000, but then declined sharply. As income rose, the proportion favoring fixed-yield assets first fell rapidly but eventually climbed back to its earlier levels, reflecting the popularity of tax-exempt municipal bonds among those with the highest incomes.

Changes in Portfolio Composition

How has the relative popularity of stocks, bonds, and other forms of assets changed in the last few years? What groups in the population have been most active in changing from one type of asset to another?

Past Changes

We reminded our respondents about the three major categories of assets—common stocks, fixed-yield assets, and interests in real estate and unincorporated businesses—and then asked:

> How does your present distribution among these categories differ from the distribution five years ago?

Two-thirds of the high-income respondents said that their distribution among the three categories had not changed appreciably. Of those who had experienced some change, about half were more concentrated than previously in common stock, about one-third were more concentrated in fixed-yield assets, while about one-fourth were more concentrated in real estate or unincorporated business interests. On the basis of this evidence alone, it would seem that the aggregate value of stockholdings has been increasing more rapidly than the values of the other asset types.

The reasons for the shifts in portfolio composition have been discussed in Chapter IV. Here the particular groups in the population who were responsible for those shifts are noted. It was found that the frequency and type of changes in portfolio composition did not vary according to income, portfolio size, or the expressed preference between capital gains and current yield. However, there was a tendency for the older respondents, particularly the rentiers, to have made more changes in the composition of their portfolios, and for these people to have shifted out of common stock and into fixed-yield assets to a greater degree than did the rest of the high-income population.

Most strikingly, it was found that there were sharp distinctions between informed and uninformed investors in the frequency and type of changes in portfolio composition. Among those classified as "very highly," "highly," or "fairly well" informed, nearly one-half had made changes, and this group had usually moved into common stock, next most often into fixed-yield assets, and least often into real estate or unincorporated businesses. But among those classified as "somewhat informed," "relatively uninformed," or "uninformed," less than one-third had made changes, and this group had generally moved into real estate or unincorporated businesses, next most often into stock, and least often into fixed-yield assets. The relatively high popularity of fixed-yield assets among the well informed investors presumably reflects the tax advantages of municipal bonds.

Planned Changes

To find out what further changes in portfolio composition were being planned, we asked the following questions:

> Are you generally satisfied with the way your money is now distributed among these (three) categories, or are there some changes you have been thinking of making?
>
> (If any changes) What changes have you been thinking of making?

About three-fourths of the high-income respondents said that they were satisfied with the present composition of their portfolios. The one-fourth who were dissatisfied and planning to make changes favored common stocks the most, interests in real estate and unincorporated businesses next, and were least favorable toward fixed-yield assets. (The reasons for these plans have been discussed in Chapter IV.)

Which groups in the population were dissatisfied? Mainly it was the younger and more active investors. Dissatisfaction was not related to income, portfolio size, or the expressed preference between capital gains and current yield. But those investors who showed the greatest sophistication in terms of tax consciousness, who had been the most active in buying and selling in the investment market, and who had actually changed the broad composition of their portfolios in recent years did show the most dissatisfaction with their present situation. Being knowledgeable and active in portfolio management did not always bring contentment, and many of these investors continued to search for further improvements.

The dissatisfied investors tended also to be young. Among all high-income respondents under thirty-five years of age, two out of five expressed dissatisfaction, but among those sixty-five or over, only one in eight did so. These age differences were reflected in the differences among occupational groups. Rentiers were overwhelmingly satisfied with their present positions, while employees (who were usually younger than the self-employed) were often dissatisfied. In one respect, however, occupation as such did appear to have some influence. Those working in the financial sector, both self-employed and employees, were in almost all cases well satisfied with their own portfolio composition—understandably so, since these investors were in the course of their daily work continuously supplied with information about new investment opportunities.

The changes that the dissatisfied investors intended to make in the composition of their portfolios are shown in Table 5.3, which also shows the links between past changes in portfolio composition and planned changes. The dissatisfied investors who had been moving into common stock and interests in real estate and unincorporated businesses tended to feel that they should move even more in the same direction and away from fixed-yield assets. Those who had

TABLE 5.3. Past and Planned Changes in Portfolio Composition

(Percentages of the aggregate income received by those with 1961 adjusted gross income over $10,000)[a]

Change in portfolio composition during last five years		*Present attitude toward portfolio composition*		*Future changes in portfolio composition planned by those dissatisfied with present composition*					
				More in:			*Less in:*		
Type of change	*Percentage distribution*	*Satisfied[b]*	*Dissatisfied*	*Stock*	*Bonds*	*Realty, etc.*	*Stock*	*Bonds*	*Realty, etc.*
More in stock	16.5	11.5	5.0	2.0	2.0	0.5	0.5	1.0	0.5
More in bonds	10.0	6.0	4.0	1.5	0.5	0.5	0.5	0.5	0.5
More in realty, etc.	8.0	5.5	2.5	0.5	0.0	1.0	0.5	0.5	0.5
No change[c]	67.5	55.0[d]	12.5	5.0	2.0	2.5	1.5	1.5	1.0
Total[e]	100.0	76.5	23.5	8.5	3.0	4.0	2.5	3.5	2.5

[a] The groups shown in each of the columns are not mutually exclusive. Throughout the table "stock" refers to common stock including mutual fund shares, "bonds" refers to nine types of fixed-yield assets (corporate bonds, U. S. savings bonds, U. S. bonds paying interest currently, Treasury bills and notes, state and local government bonds, preferred stock, mortgages and land contracts, savings accounts, and credit union deposits), and "realty, etc." refers to interests in real estate and unincorporated businesses. Percentages are shown to the nearest 0.5 percent.

[b] Includes those who were "satisfied" or "satisfied, with qualifications" and those (numbering 2 percent of the entire sample) who did not report whether or not they were satisfied.

[c] Includes those (numbering 6 percent of the sample) whose change was not ascertained and those (another 6 percent) whose total "savings, investment, and reserve funds" were under $1,000.

[d] Includes all those whose total "savings, investments, and reserve funds" were under $1,000. These cases were not asked the relevant questions.

[e] Totals for the entire sample, without double counting.

been moving into fixed-yield assets were, first, more likely than the other groups to be dissatisfied with their experience and, second, when they were dissatisfied, usually planning to move out of bonds and into stock.

All of these patterns, however, were reversed for the wealthiest and most sophisticated investors. Among those with the highest incomes and largest portfolios, and among those who showed the greatest degree of tax consciousness, the prevailing intention was not to move from bonds into stock but from stock into bonds. Doubtless this intention stemmed partly from a judgment on the part of the more knowledgeable investors that the stock market in the spring of 1964, when the interviews were taken, was "too high."

Finally, a clear relationship was observed between a respondent's age and his plans to change the composition of his portfolio. The young favored stocks—thus exhibiting again their strong interest in growth investments—while the old favored bonds. At the extremes, none at all of those in the sample under thirty-five years of age planned to decrease their stockholdings, and none at all of those aged seventy-five or over planned to decrease their bondholdings.

Summary

• One-third of the high-income respondents owned stock in a corporation in whose management they were active, and one-fourth had money invested in an unincorporated business.

• Three-fourths of the high-income respondents owned common stock, and one-half owned real estate (other than their own homes).

• The ownership of certain fixed-yield assets—in particular, savings accounts, U.S. savings bonds, credit union deposits, and mortgages and land contracts—became less frequent as income rose beyond $150,000.

• By contrast, the ownership of tax-exempt municipal bonds was confined almost exclusively to those with the highest incomes. Among the wealthiest investors, "municipals" were owned mostly by those who were better informed and older than the average.

• More than half of the high-income respondents were covered by group term life insurance, and six out of seven held ordinary life insurance. Many respondents held a poor opinion of life insurance as a method of saving.

• Three-fifths of the high-income group were covered by a private pension plan.

• Among the three broad asset types considered, common stocks were the largest component of the portfolio for one-half of the high-income respondents, fixed-yield assets were the largest component for one-fourth, and interests in real estate and unincorporated businesses were the largest component for the remaining one-fourth.

• One-third of the respondents had experienced, in the previous few years, a change in the distribution of their assets among the three broad categories mentioned. Usually the changes had involved a greater proportion of their assets being held in the form of common stock.

• One-fourth of the high-income respondents—usually the younger and more active investors—were dissatisfied with the present composition of their portfolios. Generally they planned to substitute stock for fixed-yield assets.

CHAPTER VI

Information Sources and Market Activity

IN CHAPTER III it was noted that most high-income persons appeared to manage their investments themselves. There were relatively few cases where the respondent had delegated to others all responsibility for the management of his portfolio. The question naturally arises as to whether the investors were performing competently in managing their own assets—whether they were making good use of the various sources of information available to them, for example. It is not only individual investors, of course, who should be concerned about whether their personal decisions are well informed. The entire economy has an important stake in ensuring the efficient allocation of scarce money capital among competing uses.[1]

In the survey we asked certain questions about the sources of information used by investors. We also asked about their recent transactions in the capital market, and in this way we were able to ascertain whether or not the most active and influential investors

[1] All the data in this chapter refer to proportions of the aggregate income of those with 1961 incomes over $10,000.

were also the best informed. Furthermore we asked about the motives underlying some of the transactions and can thus infer how investors would respond to various changes in their environment, including those changes brought about by public policy.

Information Sources

We asked investors about two types of information sources: verbal advice and written publications. The use made of these two sources then enabled us to classify investors according to how well informed they were.

Verbal Advice

Concerning the verbal advice, we asked:

In handling the investments which you manage yourself, do you get advice from other people?

For what kinds of investment decisions do you usually get advice?

Do you get advice from a stockbroker, a business colleague, or whom?

What special information are you able to get?

About three-fourths of the high-income respondents who managed their own assets said that they got advice from others in making their investment decisions. One in three of those seeking advice said that they "always" sought advice when investing, while two out of three said they did "occasionally." Several were emphatic about the necessity of consulting experts:

I don't do anything without investigating. I seek advice on everything, and I make my own decisions to buy and sell.

I think a person should never be too big to ask for advice or opinions. I don't always follow it, but I have friends in every walk of life: attorneys, philanthropists, bankers, accountants, politicians. When I have something on my mind, I go to them, depending on the advice or information I need. They talk it through with me. Tonight, for instance, I am having dinner with the state attorney general.

The advice was usually sought for common stock transactions;

about two-thirds of those seeking advice gave this reply. Only one-sixth of the group said that they usually sought advice for fixed-yield investments, while about one-third mentioned seeking advice for investments in real estate and unincorporated businesses, like the respondent who said:

> I try to get all the information I can about what I am looking for. Right now, I'm interested in buying a ranch for a grandson.

The persons consulted by the investors were most often qualified professionals, like stockbrokers and investment counselors. About four-fifths of those seeking advice gave this reply, including those who said:

> My wife was a stockbroker in New York. We call her associates in New York. She handles most of our stock decisions.
>
> It is my thought not to get advice from brokers. Investment counselors and bankers, yes.

Some of the experts consulted were located in unlikely places:

> I don't want advice from stockbrokers. I use a professor from New York University, through his publications and by correspondence and by telephoning him in person.

As would be expected, those respondents who worked in the financial sector made extensive use of expert advice:

> I get advice mostly from the trust departments of banks. This is available to me as a director of a bank and as a member of its trust committee.

> I get advice from brokers, also from several security analysts who come in to see me. I am a director of several mutual fund corporations and see these men quite frequently.

About one-third of those seeking advice said that they consulted other people besides qualified professionals—usually business colleagues:

> I talk with some business associates. It's just a general exchange of ideas rather than advice.

I have an associate in the office whom I respect very highly, and I talk to him occasionally.

This "nonprofessional" advice was more likely to be concerned with investments in real estate or unincorporated businesses than was the advice sought from professionals.

The kinds of information sought by the investors usually concerned features of specific investments rather than general advice about an entire industry or the economy as a whole. A few respondents explicitly said that they sought information about tax considerations:

They advise me as to what taxes are involved—the tax situation. The rest of the investing I can figure out for myself.

I get advice from a stockbroker and a lawyer. From the stockbroker I get the history of the stock so I can make my own decision. The legal advice is more pertaining to tax angles—that, rather than business judgment.

But only one in thirteen of those seeking advice wanted information about taxes. The few references to tax features were almost entirely confined to investments in real estate or unincorporated businesses, as distinct from bonds and common stock. The relationships among various social and economic variables and the readiness to seek investment advice produced no surprises. Those who "always" or "occasionally" sought such advice tended to have the higher incomes and the larger portfolios; they tended to be well educated and highly tax conscious; they were usually more active in the investment market than were those who did not seek advice. Among occupational groups there were two that conspicuously sought investment advice: female rentiers and those employed in the financial sector. In both groups nine out of ten "always" or "occasionally" sought advice when investing. Presumably of all groups the female rentiers had the least confidence in their own judgment about investments, while those working in the financial sector had the easiest access to expert opinion.

Publications

To find out what sources of information other than verbal advice are used by investors we asked the following questions:

Do you try to keep informed about various kinds of investments? What would you say are your main sources of information?

Two-thirds of the investors said that they tried to keep informed, and some were very thorough about it:

I am inquisitive. I have a wide acquaintance among bankers, customers' men, friends who are substantial investors. I talk with them often. I read a great deal, and if there is anything of interest, then I dig it out for myself. I'll read everything that I can dig out on the item. I read the company's reports, *Standard and Poor's,* copies of newspapers, annual reports. I have just invested in a stock. I even flew out to the company's headquarters in Boston, talked with the president of the company, and got a complete rundown before making my investment, since it was a substantial one.

Those who said that they tried to keep informed tended to have the higher incomes and the larger portfolios. They also tended to be more active in the investment market. Among occupational groups, those employed in the financial sector were well ahead of all others in the proportion saying that they tried to keep informed.

As for the particular sources of information, more than half of those trying to keep informed made use of "business magazines." These included periodicals like *Business Week* and *Fortune,* whose emphasis is on general business news rather than specific advice to investors. (The *Wall Street Journal* was included in this category, as a newspaper specializing in business news.) Two-fifths of those trying to keep informed referred to newspapers (other than the *Wall Street Journal*). A like proportion reported making use of investment advisory publications like *Value Line* or *Barron's.* Only one-tenth of those trying to keep informed said that they read the financial statements and other reports issued by the corporations in which they were considering an investment.

In their choice of information sources, those with the higher incomes and larger portfolios tended to rely more on investment advisory publications and less on newspapers and other unspecialized sources. The advisory publications were also popular, relative to other information sources, among those working in the financial sector and those who were most active in buying and selling assets. It was found too that the specialized information provided by the advisory publications was not used as a substitute for the personal advice discussed in the preceding section. Those who sought advice from experts tended also to consult the specialized written publications, while those who did not seek verbal advice were likely to be content with the casual, less detailed information supplied by newspapers, insofar as they did try to keep informed.

The Level of Investment Information

Our inquiries into the use made of oral advice and written publications provided us with a means of classifying investors according to their level of investment information. In making this classification we also made use of answers given later in the interview to the following questions:

> Have you heard about some special income tax advantages of investing in real estate?
>
> Are there other features of the income tax laws that affect the way you invest your savings?[2]

Investors were allotted points according to their answers to these questions and the ones quoted earlier in this chapter. One point was given if the respondent reported that he sought advice in making his investments; an additional point was given if he "always" rather than "occasionally" sought such advice, and he received another point if the advice was sought from persons who appeared to be qualified professionals; one point was given if he tried to keep informed by reading business magazines, investment advisory publications, or corporation reports (no points were allotted for reading more casual sources such as newspapers); one point was given if he either had heard of special tax advantages of investing in real estate or claimed to be affected by other features of the income tax in investing his savings, on the grounds that awareness of tax matters indicated some sophistication in the management of investments. Finally, four points were allotted if the respondent worked in the financial sector, on the grounds that his daily work presumably provided him with abundant information on investment matters.[3]

Each respondent having been scored in this manner, an attempt

[2] The answers to these questions are discussed fully in Chap. XI.

[3] The four points were not allotted if the total assets owned by the respondent were worth less than $1,000.

was made to give verbal descriptions to the various point totals, and the following distribution of cases was obtained:

	Percentage of aggregate income of those with 1961 incomes over $10,000
Very highly informed (5 points or more)	15
Highly informed (4 points)	21
Fairly well informed (3 points)	18
Somewhat informed (2 points)	17
Relatively uninformed (1 point)	11
Uninformed (0 points)	10
Other cases (total assets less than $1,000, or all investment decisions delegated to others)	8
	100

A multivariate analysis was performed in order to identify the personal characteristics of investors classified as "highly informed" or "very highly informed." The results are presented in Chart 6.1.

The analysis showed that the well informed investors tended to be the ones who were most active in the investment market. Among fairly active investors, more than half were well informed, compared with less than one in five of the others in the sample. The analysis also showed the close link between a high level of investment information and a high level of tax consciousness. The latter variable appeared twice in the analysis as an explanatory factor. It is clear that seeking information about investment possibilities led investors to become aware of the tax situation, and vice versa.

As was said earlier, our analysis of the sources of information used by investors revealed few surprises. It is reassuring perhaps for the functioning of the capitalist system that investors who controlled the largest volume of assets and were the most active in shifting funds from one investment to another were usually among the best informed, but our questioning also revealed that considerable investing was done by persons who did not make use of the information and advice available to them.

Market Activity

In studying the behavior of the investor in the capital market, we asked questions about the frequency of his transactions in

CHART 6.1. Factors Associated With a High Level of Investment Information

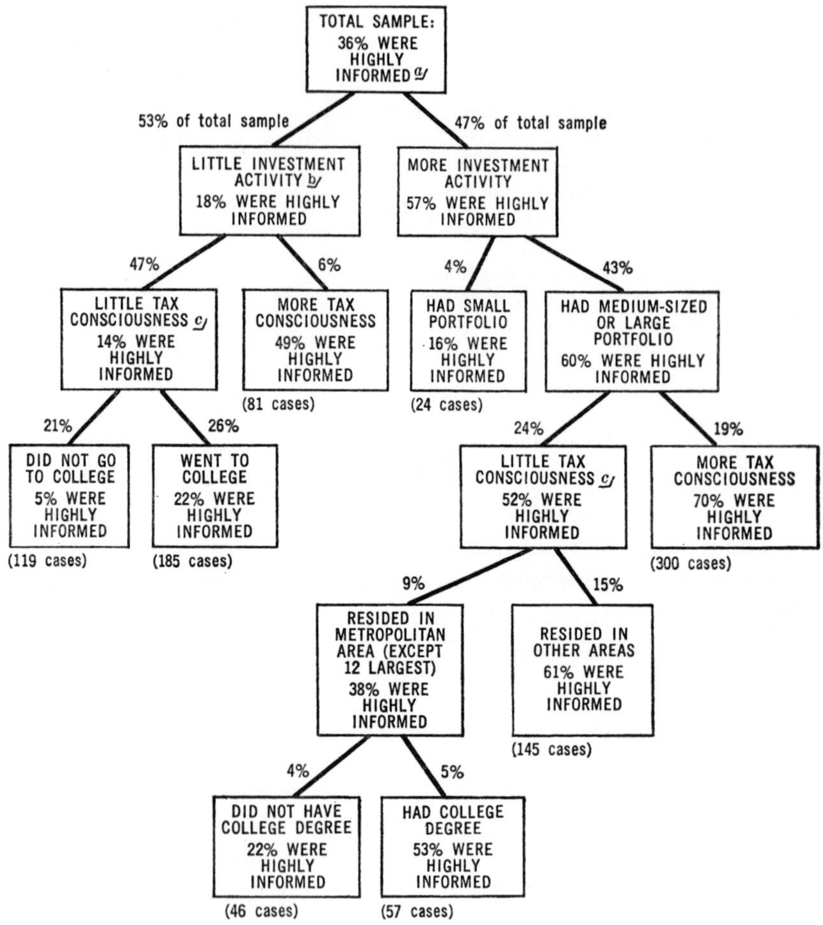

[a] Respondents classified as "highly" or "very highly" informed.
[b] Investment activity index of 2 or less.
[c] Tax consciousness index of 0 or 1.

NOTES: For explanation, see notes to Chart 4.2. In this chart the following predictors were used, listed in order of their explanatory power with a single split over the whole sample: (1) level of investment activity (for definition, see the last section of this chapter); (2) tax consciousness (for definition, see Chap. XI); (3) 1963 adjusted income; (4) education; (5) whether lived in a metropolitan area; (6) age. The eight final groups at the ends of the branches accounted for 26 percent of the total variance.

In other analyses of the level of investment information, the following variables were used in addition to those listed above and were found to have weak explanatory power: occupational group (except for the definitional relationship between having a high level of information and working in the financial sector), portfolio diversification, and the average number of hours worked per week.

bonds, common stock, and interests in real estate and unincorporated businesses. We also asked about the motives for some of these transactions. Much of this information was then used to construct an "index of investment activity," which was subjected to multivariate analysis. The details of the individual transactions are discussed first.

Purchases of Bonds

Concerning bond purchases we asked:

> Have you (or your immediate family) bought any bonds or preferred stock in the last few years?
>
> When was the last time?

Two-fifths of the high-income respondents had purchased bonds or preferred stock "in the last few years," and nearly one-third had purchased such securities during the fifteen months preceding the interview. Those who had purchased recently tended to have the higher incomes and the larger portfolios. Among occupational groups, those most likely to have purchased bonds or preferred stock recently were the owner-managers in the financial sector—such as bankers and stockbrokers—and the rentiers, both men and women. Self-employed professionals showed distinctly less interest in buying these kinds of securities.

Sales of Bonds

We asked about sales of bonds as follows:

> Have you (or your immediate family) ever sold any bonds or preferred stock?
>
> When was the last time?
>
> What did you do with the money?

More than half of the high-income group had never sold any bonds or preferred stock, and only one in eight had sold such securities during the fifteen months before the interview. As was expected, those who had sold recently tended to have the higher incomes and the larger portfolios. Also the recent sellers of bonds and preferred stock and the recent purchasers were mostly the same people. One-fifth of the high-income group were "active bondholders" in the sense that they had both bought and sold these securities during the previous fifteen months. At the other extreme was a group numbering more than a third of the sample who had never sold any bonds or preferred stock and had made no purchases "in the last few years."

Among those who had sold bonds or preferred stock at some time in the past, slightly fewer than one-half had used some or all of the proceeds to buy other earning assets, such as common stock or other bonds. When earning assets had been purchased with the proceeds, common stock had been preferred to fixed-yield assets in a ratio of two to one. The remaining sellers had used all of the proceeds to meet consumption expenses or to pay off a home mortgage.

The "active" and "inactive" bondholders, as distinguished by the date of their most recent sale, differed significantly in what they did with the proceeds of their sales. Those who had recently sold bonds or preferred stock tended to use the sale proceeds for the purchase of other earning assets rather than for consumption expenses, and they were as willing to buy fixed-yield assets as common stock. But those who had not sold any bonds or preferred stock recently had predominantly used the proceeds of their last sale for consumption expenses, and on the few occasions when they had bought earning assets, they overwhelmingly preferred common stock to fixed-yield assets. Thus there was a clear distinction between the "active" group, whose bond transactions were undertaken generally to improve their portfolio position and who were prepared to remain in the bond market in making subsequent purchases, and the "inactive" group, whose bond sales were usually not associated with the purchase of other financial investments and who were apparently reluctant to remain in the bond market.

Responses of Savings Account and Checking Account Balances to Changes in Interest Rates

Transactions involving fixed-yield assets are often undertaken because of a change in the rate of return on such assets relative to that on other investments. Such a change took place in January

1962, when the maximum rate that insured banks were permitted to pay on deposits held for a year or more was raised from 3 to 4 percent. Another change took place during the year immediately preceding the survey, when some of the funds held for periods of less than a year were also made eligible for the 4 percent rate. These changes were accompanied by a marked increase in the rate of growth of time and savings accounts in banks relative to those in savings and loan associations.[4] We wondered whether our respondents had contributed to this growth, and we asked them whether their use of savings accounts had been affected by interest rate changes.

We also asked about the changes that had occurred in recent years in the average balances maintained by the respondents in their checking accounts, and noted which respondents said that their checking account balances had been affected by changes in interest rates available on alternative types of assets (such as time deposits).

Concerning savings accounts, we asked:

Have the changes in interest rates on savings accounts had any effect on where you keep your money?

In what way?

Only 22 percent of the high-income respondents said that their use of savings accounts had been affected by changes in interest rates. One half of these had reacted by shifting funds from one savings account to another, a transaction that usually involved taking money out of one bank or savings and loan association and putting it in another. Sometimes large transfers were made in this way:

I have moved several hundred thousand from one bank to a bank in another town because it paid a higher rate of interest. I realize this seems to refute what I said back there about a high rate of return not being too important. . . . I have tried to keep liquid so that if anything happened to me, there would be enough cash for my wife to pay Uncle Sam. Young lady [added this respondent in talking to the interviewer], I'm telling you more than I ever told anyone before.

[4] Board of Governors of the Federal Reserve System, *Forty-Ninth Annual Report* (1962), p. 15.

Sometimes the lure of a higher interest rate was only one reason among many for shifting funds:

> The change from one savings and loan to another was made also on the basis of the soundness of the company and its management and investments also. I can also write checks on it, and if money is restored to the account within thirty days, I lose no interest.

Only a fourth of those who had reacted to the changes in interest rates—that is, only 6 percent of the entire high-income group—said that increasing interest rates had induced them to keep more of their total assets in savings accounts. Thus, if we take our respondents' reports at their face value, the recent rises in the interest rates paid on savings accounts have apparently redistributed funds among competing banks and savings and loan associations, but the total of funds placed in this form of investment has not been much augmented thereby.

Among the several possible explanatory variables inspected, only two—income and region—appeared to be related to the responsiveness to changes in interest rates on savings accounts. Those at the lower and upper extremes of the income scale reacted less than did those in the middle. When income was between $10,000 and $15,000 or alternatively above $300,000, only one in seven reacted in some way to the changes in interest rates, but at intermediate incomes one in four did. The variations among regions are more readily understandable than the variations among income groups. It was found that those living in the West were much less likely to have reacted by keeping more of their total funds in savings accounts and much more likely to have switched their funds between competing accounts. This presumably reflects the well-advertised competition between banks and savings and loan associations in that region, particularly in California.

No other variables shed any light on the characteristics of the persons who reacted to interest rate changes. A multivariate analysis, which made use of nine explanatory variables, produced almost nothing of significance.[5] Young and old, rentier and entrepreneur,

[5] The variables were 1963 adjusted gross income, age, size of total portfolio, occupational group, education, level of investment information, whether or not the respondent lived in a metropolitan area, preference between capital gains and current yield, and portfolio diversification.

well-informed and ill-informed, wealthy and less wealthy—all reacted to the changes in about the same limited degree. There was no special responsiveness observed even among those who had said earlier in the interview that they preferred current yield to capital gains.

The issue of whether checking account balances are influenced by interest rates was explored more indirectly. We asked the following questions:

> Would you say that you keep more money in your checking account now than you did a few years ago, or less, or what?
>
> (If any change) Why is that?

Out of every ten high-income respondents, five said that their checking accounts were larger than previously, three said there had been no change, and only one reported a reduction. Where changes in checking account balances had occurred, the reasons usually involved changes in income or wealth, living expenses, or business outlays. One-fourth of those whose accounts had become smaller (2½ percent of the entire high-income group) implied that the general rise in interest rates in recent years had induced them to leave fewer funds in checking accounts:

> Well, it used to just sit. I decided this was silly, so I got busy and transferred a few accounts to commercial banks. There at least I get 3½ to 4 percent. Some I reinvested in other things. Now I just keep enough . . . for my requirements.
>
> It wasn't working for me. It works for the bank! I keep only the minimum amount I need. When I need more I go get it and put it into the checking account.

A few respondents recognized that they were sacrificing yield by keeping large sums in their checking accounts but were not inclined to do anything about it:

> I'm getting old and lazy and I want a better cushion. Added investing doesn't yield a cent. The income on $15,000 is worth $15 to me—after taxes (*sic*).

The possibility that higher interest rates caused a withdrawal of funds from checking accounts was of course not confined to those few whose balances had actually declined in absolute terms. Some of those ending up with larger balances may have been affected by rising interest rates, but in their case the effects of the rising rates were more than offset by other factors.

Purchases of Stock

Concerning purchases of common stock, we asked:

Have (any of) you bought any common stock in the last few years?

Was the last purchase made in 1963 or 1964, or was it in 1962 or earlier?

About how frequently do you buy stock on the average—every few weeks, a few times a year, or what?

One-half of the entire high-income group had bought some common stock during the fifteen months before the survey; one-third had not bought any stock "in the last few years." Out of every twelve high-income respondents, one said that "on the average" he bought stock once a month or more frequently; another three out of twelve said that they bought stock "a few times a year."

As was expected, those who "on the average" bought frequently and who had actually bought in the recent past tended to have the higher incomes and the larger portfolios. Most of these respondents said elsewhere in the interview that they followed the stock market closely. Among occupational groups, the most frequent purchasers were those working in the financial sector, both owner-managers and employees. Three-fourths of these respondents had purchased stock during the preceding fifteen months. Business owner-managers (other than those in the financial sector) were relatively inactive as stock purchasers. Female rentiers were also inactive, only a third of this group having bought any stock during the preceding fifteen months.

Sales of Stock

We asked the following questions about sales of common stock:

Have (any of) you sold any common stock in the last few years?

When was the last time?

How did you happen to sell at that time?

One-third of the high-income group had sold some stock in the fifteen months preceding the survey, while one-half had sold none at all "in the last few years." Those who had sold recently tended to have the higher incomes and the larger portfolios, and most of them reported also having purchased stock in the recent past.

The chief reason given for the most recent sale was that the stock looked like a poor prospect. One-third of the sellers gave this kind of reply, including the respondent who said:

> I wanted to raise some cash for oil wells, and also I had lost faith in the progress of those companies.

The next most common reply, given by one-fifth of the sellers, was that the time for profit-taking had arrived:

> I had a nice profit. I take my profit when it's there in some cases, then reinvest the whole thing. As you've guessed by now, I'm a wild speculator on my own.

One out of every seven sellers said that he had sold the stock in order to transfer his funds to other more promising issues. A similar proportion said that their sale had been motivated by tax considerations:

> I took advantage of a loss and bought it back again. I bought the stock back after thirty days. I used the loss against capital gains and had to own the stock six months prior to the first of the year.

Another fairly common purpose for the sale was to raise funds for consumption expenses. About one out of every six sellers gave this reply.

The frequent sellers of stock and the infrequent sellers, as distinguished by the date of the most recent sale, differed somewhat in the motives for their sales. The frequent sellers were more likely to talk about "profit taking," more likely to talk of transferring funds to stocks with better prospects, and less likely to mention tax considerations.

Purchases and Sales of Interests in Real Estate and Unincorporated Businesses

Our final questions about investment transactions were:

> Have you (or your immediate family) bought or sold any interest in a business, farm, or real estate in the last few years (excluding your home)?
>
> When was the most recent transaction?
>
> What kind of thing did you buy or sell?
>
> What were your main reasons for doing that?

Only one-seventh of the high-income group had bought or sold such interests during the fifteen months preceding the interview. A large majority of the group—about three-fourths—had neither bought nor sold any such interest "in the last few years." Of every ten transactions mentioned, six involved real estate, two an unincorporated business, and one a farm. The most recent transactions were usually associated with those respondents having the higher incomes and the larger portfolios. Among occupational groups, the most active in this respect were the business owner-managers, but now those outside the financial sector were more active than those working in that sector—a reversal of the situation in transactions in common stock and fixed-yield assets. At the other extreme, female rentiers showed almost no interest in buying or selling "nonfinancial" investments.

The Use of Speculative Balances

Investors who are active in the capital market can be expected to hold some funds idle so that they will have cash available at short notice when promising "deals" arise. To find how prevalent such holdings were, we asked:

> Do you have some funds which you have set aside just to take advantage of opportunities that may come along, even if they are a bit speculative?

Two out of every five high-income respondents said that they did have such funds. As one respondent remarked:

I keep a lot of cash for that very reason, so I'm always able to pick up distress deals.

Those holding speculative balances tended to have the higher incomes and larger portfolios. Most of them were active in buying and selling investments, and a large proportion worked in the financial sector.

An Index of Investment Activity

Our information on specific investment transactions was used to define each respondent's degree of "investment activity." Points were allotted to each respondent as follows:

	Number of points
If last bought bonds or preferred stock in 1964[6]	2
If in 1963	1
If last sold bonds or preferred stock in 1964	2
If in 1963	1
If last bought common stock in 1963 or 1964	2
If "on the average" bought common stock every month or more frequently	2
If "on the average" bought common stock every few months	1
If last sold common stock in 1964	2
If in 1963	1
If last bought or sold interests in real estate or unincorporated businesses in 1964[7]	4
If in 1963[7]	2
Maximum score	14

Fully one-third of the high-income respondents scored zero on this index, indicating that they had neither bought nor sold any of the relevant assets during the fifteen months before the survey. For all respondents, the median score was only two. The median score, or the degree of activity, tended to increase as income rose, but quite quickly reached a ceiling. At an income level of $100,000 the median reached five, and at incomes exceeding $300,000 it was no higher. Our results suggest that the very rich may have more assets

[6] Interviewing took place from March to May in 1964.

[7] Higher scores were allotted for transactions involving these assets because fewer questions were asked about them.

to manage, but are engaged no more actively in managing their assets than are those with somewhat lower incomes.

A multivariate analysis was performed to identify the personal characteristics of those respondents classed as "highly active investors," that is, those with a score of seven or more. Nine explanatory variables were used, and the results are presented in Chart 6.2.

CHART 6.2. Factors Associated With a High Level of Investment Activity

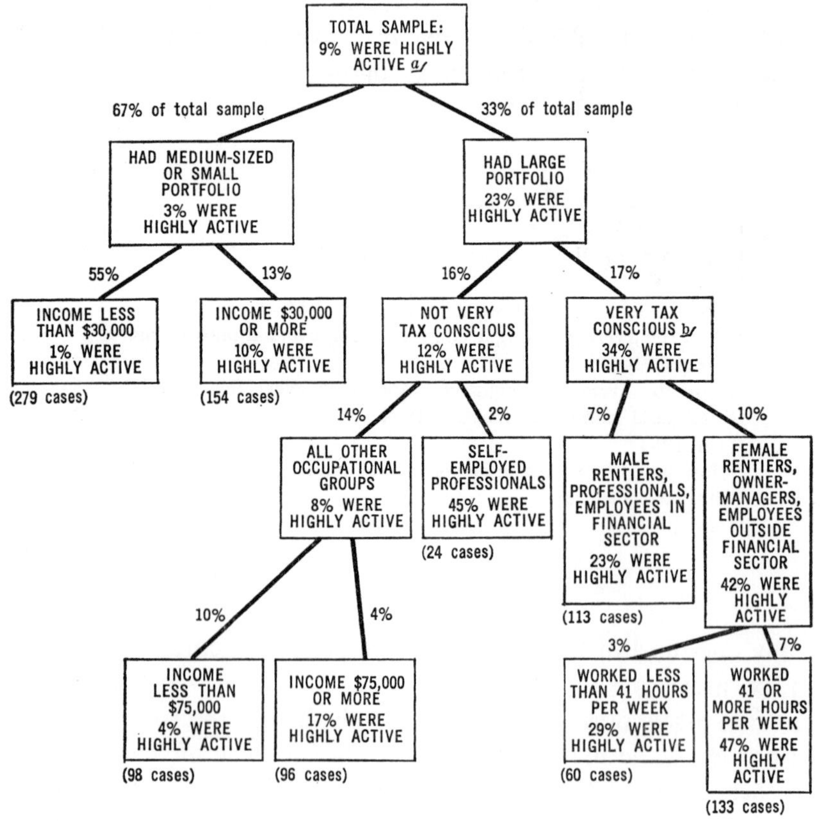

[a] Respondents with an investment activity index of 7 or more.

[b] Tax consciousness index of 2 or more.

NOTES: For explanation, see notes to Chart 4.2. In this chart the following predictors were used, listed in order of their explanatory power with a single split over the whole sample: (1) size of total portfolio (for definition, see Table 5.2); (2) 1963 adjusted gross income; (3) tax consciousness (for definition, see Chap. XI); (4) occupational group; (5) preference between capital gains and current yield; (6) education; (7) percentage of assets from gifts and inheritances; (8) average number of hours worked per week; (9) whether lived in a metropolitan area. The eight final groups at the ends of the branches accounted for 10 percent of the variance.

The analysis showed that the variable most important in explaining market activity was the size of the investor's portfolio. Among those with smaller portfolios, income was the variable which best discriminated between the highly active investors and the remainder. Among the respondents with large portfolios, those with a high level of tax consciousness were seen to be unusually active in the investment market. It is also interesting that in at least one subgroup of the population—the tax-conscious business owner-managers with large portfolios—there appeared to be no conflict between working long hours at one's primary occupation and devoting substantial time to the management of one's portfolio. In this subgroup those working the longest hours at their jobs also tended to be the most active in the investment market.

Summary

• In managing their assets, three-fourths of the high-income respondents usually obtained advice from other people. Generally they consulted stockbrokers, bank officers, and other qualified professionals, and such advice was sought chiefly for transactions in common stock.

• A majority of the high-income group read business magazines or investment advisory publications in an effort to keep informed about the investment market.

• The investors who were most active in buying and selling assets tended to be well informed.

• The buying and selling of common stock was far more frequent than the buying and selling of bonds and preferred stock. Both types of transactions were concentrated among those with the higher incomes and larger portfolios and among those working in the financial sector. There was also a positive association between activity in the investment market and the degree of tax consciousness.

• There was little evidence from our questioning that the rising level of interest rates on savings accounts in recent years has had much effect either on the total amount of funds maintained in savings accounts or on balances kept idle in checking accounts. To a limited extent the rising rates have stimulated transfers among savings accounts in competing financial institutions.

CHAPTER VII

Inheritances and Gifts Received

ECONOMISTS HAVE ALWAYS been interested in the transfer of assets from one generation to another.[1] The inheritance, estate, and gift taxes have enjoyed wide acclaim as mechanisms for altering the distribution of income and wealth with minimum effects on incentives or resource allocation. However, these taxes have never managed to strike more than a small fraction of intergenerational asset transfers.[2]

The potential importance of transfer taxes depends on the aggregate importance of gifts and inheritances in the accumulation of wealth in this country. The only previous studies of this topic have been based on estate tax data, which provide a markedly incomplete picture of wealth transfers.[3]

[1] All the data in this chapter refer to proportions of the aggregate income of those with 1961 incomes over $10,000.

[2] John Bowen, *Some Aspects of Transfer Taxation in the United States* (unpublished doctoral dissertation, The University of Michigan, 1958); and Carl S. Shoup, *Federal Estate and Gift Taxes* (Brookings Institution, 1966).

[3] Horst Mendershausen, "The Pattern of Estate Tax Wealth," in Vol. III of *A Study of Saving in the United States* (Princeton University Press, 1956);

The major problems with such data arise from gifts inter vivos, which never appear in the estate tax returns, and the difficulty of estimating age-specific death rates for wealthy people.[4]

The Receipt of Gifts and Inheritances

Sources of Current Wealth

Even with complete and detailed factual information, it would be impossible to provide a simple, definite picture of the sources of an individual's wealth. The value of gifts or inheritances or accumulations of unspent income can be established at the time of acquisition, but to identify that part of current wealth which consists of the accumulated interest, rent, profit, and capital gains on some earlier acquisition is practically impossible. Money mingles, and only in a colloquial sense can anyone say what happened to a particular part of the assets one has accumulated in the past.

Our first method of determining the sources of an individual's current wealth was simply to ask the respondent for his own impression:

> Would you say that most of your present assets are from gifts or inheritances, or savings out of income, or the result of assets that went up in value, or what?

A substantial fraction mentioned more than one of the three sources. Only 7 percent mentioned gifts and inheritances alone. Ten percent said appreciation alone was the source of most of their assets. Of course, anyone mentioning appreciation alone had to have an asset to start appreciating, but it may have started appreciating long ago, or he may have made an extremely fortunate investment.

Nearly half mentioned savings out of income as a major source of their assets, but most of this group had incomes under $75,000. Chart 7.1 shows that as income increased, there was a dramatic de-

---

Thomas R. Atkinson, *The Pattern of Financial Asset Ownership of Wisconsin Individuals, 1949* (Princeton University Press, 1956), based on Wisconsin income tax returns; Robert J. Lampman, *The Share of Top Wealth Holders in National Wealth, 1922-1956* (Princeton University Press, 1962).

[4] James N. Morgan, "Goldsmith's Study of Saving in the United States," *American Economic Review*, Vol. 46 (June 1956), pp. 370-84, especially pp. 381-83.

crease in the proportion who said most of their assets resulted from savings out of income.[5]

CHART 7.1. Main Source of Present Assets by Income Classes

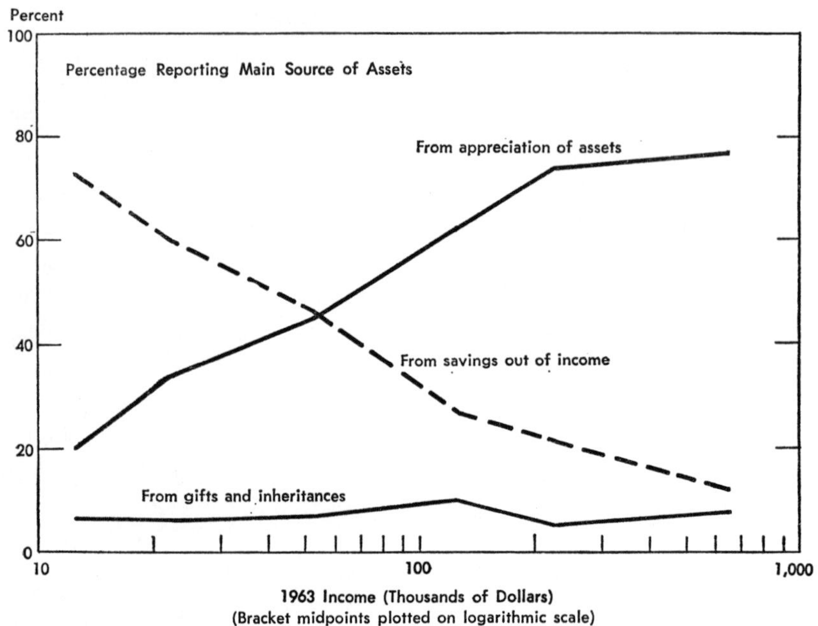

On the other hand, as Chart 7.1 shows, the importance of appreciation increased dramatically with income. The proportion mentioning appreciation, either alone or in combination with savings out of income or gifts and inheritances, increased to more than half for those with incomes over $75,000. The clear implication is that most of those with substantial assets had benefited from capital gains, and saw them as the most crucial element in the further accumulation of wealth. These findings, it must be remembered, came after many years of almost uninterrupted prosperity and some inflation. In other times and places inheritance might be a far more important source of wealth, relatively speaking.

If one is willing to make some crude assumptions, it is possible to derive some rough estimates of the quantitative importance of

[5] In this colloquial use, "savings out of income" was assumed to exclude (a) capital gains even though they are technically part of both income and saving, and (b) savings out of the cash income generated by gifts and inheritances.

inheritances as a source of aggregate wealth. Assuming, for instance, that each individual's wealth was derived solely from the main source or sources mentioned, and that the value of assets was a constant multiple of income, then it can be estimated that:

1. The proportion of aggregate wealth derived from savings (unspent current income) varied from three-fourths at incomes of $10,000-$15,000 down to one-third for those with incomes over $300,000.
2. The proportion derived from appreciation rose from one-eighth at the $10,000-$15,000 level to more than half at the highest incomes.
3. The proportion from inheritances and gifts (excluding appreciation thereon) was about one-seventh at all income levels.
4. For the entire high-income group three-fifths of aggregate wealth came from savings, one-fourth from appreciation, and about one-seventh from inheritances and gifts.

A second estimate can be made on the basis of some more explicit questions:

> Speaking of the gifts, about what fraction of your total assets today do they account for?
>
> Now speaking about the inheritance, about what fraction of your total assets today does it account for?[6]

The estimates of the proportion of wealth derived from gifts and inheritances, which can be obtained from the replies to these two questions, are within a couple of percentage points of the first estimates made above, except for the highest incomes, where, according to our second estimate, nearly a fifth of total assets were reported as resulting from gifts and inheritances. A few respondents may, however, have added appreciation to the value of the original inheritance, thus exaggerating its original importance, and some may have omitted appreciation from both the original inheritance and total assets.

A third estimate of the importance of gifts and inheritances can

[6] Interviewers were instructed that the question was intended to elicit the ratio of the *original* value of the gift or inheritance to the *current* value of total assets. Editors and coders were also instructed to make this definition prevail.

be made by returning to the earlier questions about the sources of wealth and allocating the appreciation between inherited assets and those assets accumulated by not spending current income. A correct allocation of the appreciation would require information about the timing of the gifts, inheritances, and savings.

Respondents were asked when they had received their gifts or inheritances, though not, of course, when they had accumulated assets from savings out of income. Gifts and inheritances were usually received at more than one point in time, and in the whole high-income sample the dates when those transfers had been received were evenly scattered between the recent past and the distant past. Hence, these assets had not all enjoyed a uniformly long period of appreciation. On the other hand, most of the people with substantial assets were fairly old and thus had had many years to accumulate assets out of income and have them appreciate in value. It would seem reasonable, therefore, to allocate capital gains proportionately between those on inheritances and those on assets saved out of current income.

If this is done, we estimate that more than four-fifths of the total wealth of the entire high-income group was derived from savings out of current income plus the capital appreciation of the assets resulting from that thrift and less than one-fifth from gifts and inheritances plus their appreciation.

Even at incomes over $300,000, the proportion of total assets from gifts and inheritances and their capital appreciation is less than three-tenths. And the proportion of total assets from savings out of current income and capital appreciation thereof appears to be more than seven-tenths. Thus even allocating some appreciation to gifts and inheritances leaves them significantly less important than other sources of wealth.

But it is not necessarily true that most of the wealth of the entire high-income sample was self-made rather than received through gifts and inheritances. It should be remembered that the distribution of aggregate wealth is skewed and that the situation changes at different wealth levels. Those with very large portfolios ($500,000 or more in common stock) were much more likely to report having received gifts or inheritances, particularly inheritances. Among the respondents with these very large portfolios, 28 percent said that one-half or more of their total assets reflected gifts or inheritances as distinct from appreciation and savings. Thus by looking at people with very large portfolios rather than those with the highest incomes one gets the impression that perhaps inherited wealth is more important than it seemed at first. Our oversampling of those with very high incomes is therefore not a substitute for the oversampling of those with very large assets that would be necessary to provide a precise estimate of the relative importance of thrift versus transfers in the accumulation of wealth. Unfortunately there is no reasonably effective way of sampling people according to their wealth.

Gifts Received

Almost half of the high-income individuals reported having received gifts and inheritances at some time in the past. Inheritances were far more frequently reported than were gifts. Only one-fifth of the sample reported receiving gifts, and half of these also received inheritances.

The most common forms in which gifts were received were cash or fixed-yield assets, followed closely by common stock, with interests in real estate or unincorporated businesses the least common forms.

Gifts had usually been received over a period of years, rather than in a single year only. As income increased, however, the individual was more likely to have received gifts in the distant past. Of course, the higher-income people were also older. Of those with incomes between $10,000 and $15,000, only 13 percent reported having received gifts before 1950, compared with 69 percent of those with incomes over $300,000.

Those with higher incomes or larger portfolios were more likely to have received gifts, but only 4 percent of the entire high-income group said that the gifts accounted for more than 15 percent of their total assets. Even among those with the highest incomes or those with large portfolios, no more than one-fourth reported having received any gifts at all. It is interesting to note, however, that among those with very large portfolios ($500,000 or more), 5 percent (one-half of 1 percent of the high-income sample) reported that more than half their assets had been acquired through gifts.

There was no relationship between the amount of the gifts (relative to total assets) and the amount of total assets held. Nor was there any relationship between the amount of the gifts and when they were received, nor the form in which they were received. But gifts that formed a large fraction of an individual's total assets were much more likely to have been received in the form of common stock, and those forming only a small fraction of total assets had usually been received in the form of cash or bonds.

Inheritances

Even though inheritances did not account for a substantial fraction of assets for most people, the higher an individual's current income the more likely he was to report having received an inheritance. The proportion rose from one-third for those with incomes between $10,000 and $15,000 to about one-half for those with incomes of $75,000 and higher.

Inheritances as a percentage of current total assets did not vary systematically with income. Less than one-tenth of the high-income group reported that more than half of their total wealth was from inheritances. Three-fifths reported no inheritance at all, and another fifth said that inheritances amounted to less than 15 percent of their total assets.[7] Among those with the largest portfolios ($500,000 or more), however, nearly one-fourth reported that more than half of their current total assets resulted from inheritances. Hence, the extreme skewness of the distribution of wealth makes it very difficult to measure the aggregate importance of transfers of wealth, even with our high-income sample.

Inheritances were somewhat more likely than gifts to have been received in the form of real estate or interests in unincorporated businesses. The higher the individual's income the more likely it was that the inheritance was received in the form of common stock, rather than in cash or fixed-yield assets.

The higher the current income and the older the respondent, the longer ago the inheritance was likely to have been received. Of those who had received an inheritance and who had current incomes between $10,000 and $15,000, only 35 percent had received the inheritance before 1950. Among those with incomes of $300,000 and over who had received an inheritance, 70 percent had

[7] Respondents were asked to relate the original value of the inheritance to the current value of their total assets.

received it before 1950. Of course, these people were generally older as well.

However, inheritances that represented a large fraction of current total assets had not been received longer ago than those representing a small fraction. The form of the inheritance bore no relation to when it had been received nor to its size relative to the heir's total assets.

With regard to inheritances, it is interesting to compare the high-income sample with a representative national sample of heads of spending units who were asked these questions in 1960:

> Have you ever inherited any money or property?
> (If yes) When was that?
> What was it worth?

Less than one-fifth of the representative national sample reported having received an inheritance. That is, inheritances were only half as common in the whole population as in the high-income group. In the 1960 representative national sample the frequency of those having received an inheritance did increase with age. One-third of those aged sixty-five and older reported having received an inheritance. The size of the inheritances was small, only three in a hundred having reported inheritances of $10,000 or more.[8] A similar question was used in a later representative national sample in the *1963 Survey of Consumer Finances:*

> Did you people ever receive any inheritance?

Again, the proportion of this representative national sample who reported having received an inheritance was about one-fifth, but the proportion was more than one-third for those sixty-five or older.

The Disposition of Gifts and Inheritances Received

Since nine-tenths of the high-income sample who had received gifts or inheritances reported no restrictions on their reinvestment,

[8] James N. Morgan *et al., Income and Welfare in the United States* (McGraw-Hill, 1962), p. 89.

it is interesting to note whether these assets were reinvested, and why.

Disposition of Gifts

Three-fifths of those who received unrestricted gifts reported having reinvested some or all of them. Cash or fixed-yield assets were more likely to have been reinvested than was common stock. A gift or inheritance received in the form of real estate or an interest in an unincorporated business was unlikely to have been liquidated and reinvested.

Nearly two-thirds of those who had not reinvested an unrestricted gift explained that no better investment opportunity had been found. Less than one-tenth mentioned a desire to manage the assets received (usually an interest in a business), and only one-twentieth mentioned family constraints, such as the desires of relatives. Only one respondent—whose income was under $30,000—mentioned tax considerations as a reason for not reinvesting the gift he had received. In view of the fact that the donee's basis for purposes of the capital gains tax is carried over from the donor, this is a rather startling result that does not support the hypothesis that investors tend to be "locked in" their investments by the prospect of capital gains tax liability.

The reasons for not reinvesting gifts varied neither with the value of the gift relative to current total assets, nor with the form in which the gift was received, nor with the length of time since the gift was received. It must be remembered, however, that only 6 percent of the high-income group (66 cases) had received unrestricted gifts and failed to reinvest them, and so an analysis of these cases cannot proceed very far.

Those who did reinvest their gifts were asked when they did so and why. Two-thirds of those who had received unrestricted gifts reported having reinvested them. Of this group, which is only 10 percent of the entire high-income sample, nearly half had put some or all of their gifts into common stock. This proportion varied substantially with income, from one-fifth for those with incomes between $10,000 and $15,000 to three-fourths for those with incomes of $300,000 and over. More than one-fourth of those who reinvested gifts reported using the gift for some consumption expenditure or to reduce a mortgage, and most of these had incomes under $30,000. About one-sixth said they had purchased real estate or an interest in an unincorporated business, and nearly as many said they had purchased bonds or other fixed-yield assets.

What were the reasons for reinvesting? Most frequently mentioned was some advantage of the new investment. In view of this, it is interesting to note that those whose gifts had been received in the form of cash or fixed-yield assets were the most likely to have spent the proceeds wholly on consumption items. Those who had received gifts in the form of common stock, real estate, or an interest in an unincorporated business generally reinvested them in the same type of investment. Reinvestment usually took place soon after the receipt of the gift. The larger the gift relative to current total assets, the more likely the reinvestment was to be in the form of common stock, and the less likely it was to be spent wholly on consumption items.

Disposition of Inheritances

As with gifts, two-thirds of those who received inheritances without restrictions reinvested part or all of them. The proportion reinvesting varied little among income groups, the chief determinant being the form in which the inheritances were received. Three-fourths of those who received cash or bonds reinvested them, but only one-half of those who inherited stock or real estate or an interest in an unincorporated business reinvested the inheritance.

Again, the only reason nearly half of these who had not reinvested could give was that they had not found any better investment opportunity. Four percent mentioned a desire to manage the asset, and 6 percent mentioned family restraints as reasons for not reinvesting the inheritance. Only 2 percent mentioned tax considerations, and none of these individuals had incomes of more than $75,000. About one-fifth could give no reason for their inaction, and they were generally those who had inherited cash or fixed-yield assets!

Most reinvestment took place shortly after receipt of the inheritance, with inheritances of the distant past somewhat more likely to have been reinvested than those received in the past few years. One-fourth of the entire high-income sample had reinvested an inheritance. Half of these heirs said they had reinvested in common stock, the proportion being lower for those with current incomes between $10,000 and $15,000 and higher for those at the upper income levels. One-fourth reinvested in fixed-yield assets; 14 percent reinvested in real estate or unincorporated businesses; and 15 percent used the money to help pay off a mortgage or to buy consumption items.

When asked why they had reinvested, most gave as their reason the desire to secure a better yield. Only a few mentioned tax considerations.

The larger the inheritance as a proportion of current total assets, the more likely it was to have been reinvested in the form of common stock; and the smaller the inheritance, the more likely it was to have been spent wholly on consumption items. Common stock was the most favored form of reinvestment. The shifts in the form of investments were largely from cash or fixed-yield assets to common stock, and those who had inherited common stock or real estate or unincorporated businesses generally reinvested in the same type of asset. It may well be that familiarity with real estate or a particular kind of business keeps people in one or the other, but a switch to a variable-yield asset from fixed-yield assets or cash is usually a switch to common stock, which requires no special expertise or management skill. Moreover, interests in unincorporated businesses are frequently not readily marketable, and more sentiment may attach to such businesses and real estate than to financial assets.

Summary

• The receipt of gifts and inheritances accounted for a relatively small fraction of aggregate wealth, even if one attempts to take account of appreciation in these assets.

• Both gifts and inheritances tended to be received in the form of cash or fixed-yield assets.

• Among those individuals who had received gifts or inheritances very few reported any restrictions on their disposition or reinvestment.

• Where there were no restrictions, about two-thirds of the receivers had reinvested their gifts or inheritances, generally in stock or some other variable-yield investment.

CHAPTER VIII

Gifts and Estate Planning

AMONG HIGH-INCOME INDIVIDUALS, gratuitous transfers of wealth at death or by inter vivos gift assume major proportions each year.[1] In 1961, for example, the gross value of assets reported on federal estate tax returns (required only when the gross estate exceeds $60,000) amounted to $14.6 billion, all but about $1 billion of which passed to heirs other than charitable institutions.[2] Those who filed gift tax returns in the same year (required only when gifts to *any one* donee exceed $3,000 in value) reported total gifts of $2.3 billion, of which $300 million went to charitable institutions.[3] In addition, income taxpayers with incomes of $10,000 or more in 1960 claimed deductions for charitable contributions of $2.7 billion.[4] Thus estate, gift, and income tax returns suggest that during 1960 the well-to-do gave or passed on at death net assets worth

[1] All the data in this chapter refer to proportions of the aggregate income of those with incomes over $10,000.

[2] U.S. Treasury Department, Internal Revenue Service, *Statistics of Income, 1960, Fiduciary, Gift, and Estate Tax Returns Filed During Calendar Year 1961,* p. 46. Debts outstanding plus deductible funeral and administrative expenses reduced the sum indicated in the text as passing to heirs by $1.3 billion.

[3] *Ibid.,* pp. 33-34.

[4] U.S. Treasury Department, Internal Revenue Service, *Statistics of Income, 1960, Individual Income Tax Returns for 1960* (1962), p. 12. By 1962 the amount deducted by this group had climbed to $3.4 billion. *Statistics of Income, 1962* (1965), p. 6.

at least $18 billion, a sum that does not include gifts of less than $3,000 to any one noninstitutional donee or nondeductible contributions to political parties, causes, and candidates, etc.

Factors Affecting Wealth Transfers

Whatever other considerations may motivate people to give away portions of their asset holdings, it would seem a priori that income, estate, and gift taxes play a major role. Gifts to relatives and other potential heirs can reduce substantially the tax liability incurred under federal and state wealth transfer taxes. The federal tax laws provide exemptions under the gift tax of $3,000 per donee per year ($6,000 if the donor is married) plus a specific exemption of $30,000 ($60,000 for husband and wife). The sums thus exempted would otherwise be taxable under the estate tax if transferred at death, at the highest marginal rates applicable to the estate, up to a maximum of 77 percent. In addition, further tax savings are available because the gift tax rates are only three-fourths as high as the estate tax rates; the gift tax base, unlike that of the estate tax, does not include the tax liability on taxable gifts; and the separation of the two taxes permits "splitting" of the estate and application of the lower range of marginal rates under each of the two schedules. Moreover, only 12 of the 50 states tax gifts at all, whereas 49 states tax estates or inheritances.

Gifts to relatives, particularly to dependent children, may also carry important income tax advantages. In effect, such gifts permit multiple splitting of income and, consequently, very much lower effective rates of tax. For example, in 1963 an individual subject to a 75 percent marginal tax rate (taxable income in the case of a married taxpayer of $100,000 to $120,000) needed $12,000 of pre-tax income in order to meet college expenses of $3,000 incurred on behalf of a child. On the other hand, approximately $3,600 in pre-tax income, if received by the child, directly or as beneficiary of a trust, would have provided for these college expenses. Thus an income tax saving of about $2,159[5] could have been effected by transferring, say, $60,000 in assets yielding 6 per-

[5] The father saves $2,700 in tax on $3,600 of income, and the child's tax liability is $541, assuming that the child continues to qualify as a "dependent." Otherwise the net tax saving is only $1,709.

cent as a gift to the child or to a trust of which he was the beneficiary. Nor need any offsetting gift tax liability have arisen even if the gift had been made in one year, provided the donor's wife consented and $54,000 of the specific husband-wife exemption was still available.

If the assets transferred to the child had appreciated substantially in value since their acquisition by the donor and if it were contemplated that they might ultimately be sold by the donee and potential heir, their transfer by gift rather than at death would involve some partially offsetting tax disadvantage. This follows from the quirk in the tax laws under which the basis for capital gains tax purposes is the value as of the date of transfer in the case of property passing at death but the donor's basis is carried over from donor to donee in the case of gifts. How important this is depends, of course, on the relation between cost and value at the time of the contemplated gift and on the expected marginal estate tax rate relative to the capital gains tax rate to which the heir or donee might be subject. (Since 1942 the maximum capital gains tax rate has been 25 percent, compared with estate tax rates ranging from 3 to 77 percent.)

Philanthropic gifts or contributions, deductible under the individual income tax in amounts up to 30 percent of income, could be made at a net after-tax cost to the donor of as little as "9 cents on the dollar" under tax rates prevailing between 1954 and 1963. In 1962, 5.3 million taxpayers with incomes of $10,000 and over reported deductible contributions of $3.4 billion, or 3.6 percent of income. At income levels of $100,000 and over this proportion rose to 9 percent of income.[6]

For high-income taxpayers contributions of appreciated property are particularly attractive because the amount of the appreciation is not reportable as income, while the full market value may be deducted. Suppose, for example, that a share of corporate stock acquired at a cost of $100 is contributed to a charitable organization when its value is $1,000. In the case of a taxpayer subject (under the pre-1964 schedule) to a marginal tax rate of 75 percent this gift would have reduced his tax liability by $750. Had he sold the stock, his gain of $900 would have been taxed at the 25 percent capital gains maximum rate, leaving him with $775 in cash, or only

[6] *Statistics of Income, 1962.*

$25 more than the increase in his after-tax income that would have resulted if he had contributed the stock to charity. In the extreme case, if the taxpayer's marginal rate were 91 percent, his after-tax income actually would have been $135 higher if he had chosen to make the contribution instead of selling the stock.[7] Of course, the taxpayer would be "better off" if he neither sold nor gave away the stock during his lifetime. In this event he would retain the $1,000 asset, and income tax might never be paid on the appreciation because its "cost basis" in the hands of his heirs would generally be its value at the time of his death. If we assume that the asset would then be taxable under the maximum marginal estate tax rate of 77 percent (applicable to that part of the taxable value of the estate in excess of $10 million), the net amount retained would be only $230. This sum is, nevertheless, larger than 23 percent (1 —0.77) of the maximum tax saving ($910) realizable during the taxpayer's lifetime by donating the asset to charity.

Factors other than the tax laws certainly influence the giving of large gifts to relatives and to philanthropic organizations. Whether or not it is in fact "better to give than to receive," people do derive pleasure, satisfaction, and sometimes enhanced status and prestige from giving. Large gifts to children and other close relatives may be inspired by the desire to permit them to enjoy a higher standard of living, may be in the nature of basic support payments, or may be made to enable and require children to assume property management responsibilities under the guiding hand of the donor.

Philanthropy appealed to the wealthy long before the development of modern income and wealth transfer taxation.[8] There is satisfaction to be gained from contributing to the furtherance of "good works"—whether charitable, educational, religious, scientific, or medical. Through such contributions people may help seek comfort for the unfortunate, a "better world," or moral sanctity for themselves. Philanthropy enjoys biblical and social approbation and provides a means of building monuments to oneself, literally and figuratively. Thus it may appeal to both altruistic and selfish mo-

[7] The gift reduces his tax liability by $910, compared with the net amount of $775 realizable upon sale of the stock and payment of the capital gains tax on the appreciation of $900.

[8] Merle Curti, "American Philanthropy and the National Character," *American Quarterly* (Winter 1958), pp. 420-37.

tives and hence enjoys wide support quite independently of tax considerations.

Much of the activity under the heading of estate planning involves efforts to minimize tax liabilities. However, concern for the welfare of one's heirs ordinarily transcends tax considerations; or the latter may play a major role only if the actions indicated are compatible with other objectives. Estate planning may consist in large part of switching assets into forms that are manageable by potential heirs, establishing trust arrangements that will put assets under the control of experienced management, or of shifting assets gradually over to potential heirs during the owner's lifetime so as to permit the heirs to enjoy the income earlier and to gain experience in asset management while the counsel of the donor is still available.

A series of questions on gift-making and estate planning was asked of our high-income sample.

Gifts to Relatives and Philanthropic Organizations

We asked:

> Within the last couple of years, have you (or your immediate family) made any large gifts, in cash or property, either outright or in the form of a trust, or some other way?
>
> Were the gifts made to individuals, or to churches or charitable organizations, or what?

Twenty-eight percent of the entire high-income sample reported having made large gifts. The making of gifts appeared to be closely related to income, the proportion responding affirmatively rising from only 14 percent in the income bracket \$10,000-\$15,000 to 88 percent among those with incomes of \$300,000 and higher.

Donors were equally divided between those who gave to relatives and those who gave to charitable organizations, but donors with higher incomes were more likely to have made gifts to charity. Sixty-two percent of the donors with incomes between \$10,000 and \$15,000 reported having contributed large amounts to charity, whereas at income levels above \$300,000 the proportion was 88 percent.

Gifts to Relatives

For the high-income sample as a whole, 18 percent had made large gifts to their children or other relatives in the previous two years. The principal factors associated with the giving of gifts to relatives were the size of total portfolio, 1963 income, and tax consciousness. Of secondary importance were age, portfolio diversification, occupational group, whether or not there were independent children, the holding of assets with accumulated unrealized capital gains, and the proportion of total assets that had been obtained through gift or inheritance.

As Chart 8.1 shows, whereas 18 percent of the total high-

CHART 8.1. Factors Associated With Making Large Gifts to Relatives

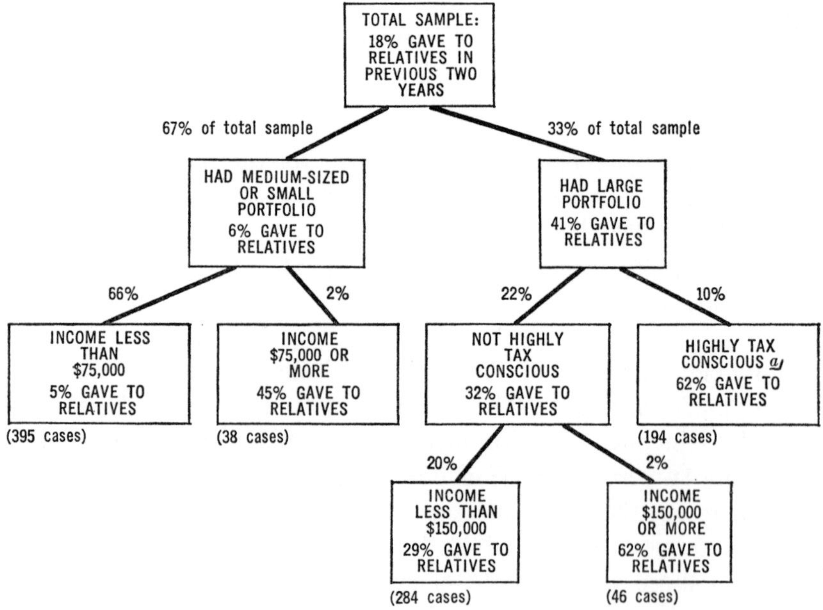

[a] Tax consciousness index of 3 or more.

NOTES: For an explanation, see notes to Chart 4.2. In this chart the following predictors were used, listed in order of their explanatory power with a single split over the whole sample: (1) size of total portfolio (for definition, see Table 5.2); (2) 1963 income; (3) tax consciousness (for definition, see Chap. XI); (4) age; (5) whether any unrealized capital gains; (6) whether any independent children; (7) percent of assets from gifts and inheritances; (8) whether any dependent children; (9) education; (10) frequency of church attendance. The five groups at the ends of the branches accounted for 26 percent of the total variance.

income sample made gifts, the split between those with large portfolios and medium-sized or small portfolios shows that 41 percent of the former and only 6 percent of the latter group gave gifts to relatives. Of those with large portfolios, the highly tax conscious were almost twice as likely to make gifts to relatives as were those who were not highly tax conscious, suggesting the importance of tax minimization in estate planning. Among those with medium-sized or small portfolios, income provides a sharp split, with 45 percent of respondents with incomes of $75,000 or more having made large gifts in contrast to only 5 percent for those with incomes of less than $75,000. Income also makes a difference on this score among those with large portfolios who are not highly tax conscious.

Chart 8.1 can be summarized by saying that either substantial assets or high income can lead to large gifts to relatives, but that it takes a combination of a large asset portfolio *and* either high tax consciousness or high income to lead a majority to make such gifts in a two-year period.

Of the respondents who had made gifts to relatives, 84 percent had given property to their children and 15 percent to their grandchildren. These proportions varied with income, however. Among donors with incomes of over $300,000, 38 percent had made gifts to grandchildren, a proportion that reflects, of course, the higher average age of this income group.

In more than two-thirds of the cases of gifts to relatives the assets were transferred directly to the donees. Among donors with incomes in excess of $300,000, however, the proportion who resorted to trust arrangements approached 50 percent.

Common stock was the kind of asset most frequently reported as having been given to relatives, 58 percent of the donors having included it in their gifts. Cash or fixed-yield assets appeared almost as frequently as common stock. However, only 4 percent of the donors gave real estate or interests in an unincorporated business. The level of the donor's income again appeared to be a major influence, those with the highest incomes having been far more likely to give common stock. Thus of donors with incomes between $10,000 and $15,000 only 11 percent gave stock, compared with 63 percent of those with incomes of $300,000 and higher.

To get information on motives for giving large gifts to relatives we asked donors:

What particular reasons did you have for making the gifts at that time?

Tax considerations were the most frequently reported reason, with the needs of the donees mentioned less than half as frequently. The importance of tax considerations rose only moderately with income. They were mentioned by 40 percent of donors with incomes of $10,000 to $15,000 and by 57 percent of those whose incomes exceeded $300,000. Tax factors persisted as the dominant motive irrespective of whether the donees were children, grandchildren, or other relatives.

The relevance of tax considerations may perhaps best be illustrated in the words of the respondents themselves. For example, donors answered the above question as follows:

Only one reason—to avoid inheritance taxes. [He then added, perhaps as an afterthought] My love for my children prompted it.

Estate taxation.

Part of a long-range program to avoid inheritance taxes.

Because of high inheritance taxes—because of high income taxes.

It's a personal thing. It seemed like an appropriate time. I felt I'd better do it while the spirit moved me, and at the time the securities had appreciated greatly so there were large taxable gains on them. The recipients were not in the tax bracket that I was, so that was the time to do it.

Gifts to Philanthropic Organizations

As we have noted, large gifts to philanthropic organizations occurred with about the same frequency as gifts to relatives, the most important factors associated with philanthropic gifts being income and size of total portfolio. Reference to the second and third rows of boxes from the top of Chart 8.2 makes this clear—38 percent of those with large portfolios made charitable gifts, compared with only 8 percent for those with medium-sized or small portfolios. Among the holders of large portfolios, those with incomes of $150,000 or more gave to charitable organizations with twice the frequency reported by respondents with lower incomes.

Even among those with small or medium-sized portfolios, in-

CHART 8.2. Factors Associated With Making Large Gifts to a Church or Charity

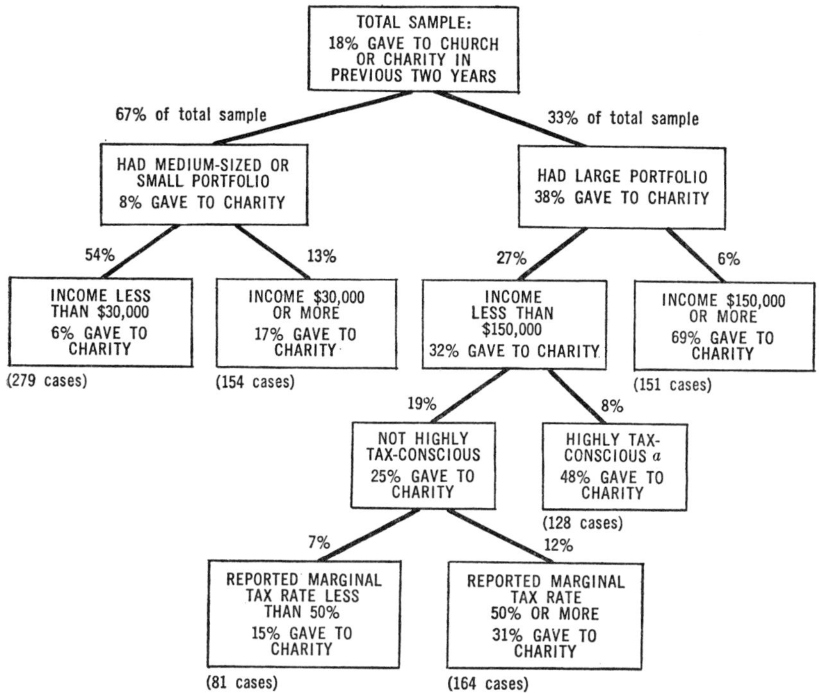

[a] Tax consciousness index of 3 or more.

NOTES: For an explanation, see notes to Chart 4.2. In this chart the following predictors were used, listed in order of their explanatory power with a single split over the whole sample: (1) size of total portfolio (for definition, see Table 5.2); (2) 1963 income; (3) tax consciousness (for definition, see Chap. XI); (4) reported marginal tax rate; (5) percentage of total assets from gifts and inheritances; (6) whether any unrealized capital gains; (7) age; (8) political preference; (9) education; (10) whether any independent children; (11) whether any dependent children; (12) size of place of residence; (13) religious preference. The six final groups at the ends of the branches accounted for 22 percent of the total variance.

come made a difference; those with incomes of $30,000 or more reported gifts to church or charity nearly three times as frequently as those with lower incomes.

Of those with large portfolios, but with current income of less than $150,000, the highly tax conscious—those who mentioned taxes voluntarily three or more times—were more likely to contribute to charity than were the less tax conscious. Finally, among respondents with large portfolios and incomes of less than $150,000 who were not highly tax conscious, those who said that their marginal tax rate was 50 percent or higher were twice as likely to make large gifts to a church or charity as were those subject to lower tax rates.

The other factors that were introduced into the analysis are listed in the notes to Chart 8.2. Religious preference was the least important among those listed. Having inherited assets or owning unrealized capital gains was of some importance taken singly over the whole sample, but became insignificant when the analysis took account of portfolio size and income. In an earlier analysis, the respondent's activity in church or civic groups was used and appeared to be quite important; but this relationship seemed circular, and the variable was omitted.

Gifts of Appreciated Assets to Charity

The tax advantages of giving appreciated assets to charitable organizations, as was pointed out earlier in this chapter, were expected to be of major interest to our sample of high-income people. Thus we asked:

> Have you ever given to church or charity an asset that was worth more than you had originally paid for it?

Somewhat surprisingly, only 13 percent answered yes, although the proportion of affirmative answers did rise sharply with income, from 3 percent at incomes of $10,000-$15,000, to 32 percent in the $75,000-$150,000 bracket, and to 62 percent among those with incomes over $300,000.[9]

The term "church or charity" may have been interpreted by some as excluding educational institutions, museums, hospitals, symphony orchestras, etc. Nevertheless, neither the frequency of church attendance nor religious affiliation appeared to be strongly related to the donation of an appreciated asset to "church or chari-

[9] For the tax year 1962 the U.S. Internal Revenue Service has compiled data on deductible contributions of appreciated property. These data show that only 1,179 out of 199,590 taxpayers with incomes of $10,000 and over who made contributions of property gave assets worth more than "cost or other basis." As the IRS notes, however, "the data . . . at best represent only those contributions of property which could be clearly identified in the process of statistical editing. The taxpayer was not required to enter the description and cost or other basis of property contributed on the return form itself, but was instructed to enter that information on a separate statement. To the extent that taxpayers failed to file a statement, the data . . . are understated." U.S. Treasury Department, Internal Revenue Service, *Statistics of Income, 1962, Individual Income Tax Returns,* p. 8.

ty," and this suggests that the response might not have been notably different had the intended meaning of the question been clearer.

Chart 8.3 presents quite dramatically the influences of income and portfolio size. Whereas only 13 percent of the total sample reported having contributed an appreciated asset to church or charity, the proportions were 43 percent for those with incomes of $75,000 or more and 8 percent for those with incomes less than $75,000. Similarly, within each of the two income groups a split was obtained on the basis of the size of the total portfolio. For those with

CHART 8.3. Factors Associated With The Donation of an Appreciated Asset to Charity

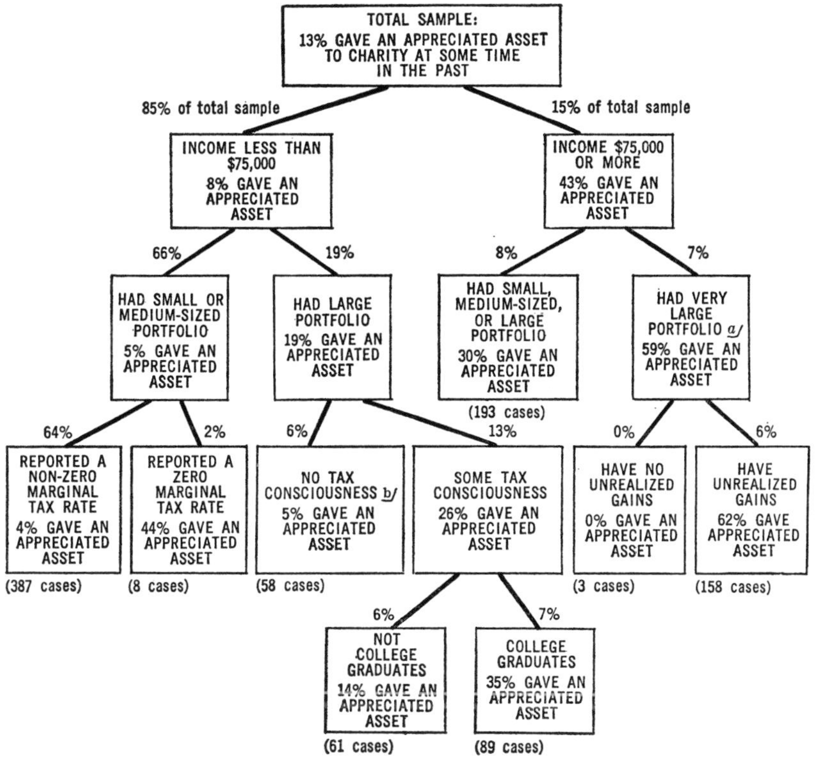

[a] Owned common stock worth more than $500,000.

[b] Tax consciousness index of 0.

NOTES: For an explanation, see notes to Chart 4.2. In this chart the following predictors were used, listed in order of their explanatory power with a single split over the whole sample: (1) income; (2) size of total portfolio (for definition, see Table 5.2); (3) tax consciousness (for definition, see Chap. XI); (4) education; (5) whether owned any unrealized capital gains; (6) reported marginal tax rate; (7) age; (8) whether any independent children; (9) percent of total assets from gifts and inheritances; (10) whether any dependent children; (11) religious preference; (12) size of place of residence; (13) political preference. The eight final groups accounted for 24 percent of the total variance.

lower incomes but substantial portfolios, giving appreciated assets was more common among tax-conscious respondents, particularly if they were also college graduates. Two unusual small groups were isolated. Eight cases with lower incomes and smaller portfolios reported a zero marginal tax rate, and half of them had given appreciated assets. The zero rate may have been attributable to the gifts. Three cases with high incomes and large portfolios said they had no unrealized capital gains and had not given any appreciated assets to charity.

The unexpectedly low frequency of reported gifts of appreciated assets may reflect some understatement resulting from lack of clarity in the question. The tax incentives for such gifts are strong. But it is also entirely possible, of course, that a misleading impression of the prevalence of gifts of appreciated assets may have been given by the well-publicized efforts of some colleges and other institutions to encourage such gifts and by the publicity given to the occasional large contributions that take this form.

Estate Planning

As has been seen, gifts to relatives are made for tax reasons, among others, as an integral part of estate planning. But what of other activities related to estate planning? To what extent is the high-income population concerned with them? We asked a series of questions on this subject, the first of which was:

> Have you given some thought to how your estate will be handled when you die?

To this question the overwhelming majority of our sample—83 percent—answered "Yes," while more than one-third of the others were among those who reported having no savings, investments, or reserve funds. People with incomes of over $75,000 virtually all indicated that they had in fact thought about the problem of how their estates would be handled upon their death.

The foregoing question was followed by three more, designed to provide information on the nature of, and reasons for, such actions as had been taken in connection with estate planning.

Have you already made any changes in your asset holdings because of this?

What have you done?

What reasons did you have for doing that?

There is apparently a big difference between "thinking about" the handling of one's estate and "doing something" about it. Only 16 percent of the entire sample of high-income people reported having made any changes in asset holdings for estate planning purposes. As was to be expected, the proportion of those who did make changes increased with income, from 8 percent among those with incomes between $10,000 and $15,000 to 35 percent among people with incomes of over $300,000. The latter proportion appears to be small when one considers that most of the people with very high incomes are relatively old.

In general, the proportion of those who had made asset changes for estate-planning purposes also increased with the size of the total portfolio and with age. Of those with small portfolios only 7 percent had made changes in asset holdings, contrasted with just under 30 percent among those with very large portfolios ($500,000 or more in common stock). The expected influence of age is seen in the fact that asset changes were made by a scant 2 percent of those who were under thirty-five, the proportion rising to 14 percent for those forty-five to fifty-four and to 25 percent for individuals seventy-five or older.

Tax consciousness also appears to have played a major role in determining the frequency with which asset changes for estate planning purposes were reported. Among those who were not tax conscious (index of 0), only 7 percent reported having made such changes, whereas for the highly tax conscious (index of 4 or more) the proportion rose to 45 percent.

Of those who did report having engaged in estate planning activities, approximately one-fourth had established trusts or life estates for their children; about one-fifth had transferred assets by gift directly to their children; about one-twelfth had increased the liquidity of their estates—by selling a family business, for example; and about one-tenth had acquired more life insurance. Very few respondents mentioned having set up any trusts other than for their children. There were no striking differences among income groups in the nature of the actions taken.

The relative importance of gifts and changes to increase liquidity tended to rise with increasing age. On the other hand, the importance of increased insurance fell with increasing age, while the frequency with which respondents had set up trusts for children first rose, peaking for those aged forty-five to fifty-four, and then fell off.

The size of the total portfolio was also related to the kinds of asset changes made. Gifts and liquidity-increasing arrangements increased in relative importance with rising portfolio size, while trusts in behalf of children first rose and then fell at the higher levels.

Again, as in the case of gifts to children and other relatives, the most important single motivating factor in estate planning was tax considerations. Fully half of those who reported having made changes in asset holdings said that they did so in order to minimize or to avoid taxes. Our index of tax consciousness was closely associated with the extent to which inter vivos transfers of assets were a part of estate planning activities, the two rising together. Similarly the frequency with which the establishment of trusts for children was reported rose with increasing tax consciousness, as did, to a lesser extent, asset changes to increase liquidity. It should be emphasized, however, that even at the highest incomes, the planning of estates to avoid taxes was far from widespread. Among all respondents with incomes over $300,000, less than one-fifth mentioned taxes as a reason for whatever estate planning activity they had undertaken.

Only 7 percent of the estate planners mentioned increased liquidity as a reason or goal, and even some of these may have had tax considerations in mind. Most surprisingly perhaps (although conceivably considered by many as too obvious to be worth mentioning), only 15 percent of the group said that their actions had been motivated by a desire to make the estate easier to manage for their heirs. And 13 percent indicated that they had acted to reduce the risks that the heirs would have to face.

Expressed reasons for estate planning activities are, of course, difficult to quantify. Their flavor may, perhaps, best be appreciated through some of the responses from those who were interviewed:

I'm trying to take advantage of recent government regulations.

To provide for management of assets for wife and children and for continuity of income.

Redistribution of assets based on tax considerations.

This is being done for tax reasons.

They're going to get it some day [the children to whom he had made large gifts]. They should learn what to do with it. At least they'll get what those swine in Washington leave for them. And the average stupid citizen doesn't even know what he's doing to himself and all of us when he votes for that outfit, or doesn't vote at all.

The principle of the advantage is death-tax savings. The object of the change in wills [the respondent's and his wife's] is to minimize death taxes and see that assets are distributed as we desire.

Perhaps one of the most surprising findings, in view of the importance of tax considerations, is the relatively minor role played by increased life insurance in estate planning on the part of high-income people. Many states exempt life insurance proceeds in whole or in part under their estate or inheritance taxes, and even under the federal laws it is possible to achieve one's tax-avoidance objectives in estate planning through life insurance if the estate owner is willing to give up certain elements of ownership in the insurance policies.

Summary

- More than one-fourth of the high-income group had made large gifts to relatives or philanthropic organizations in the two years preceding the survey.
- Motives for making large gifts to relatives were dominated by tax considerations.
- The making of gifts to relatives and to charity increased in frequency with rising portfolio size and income.
- Comparatively few people in our sample, only 13 percent, had *ever* used the tax-avoidance device of giving an appreciated asset to a church or charity, although at very high income levels (over $300,000) the proportion approached two-thirds.
- While most respondents had given some thought to how their estates would be handled at their deaths, very few had actually

made changes in asset holdings for estate planning purposes.

• As in the case of gifts to relatives, the most important factor affecting those who did engage in estate planning activities was the effort to minimize or avoid taxes.

• The most commonly reported kinds of activities associated with estate planning were the creation of trusts for the benefit of children and the giving of large gifts to children.

CHAPTER IX

Capital Gains and Losses

CAPITAL GAINS[1]—appreciation in the value of assets other than those held for resale—represent a major objective of investors and a principal source of the current value of wealth holdings.[2] Capital gains reported for tax purposes, in the ten years 1953-62, ranged from a low of about $5 billion in 1953 to a high of over $16 billion in 1961.[3] What fraction of annual appreciation in the value of as-

[1] All the data in this chapter refer to proportions of the aggregate income of those with 1961 incomes over $10,000.

[2] On the importance of capital gains as an objective sought by investors see Chap. IV, and on capital gains as a source of wealth, see Chap. VII. For tax purposes capital gains are defined in the law in considerable detail. They include only "realized" gains, realization being held to take place generally upon the occurrence of certain types of "conversions." The tax laws also confer capital gains status on various kinds of "ordinary income," such as coal and iron ore royalties, patent royalties, certain lump sum payments to employees, etc. See *Internal Revenue Code,* sections 1201-41, 631, 341, 402-403, and 522 (a); and Stanley S. Surrey, "Definitional Problems in Capital Gains," *Tax Revision Compendium, Compendium of Papers on Broadening the Tax Base, Submitted to the Committee on Ways and Means,* 86 Cong. 2 sess., Vol. II (1959), pp. 1203-32. See also Lawrence H. Seltzer, *The Nature and Tax Treatment of Capital Gains and Losses* (National Bureau of Economic Research, 1951), particularly Chap. 9.

[3] U.S. Treasury Department, Internal Revenue Service, *Statistics of Income, 1962, Individual Income Tax Returns* (1965), p. 162. The figures presented in the text are roughly double the amounts reported in *Statistics of Income.* The latter gives as "net gain from sale of capital assets" the amounts included by taxpayers in "adjusted gross income," which amounts are only 50 percent of total gains in the case of assets held over six months.

sets these figures represent is not known, but given the fact that only a small proportion of assets on which gains may accumulate turns over each year, it is safe to assume that total appreciation is a substantial multiple of realized gains.[4]

Capital Gains as Income

In 1962 individual taxpayers reported net capital gains of $6.8 billion,[5] which was approximately 50 percent of their actual reported gains of more than $13 billion. The latter amount was less than 4 percent of total adjusted gross income (plus the 50 percent of excluded capital gains on assets held more than six months), and only 4.3 million taxpayers out of a total of 62.7 million reported net gains on capital assets. Almost three-fourths of the gains were realized by taxpayers with adjusted gross incomes of $10,000 and over. For all taxpayers in this group, reported realized gains amounted to double the average proportion of income, or 8 percent, and where adjusted gross income exceeded $50,000, the proportion was 30 percent.

Thus, even apart from the question of nonreporting, and taking into account only realized gains rather than actual annual appreciation, capital gains comprise an appreciable part of the income of high-income people.

Advantages of Capital Gains

Since 1922 capital gains have received favorable treatment under the federal income tax. Many changes have been enacted in

[4] Studies made for the New York Stock Exchange estimate that, of total stock values held by individual investors in 1965, 54 percent represented unrealized capital appreciation, compared with 40 percent in early 1960. (Reported in the Personal Investing section of *Fortune* [February 1966], p. 207.) Moreover, it has been estimated that only about two-thirds of the gains realized by individuals on corporate stock are reported on tax returns. See Harley H. Hinrichs, "Unreporting of Capital Gains on Tax Returns or How to Succeed in Gainsmanship Without Actually Paying Taxes," *National Tax Journal* (June 1964), pp. 158-63. If Hinrichs is reasonably correct, and if his estimate of nonreporting is applicable to gains other than those realized on corporate stock, our revised estimates of realized capital gains would range from $7.5 billion in 1953 to $24 billion in 1961.

[5] *Statistics of Income, 1962,* p. 36. Taxpayers also reported net losses of $1.1 billion.

the past 45 years, but in general terms the rules now applicable were established by the Revenue Act of 1942. The law[6] distinguishes between "short-term" and "long-term" gains, the latter being defined as gains on assets held more than six months. In computing the amount subject to tax, the taxpayer must first offset any short-term losses against short-term gains and similarly calculate net long-term gains. If there are net gains in both categories, the amount used to determine taxable income is net short-term gains plus *50 percent* of net long-term gains. But whereas the marginal tax rates applicable to ordinary income between 1954 and 1963 ranged from 20 to 91 percent, in the case of includable long-term capital gains the maximum rate was 50 percent. In effect, tax rates on long-term capital gains ranged from 10 to 25 percent.[7]

Although net short-term gains are subject in full to ordinary income tax rates, the realization of net long-term capital losses is permitted, dollar for dollar, to offset short-term gains (as well as ordinary income up to a maximum of $1,000 annually). For example, a taxpayer who realized only short-term gains, which otherwise would have been taxed at rates as high as 91 percent, could escape the tax entirely by realizing net long-term losses in an equal amount. Thus realization of such losses, appropriately timed, can be very attractive as a tax-saving device. Long-term losses realized when the taxpayer had equal or greater long-term gains could, on the other hand, only have resulted in a tax saving of a maximum of 25 percent of the long-term gains, contrasted with a maximum of 91 percent of short-term gains in the preceding case. It seems that the tax-saving possibilities inherent in these aspects of the law would be extremely attractive to high-income people with substantial asset holdings. We tried, therefore, to get information on the extent to which individuals in our sample in fact responded to these possibilities. Our findings are presented below in the section on "Realization of Capital Losses."

Individuals holding assets that have appreciated in value, however, need not resort to realizing offsetting losses in order to avoid

[6] For references to the *Internal Revenue Code,* see note 2 to this chapter.

[7] Under the Revenue Act of 1964, the rate schedule for 1965 and subsequent years begins at 14 percent and rises to 70 percent. The maximum rate of 25 percent (50 percent of 50 percent) on long-term capital gains was not changed, so the new range of effective rates is from 7 to 25 percent.

taxation of the gain. As we have noted, it is only *realized* gains that are taxable, and realization is defined as not including the transfer of assets by *inter vivos* gift or at death. In the case of gifts, the donee, upon sale of the assets, computes his gain as the difference between the net sale price and the cost or other basis of the donor.[8] When assets are transferred at death, on the other hand, the heir's basis for computing gain or loss is generally the value at the time of death.[9] It is possible, therefore, for a family's wealth to increase without limit through appreciation in the value of its asset holdings without such appreciation *ever* giving rise to income tax liability.

This points up the great difference between the accumulation of wealth out of income subject to tax rates that ranged up to 91 percent between 1954 and 1963 and the accumulation of wealth out of "unrealized" (though often readily realizable) capital gains. There are, in effect, three levels of income tax, ranging from zero under the circumstances just described, through capital gains rates of half the ordinary rates (with a maximum of 25 percent), and up to the ordinary income tax rates. The differences among them are so great that one would expect people to respond significantly to them, at least when they have the opportunity to do so. Indeed, the tax treatment of capital gains, given the income tax rates that have prevailed since World War II, has made possible the accumulation of a large proportion of the private wealth amassed in the past 25 years. Professor Seltzer has suggested that an important reason for this treatment is a matter of "sentiment." As he explains:

> Few persons like to see a baseball game in which there are no runs, no hits, and no errors; or a football game in which no one makes a touchdown. Many Congressmen and other persons have a similar feeling about the tax system and the chances of achieving outstanding financial

[8] Or last prior holder who had obtained the asset or assets other than by gift. In certain cases the donee may realize neither gain nor loss for tax purposes. This situation arises when the selling price realized is less than the donor's cost or other basis but more than the value of the assets as of the date of the gift. In other words, the basis in the event of a loss is the lower of the donor's basis or the value as of the date of the gift. *Internal Revenue Code,* Section 1015.

[9] *Internal Revenue Code,* Section 1014. When the estate is valued for estate tax purposes as of a date other than the date of death, the alternative valuation date applies as well in determining the basis of the property in the hands of the heir for capital gains purposes.

success. They do not want an airtight tax system. They want to preserve the opportunity for a man to make a financial homerun, a touchdown, a killing. The preferential tax treatment of capital gains has the virtue, in their minds, of offering just such an opportunity.[10]

Capital gains might be expected to be a preferred form of property income for many people even in the absence of tax considerations. In effect, it provides costless reinvestment of earnings, as contrasted, say, with cash dividends, the investment of which involves brokerage fees and the costs of decision making. Some people may need to exercise a great deal of self-discipline in order to refrain from consumption and to save and accumulate. When capital gains accumulate, the saving is "automatic." Consuming the income would require a specific decision to liquidate part of one's holdings, and self-discipline is thus aided by inertia. Also capital gains are associated with investments that are relatively inflation-proof. Hence there are some important nontax reasons for preferring capital gains to other forms of property income.

Preferences among different forms of income as expressed in people's investment policies were discussed at length in Chapter IV. Here experiences in holding or selling assets on which capital gains or losses have accumulated will be analyzed.

Holdings of Appreciated Assets

How widespread among high-income people is the holding of assets that have appreciated substantially in value? Part of the answer to this question was provided in the discussion of the sources of wealth,[11] where it was seen that capital appreciation had been a major source of wealth for those who had accumulated large portfolios. Further evidence is available in the responses to the question:

Looking at the investments which you (and your immediate family) now have—such as your business, or your common stock—are any of them currently worth a great deal more than when you got them (excluding your home)?

[10] Lawrence H. Seltzer, "Capital Gains and the Income Tax," *American Economic Review* (May 1950), p. 378.

[11] See Chap. VII.

Fully two-thirds of the high-income group reported owning some assets that had appreciated "a great deal." The proportion so reporting rose with income until at incomes in excess of $75,000 almost everyone—more than 90 percent—replied affirmatively.

The kind of asset most likely to have appreciated in value was common stock. Of those holding assets that had appreciated substantially, 76 percent reported that these assets consisted wholly or in part of common stock. Forty percent of those holding appreciated assets reported that their interests in real estate or unincorporated businesses had gone up substantially in value, while only 5 percent said that they held appreciated assets in the form of fixed-yield securities. The relative importance of appreciated interests in real estate and unincorporated businesses declined as income rose, from 45 percent for persons in the $10,000-$15,000 income bracket with appreciated assets to 31 percent for people with incomes above $300,000.

Reasons for Not Selling Appreciated Assets

There has been a great deal of discussion over the years about the extent to which people feel free to sell assets that have appreciated in value, but it has been largely speculative and has turned primarily on the question of the influence of tax considerations in producing a "lock-in" effect.[12] To get some insight into the mobility of the capital owned by high-income investors, we asked the following questions:

Have you considered selling any of those assets that are worth more than when you bought them?

[12] See, for example, Lawrence H. Seltzer, *The Nature and Tax Treatment of Capital Gains and Losses* (The National Bureau of Economic Research, 1951), pp. 16-18, 283-84, and 287-88; Walter W. Heller, "Investors' Decisions, Equity and Capital Gains," and Jonathan A. Brown, "'Locked-In' Problem," in U.S. Congress, Joint Committee on the Economic Report, *Federal Tax Policy for Economic Growth and Stability* (Washington, 1955); Harold M. Somers, "Reconsideration of the Capital Gains Tax," *National Tax Journal* (December 1960); and Charles C. Holt and John P. Shelton, "The Lock-In Effect of the Capital Gains Tax," *National Tax Journal* (December 1962). For the findings of a survey of "active investors" that dealt with the timing of effects of the capital gains tax on investment transactions, see J. Keith Butters, Lawrence E. Thompson, and Lynn L. Bollinger, *Effects of Taxation: Investments by Individuals* (Harvard University, Graduate School of Business Administration, 1953), pp. 339-46.

(If yes) Why is it that you haven't sold the asset?

(If no) Why haven't you considered selling it?

That people are indeed closely wedded—if not "locked-in"—to their holdings of appreciated assets is indicated by the fact that 64 percent of those owning such assets reported that they had never considered selling them. The proportion so reporting declined as income rose, falling to a still remarkably high 44 percent at incomes above $150,000.

In most cases the attachment to appreciated assets appeared to have been due to considerations other than the desire to avoid taxes on the appreciation. The reason most frequently given for not selling or for not having considered selling was the feeling that there were no better investment opportunities available. Sixty-one percent of those who owned appreciated assets offered this explanation. A small group—3 percent—said that the asset in question was not readily marketable; another group of approximately the same size were restricted in their freedom of action by family considerations; 8 percent said that they were too interested in managing the assets to sell or consider selling them; and 19 percent reported that tax considerations—presumably the capital gains tax—blocked the sale of their appreciated assets. At incomes over $300,000, tax reasons for holding onto appreciated assets were only slightly more prevalent than among the entire high-income sample: 23 percent as opposed to 19 percent.

The influence of tax considerations, moreover, was confined almost exclusively to those whose appreciated assets took the form of common stock. Approximately one-fourth of the respondents with substantial appreciation in their common stock holdings cited taxes as a reason for not selling, whereas virtually no one with appreciated assets in the form of real estate or interests in unincorporated businesses mentioned the tax factor. Some of the tax-inspired reactions to the question of why the asset had not been sold or why selling had not even been considered were the following:

Because I don't want to pay capital gains tax.

I'd have to pay so much tax. They have grown so much in value.

Well, if I sold, it would be at a substantial gain—a capital gain. If my death precedes my wife's, she inherits at the market value. Then when she disposes of it she doesn't have to pay a high tax because the value to her would be at the date she received it.

While only the last of the above replies—offered by a high-level executive with an income of $100,000 who was concerned with the financial management of a major industrial firm—explicitly notes the possibility of avoiding capital gains tax by transferring assets at death, this escape route is clearly implicit in the other replies quoted, as well as in virtually all of the other responses that mentioned taxes.[13] It may be the ultimate availability of a zero tax rate that matters rather than the opportunity to postpone tax liability. It is therefore questionable that even a substantial reduction in the capital gains tax rate would make much difference in asset mobility, as long as the tax-free alternative remained.

Moreover, as we have noted, tax considerations were not viewed as a major reason for holding onto appreciated assets—even in the case of common stock.[14] Far more frequently offered were such explanations as the following:

> It's a question of whether I could reinvest more advantageously and with greater security.
>
> I guess the fact is that I can't reinvest it in safer and better investments.
>
> Because they will be worth more in the future.
>
> It would be foolish at this time with their contemplated growth. Money doesn't grow, investments do.

Investors apparently feel that there is much to be said for holding assets with which one feels "comfortable." Changes in asset holdings involve the costs of arriving at new decisions; changes involve new and unfamiliar uncertainties and new and different risks. This attitude was expressed quite often, as for example:

[13] This finding contrasts with that of Butters, Thompson, and Bollinger. They were "surprised" to find that "In no instance was any reference made to the fact that gains on assets held until death permanently escape taxation." *Op. cit.*, p. 346.

[14] The authors are not convinced by the finding of two Harris polls for the New York Stock Exchange that substantial numbers say they would sell assets if the capital gains tax were lower. The responses to such "iffy" questions are generally not good predictors of behavior.

I just like to hold them I suppose. Good comfortable holdings are just good business too. In fact in the long run they're the best. That's what my business really is as a broker for others—to get them solid holdings that are dependable.

Realization of Capital Gains

Although it would appear that most high-income people who held appreciated assets wanted to keep at least some of them, a similar proportion—63 percent—of the entire high-income sample reported having realized a capital gain at some time in the past. In fact more than half of this group said that they had last realized a capital gain within about 15 months of the interview. As income rose, the proportion of people who had realized a capital gain at some time in the past increased, from 36 percent in the $10,000-$15,000 bracket to almost 90 percent of those with incomes of more than $300,000.

Type of Assets Most Recently Sold

The kind of asset most recently sold at a gain was usually common stock. Of those who had realized capital gains in the past, 68 percent reported that their latest gain had come from the sale of common stock, whereas only 22 percent reported that the sale of real estate or unincorporated business interests had produced their most recent gain.[15]

[15] At first glance, the proportion reporting that their most recent asset sale involved common stock appears to be inordinately high. In 1959, the latest year for which such data are available, of 4.6 million individual tax returns on which long-term capital gains were reported, only 1.6 million, or a little over one-third, reported capital gains from the sale of corporate stock. But more than 1 million individual taxpayers reported long-term capital gains in the form of distributions from regulated investment companies, and, although a precise breakdown is not available, it is likely that an additional million reported capital gains realized in ways other than by selling assets. (These would include long-term capital gains in the form of lump-sum pension distributions, coal royalties, patent royalties, liquidating dividends, etc.) Subtracting 2 million returns from the total of 4.6 million leaves 2.6 million, of which the 1.6 million who reported long-term capital gains on corporate stock comprise a proportion that is reasonably close to our comparable figure of 68 percent. For data derived from income tax returns see U.S. Treasury Department, Internal Revenue Service, *Statistics of Income, 1959, Supplemental Report: Sales of Capital Assets Reported on Individual Income Tax Returns for 1959,* p. 10. It is not possible from our data to estimate the relative

Fixed-yield assets were reported by a scant 6 percent—virtually all of whom had incomes of less than $150,000—as their most recent source of capital gains. Since high grade corporate bonds yielded approximately 4½ percent in early 1964, compared with substantially less than 3½ percent for the 15 years preceding 1952, it has been possible to buy such bonds in the market at well below par and by "riding the yield curve" realize much of one's income in the form of capital gains. The tax advantages of doing so are, of course, especially attractive to those in the highest income brackets. It is interesting, therefore, to find that fixed-yield assets rarely appeared as the source of capital gains most recently realized by those in the highest income brackets in our sample. We can offer no definite explanation of this and can only suggest that perhaps there is a wide variety of even more attractive and profitable ways of avoiding the high marginal tax rates that apply to "ordinary" income. Alternatively, or additionally, since we asked only when and what kind of asset people had *sold* at a gain, we may well have missed some instances in which individuals purchased bonds in the market at a price well below par and held them to maturity.

Respondents' Judgments of Their Own Selling Performance

Investors who had sold assets at a gain generally felt that they had done well to sell when they did. This opinion was held by 74 percent of the group, with another 5 percent indicating that they were unsure or undecided on this point. Of those who believed that they ought not to have sold when they did, almost three-fourths cited the behavior of the market subsequent to the sale as justifying this feeling. This was also the reason most commonly offered by those who believed that they had done well to sell when they did, but their explanations were in general much more diverse, and only 29 percent cited market behavior.

In only 5 percent of the cases did tax considerations enter into respondents' judgments on the wisdom of selling at a gain—and almost always as a reason for believing that they had done well. We have no direct evidence as to why people should have believed that tax considerations justified their selling an asset at a gain. The re-

---

dollar volume of various kinds of capital gains. The stock sales may have been in smaller amounts, but also more frequent, so that the *last* sale of many individuals would have been a stock sale.

sponse would be entirely reasonable, of course, if offsetting capital losses or capital-loss carryovers were realized or available in the year in question, or if total income in that year was unusually low—low enough to subject the capital gain to an income tax rate of less than the maximum 25 percent capital gains tax rate.

Holding Period for Assets Sold at a Gain

Of those who had realized capital gains at some time in the past, 71 percent reported that their most recently realized gain was from the sale of an asset they had held for two years or more, and in one-third of these cases the asset had been held for ten or more years.

Only 5 percent of the group reported that the asset had been held for less than six months. In these cases the gain would not have qualified for favorable tax treatment. The relative number of replies indicating short-term capital gains differed radically among income groups. It was more than three times as common at income levels below $75,000 as above, where the differential between ordinary and capital gains tax rates was as high as 66 percentage points before 1964. Moreover, the frequency with which the latest capital gain had been realized on an asset held between six months and one year was 50 percent higher at incomes over $75,000 than it was in the $10,000-$75,000 range. At least at the margin, therefore, it appears that the timing of the realization of capital gains is influenced by tax considerations.

Disposition of the Proceeds of the Sale of Assets

Respondents were asked, with respect to the proceeds from their most recent sale at a gain:

> Did you reinvest the money, or spend it, or what?

By far the most commonly reported disposition was reinvestment of the proceeds in other earning assets. Almost three-fourths of those who had realized gains said that they had followed this course. On the other hand, more than one-sixth of the group used all of the proceeds for consumption purposes. The latter tended to be in the lower income range. A few people accelerated payments on a home mortgage, and some still held the proceeds in bank accounts.

The evidence we have does not permit a precise comparison of the uses of capital gains income with those of "ordinary" income; but it does suggest that the former is more likely to be saved and reinvested. However, since income as well as money "mingles," it is possible that what appears to be saving in the form of realization and reinvestment of capital gains may serve as a substitute, at least in part, for saving and investment out of other sources of income. In other words, the *net* increase in the value of asset holdings attributable to realized capital gains may be smaller than the *gross* increase.

Realization of Capital Losses

As has been pointed out, the realization of capital losses may carry with it some important tax advantages. There are, of course, important nontax reasons for realizing capital losses through the sale of an asset that has depreciated in value, including a desire to cut one's losses, to obtain cash for reinvestment in more attractive assets, or to finance consumption. In any event, we find that among our sample of high-income people, the proportion that had realized a capital loss at some time in the past was about the same as the proportion that had realized a capital gain. Fifty-two percent of the entire sample had realized a capital loss, the proportion rising from 28 percent of those with incomes between $10,000 and $15,000 to 78 percent of those whose incomes exceeded $300,000.

In contrast to the situation with realization of capital gains, however, there was only a slight tendency for the higher-income people to have realized their most recent capital losses at a later date than those with lower incomes. This undoubtedly is because the number of capital transactions increases with income, and gains and losses are not randomly distributed among income groups—in part, of course, because capital gains and losses themselves constitute elements of income. The higher the individual's income, the less likely it is that one loss or even a series of losses will force or induce him to leave the market or seek assets involving less risk. Hence the likelihood, borne out by our findings, is that as income rises the ratio of those having realized a loss recently to those having realized a gain will fall.

Further insights into the experience of high-income people with capital losses are available from our specific analysis of losses during the 15 months preceding our survey. Twenty-eight percent of the entire high-income group reported having realized a capital loss in 1963 or the first three months of 1964. As Chart 9.1 indicates, whether or not a capital loss had been realized recently was determined chiefly by whether or not capital gains had been realized in the same period. Recent losses were not always explicable, however,

CHART 9.1. Factors Associated With The Recent Realization of a Capital Loss

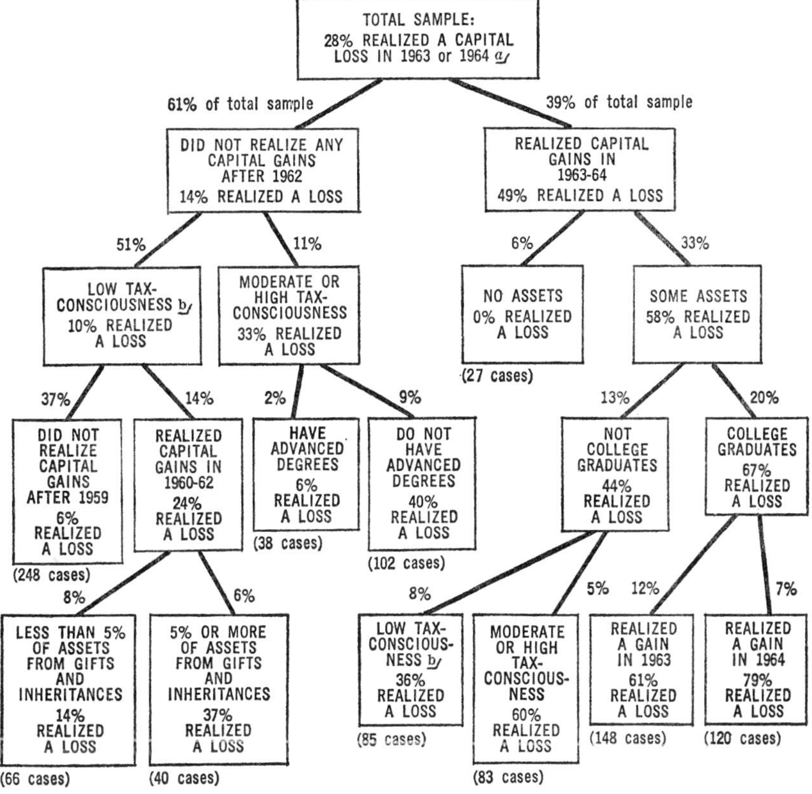

[a] Interviewing took place in the period from March to May 1964.
[b] Tax consciousness index of 0 or 1.

NOTES: For an explanation, see notes to Chart 4.2. In this chart the following predictors were used, listed in order of their explanatory power with a single split over the whole sample: (1) when last realized any capital gains; (2) tax consciousness (for definition, see Chap. XI); (3) whether owned any unrealized capital gains; (4) 1963 income; (5) size of total portfolio; (6) education; (7) percentage of assets from gifts and inheritance; (8) reported marginal tax rate; (9) age. The ten final groups at the ends of the branches accounted for 27 percent of the total variance.

in terms of offsetting gains. For example, among a group of respondents with little tax consciousness, those who had last realized capital gains in 1960-62 were more likely to have realized a loss in 1963-64 than were those who had realized no gains after 1959. Investment activity is apparently the clue. But we could not use our index of investment activity to explain realizing capital losses, because realizing a loss was one of the activities that underlay the index.

It is interesting that educational attainment was associated with a greater tendency to realize losses when there were offsetting gains and also with a lesser inclination to realize losses when gains had not been realized.

Tax consciousness was associated with realizing a loss, but may have been a result rather than a cause. Indeed, one place where the respondent could indicate that he was tax conscious was in his answer to the question why he thought he had done well or badly to sell an asset when he did. Finally, among the group of people who had not recently realized a capital gain and who showed little tax consciousness, those who had inherited a substantial part of their assets were more likely to have realized a loss—perhaps because they were more likely to have an investment that had turned over.

One gets the impression from Chart 9.1 that those who realized a capital loss were active investors who had capital gains to offset, were tax conscious, and were perhaps highly educated. A more restrictive (additive) multivariate analysis not presented here showed similar results.[16] In addition it showed that those with gains still unrealized were more likely to have realized losses, and that people at *both ends* of the education scale were more likely to have realized losses—even when other variables were taken into account simultaneously.

Type of Assets Most Recently Sold at a Loss

As in the case of capital gains, most capital losses were realized on the sale of common stock.[17] Of those who had realized capital

[16] This analysis took the form of multiple regression, which assumes a set of additive and universal effects: that is, each variable is assumed to affect everyone in the population, and to the same extent. See Appendix F.

[17] This finding is consonant with the data derived from individual income tax returns for 1959. See reference cited in note 15 to this chapter.

losses in the past, 78 percent reported that their most recent loss had been from the sale of common stock; for 11 percent of the group the loss involved the sale of real estate or unincorporated business interests; and only 3 percent reported that their most recent loss had been from the sale of a fixed-yield asset.

Respondents' Evaluations of Loss Realizations

As with sales of assets on which gains were realized, we asked:

Do you think you did well to sell it when you did?

Of those who had realized losses in the past, 72 percent felt that they had done well to sell the asset on which they had most recently realized a loss. Thus, satisfaction with sales on which losses were taken was almost as widespread as it was with sales of assets involving gains. The proportion expressing such satisfaction was roughly the same in each income group.

When asked why they thought they had or had not done well to sell the asset at a loss, respondents usually cited the behavior of the market for the asset following the sale. Forty-five percent of those who felt that they had done well to sell and 70 percent of those who felt that they had not gave this reason. Nineteen percent of those who had sold an asset at a loss at some time in the past cited tax considerations as a factor in their judgment of the sale. This is *four times as large a proportion as in the case of capital gains.* Tax considerations, moreover, were mentioned almost exclusively by those who felt that they had done well to sell at a loss, presumably because losses may be used to offset gains and, to a limited extent, ordinary income, thus reducing income tax liabilities. This inference is supported by the evidence in Chart 9.1, which shows that recent losses were closely associated with recent gains.

Summary

- Two-thirds of all high-income people held assets that had appreciated greatly in value. Most of these assets were common stock.
- Almost two-thirds of those who held appreciated assets had never considered selling them, usually because no better investment opportunities were available.

• About one-fifth of those with appreciated assets were deterred from selling them because of tax considerations.

• Approximately three-fourths of those who had realized a capital gain in the past (63 percent of the entire high-income sample) reported that their most recent gains had been realized on the sales of assets that they had held for two years or more—common stock in the vast majority of cases.

• For the most part the proceeds from the sale of appreciated assets were reported as having been reinvested rather than spent on consumption items.

• More than half of the high-income respondents reported having realized a capital loss at some time in the past.

• A large majority of those who had sold assets—close to three-fourths—thought that they had done well to sell when they did, primarily because of observed market behavior following the sale. This held true irrespective of whether the sale produced a gain or a loss.

CHAPTER X

Working Behavior

THE VIEW IS WIDESPREAD THAT rich men are successful largely because they work extremely hard. The hard-driving tycoon is closer to the popular American notion of a rich man than is the languid Sybarite. Another common view, somewhat contradictory to the first, is that the economy has suffered serious losses because the high rates of the income tax have discouraged rich and talented men from supplying their valuable services in full measure. Both of these beliefs were explored in the survey, and the results show that the popular view was nearer to the truth in the first instance than in the second.[1]

The view that high income tax rates seriously deter work effort has been advanced for many years by such businessmen's associations as the National Association of Manufacturers and the U.S. Chamber of Commerce and by many others. At first glance it seems reasonable to argue that when taxation reduces the reward for extra effort by as much as 91 percent (the top income tax rate in effect before the 1964 tax cut), then that extra effort will not be forthcoming.

But further reflection raises some doubts on this point.[2] Taxa-

[1] All the data in this chapter refer to proportions of the aggregate income of those with 1961 incomes over $10,000.

[2] For a more detailed review of the theoretical reasoning and empirical studies relating to income taxation and work effort, see Earl R. Rolph and George F. Break, *Public Finance* (Ronald Press, 1961), pp. 151-57.

tion reduces the reward for extra effort, but it also reduces disposable income and thus may lead the taxpayer who is anxious to maintain his living standard to work even harder. This effect is particularly strong when the taxpayer has to meet large contractual obligations, such as the repayment of a debt. Next, many workers are not in a position to vary their work hours in response to taxation or any other factor; they are hired to work a standard number of hours a week and have little discretion in varying that amount. Further, many of those who are able to vary their work effort may also be able to shift their tax liability onto the buyers of their services. For example, many doctors and lawyers may be in a position to raise their fees when they move into higher tax brackets. The higher bracket may serve to justify to them and to their clients a fee which earlier would have seemed exorbitant. Finally, there are other motives for working besides the earning of after-tax income. Many jobs give their occupants a sense of belonging, or a sense of power, or social status, or the satisfaction of meeting self-imposed standards of performance. Such jobs mute the effects of taxation by providing abundant "income" in a nonmonetary—and nontaxable—form. And even when the individual regards his monetary income as an important index of success, he is often focussing on his gross, before-tax income rather than on what he has available for spending.

In the past there have been a few personal-interview studies of the effect of income taxation on work effort, and it is significant that despite their diverse methodologies and the diverse nature of the populations studied, these investigations have concluded unanimously that the disincentive effects of the progressive income tax are indeed minor. These include Sanders' study of 160 American business executives, Break's study of 306 British lawyers and accountants, the survey of 1,429 British industrial workers by the Royal Commission on the Taxation of Profits and Income, and Strümpel's study of 1,000 German businessmen and professionals.[3]

[3] Thomas H. Sanders, *Effects of Taxation on Executives* (Harvard University, Graduate School of Business Administration, 1951); George F. Break, "Income Taxes and Incentives to Work: An Empirical Study," *American Economic Review* (September 1957), pp. 529-49; Royal Commission on the Taxation of Profits and Income, *Second Report,* Cmd. 9105 (London: Her Majesty's Stationery Office, 1954), pp. 91-124; and Buckhard Strümpel, *Steuermoral und Steuerwiderstand der Deutschen Selbständigen—ein Beitrag zur Lehre von den Steuerwirkungen* (Köln und Opladen: Westdeutscher Verlag, to be published in 1966).

In addition there have been some empirical studies that used less direct techniques than the personal interview, and all of these have likewise concluded that tax disincentives are unimportant. In this category are the studies by Rolfe and Furness, by Long, and by Buck and Shimmin.[4] The present survey does not break the record of unanimity so far established.

Occupations

Nine out of ten in the high-income group were working as members of the labor force, most of the rest being retired. The occupations followed by the high-income persons and the changing importance of those occupations at different income levels are shown in Table 10.1.

Those working in the labor force were evenly divided between employees and owner-managers. The latter group included self-employed professionals, owner-managers of unincorporated businesses and closely held corporations, presidents and chairmen of larger corporations, and other corporate officers who held stock in the enterprises they served. At the lower income levels, owner-managers were far outnumbered by employees; but at the highest incomes, those in the labor force were almost exclusively of the owner-manager class.

There was some variety in the average incomes of the different owner-manager groups. The self-employed professionals as a group were no more numerous relatively at incomes over $300,000 than they were at incomes between $10,000 and $15,000. They represented about 5 percent of each of these income groups. But at an intermediate income level of about $100,000 they comprised nearly a fourth of the group. This nonlinearity was caused chiefly by the earnings situation of doctors, most of whom earned incomes well above $15,000 but few of whom could earn much over $100,000.

[4] Sidney E. Rolfe and Geoffrey Furness, "The Impact of Changes in Tax Rates and Method of Collection on Effort: Some Empirical Observations," *Review of Economics and Statistics* (November 1957), pp. 394-401; Clarence D. Long, "Impact of the Federal Income Tax on Labor Force Participation," in U.S. Congress, Joint Committee on the Economic Report, *Federal Tax Policy for Economic Growth and Stability,* 84 Cong. 1 sess. (1955), pp. 153-66; Leslie Buck and Sylvia Shimmin, "Is Taxation a Deterrent?," *Westminster Bank Review* (August 1959), pp. 16-19.

TABLE 10.1. Distribution of Occupations at Different Income Levels, For Entire High-Income Sample

Occupation	*Percentage distribution of aggregate income of persons with 1961 incomes over $10,000*		
	All cases[a]	*1963 incomes between $10,000 and $15,000*	*1963 incomes over $300,000*
Working in labor force:			
Owner-managers			
Professionals	12	5	5
Physicians	5	1	0
Lawyers	4	1	5
Engineers, architects, and scientists	3	3	0
Financial sector[b]	7	4	25
Other businesses	26	17	47
Realtors and contractors	3	2	1
Farmers and ranchers	2	3	1
Others	21	12	45
Employees			
Professionals	14	19	1
Physicians	0	0	0
Lawyers	2	2	1
Engineers, architects, and scientists	12	17	0
Financial sector[b]	4	2	6
Other businesses	28	43	0
Rentiers:			
Males	7	9	15
Females	2	1	1
Total	100	100	100

[a] The column headed "All cases" should be read as follows: of the aggregate income of those with incomes over $10,000, 5 percent was received by physicians, 4 percent by lawyers, and so forth.
[b] Banking, insurance, stockbrokerage, and accountancy.

At the highest income levels the group of "self-employed professionals" consisted almost entirely of lawyers.

As between the other two broad groups of owner-managers, it is interesting to note that those in the financial sector—the bankers, investment counselors, stockbrokers, and other "financiers"—enjoyed more financial success than their counterparts elsewhere in the business world. In the income class from $10,000 to $15,000, only one in six owner-managers was a "financier," but at incomes over $300,000 the proportion so employed rose to one-third.

Second Jobs

It is always difficult to classify people precisely according to occupations. Formal job titles are often misleading; some jobs oblige their holders to perform several different economic roles almost simultaneously. For example, the small-scale contractor must be at once engineer, entrepreneur, and laborer. Some persons move frequently from one occupation to another, sometimes as a way of life; others engage in "moonlighting." The difficulties of classification are perhaps greater for those with the higher incomes.

To obtain information on the complexity of working roles among the high-income group, we asked the following questions:

> Do you have more than one kind of work at which you earn money?
>
> What is your other work?
>
> Is that an occupation where you work for yourself, or for someone else, or what?

Among those working in the labor force, one in five had a second job. The most typical second job was that of a lawyer with a substantial income who doubled as a corporation official. Two out of every five lawyers reported holding a second job; all of the other occupational groups defined in Table 10.1 lagged far behind in this respect. And the higher the income, the more frequently were second jobs reported. At an income level of $12,000, only one in eight of those in the labor force held a second job; but at an income level of $200,000, three in eight did.

The second jobs reported by the high-income respondents were fairly similar in nature to their primary jobs, both in the aggregate and on an individual basis. Many persons reported holding two separate jobs within the same general occupation. There was, however, some crossing of occupational lines: several lawyers reported that they held second jobs as corporation directors; some realtors and contractors were also in farming. And naturally there were some occupations that were very rarely secondary ones. In particular, medical and legal positions were almost never second jobs. Finally, we may note that nearly two-thirds of those with second jobs regarded themselves as being self-employed in those jobs.

Perhaps the most interesting finding here is that the second jobs were generally held by those with the higher incomes. It is not easy to trace causation in this area. Nevertheless a picture begins to emerge of high incomes being linked with hard work—of the rich being far from idle. These impressions were confirmed by the findings on hours of work, which are reported next.

Work Effort

In attempting to measure work input one is bedeviled by problems of classification. For example, should weekend hours spent golfing with a client be classed as work or leisure? In the survey we left those problems for the respondents to cope with and simply asked the following questions:

> About how many hours per week do you work ordinarily?
> How many weeks did you work last year?

The high-income workers showed themselves to be an industrious group. Their median work week was 48 hours. One in four claimed to be working 60 hours a week or more. The workers who put in the longest hours on the job tended to be the youngest, those with the higher incomes, and those in the owner-manager class. As age increased, the median work week gradually declined, from 52 hours for the high-income respondents aged under thirty-five to 40 hours for those aged sixty-five and over who were still working. Higher incomes were associated with longer work weeks—although here again the nature of the causation is not easily discerned. At an income level of $12,000, only one in six of those in the labor force worked 60 hours a week or more, whereas at an income level of $200,000, more than one in three did. At still higher incomes, the proportion working very long hours began to decline.

Among occupation groups the owner-managers outside the financial sector worked the longest hours. The median work week for the self-employed professionals was 53 hours, and for other business owner-managers outside the financial sector the median work week was no less than 55 hours. In this latter group two out of five worked 60 hours a week or more. By contrast, the owner-managers in the financial sector reported a median work week of only 46 hours. Thus there seems to be some substance to the hoary jibes about "bankers' hours."

As for vacations, the high-income respondents were far from being self-indulgent. Of every twelve workers, seven took vacations of no more than two weeks during the year, another three took between two and four weeks, and only two vacationed for a total of more than four weeks. However, while higher incomes were associated with longer work weeks, they were also associated with longer vacations. At an income level of $12,000 only one in seven workers took vacations of more than four weeks, but this proportion rose to one in three at an income level of $400,000. The richest men seem to have both worked hard and played hard.[5]

No attempt was made in the survey to measure the relationship between wage rates and work effort, that is, to determine the shape of the supply-of-labor curve at these high levels of wage rates. Such an exercise was rendered impossible by our decision not to collect information on labor income as distinct from other forms of income. Cross-sectional studies of lower-income groups have suggested that there is a negative relationship between wage rates and the total number of hours worked during the year.[6] In view of the strong connection observed in our survey between longer work weeks and higher incomes, there is reason to believe that the relationship prevailing at lower wage rates does not also prevail at higher wage rates. It is possible that the supply-of-labor curve, far from being backward-bending, may actually be forward-bending. But it must be admitted that the need to adjust our data to take ac-

[5] For other empirical studies which show that high-income people devote a lot of time to their jobs, see F. W. Taussig and C. S. Joslyn, *American Business Leaders* (Macmillan, 1932); Mabel Newcomer, *The Big Business Executive—The Factors That Made Him, 1900-1950* (Columbia University Press, 1955); W. Lloyd Warner and James C. Abegglen, *Occupational Mobility in American Business and Industry, 1928-1952* (University of Minnesota Press, 1955); W. Lloyd Warner and James C. Abegglen, *Big Business Leaders in America* (Harper and Brothers, 1955).

[6] See especially the multivariate analysis in James N. Morgan *et al., Income and Welfare in the United States* (McGraw-Hill, 1962), pp. 76-77. See also James N. Morgan, "Time, Work, and Welfare" in M. J. Brennan (ed.), *Patterns of Market Behavior* (Brown University Press, 1965), p. 97.

count of nonlabor income and vacation time, and the dangers of deriving spurious conclusions from simple correlations between two variables, make it impossible to be definite on this point.

Factors Affecting Work Effort

In order to discover what factors in general affected work effort, we asked the following series of questions:

> Do you have opportunities to earn additional income by working more or taking on extra work?
>
> (If yes) How do you decide how much work to do then?
>
> Do you spend more time at your work than you did a few years ago, or less, or what?
>
> (If any change) What are the main reasons for this change?

Two out of every five high-income workers said that they had opportunities to work more. Perhaps contrary to expectations, those with the lower incomes were the most likely to report having such opportunities. This finding presumably reflected the shorter hours typically worked by those with lower incomes; the hardworking people with the higher incomes tended to regard themselves perhaps as already working to the limit and hence as having no chance to work more.

As would be expected, the owner-managers saw themselves as having more opportunities to do additional work than did the employees (when account is taken of the difference in work hours between the two groups). Within the group of owner-managers, those in the financial sector and the self-employed professionals reported having the greatest flexibility. Again, this result presumably stemmed from the fact that these persons typically worked shorter hours than their compulsive brethren elsewhere in the business world.

The high-income respondents who reported having opportunities to work more were then asked how they decided on the amount of work to do. Remarkable in the answers here was the relative unimportance of the workers' own preferences. In fully one-half of the answers the respondents said that they were driven by the demands of their job or that they worked to the limit of their physical capacity. Typical of such comments were the following:

> I work till I start to get too tired from traveling. When I get so tired that I'm not doing a good job, I stop or back off.
>
> I work till I'm tired, till I'm through.
>
> I give this [job] everything I've got. I've turned down outside directorates because I felt they would take time which my company was entitled to. However, it's a good thing everybody doesn't feel this way or we would have a hard time getting a Board of Directors.

Other kinds of answers were much less common. One in six of those who were asked the question gave the uninformative reply that they worked as much as they wanted to. One in twelve mentioned having to leave some time for leisure activities. Only 3 percent of the group (that is, 1 percent of the entire high-income sample) reported that they limited their work because of tax disincentives. At the same time, none at all said in this context that taxes made them choose to work harder. And only 4 percent of the group claimed to be driven by the need to earn additional income in order to meet expenses. All of these people had relatively low incomes.

The occupational groups differed considerably in the explanations that they gave for their work effort. The references to physical constraints were most frequent among the nonprofessional owner-managers, who, as has been seen, tended to work the longest hours. This same group was also the least likely to say that leisure needs determined the amount of work they chose to do. Thus our earlier impression is confirmed that the entrepreneur is the most compulsive of workers.

By contrast, the professionals, both employees and self-employed, talked little of physical constraints and seldom reported that they worked as much as their business demanded. There is a suggestion in our data that feelings of "company loyalty" were weakest among the professionals, many of whom may have regarded their membership in a particular business organization as being less important than their membership in a profession. At the same time, the professionals, particularly the self-employed, made the most references to tax disincentives.

A further perspective on the factors governing work effort was provided by the questions about the changes that had occurred in the individual's work effort during the previous few years. Judging from the answers, there does not seem to have been any upward or downward trend in recent years in the total work input of high-income persons. One-fourth of those in the labor force said they were working more than previously, one-fourth said that they were working less, and one-half reported no change. Not surprisingly the individual's age chiefly determined his answer to this question. The younger respondents tended to work harder than previously, while the older ones were slowing down.

The reasons given for the change in work effort echoed those given earlier in answer to the question about decisions on how much work to do. Of those who were working more than previously, about two-thirds explained the change by referring to the demands made upon them by their jobs. They said that they had been given more responsibility, that business was better than it used to be, etc. None said in this context that he was working more in order to earn enough to pay taxes.

Similarly those who were working less than previously most often gave explanations that had little to do with their own preferences. They cited advancing age, deteriorating health, or the fact that less work was available. A few mentioned the desire for more leisure or time to travel. A few mentioned tax disincentives, such as the respondent who said, "I got tired of working for the government and paying taxes," but these numbered only 3 percent of those who were working less (that is, 1 percent of the entire high-income sample). Once again a high proportion of the references to tax disincentives came from the self-employed professionals.

Tax Disincentives

Our inquiry into the delicate issue of tax disincentives proceeded in two stages. We first asked general questions about work effort. While these did not explicitly suggest the question of tax disincentives, the respondent could properly have talked about taxes in his answer. The results of that inquiry have been presented in the preceding section. Very few of the high-income respondents—not many more than 1 percent—mentioned tax disincentives at that stage.

We then asked some direct questions about tax disincentives:

If you (or your wife) earned any extra money, about what fraction of it would be taken in extra income taxes?

Has the income tax had any effect on how much work you (or your wife) do?

(If yes) In what way?

Would you give me a specific example?

Even at this stage the vast majority (seven out of eight) of the high-income respondents gave no indication that their work effort had been reduced by income taxes. (This group included the 1 percent of the sample who said in answer to the direct questions quoted above that they worked harder because of income taxes.) But for one in eight—the disincentive group—the question clearly touched a raw nerve:

I quit trying to get rich. Somebody in Washington grabs it before you get it. I used to turn everything I could think of to make a dollar. Now I quit when I get to the place where it really costs to make it. Why bother?

I have curbed my ambitions. I regret to have to say that. Why expand and take on more? Why run the risk? Why work so hard?

I'd work more, take on a few more opportunities that come along. I could have gone in on a deal a few weeks ago, but it would have required a lot of effort and time and besides there was the tax disadvantage. . . . I could cite you at least twenty examples of men who are semi-retired at an early age because of income tax reasons.

Not all of those claiming to work less because of income taxes gave fully logical answers. Some seemed to be saying that the alternative to a decline in work effort caused by the income tax would be some sort of physical overstrain (which presumably would in time cause an even more drastic decline in work effort!):[7]

There's no point in having the government as my 50 percent partner in killing myself. Many of my younger friends are dropping dead of heart attacks from overwork.

[7] Rolph and Break have proposed that for this reason the progressive income tax should be regarded as a useful public health measure. *Op. cit.*, p. 157.

CHART 10.1. Factors Associated With Reported Tax Disincentives

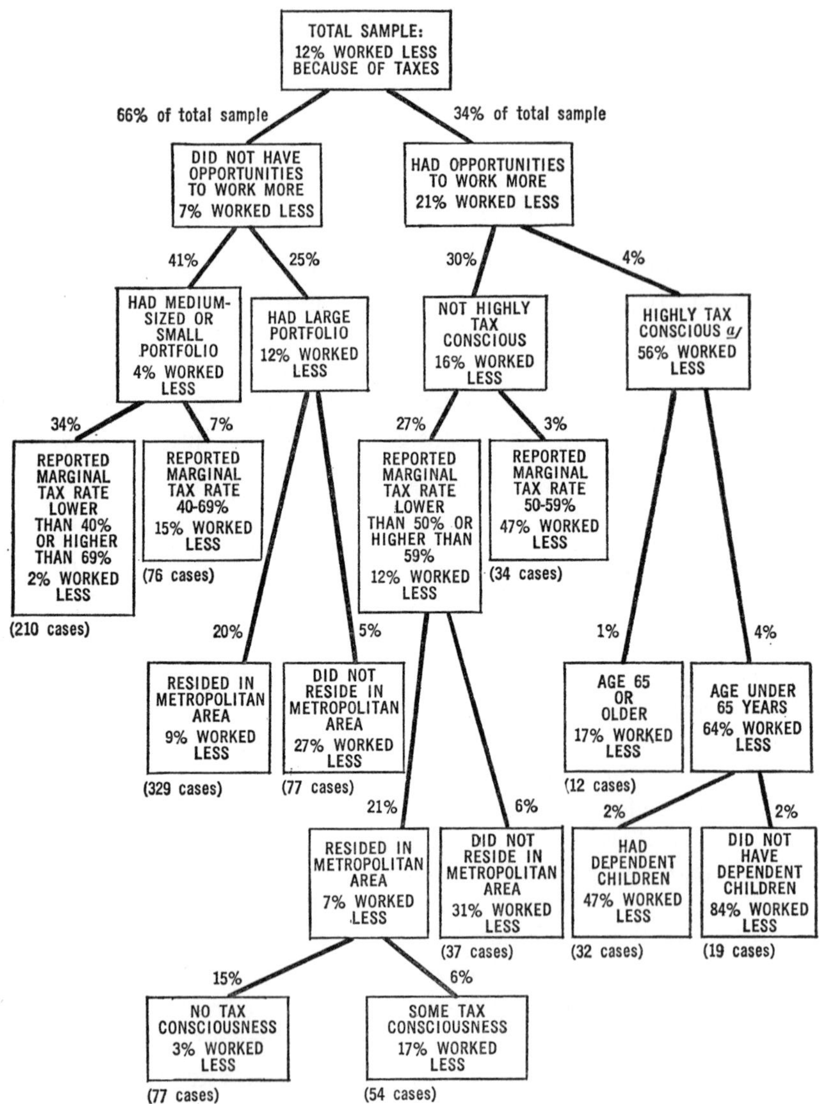

[a] Tax consciousness index of 3 or more.

NOTES: For explanation, see notes to Chart 4.2. In this chart the following predictors were used, listed in order of their explanatory power with a single split over the whole sample: (1) whether any opportunities to work more; (2) tax consciousness (for definition, see Chap. XI); (3) occupational group; (4) reported marginal tax rate; (5) size of total portfolio; (6) whether lived in a metropolitan area; (7) 1963 adjusted gross income; (8) education; (9) age; (10) political preference; (11) whether any dependent children. The eleven final groups at the ends of the branches accounted for 22 percent of the total variance.

I stopped Saturday morning work because the rate of tax was evidently going to take such a percentage out that it wasn't worth the additional physical work or the possible results from overwork.

Apart from the doubts raised by such answers as these, there are several grounds for our reluctance to believe that so significant a fraction as one-eighth of the high-income group really worked less because of income taxes. First, many of the one-eighth claiming to suffer a disincentive had reported earlier in the interview that they had no opportunities to work more, and so the nature of the disincentive in these cases must remain obscure. Second, as was noted above, very few in the disincentive group had voluntarily mentioned tax considerations in answer to the earlier general questions about work effort. Third, it was found that the one-eighth claiming a disincentive worked on the average about as many hours a week and as many weeks a year as did the seven-eighths who said that their work effort was unaffected by taxation. The median work week for the disincentive group was 47 hours, and for the unaffected group it was 48 hours; for both groups the median number of weeks worked during the year was 50.[8]

Estimated Extent of Tax Disincentives

A more plausible estimate of the extent of tax disincentives can be made by assuming that the reported disincentives were illusory or negligible in the case of those who had no opportunity to work more and in the case of persons who were already working 60 hours a week or more. If this assumption is made, then it can be estimated that one-sixteenth, not one-eighth, of the high-income group had suffered a tax disincentive.

Since so much political and intellectual concern has been focussed on the individuals made idle by taxation, it is interesting to examine their personal characteristics. A multivariate analysis was performed in order to identify the social and economic factors predisposing an individual to report a tax disincentive.

No distinction was made here between "plausible" and "implausible" cases. Eleven explanatory factors were used in the analysis. The results are summarized in Chart 10.1.

[8] About one-tenth of both the disincentive group and the unaffected group were retired. These cases were excluded from the calculation of the medians cited here.

With one or two exceptions the findings were as expected. The most important factor in explaining the occurrence of a tax disincentive was whether the individual had opportunities to work more. For those with some flexibility in their work effort, among whom 21 percent reported a disincentive, the next most important factor was the level of tax consciousness. In the subgroup of highly tax-conscious individuals with some work flexibility, more than one-half reported a disincentive. A further analysis of this subgroup identified the part of the population where tax disincentives were almost universally reported. Among those in the subgroup who were under sixty-five years old and without dependent children, 84 percent said they worked less because of taxes. The association between the lack of dependent children and the prevalence of tax disincentives could be explained as follows: those without dependent children were under less social and family pressure to maintain particular living standards, and hence the "income effect" of taxation —the tendency for persons to work harder in order to make up for the income paid out in taxes—would be weaker in these cases.

For the subgroup who were less tax conscious but nevertheless had some work flexibility, there were other factors that explained the presence of tax disincentives. First in importance was the individual's marginal income tax rate. But surprisingly enough, those with the highest rates were not the most likely to suffer disincentives. Rather, the disincentives were concentrated among those with marginal rates between 50 percent and 59 percent. In this group about half reported a disincentive, whereas among those in higher or lower tax brackets only one-eighth did. One is inclined, of course, to dismiss this finding as a statistical accident.[9] But, as will be seen in Chart 10.1, a similar phenomenon occurred elsewhere in the analysis. Indeed, inspection of the data from several points of view showed the "peaking" to be very conspicuous and unlikely to have been caused by pure chance.

Further details about the peaking are given in Table 10.2. The first column shows that for the entire sample (excluding the rentiers)

[9] The finding differs from that of Break (see note 3 to this chapter), who observed from his British sample that disincentives were reported most frequently by those with the highest marginal tax rates. Break has presented his finding in Congressional testimony. See *Income Tax Revision,* Panel Discussions before the House Committee on Ways and Means, 86 Cong. 1 sess. (1960), pp. 1199, 1212, and 1221.

TABLE 10.2. Tax Disincentives and Marginal Tax Rates, For High-Income Sample, Excluding Rentiers

Reported marginal income tax rate (Percent)	*Percentage of each tax bracket's aggregate income received by those who said they worked less because of taxes*	*Percentage after adjustments to remove the effects of nine other variables*[a]
Zero	0	−8
1–19	12	14
20–29	7	11
30–39	9	12
40–49	17	12
50–59	24	20
60–69	24	18
70–79	18	6
80–89	18	6
90 or more	6	8
Not ascertained	8	9

[a] The figures in this column are derived from coefficients for the tax brackets in a multiple regression equation in which each bracket is a separate (dummy) explanatory variable and in which the other explanatory variables consist of classes of the following nine characteristics: whether any opportunities to work more, tax-consciousness, whether lived in a metropolitan area, occupational group, education, age, whether any dependent children, 1963 income, and size of total portfolio.

the proportion reporting a disincentive first rose along with the marginal tax rate and then declined. The figures in this column show the relationship between disincentives and the tax rate without any account being taken of other factors. The second column shows how this relationship changes when account is taken of several other factors. Each percentage in the second column indicates what the frequency of disincentives would have been if the respondents in that tax bracket had been identical to the rest of the sample in their age distribution, occupational distribution, etc. In this way the effects of age, occupation, and seven other variables are accounted for or "held constant." It can be seen that the peaking survives even this more rigorous analysis.

We therefore accepted the finding and offer the speculation that when a person's income reaches the level where the federal government becomes for the first time the major partner in extra earnings, resentment of the tax becomes intense and disincentives are strong. But after a while the high-income taxpayer becomes used to having only a minority interest in his own extra earnings, and from then on disincentives weaken. An alternative explanation might lead to the policy suggestion that the government should remove the offending percentages from the schedule of tax rates, just as the superstitious management of a skyscraper hotel omits the thirteenth in numbering the floors.

Elsewhere in the analysis, the population of the area where the respondent lived also seemed to be an important explanatory factor, disincentives being most widespread in the nonmetropolitan areas. This result is similar to one reported by Break in his study of British lawyers and accountants.[10] Break offers the explanation that social pressures to maintain particular living standards might have been weaker in the rural areas and smaller towns and hence the "income effect" of income taxation might have been weaker in those places. An alternative explanation might be that many businessmen in the smaller communities, being spatial monopolists, were less subject to competition from rivals. Hence one influence leading to intense work effort was largely absent.

In Chart 10.1 we turn finally to the group that had no opportunities for working more. Only 7 percent of these individuals claimed to suffer a tax disincentive, and, as has been suggested above, the actual existence of this kind of disincentive must remain in some doubt. But it is noteworthy that the multivariate analysis of this group duplicates the other results which showed disincentives to be strongest among those at the middle of the tax rate schedule and among those who lived in nonmetropolitan areas. In addition the analysis showed that for this part of the population, tax disincentives were more prevalent among those with the large portfolios. This result confirms the theoretical proposition that the "income effect" of taxation is weaker in cases where large capital incomes are received.

Some other variables were included in the multivariate analysis besides those appearing in the chart, but all turned out to have negligible value in explaining why some persons worked less because of income taxes while others were unaffected. These other variables included 1963 income, occupational group, education, and political preference. Although occupation as such had little to do with the occurrence of tax disincentives, it is worth noting that nearly half of what we called the "plausible" disincentive group consisted of

[10] *Loc. cit.* in note 3 to this chapter.

professionals. Their appearance in such large numbers in the disincentive group was due to the fact they usually had opportunities to work more; and it is this latter factor which the multivariate analysis revealed to be the most crucial in determining whether there was likely to be a tax disincentive.

Losses Caused By Tax Disincentives

We can use the survey findings to make a rough estimate of the loss of annual output suffered by the economy as a result of the work disincentives caused by the pre-1964 progressive income tax. Not all of the data needed for an accurate estimate are available from the survey, and therefore the following simplifying assumptions will be made:[11]

1. Among those with incomes under $10,000 the work effort effects of replacing the pre-1964 progressive income tax with some feasible alternative with minimal disincentive effects—such as perhaps a proportional or mildly progressive income tax—would have been negligible. At these income levels the rates of income taxation, both average and marginal, were low.
2. Among the population with incomes over $10,000 those claiming to be unaffected by income taxation would not have changed their work effort if the progressive income tax had been replaced by the feasible alternative, while those claiming to suffer a disincentive because of the progressive income tax would have worked as much as the first group if that tax had been replaced.
3. The disincentives claimed by those with no opportunities to work more and by those already working 60 hours a week or more were negligible.
4. If work effort had increased by 1 percent and had not been accompanied by any increase in capital inputs, then output would have increased by two-thirds of 1 percent.

The survey revealed that those reporting a plausible disincentive received 6 percent of the aggregate income of the high-income

[11] Among the considerations ignored in the following computations are (a) the effects of taxation on choices among occupations, and (b) the effects of taxation on investment in human capital.

group, or about 2.5 percent of total income in the economy. The survey also revealed that those reporting a plausible disincentive worked on the average about five-sixths as many hours during the year as did the rest of the high-income persons in the labor force. Thus on the basis of the assumptions cited above, it follows that the total loss of annual output in the economy in 1963 due to the existence of the progressive income tax instead of some feasible alternative may have been of the order of one-third of 1 percent.

Retirement Decisions

Seven percent of the high-income group were retired, and a series of questions inquired first into the factors affecting the timing of their retirement and, second, into the opportunities they had had for working since that time. About the timing of their retirement we asked:

> When did you retire?
> How did you happen to retire when you did?

The most common answer, which was given by only one in six, however, was that a compulsory retirement age had been reached. One in seven referred to bad health, and one in nine said that others in the business were by that time ready to take over. Virtually none in the group reported having retired early because of high taxes. At the same time there was no evidence that taxes had caused a postponement of retirement by lengthening the time necessary for the accumulation of an estate of a given size. None of the retirees stated that they had retired at that particular time because they had by then accumulated enough savings. Thus some doubt is thrown on the separate findings of Sanders and Break that the most conspicuous effect of taxation on work effort lay in the postponement of retirement.[12] It should be noted, however, that the conclusions of Sanders and Break were derived from the forecasts, as it were, of younger men still at work, whereas our conclusions were derived from questioning the retirees themselves.

About work after retirement we asked:

[12] Sanders, *op. cit.;* Break, *loc. cit.* in note 3 to this chapter.

Have you had opportunities to work for money since your retirement?

What opportunities have you had?

Have you accepted any of them?

What were your main reasons for doing that?

About half of the retirees reported having had opportunities to work after retirement, mostly involving skills roughly equivalent to those used in their previous work. Such opportunities were reported most frequently by those who had worked as engineers or in the financial sector, and least frequently by those who had worked as lawyers, realtors, contractors, or farmers.

Of those who had had opportunities for paid work after retirement, one-half reported having accepted the offers, this proportion being about the same at all income levels. Where offers had been accepted, the reasons given were usually that the work promised to be interesting or provided an escape from boredom. Financial inducements were scarcely mentioned at all. Where offers had been rejected, most explained simply that they preferred to remain men of leisure. Two of the twenty-four retirees who rejected work offers mentioned tax considerations.

Employment of Wives

In the lower-income population it is very common for wives to have paid jobs, and financial necessity plays a large part in their decisions to work.[13] Among the wives of high-income persons, paid jobs were fairly common, but it appeared that financial necessity was seldom an important influence on those wives who did work.

The survey indicated that there was a threshold at a family income of about $30,000 beyond which the wives' participation in the labor force became markedly reduced. Where income was between $10,000 and $30,000, four-tenths of all wives (aged under sixty-five) held paid jobs at the time of the survey; but at higher in-

[13] See Morgan *et al., op. cit.*, pp. 106*ff*. and references therein; Morgan, *op. cit.* in note 6 to this chapter; F. Ivan Nye and L. W. Hoffman, *The Employed Mother in America* (Rand-McNally and Co., 1963); Jacob Mincer, "Labor Force Participation of Married Women: A Study of Labor Supply," in *Aspects of Labor Economics,* a Conference of the Universities-National Bureau Committee for Economic Research (Princeton University Press, 1962).

comes less than one-tenth of all wives did. At the lower incomes four out of every five employed wives worked full time, but at the higher incomes, only two out of every five. At the lower incomes one out of every four wives who were not currently employed intended to go to work at some time in the future; but at the higher income level, only one in nine of those not currently employed had that intention.[14]

It may appear from these results considered alone that the wives in high-income families worked mainly for economic reasons. But the answers to other questions suggested otherwise. Concerning wives who were currently at work we asked the following questions:

How long does she plan to keep on working?
Why is that?

The most common reply, given by one-third of the respondents to whom the question was put, was simply that the wife would continue working indefinitely because she enjoyed the job. One in eight said that the wife would continue working until she reached a compulsory retirement age. Only one in six gave the specifically "economic" reply that the wife would continue working for as long as the family needed her earnings.

A further question inquired into the reasons for wives withdrawing from the labor force. Concerning those wives who were not currently at work but who had held a job at some time during the previous ten years, we asked:

How did she happen to give up her job?

About half of the answers referred to family responsibilities of various kinds, such as the need to care for children. There were virtually no references to tax disincentives in this context.

Finally, we inquired into the plans for wives to enter the labor force at some time in the future. Concerning wives aged fifty or under

[14] In contrast, other studies by the Survey Research Center and the U. S. Bureau of the Census show that among families with incomes under $10,000, there is a *positive* relationship between family income and the wife's participation in the labor force. But this result is partly circular, since the wife's earnings are a component of family income. The effect of the husband's earnings is negligible below $5,000 and negative above that. See Morgan *et al., op. cit.,* Chap. 9.

who were not currently at work we asked the following questions:

> What about the future? Do you think she will go to work for money sometime in the future?
>
> Why is that?

Among those who thought that their wives would go to work in the future, two out of three said that this was because their wives would find the work interesting or would be bored otherwise. One in three explained that the departure of children to school or elsewhere would make it possible for the wife to work. Only one in eight said that their wives would work because the family needed more money.

As for those who did not think that their wives would go to work, about half explained that the family did not need the extra earnings, and most of the remainder explained simply that their wives did not want to work. Virtually none in the group mentioned high taxes as a reason for their wives not working in the future.

Thus despite the strong negative relationship observed between family income and the participation of wives in the labor force, the factors mentioned by respondents as affecting that participation were mainly noneconomic. It is possible of course that some of the replies were biased. Many of the respondents gave the interview apart from their wives, and some of them may have been reluctant to admit to the interviewer that the family was dependent, even if only to a small degree, on the wife's earnings. Otherwise, one may conjecture that most of the wives in high-income families felt a need to keep busy and make worthwhile contributions to society; but whereas at the lower incomes within the group there was some pressure to combine these primary objectives with the secondary objective of earning extra money, at the highest incomes that pressure was mostly absent, and in those families the women accordingly felt more free to occupy themselves with voluntary unpaid activities.

Summary

- The average high-income person worked 48 hours a week and took only two weeks' vacation during the year.

• High-income individuals were far from being free agents in deciding how much work to do. Among the most important influences on their work effort were the inescapable demands of the job and the limits of their physical endurance.

• Seven-eighths of the high-income respondents explicitly stated that they had not curtailed their work effort on account of the income tax. Many of the tax disincentives reported by the remaining respondents seemed implausible in the light of other information.

• On the basis of some simplifying assumptions, it appeared that the loss of annual output in the economy due to the existence of the progressive income tax instead of some feasible alternative was extremely small.

• Income taxes did not appear to have had a significant effect either on the timing of retirement or on the participation of wives in the labor force.

CHAPTER XI

Tax Consciousness

TAX CONSCIOUSNESS IS promoted in the United States by the combination of high marginal individual income tax rates (ranging from 20 to 91 percent in 1963) and many kinds of preferential treatment accorded to selected sources, forms, and dispositions of income.[1] On earned income, for example, cash compensation currently received is fully taxed, whereas "fringe benefits" are often taxed lightly or not at all. Such benefits may be in the form of employer-financed group term life insurance, medical and hospital insurance, deferred compensation, employer contributions to pension and profit-sharing plans, employee stock options, or "perquisites of office" in the form of the privilege of using company-provided dining rooms, automobiles, yachts, hunting lodges, and other entertainment facilities.

Those who own property have many opportunities to realize investment income that is either tax free or taxable at only a fraction of "ordinary" rates. In addition to those opportunities discussed in Chapter IX under the heading of capital gains, there is tax-free interest on state and local bonds, tax-exempt accumulations of interest on life insurance policies that are paid at the death of the insured, deductibility of "losses" incurred by "hobby" farms and

[1] All the data in this chapter refer to proportions of the aggregate income of those with 1961 incomes over $10,000.

other enterprises (such as the owning and running of a stable of race horses), rental real estate on which book losses are accompanied by large cash payouts (a combination made possible by excessive depreciation allowances), generous depletion allowances unrelated to capital costs, coupled with the immediate expensing of many such costs in oil and gas production, and many others.[2]

Tax liabilities may be substantially reduced by distributing income-producing property among the several members of one's family (either by outright gift or through the creation of trusts), by forming specious partnerships,[3] and by establishing corporations whose primary function is to receive property income so that it will be taxed at rates far lower than it would be if it were taxed to high-income individuals.

People of wealth may indulge their tastes for certain forms of consumption and at the same time thereby avoid income taxes. Before the law was changed in 1964, a person could buy a work of art, enjoy it in his home during his lifetime and yet deduct much of its value as a charitable contribution if he signed an agreement under which it would go to a museum at his death. Similarly, prominence in church, hospital, performing arts, and educational circles may be enjoyed at the price of contributions deductible for tax purposes, a price that may be very small indeed if the contribution takes the form of appreciated property. A great deal of traveling can be, and is, undertaken under the guise of tax-deductible "medical treatment."

It has generally been assumed in recent discussion that many taxpayers are in fact heavily preoccupied with the income tax and that their economic decisions—to assume or to avoid risk, to invest in one asset rather than another, and to work more or to work less—are governed in large part by tax considerations. Thus in 1963 when urging the Ways and Means Committee of the House of Representatives to accept President Kennedy's tax reform proposals,

[2] In recent years attention has been called by indignant authors of popular treatises to the many ways in which tax liabilities may be reduced. See, for example, Louis Eisenstein, *The Ideologies of Taxation* (Ronald Press, 1961); Jerome R. Hellerstein, *Taxes, Loopholes, and Morals* (McGraw-Hill, 1963); and Philip M. Stern, *The Great Treasury Raid* (Random House, 1964). A more technical and dispassionate analysis may be found in Richard Goode, *The Individual Income Tax* (Brookings Institution, 1964).

[3] Under the law even the taxpayer's infant child may be a business partner if property held in the child's name can be said to contribute substantially to the earnings of the business.

Treasury Secretary Dillon said that "the primary objective is to release our economy from the shackles of an overly repressive income tax rate structure . . ." and that rate reduction "will restore incentives for risk-taking, initiative, and extra effort,"[4] as well as "minimize the diversion of energy from productive activities to tax avoidance. . . ."[5] Selected cases in which investors appear to have been motivated in their choice of investments by tax considerations are readily found, and men whose views are given much public attention have frequently insisted that high income tax rates are destroying work incentives. However, funds do continue to be attracted to the more mundane (from a tax viewpoint) industries, high risks are assumed in new and venturesome enterprises, and corporate executives subject to very high marginal tax rates appear to be among the hardest working of people.

In this chapter the evidence from our survey is presented in an effort to cast light on the tax consciousness of high-income people. It is by no means self-evident (1) that individuals are keenly aware of the actual or potential impact of the income tax and the means of escaping it, or (2) that if they are aware they are moved to change their behavior in response to tax considerations.

Measures of Tax Consciousness

Tax consciousness may be gauged in a number of ways. We have first an "index of tax consciousness," the number of times during the interview the respondent mentioned tax considerations (without their being suggested) as a reason for action, inaction, preference, satisfaction or lack of satisfaction with past actions or present circumstances, or as a reason for specified behavior, such as retiring at a particular time, incorporating a business, giving large gifts to relatives, etc.

A second measure of tax consciousness is provided by the answer to the question whether or not the respondent knew his marginal income tax rate or at least could state a rate which appeared

[4] *President's 1963 Tax Message along with Principal Statement, Technical Explanation, and Supporting Exhibits and Documents Submitted by Secretary of the Treasury Douglas Dillon,* Statement before the House Committee on Ways and Means on the President's Special Message on Tax Reduction and Reform (1963), p. 25.

[5] *Ibid.*, p. 29.

plausible in light of his declared income and wealth position.

Finally, we measured tax consciousness in terms of the respondent's awareness of opportunities that the law affords for avoiding high marginal tax rates.

An Index of Tax Consciousness

During the course of the interview there were as many as 39 opportunities to mention taxes, not counting the questions that referred explicitly to tax matters.[6] The actual number of such opportunities open to any one respondent was somewhat less than 39 and varied with his circumstances. The married man still in the labor force, for example, had more opportunities to mention taxes than did the retired widower, for whom many questions that might

[6] These opportunities arose in connection with questions having to do with the following (the percentage of respondents who mentioned taxes appears in parentheses; [*] means less than 0.5 percent): Matters considered in making investment decisions (*6*); why dissatisfied with investment portfolio (*1*); factors of importance in portfolio management (*4*); why investments jointly owned (outside of immediate family) (*1*); policy followed by persons to whom asset management delegated (*); nature of advice sought concerning investment (*4*); basis for choice among retirement plan options (*1*); basis for choice of amount paid into retirement plan (*); opinion on life insurance as a savings medium (*1*); preference between growth and income stocks (*17*); factors affecting distribution of earnings of corporation of which respondent was owner-manager (*2*); reasons for most recent sale of stock (*7*); factors affecting distribution of earnings of unincorporated business (*2*); motives for holding real estate (*); reasons for not incorporating interests in unincorporated business or real estate (*4*); reasons for latest sale or purchase of interest in unincorporated business or real estate (*1*); reasons for past changes in portfolio composition (*2*); reasons for planned changes in portfolio composition (*3*); why gifts received were not reinvested (*); why gifts received were reinvested (*); why inheritances were not reinvested (*); why inheritances were reinvested (*1*); reasons for having made large gifts to relatives (*8*); reasons for change in assets for estate planning purposes (*7*); reasons for not having sold an appreciated asset (*13*); judgment of own performance in latest sale of an asset at a gain (*3*); judgment of own performance in latest sale of an asset at a loss (*10*); choice between fringe benefits and current cash compensation (*1*); decision on how much work to do (for those who had opportunities to work more) (*1*); reasons for working more now than a few years earlier (*); reasons for working less now than a few years earlier (*1*); timing of retirement (for those who had retired) (*); reasons for having accepted work opportunities after retirement (*); reasons for having rejected work opportunities after retirement (*); reasons for single, female head of household having stopped working (*); reasons for single, female head of household not having taken a job (*); reasons for wife having left the labor force (*); reasons for wife's intention to enter labor force (*); reasons why wife would not enter labor force (*).

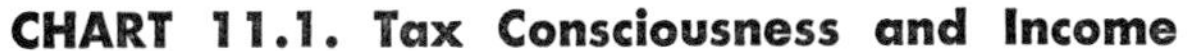

CHART 11.1. Tax Consciousness and Income

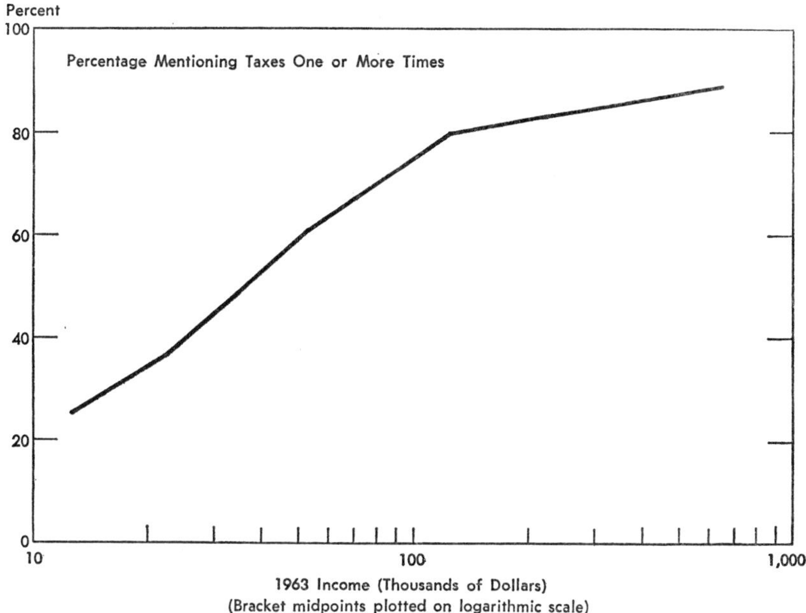

otherwise have led to a reference to taxes were not relevant.[7] Nevertheless, in virtually all cases there were several opportunities.

Our index of tax consciousness is simply the number of times the respondent mentioned taxes. We regard the respondent as being tax conscious if he mentioned taxes at least once (index of 1 or more), and "highly" tax conscious if he mentioned taxes at least 4 times (index of 4 or more).

Forty-five percent of the entire high-income sample mentioned taxes at least once. As is seen in Chart 11.1, the proportion of those who were tax conscious in that sense rose sharply with income up to an income level of about $100,000, where it reached 80 percent, compared with only 24 percent at the $12,000 income level and 36 percent for those with incomes of around $20,000.

It appears, however, that tax consciousness is not so much a function of income as of the size of the respondent's total portfolio. This is well demonstrated in Chart 11.2, where it may be seen that portfolio size provides the best single "split" in our data analysis, followed closely by whether or not the respondent reported having

[7] The listing given in note 6 above makes this clear.

CHART 11.2. Factors Associated With Tax Consciousness

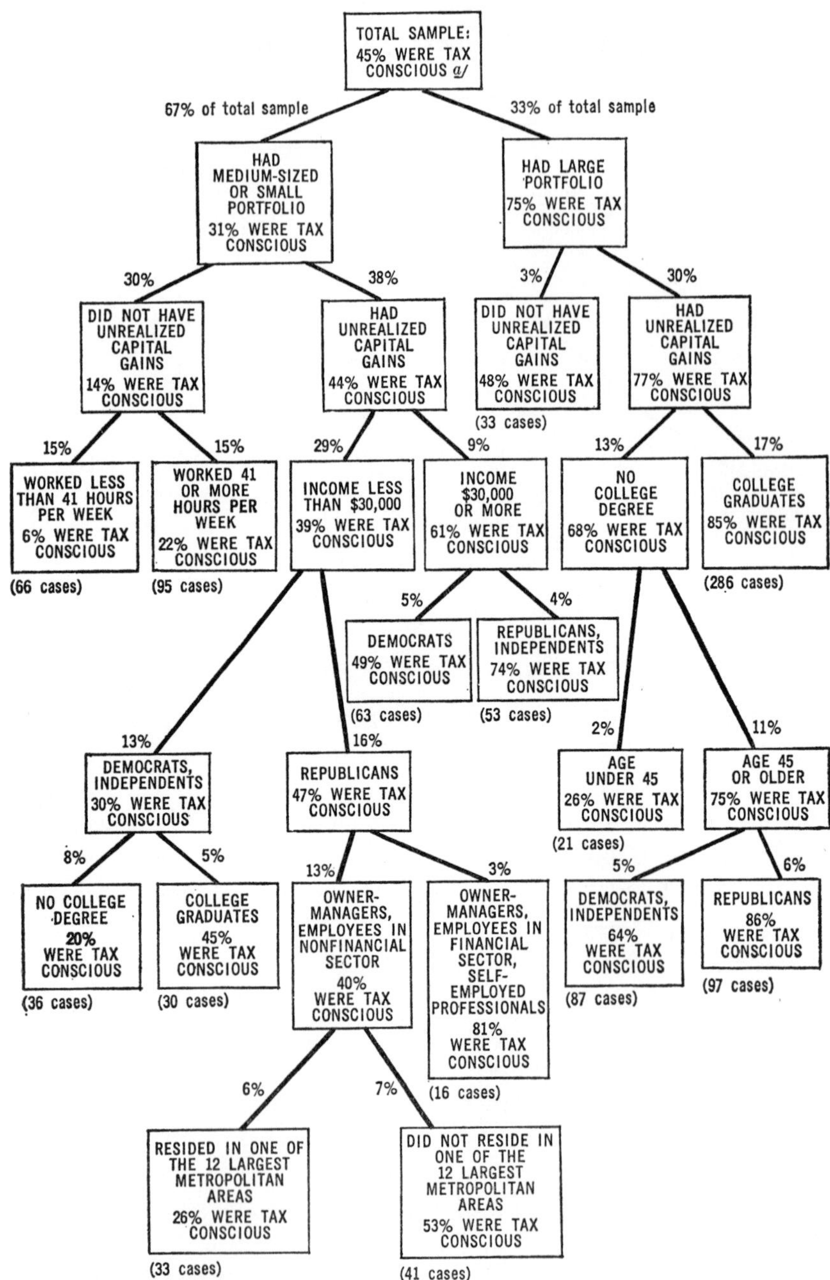

[a] Tax consciousness index of 1 or more.

NOTES: For explanation, see notes to Chart 4.2. In this chart the following predictors were used, listed in order of their explanatory power with a single split over the whole sample: (1) size of total portfolio (for definition, see Table 5.2); (2) whether any unrealized capital gains; (3) 1963 adjusted gross income; (4) occupational group; (5) political preference; (6) education; (7) percentage of total assets from gifts and inheritances; (8) age; (9) average number of hours worked per week; (10) whether lived in a metropolitan area. The fourteen final groups at the ends of the branches accounted for 29 percent of the total variance.

unrealized capital gains. This finding is consistent with the fact that opportunities to avoid taxes on property income are far more prevalent than they are in the case of earned income. Arrangements that permit substantial fractions of earned income to be subject to favorable tax rates are generally complex and difficult to set up, whereas with respect to property income the substitution of capital gains for "ordinary" income is comparatively easy. Even ordinary income may be subject to low effective tax rates because of generous depreciation and depletion allowances or even outright exemption, as in the case of municipal bond interest and most interest accumulated on life insurance.

The remainder of Chart 11.2 points up the association between tax consciousness and income, education, age, political preference, hours worked, place of residence, and occupational group. As with the variables representing portfolio size and unrealized capital gains, the splits provided by these factors offer no surprises.

Of the total sample, 7 percent mentioned taxes four or more times. Again the factor most important in producing a "high" level of tax consciousness was the size of the total portfolio. (See Chart 11.3.) Among those with large portfolios, one-fifth were "highly tax conscious," contrasted with only 1 percent for the two-thirds of the sample with medium-sized or small portfolios.

For the highly tax conscious with large portfolios, a high level of tax consciousness appeared twice as frequently among those who had inherited 15 percent or more of their assets as among those who had inherited less than 15 percent of their total assets.

Male rentiers were more likely than other respondents to be highly tax conscious, as were people who had not retired but whose incomes exceeded $75,000. Education and political preference again appeared to be significant factors.

Awareness of Marginal Tax Rates[8]

If the income tax is to influence an individual's economic behavior, presumably he must be reasonably well aware of the incremental tax costs. Exceptions may occur in the case of those who delegate to others responsibility for managing their assets,[9] and it is

[8] For a somewhat more detailed analysis, see Bruce L. Gensemer, Jane A. Lean, and William B. Neenan, "Awareness of Marginal Income Tax Rates Among High-Income Taxpayers," *National Tax Journal* (September 1965), pp. 258-67.

[9] Very few high-income people do delegate this responsibility. See Chap. III.

CHART 11.3. Factors Associated With a High Level of Tax Consciousness

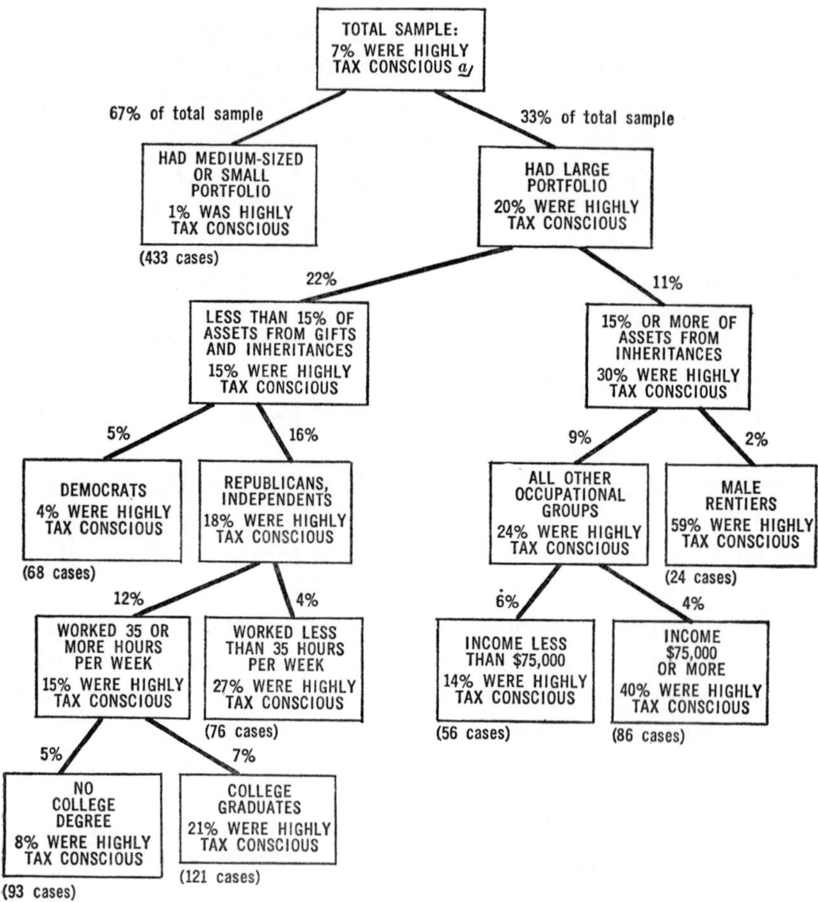

[a] Tax consciousness index of 4 or more.

NOTES: For explanation, see notes to Chart 4.2. In this chart the following predictors were used, listed in order of their explanatory power with a single split over the whole sample: (1) size of total portfolio (for definition, see Table 5.2); (2) 1963 adjusted gross income; (3) occupational group; (4) average number of hours worked per week; (5) whether any unrealized capital gains; (6) percentage of total assets from gifts and inheritances; (7) education; (8) political preference; (9) age; (10) whether lived in a metropolitan area. The eight final groups at the ends of the branches accounted for 21 percent of the total variance.

conceivable that behavior may be guided by serious misconceptions as to the levels of marginal tax rates. Nevertheless, it seems safe to conclude generally that if one is quite unaware of his marginal tax rate, that rate is not likely to affect his economic behavior.

In order to find out the extent to which high-income people were aware of their marginal tax rates we asked:

> If you (or your wife) earned any extra money, about what fraction of it would be taken in added income taxes?

The tax rates mentioned in answer to this question were classified as "definitely understated," "definitely overstated," or "conceivably correct." Those respondents who "definitely understated" their rate included only those who claimed that their marginal income tax rate (under the 1963 federal individual income tax rate schedule on earned income ranging from 20 to 91 percent) was less than 20 percent and higher than zero.[10] Those classified as "definitely overstating" their rates were respondents whose stated adjusted gross income (assuming it to be at the top of the bracket into which it fell) could not possibly have made them subject to a combined federal *and* state marginal tax rate as high as the rate reported, even if they claimed an exemption only for the taxpayer (and his wife, if he was married), took the optional standard deduction or itemized only state income taxes, and had no long-term capital gains included in adjusted gross income. All others who attempted to answer the question were classified as "conceivably correct," even where all or most of the information obtained in the interview hinted at a much higher or lower marginal rate than that reported. Thus, our findings undoubtedly exaggerated the extent of awareness of marginal tax rates. Finally, some respondents answered that they did not know their tax rates and others refused to give theirs.

Our findings on awareness of marginal tax rates are summa-

[10] A marginal tax rate of zero is plausible at any level of adjusted gross income, either because deductions and exemptions reduce taxable income to a negative figure or because the respondent's stated income did not take business losses into account. On the other hand, a marginal rate of 1 percent up to anything less than 20 percent is not plausible for people with incomes of $10,000 or more. At less than $10,000 a marginal rate of 18 percent could, strictly speaking, have been correct for those who took the optional standard deduction of 10 percent of adjusted gross income, subject to a maximum of $1,000.

TABLE 11.1. Awareness of Marginal Tax Rate

Item	*Percentage of entire high-income sample*
Definitely understated marginal tax rate	3
Conceivably correct	66
Definitely overstated	7
Did not know marginal tax rate	22
Refused to answer the question or no response recorded	2
Total	100

rized in Table 11.1. One-third of the entire sample seemed to have been in ignorance, but this proportion varied widely with income. Among those with incomes between $10,000 and $15,000, 4 percent definitely understated and 10 percent definitely overstated their marginal tax rates; 32 percent did not know their tax rates. In marked contrast, at income levels of $300,000 or higher, none either definitely understated or definitely overstated his marginal tax rate, and only 7 percent did not know the rate. The association between unawareness of marginal tax rates and income is clearly pointed up in Chart 11.4.

This association may be explained by two facts that tend to reinforce each other in producing increasing awareness of marginal tax rates as incomes rise. First, at incomes between $10,000 and $15,000, and to a declining extent as income goes up, most or even all of the individual's income tax liability is discharged through withholding. Although the taxpayer in this income bracket must file a Form 1040 and compute his tax liability, using the appropriate table of marginal rates,[11] the computation does not ordinarily result in his having to pay a substantial sum in addition to the amount already withheld. And second, opportunities to minimize tax liabilities increase with rising income as property becomes more important as a source of income, thus giving rise to increased sensitivity and awareness of tax rates.[12]

[11] In contrast to those with incomes of less than $5,000, who may file Form 1040A and have the Internal Revenue Service compute their tax liability for them.

[12] It is true also that the margin of error allowed to respondents in our scheme of classification increases as income rises because the possible variance

CHART 11.4. Unawareness of Marginal Tax Rate by Income Classes

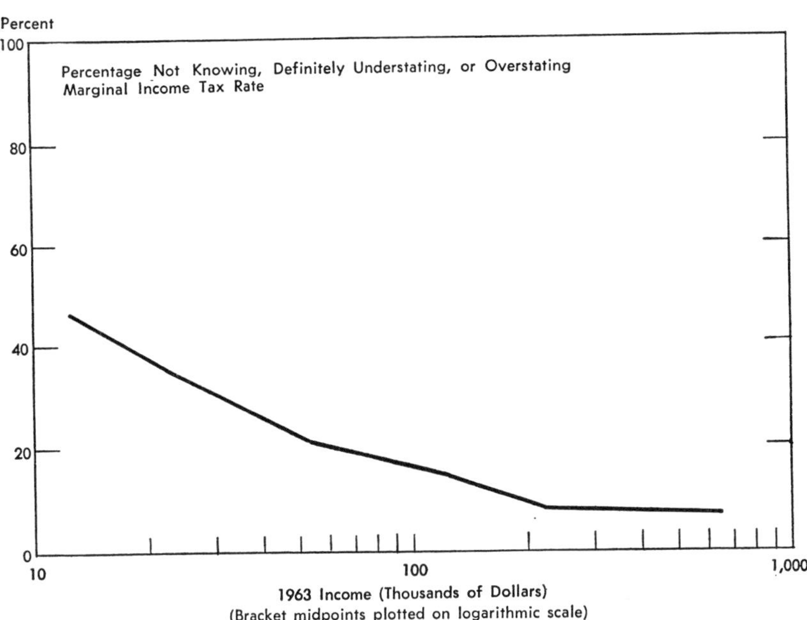

It may be argued that those who were classified as having overstated their marginal tax rates in fact had understated their incomes and therefore were "conceivably correct." If this group and the small number who refused to answer the question were omitted, the proportion of the rest of the sample who were unaware of their marginal tax rate would be reduced from 32 to 27 percent.

For this latter group we found that the close association between tax awareness and income was apparent even in a multivariate analysis. As is indicated in Chart 11.5, the proportion of respondents who were unaware of their marginal tax rates was more than twice as high for those with incomes between $10,000 and $30,000 as it was for people with incomes of more than $30,000.

---

in the marginal tax rate goes up with the level of adjusted gross income. Thus, for example, a married man with adjusted gross income of $500,000 (and positive taxable income) who files a joint return could conceivably have been subject to any marginal rate between 20 and 91 percent, but the conceivable range for a similarly circumstanced individual with adjusted gross income of $10,000 would have been from 20 to 22 percent.

CHART 11.5. Factors Associated With Unawareness of Marginal Tax Rates

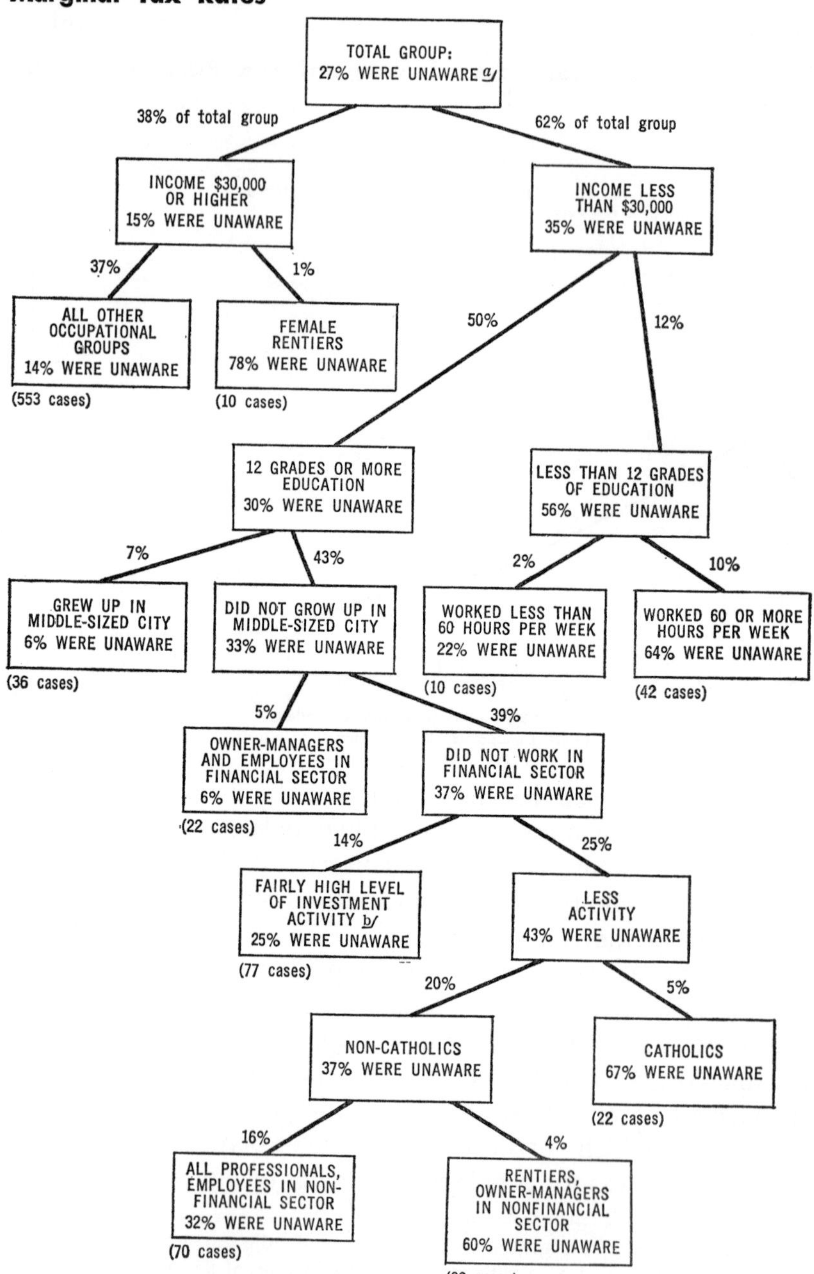

[a] Excluded from this analysis were respondents who either refused to divulge or "definitely overstated" their marginal tax rate. A case was classified as "unaware" if the marginal tax rate was either "not known" or "definitely understated."

[b] Investment activity index of 5 or more.

NOTES: For explanation, see notes to Chart 4.2. In this chart the following predictors were used, listed in order of their explanatory power with a single split over the whole sample: (1) 1963 adjusted gross income; (2) education; (3) level of investment activity (for definition, see Chap. VI); (4) occupational group; (5) average number of hours worked per week; (6) whether any opportunities to work more; (7) religious preference; (8) past and future income-change patterns; (9) size of total portfolio; (10) whether any unrealized capital gains; (11) whether active in church or civic groups; (12) size of place where grew up; (13) percentage of total assets from gifts and inheritances; (14) age; (15) whether lived in a metropolitan area; (16) political preference. The ten final groups at the ends of the branches accounted for 20 percent of the total variance.

Given the split for income, education, and the number of hours worked per week appeared as the next most important predictors of unawareness of marginal tax rates. People with less than a high school education who claimed to be working more than 60 hours a week were the most unlikely to know their marginal tax rates. Unawareness of marginal tax rates tended to be most prevalent among the better educated with incomes of less than $30,000 if they had grown up anywhere other than in a middle-sized city, were not employed in the financial sector, engaged only slightly in investment activity, and were Catholics. Among those with incomes of $30,000 or more a significant split appeared in the tree only for female rentiers, three-fourths of whom were unable to state their marginal tax rates.

Response to Preferential Tax Treatment

Attention is now directed specifically to the extent to which the high-income people were conscious of the legal means of reducing income tax liability.

LIFE INSURANCE. The proceeds of life insurance policies, including accumulated interest on the savings element, are wholly exempt from income tax when paid by reason of the death of the insured, and only a portion of the interest accrued on amounts paid during the insured's lifetime is subject to tax.[13] Nevertheless, "both pure insurance proceeds and interest earned on savings accumulated under life insurance policies may be provisionally regarded as income in the broad sense."[14] If individuals do regard pure insurance proceeds and interest as income, their tax-free status should make life insurance an attractive investment medium, particularly for people subject to high tax rates.

To find out whether this was so, we asked:

What do you think of life insurance as a way of saving money?

[13] For discussion of the issues involved in the taxation of life insurance proceeds, see Goode, *op. cit.*, pp. 130-39; William Vickrey, *Agenda for Progressive Taxation* (Ronald Press, 1947), pp. 64-75; and Harvey E. Brazer, *A Program for Federal Tax Revision* (Institute of Public Administration, The University of Michigan, 1960), pp. 7-8.

[14] Goode, *op. cit.*, p. 130. Vickrey is less equivocal. *Op. cit.*, pp. 65-66.

Opinions expressed by the total sample of respondents were about equally divided between those favorable to life insurance and those unfavorable, but only 1 percent of our respondents said that tax considerations made life insurance a good way to save. There was no systematic relation between reported marginal tax rates and opinions on life insurance, although those who reported marginal tax rates of 80 percent or higher were much more likely to favor life insurance than were people who reported lower marginal tax rates. Our index of tax consciousness was not associated with expressed views on life insurance.

These findings confirm those of the earlier Butters-Thompson-Bollinger study, which indicated that only a minor fraction of their sample of investors had added to their life insurance for tax reasons.[15] We need not seek far for the probable answer as to why this means of reducing tax liabilities was not more attractive to high-income individuals. The answer probably lies in the facts that loading charges are very heavy on life insurance, that the law and the Internal Revenue Service have cracked down on the most lucrative form of this device (disallowing the deduction of interest paid on funds borrowed to finance single-premium life insurance policies), and that other tax-exempt or tax-favored opportunities abound which do not carry the constraints or loading charges of life insurance.

INVESTMENT IN REAL ESTATE. In recent years the tax advantages of investment in improved real estate, particularly new multiple dwellings and commercial and office buildings, have given rise to the term "real estate tax shelter." These advantages arise because the law, since 1954, has permitted double-declining-balance depreciation, which in the early years of a building's life ordinarily exceeds the decline in market value, and because when the building is sold at a price higher than the depreciated basis, the excess depreciation recovered (despite having been charged against income taxable at ordinary rates) is taxed only at capital gains rates.[16] In the

[15] *Op. cit.*, pp. 319-23.

[16] The 1964 Revenue Act contains a provision that limits the recovery of excess depreciation as capital gains to straight-line depreciation plus a portion of the difference between straight-line and double-declining-balance or sum-of-the-years-digits depreciation that varies directly with the length of the period over which the property has been owned by the seller.

early years many real estate ventures produce income that is entirely offset, or more than offset, by depreciation charges, so that taxable income is zero or even negative. At the same time individuals with ownership interests in the property may receive large cash distributions that are not taxable. The property may even show a "loss," in which case the owners may be able to offset income from other sources. When depreciation charges decline to the point where they no longer absorb income fully, usually in six to ten years, the property may be sold, and depreciation which has been charged against income subject to rates as high as 91 percent under the pre-1964 law may be recovered and subjected to capital gains rates of no more than half the ordinary rates up to a maximum of only 25 percent.

Journalists and others have given wide publicity in popular magazines and in newspapers to this way of avoiding tax,[17] but are high-income people aware of it, and to what extent do they seek tax advantages through investment in rental real estate? To obtain answers to these questions we asked:

> Have you heard about some special income tax advantages of investing in real estate?
>
> Have you made any such investments, or have you thought about doing so?

Of the entire high-income sample, 48 percent reported having heard of the special income tax advantages of investing in real estate. Forty percent of this group had actually made such investments or had thought about doing so. Both of these proportions tended to increase with income, from 37 and 31 percent for people with incomes between $10,000 and $15,000 to 67 and 44 percent for those with incomes of $75,000 or higher.

At first sight it might seem surprising that so many people, even at very high income levels, had not even heard about the tax advantages associated with rental real estate and that so many of those who had heard about them had not made such investments. But many high-income people, as our evidence on work hours suggests, are very much preoccupied with their primary jobs, and the com-

[17] See, for example, Daniel M. Frieberg, "The Coming Bust in the Real Estate Boom," *Harper's* (June 1961), pp. 29-40.

plexities of depreciation, real estate syndicate organization, etc., are not readily mastered, particularly outside the large metropolitan areas. People tend to be suspicious, or at least wary, of the unfamiliar, and it takes more than just "having heard" about something to induce action.

OTHER TAX ADVANTAGES. Immediately after the specific questions relating to real estate tax shelters, the respondents were asked:

> Are there other features of the income tax laws that affect the way you invest your savings?
>
> What are they?

Approximately one-third of the entire high-income group said that there were "other" features of the income tax laws that affected their investment decisions. By far the most frequently mentioned tax feature was the favorable treatment of capital gains—mentioned at this point by 22 percent of the entire high-income sample.

The proportion of respondents who indicated that "other" tax considerations influenced their investment decisions rose sharply with income, from only 15 percent for those with incomes between $10,000 and $15,000 to 67 percent for those with incomes of $150,000 or higher.

Tax-exempt municipal bonds ranked second to capital gains among the "other" tax considerations mentioned by the respondents, but only 2.4 percent of the sample, almost all of whom had incomes over $75,000, referred to them. This proportion was far below the 19 percent that reported owning municipals, which suggests that there are additional motives for holding these securities besides their tax-exempt status.

Another 2 percent of the sample reported being influenced by the opportunities to realize ordinary income in the form of statutory capital gains through investment in such assets as standing timber and livestock, and 2 percent mentioned percentage depletion. Again these provisions were mentioned, for the most part, by only those with the highest incomes. No other features of the income tax were reported by enough respondents to warrant analysis.

It is of particular interest to note that many ways of avoiding tax that have long been familiar to students of taxation and prime targets of tax reformers—for example, the use of personal holding companies as tax shelters for the income of the wealthy—were mentioned by only a very few of our high-income respondents. The apparent indifference to or unawareness of tax advantages displayed by a large proportion of high-income people is illustrated by one respondent who said:

> I don't think I ever invested a penny because of income tax laws. I invest because the company is sound. I notice you stressed municipal-type bonds. That's all right, and the income is tax free, but they didn't appeal to me.

Income Splitting in the Family

Since 1948 husbands and wives resident in any state have been permitted to file joint returns, computing tax liability as though the income reported by the couple had accrued in equal parts to each spouse. But income may be split further within the family (defined to include dependent children) by transferring assets to minor children, outright or by creating trusts, and having the income on these assets taxable to the children at lower rates than those to which the parents are subject. Children may also, in certain cases, be given partnership interests in business.

Joint Returns of Husbands and Wives

Ordinarily the income tax liability of a husband and wife will be minimized if they file a joint return and split their income. A small proportion of couples choose to file separate returns, however. In 1962, the latest year for which data are available, 6.6 million married couples with adjusted gross incomes of $10,000 or more filed joint returns, while approximately 585,000 husbands and wives, at least one of whom had an income of $5,000 or more, filed separate returns.[18] Thus roughly 95 percent of all couples with incomes of $10,000 and over filed joint returns.

Ninety-seven percent of married respondents in our sample re-

[18] U.S. Treasury Department, Internal Revenue Service, *Statistics of Income, 1962,* p. 79.

ported having filed joint returns. The tendency to file separate returns increased with income, rising from only 1 percent of the married respondents with incomes between $10,000 and $15,000 to 5 percent of those whose income exceeded $75,000.

Among those filing separate returns more than half reported that the wife received about one-half of the family income. Under these circumstances the choice between joint and separate returns is unlikely to affect tax liability appreciably. But when the income of the couple is not received in approximately equal parts by each spouse, there is usually a tax saving to be realized by filing a joint return. Some people, however, are willing to forego this tax advantage rather than disclose the facts about their incomes to their spouses. They may be estranged, and a divorce settlement may be in the offing. They may be out of touch with one another. Or they may simply prefer to avoid disclosure even if living together amicably.

Finally, under certain circumstances there may be tax advantages to be gained by filing separate returns. For example, capital losses may be deducted from ordinary income only to the extent of $1,000 *per return* each year. This amount could be doubled if each spouse filed a separate return and claimed a capital loss. Also medical expenses may be deducted only to the extent that they exceed 3 percent of adjusted gross income. Thus a portion of these expenses incurred, say, on behalf of the wife, may be deductible only if she files a separate return.

Separate Returns of Dependent Children

Twenty-nine percent of the respondents with dependent children reported that one or more of these children filed income tax returns. That many of them were not filing returns merely in order to claim refunds of tax withheld on small earnings from after-school or vacation jobs seems clear from the fact that the proportion of respondents whose dependent children filed tax returns rose steadily with income, from 23 percent at incomes of under $30,000 to 75 percent when income was $300,000 or higher.

For the most part, however, the fraction of total family income reported for tax purposes by dependent children was small, representing less than 10 percent in more than three-fourths of all families in which dependent children filed returns. But at the highest levels of income, dependents filing separately tended to account for a larger share of family income. In the income bracket $10,000 to $15,000 none of those with dependent children filing separately reported that the dependents received over one-tenth of family income, whereas when family income exceeded $300,000, more than one-fourth of the dependents who filed separately claimed more than 10 percent of that income.

This finding shows that tax avoidance by this means becomes more common as family income increases. Our data also reveal that separate filing of tax returns by dependent children who reported more than 10 percent of family income was clearly associated with the giving of large gifts to relatives in the recent past, as well as with tax consciousness.

Tax Levels and Choice of Residence

Our sample of high-income respondents was about equally divided between those who believed that their state and local taxes were higher where they then lived than in other places where they might live and those who did not, suggesting the absence of bias in the question. Apparently in this respect, other fields do not necessarily seem greener.

Of those who did believe that their taxes were higher where they were then residing than in alternative places of residence, however, only about one-sixth had thought of moving in order to save taxes, and only one-sixth of that sixth said that they probably would move. It is interesting to note that virtually none of those with incomes of $30,000 or higher said that they probably would move.

Respondents' thoughts and intentions about moving tended to vary with the length of time they had lived in the area. Those who had been in their current localities for less than three years and who thought their taxes where higher than in alternative places were about twice as likely to have thought about moving than were people with similar observations on taxes who had maintained a residence in the same place for three years or more. Moreover, among those who had thought of moving, people with the shortest period of residence in their present localities were the most likely to declare that they probably would move.

Neither the existence of dependent children, nor the level of income, nor the size of the community appeared to affect an inclination to move because of high taxes. But professionals, both self-employed and employees, were definitely more inclined to have thought of moving and to declare that they probably would move than were those in other occupational groups. Also, as was to be expected, those aged under forty-five accounted for most of the probable movers.

Thus, in general, the relative level of state and local taxes did not appear to be an important factor in the selection of a place of residence, except to a minor extent for younger professionals who had lived in the community for only a brief period. Further pursuit of this matter might have revealed that many people recognize a connection between local tax levels and public services. But the deductibility of state and local taxes from income subject to federal tax, as well as the fact that these taxes commonly absorb less than 10 percent of income, may also play a role in producing the apparent lack of sensitivity to differences in state-local tax obligations.

The Use of Tax Consultants

Testifying to the complexity of the federal individual income tax, almost two-thirds of the entire high-income sample reported that they got expert advice in making out their income tax returns. The proportion obtaining such advice rose from 58 percent among those with incomes in the $10,000 to $30,000 bracket to 94 percent for people with incomes of $300,000 or more. With few exceptions the advice on filing income tax returns came from accountants; only 3 percent of those who got advice for this purpose consulted lawyers, and a similar proportion consulted other experts or advisers who were neither accountants nor lawyers.

Summary

- Almost half of the sample of high-income people were tax conscious, the proportion rising to 80 percent for those with incomes of around $100,000.
- Tax consciousness appeared to be primarily a function of the size of respondents' asset portfolios.

• Between one-fourth and one-third of the high-income group were definitely unaware of their marginal income tax rates, the proportion falling off sharply as income rose.

• The awareness of preferential tax treatment and the inclination to take advantage of it appeared to be confined to a small minority of high-income people, with the notable exception of the tax advantages of capital gains.

• The splitting of income with dependent children for tax purposes was quite widespread. Among respondents with incomes of more than $300,000, three-fourths of those with dependent children reported that one or more of those children filed income tax returns.

• The choice of where to live did not appear to be greatly affected by differences in state and local tax levels.

APPENDIX A

Sampling Procedures

THE UNIVERSE FOR THIS STUDY consisted of individuals who lived in the forty-eight continental states and the District of Columbia. The sample list was so compiled as to include a disproportionate number of people with higher than average (1961) incomes. To each income stratum represented in this list, a subsampling fraction was applied to select one individual for each $54 million of income, or a specified multiple of this amount. Additional stratification and subsampling by income class were performed to yield a working sample of 3,799 individuals distributed as follows by income class:

Income class	*Sampling rate in units of F*[1]	*Sample size at the specified rates*
All classes	. . .	3,799
Less than $10,000	1/20	200
$10,000 to $14,999	1/8	531
$15,000 to $24,999	1	700
$25,000 to $49,999	2	536
$50,000 to $99,999	4	778
$100,000 to $149,999	8	178
$150,000 or more	12	876

Disproportionate sampling was used to obtain an adequately large sample of individuals with the highest incomes. Since no specific information was available on the income of any one individual, inclusion in

[1] F = 1/54 million.

the sample did not mean that the individual's income was necessarily of any given size or even above any stipulated limit.

To permit adjustments in interviewer loads, and to provide for some modest geographical clustering (thus reducing interviewing costs), the sample contained about twice the number of names actually to be contacted. For reasons to be explained, the original list of 3,799 individuals was divided into ten equal subsamples. As far as possible, each contained 10 percent of the sample drawn proportionately from each income class in each geographical area.

The sample was distributed throughout the coterminous United States but not in proportion to population, since there are concentrations of high incomes in some areas. It should be noted that the conditions under which the sample was obtained precluded the use of the county as a primary sampling unit. Furthermore, it was impractical to compile more than twice the number of addresses ultimately to be used.[2] Therefore, of the Center's national sample of dwellings, the only strata that could be used were those containing either one or two Primary Sampling Units (PSU's). In the Center's dwelling unit sample, there are twelve strata with one primary area each: Baltimore, Boston, Chicago consolidated area, Cleveland, Detroit, District of Columbia, Los Angeles, New York and Northeastern New Jersey consolidated area, Philadelphia, Pittsburgh, St. Louis, and San Francisco.[3] These are the twelve largest Standard Metropolitan Statistical Areas in the country. Each was included with certainty in the dwelling unit sample and was treated similarly in this study. From the ten strata that consist of two Standard Metropolitan Statistical Areas, the five PSU's used in the dwelling unit sample were chosen: Atlanta, Houston, Minneapolis-St. Paul, Phoenix, and Seattle. Those not included were Dallas, Denver, Kansas City, New Orleans, and Portland, Oregon. This means that in each of the first five PSU's it was necessary to take twice the sample size that would have been required if the PSU had represented only itself. Therefore, in the five sample areas all sample addresses instead of only one-half were assigned for interviewing. Only small adjustments in weights were needed to keep the sample on a strict probability basis.

For the remainder of the country, a half-sample was selected by ran-

[2] A larger sample would have been an unreasonable workload. In addition, the large differences in sampling rates pose difficult technical problems, which mount with the size of the sample and the amount of subsampling that is required.

[3] Leslie Kish and Irene Hess, "The Survey Research Center's National Sample of Dwellings" (Institute for Social Research, The University of Michigan), ISR No. 2315.

domly choosing five of the ten subsamples. By this means, a proper distribution by geographic location and income class was maintained. Next this half-sample of individuals was divided into three groups: (1) those in the twelve largest metropolitan areas, (2) those within a radius of about 100 miles of one of the Center's interviewers, and (3) those farther removed from the interviewing staff.

Because of the heavy interviewing load in the 12 largest metropolitan areas, one of the five subsets from the half-sample in these areas was eliminated, using probability methods. All five subsets were retained in the areas that were roughly within 100 miles of an interviewer and in a few areas where the concentration of addresses was unusually heavy. In the remaining areas, which were more than 100 miles from the interviewing staff, two of the five subsets were eliminated from the half-sample on a probability basis. Interviewers visited the places retained in the sample.

There was one other minor adjustment to reduce field costs. In the half-sample, Montana and Wyoming were each represented by six widely scattered individuals. Rather than have interviewers cover both of these large states, a random choice resulted in the selection of the six Montana individuals to represent both Montana and Wyoming in the sample.

The distribution of sample individuals by the various subsampling procedures, the subsampling fraction applied to the 3,799 individuals, and the number of individuals assigned to interviewers are shown below:

Subsampling classification	*Sampling fraction applied to original working sample*	*Number of selections*
All groups	. . .	1,696
12 largest metropolitan areas	4:10	682
5 other metropolitan areas	about 5:10	180
Other areas within 100 miles of interviewer	5:10	753
Montana and Wyoming	2.5:10	6
Remaining areas	3:10	75

A disproportionate sample can undergo several sampling operations while remaining a strict probability sample and without introducing large increases in sampling variability. This is possible through the selection and identification of ten equal subsamples. The technique of subsampling by choosing entire subsamples means that the final sample retains proper proportions of each of the original strata.

One definite disadvantage to this sample design is that the proper weighting of the interviews requires knowledge of each individual's 1961 income, information available only from individual respondents. For some types of information, the system may work well, but income data are susceptible to response errors.

There is, however, only a relatively small possibility of damage through errors in weighting, since for all incomes over $10,000, the weights do not vary much from one income class to the adjacent one. Hence, a respondent would have to be misclassified by two or more income brackets before the weighting error would exceed a factor of three. Weighted estimates (index numbers) are quite stable under moderate changes in weights.

The sampling errors of proportions and differences between proportions were estimated by a method of replicated half-samples.[4] For this purpose, the sample was divided into 17 pairs of matched groups of individuals, the matching having given consideration to the income class and geographic stratification that had entered into the sample design. A half-sample was built by selecting one group from each of the 17 pairs. A fourth of the square of the difference between the estimates based on the selected and the rejected half-samples provided an estimate of the sampling variability in the pooled sample. To increase the stability of this estimate, the procedure was repeated 32 times, and the selection of the half-sample was carried out according to a predetermined set of balanced (orthogonal) patterns suggested by Professor Philip J. McCarthy.[5] The average of the sampling variability over the 32 replications provided a final estimate of the variability in the pooled sample. The square roots of these values for selected proportions and differentials are shown in Table A-1.

Note that the sampling error thus obtained depended on the total number of units in the cell, the strata from which the units were drawn, and the characteristic studied. The sampling error of a particular proportion *cannot* be extrapolated directly to other proportions of similar magnitude.

[4] P. J. McCarthy, "Analysis of Data from Complex Sample Surveys" (mimeo.). Also see U.S. Bureau of the Census, "The Current Population Survey—A Report on Methodology," Technical Paper no. 7 (1963).

[5] *Op. cit.*

TABLE A-1. Approximate Standard Errors for Various Characteristics

Characteristics of respondents	Owned municipal bonds		High level of investment information		Some tax consciousness		Preferred current yield to capital gains		Assets diversified rather than concentrated[c]	
	Percent	Standard error (±)	Percent	Standard error (±)	Percent	Standard error (±)	Percent	Standard error (±)	Percent	Standard error (±)
1963 income[a]										
Less than $15,000	11	2	19	1	29	12	20	2	6	3
$15,000– 29,999	8	1	31	4	38	1	18	2	13	4
30,000– 74,999	24	1	52	2	63	2	11	3	31	1
75,000–149,999	48	9	61	17	79	9	10	4	50	5
150,000–299,000	46	4	52	4	84	1	11	d	55	4
300,000 or more	63	7	50	19	90	2	9	2	65	7
Difference between $300,000 or more and $150,000–299,999	−17	10	2	22	−6	3	2	2	−9	10
Size of total portfolio[b]										
Medium-sized or small	8	7	26	6	33	19	18	11	9	4
Large	43	1	56	1	77	5	12	1	48	2
Difference between medium-sized or small and large portfolio	−35	8	−30	6	−44	25	6	10	−39	7
Occupational group										
Male and female rentiers	47	5	36	4	57	4	20	2	37	6
Business owner-managers and employees in financial sector	34	7	94	6	60	6	10	2	43	2
Business owner-managers in nonfinancial sector	18	1	34	1	57	29	15	5	23	2
Self-employed professionals	19	1	35	5	60	2	12	1	23	1
Professional employees	9	2	23	2	28	1	21	1	10	1
Employees in nonfinancial sector	11	d	23	1	35	1	16	1	12	1
Difference between rentiers and those in financial sector	13	12	−58	9	−3	9	11	2	−6	4
Total sample	19	3	35	7	47	18	16	6	21	2

TABLE A-1 (Continued)

Characteristics of respondents	Gave gifts to charity in previous couple of years		Gave gifts to relatives in previous couple of years		Investments were affected by changed interest rates on savings accounts		Realized a capital loss in 1963 or 1964	
	Percent	Standard error (±)	Percent	Standard error (±)	Percent	Standard error (±)	Percent	Standard error (±)
1963 income[a]								
Less than $15,000	8	2	5	2	15	2	13	1
$15,000– 29,999	10	[d]	10	4	26	6	26	4
30,000– 74,999	18	6	23	3	26	1	37	2
75,000–149,999	38	3	46	5	18	6	48	7
150,000–299,999	49	1	42	1	22	4	57	[d]
300,000 or more	76	8	72	2	12	3	46	13
Difference between $300,000 or more and $150,000–299,999	−26	9	−30	4	10	2	11	13
Size of total portfolio[b]								
Medium-sized or small	8	1	6	1	22	16	21	1
Large	38	2	42	2	20	2	42	3
Difference between medium-sized or small and large portfolio	−30	3	−36	2	2	18	−21	4
Occupational group								
Male and female rentiers	39	2	32	1	21	2	38	3
Business owner-managers and employees in financial sector	24	3	31	8	28	[d]	46	11
Business owner-managers in nonfinancial sector	22	4	24	5	17	[d]	29	4
Self-employed professionals	21	4	19	1	30	6	35	[d]
Professional employees	11	2	8	1	26	2	18	2
Employees in nonfinancial sector	5	1	8	[d]	17	4	20	3
Difference between rentiers and those in financial sector	15	5	[d]	9	−7	2	−8	9
Total sample	17	8	18	1	21	15	28	4

TABLE A-1 (Continued)

Characteristics of respondents	Said taxes affected work effort		Highly tax conscious		High level of investment activity		Gave appreciated assets to charity		Number of cases
	Percent	Standard error (±)	Percent	Standard error (±)	Percent	Standard error (±)	Percent	Standard error (±)	
1963 income[a]									
Less than $15,000	7	1	2	d	3	1	4	3	122
$15,000– 29,999	9	2	2	1	2	d	8	2	220
30,000– 74,999	15	d	10	d	16	1	14	1	261
75,000–149,999	23	11	23	2	25	5	30	9	198
150,000–299,999	24	1	21	1	30	1	47	4	66
300,000 or more	12	4	33	9	36	17	64	12	90
Size of total portfolio[b]									
Medium-sized or small	8	6	1	1	3	1	5	1	423
Large	19	1	20	2	24	1	31	3	524
Occupational group									
Male and female rentiers	11	1	22	4	14	2	22	1	112
Business owner-managers and employees in financial sector	18	7	11	1	18	6	25	7	116
Business owner-managers in nonfinancial sector	14	2	11	2	13	d	14	8	320
Self-employed professionals	24	2	8	1	12	2	21	3	144
Professional employees	5	2	d	d	d	d	2	1	81
Employees in nonfinancial sector	4	d	2	d	5	d	7	d	184
Total sample	11	1	7	2	9	3	13	1	957

[a] These are the income brackets after adjustment for underreporting of income. See Appendix D.
[b] For definition, see Table 5.2.
[c] For definition, see Appendix E.
[d] Less than 0.005.

APPENDIX B

Weighting of Interviews

FOR EACH INTERVIEW two sets of weights were calculated, one representing dollars of income and the other the number of "individuals" (a married couple being counted as an "individual" in this context). This was done so that analyses could be made either in terms of dollars of income represented by a particular subgroup or in terms of numbers of individuals or couples in that particular subgroup.

Statistics of Income, 1961[1] was used to determine the distribution of individuals and of aggregate income among income groups. The year 1961 was used because the list of names used for sampling purposes was derived from 1961 data.

Weighting for both individuals and dollars of income required us to account for variations in response rates for the different subselection strata since these variations turned out to be substantial. The gross response rates for the selection strata were as follows:

Selection stratum	*Response rate*
12 largest metropolitan areas	56%
5 other metropolitan areas	59
Areas more than 100 miles from interviewing staff	72
Remaining areas	68

These rates allow for all losses: bad addresses, persons who were seriously ill, deceased, or unavailable, and refusals.

[1] U.S. Treasury Department, Internal Revenue Service.

The data on aggregate income and the number of individuals in each income class (derived from the *Statistics of Income, 1961)* are shown in Table B-1.

TABLE B-1. Distribution of Individuals and Aggregate Income by Income Classes, 1961

1961 adjusted gross income	*Percentage distribution of individuals*	*Percentage distribution of aggregate income*
Less than $5,000	56.5	25.2
$5,000– 9,999	33.8	44.0
10,000– 14,999	6.7	14.7
15,000– 24,999	2.0	7.0
25,000– 49,999	0.8	5.1
50,000– 99,999	0.2	2.2
100,000–149,999	[a]	0.6
150,000–499,999	[b]	0.8
500,000–999,999	[c]	0.2
1,000,000 or more	[d]	0.2
Total	100.0	100.0

[a] 0.027.
[b] 0.019.
[c] 0.002.
[d] 0.001.

The information used in computing the two weights for each interview is shown in Tables B-2 and B-3. Note that the weights for income were adjusted so that each digit of a weight represented $5 million of income (Table B-2). The second set of weights was adjusted so that each digit represented 33,333 "individuals" (Table B-3). These adjustments were made for the purpose of obtaining two-digit weights, which would be convenient for computer operations.

Table B-4 shows that there was little difference in response rates for various regions of the country. But response rates did differ with the size of the place where the individual was contacted, being generally lower for the twelve largest metropolitan areas than for the country as a whole. The response rate for the total sample was 62 percent; for the twelve largest metropolitan areas, it was 56 percent.

The response rate in the five smaller metropolitan areas (59 percent) was also lower than that for the sample as a whole. In part this lower rate can probably be attributed to the fact that the interviewers in these areas had large assignments in relation to the time available.

The response rate for the remainder of the sample was 68 percent.

TABLE B-2. Table of Weights for Dollars of Income

1961 income	Aggregate 1961 income[a] (In billions of dollars)				Number of interviews[b]				Weights for dollars of income[c]			
	Twelve largest metro areas	Five other metro areas	Remote areas	Remaining areas	Twelve largest metro areas	Five other metro areas	Remote areas	Remaining areas	Twelve largest metro areas	Five other metro areas	Remote areas	Remaining areas
$10,000–$14,999	18.270	2.944	4.150	23.125	55	16	11	87	66	37	75	53
15,000– 24,999	10.380	1.956	1.570	9.164	87	23	9	96	24	17	35	19
25,000– 49,999	6.270	0.999	1.332	7.998	74	20	13	118	17	10	20	14
50,000– 99,999	3.161	0.702	0.625	2.774	72	23	10	79	9	6	13	7
100,000–149,999	0.851	0.314	0.059	0.775	29	11	1	33	6	6	12	5
150,000–499,999	1.515	0.114	0.234	0.831	35	4	4	24	8	6	12	7
500,000–999,999	0.365	0.142	0.290	0.256	8	1	0	7	11	28	58	9
1,000,000 or more	0.167			0.266	2	0	1	4				
Total	40.979	7.171	8.260	45.189	362	98	49	448				

[a] Data principally from U. S. Treasury Department, Internal Revenue Service, *Statistics of Income, 1961*.
[b] Distribution by income as reported by respondent (before adjustment for understating of income as described in Appendix D).
[c] The weights for dollars of income were calculated as follows: the income for each stratum was divided by the number of interviews for that stratum, and the result was then divided by five million to obtain a convenient two-digit weight.

TABLE B-3. Table of Weights for "Individuals"

1961 income	Number of individuals (In thousands)[a]				Number of interviews[b]				Weights for individuals[c]			
	Twelve largest metro areas	Five other metro areas	Remote areas	Remaining areas	Twelve largest metro areas	Five other metro areas	Remote areas	Remaining areas	Twelve largest metro areas	Five other metro areas	Remote areas	Remaining areas
$10,000–$14,999	1,559.3	246.0	346.7	1,973.2	55	16	11	87	84	45	93	69
15,000– 24,999	560.2	106.6	85.5	494.5	87	23	9	96	19	14	29	15
25,000– 49,999	187.2	30.2	40.3	238.8	74	20	13	118	8	4	9	6
50,000– 99,999	47.950	10.787	9.610	42.028	72	23	10	79	2	1	3	2
100,000–149,999	7.105	2.585	0.482	6.468	29	11	1	33	1	1	1	0
150,000–499,999	6.580	0.460	0.944	3.600	35	4	4	24	1	0	0	0
500,000–999,999	0.544	0.045	0.092	0.378	8	1	0	7	0	0	0	0
1,000,000 or more	0.126			0.200	2	0	1	4				
Total	2,369.0	396.7	483.6	2,759.2	362	98	49	448				

[a] Data principally from U. S. Treasury Department, Internal Revenue Service, *Statistics of Income, 1961.*

[b] Distribution by income as reported by respondent (before adjustments for understating of income as described in Appendix D).

[c] The weights for the number of individuals were calculated as follows: the number of individuals for each stratum was divided by the number of interviews for that stratum, and the result was multiplied by 0.003 to obtain a convenient two-digit weight.

Interviewers generally had an easier time contacting individuals in the rural areas and in the smaller urban areas than in the large metropolitan areas.

TABLE B-4. Summary of Response Rates

Region of country[a]	Number of names originally selected	Number of unusable names[b]	Number of usable names	Percent usable	Number of ill and refusals	Number of interviews obtained	Response rate (percent of names originally selected)	Response rate (percent of usable names)
Northeast	560	77	483	86	163	320	57	66
North Central	471	49	422	90	115	307	65	73
South	382	50	332	87	78	254	66	77
West	283	45	238	84	68	170	60	71
Total	1,696	221	1,475	87	424	1,051[c]	62	71

[a] The regional definitions are those used by the U. S. Bureau of the Census.
[b] Unusable names were those of individuals who were unavailable for the duration of the study, deceased, minors, or whom the interviewer could not verify or locate with certainty.
[c] Including the 94 cases with income under $10,000.

APPENDIX C

An Analysis of Nonresponse

HIGH-INCOME SAMPLES ARE generally more difficult to interview than representative cross sections. Our interviewers were often obliged to make appointments for interviews, and in some cases the appointments were tentative and subject to cancellation.

Problems Encountered in Securing Interviews

High-income people are frequently asked to donate their valuable time for giving opinions on other matters, and they are often solicited for funds by representatives of universities. Thus some individuals were suspicious of our interviewers' purposes. Special letters to such people were sent from Ann Arbor, assuring them that statistical research was our only purpose. But since these letters used names as well as addresses, it was sometimes difficult to convince the individual of the anonymity of his responses. A further difficulty was that the high-income people sometimes were reluctant to disclose financial information or attitudes to a local interviewer, no matter what the guarantees. This problem was encountered mainly in rural and small urban areas.

Some high-income individuals did not consider themselves knowledgeable about investments and hence were reluctant in many instances to be interviewed. These individuals had to be reassured by a special letter that the study was not seeking investment advice, but was concerned only with people's personal experiences with asset management.

Some of the individuals' addresses could not be verified from any public directory, but only through a name on a mailbox or on an apartment house door. (The use made of public directories is explained below.) Most often these were individuals with very high incomes who did not wish to be disturbed by solicitors or interviewers. It was thought that in these instances an interview was more likely to be secured if a letter were sent asking the person to contact the interviewer, rather than having the interviewer make the initial contact by personal visit.

Two initial explanatory letters had been sent directly from the Survey Research Center. One letter was from University of Michigan President Harlan Hatcher describing the work of the Center, and the other was from Dr. Angus Campbell, Director of the Survey Research Center, describing the nature of the study. Since these were obviously form letters (even though names and addresses were typed individually), many individuals probably discarded them without reading them, thinking that nothing would happen if they did nothing. Many individuals, when first contacted, said they had never received the letters. In these cases, it was of course necessary to send a second set of letters. It was also thought appropriate to include a personal, individually typed letter of apology for the individual's having been contacted prior to receipt of the Center's initial letters.

Some individuals responded to the interviewer's initial telephone contact by claiming to be too ill to be interviewed, and it was often not clear whether they were temporarily ill or suffering from chronic poor health. It was also thought that these people might have misunderstood what was being asked of them. A special letter was sent in these cases, with reassurances that the interview would make only minimal demands on their time and energy.

Others declined to be interviewed, but were willing to fill out the questionnaire themselves. They were advised not to do this on the grounds that they would save time if the questionnaire were administered personally by our trained interviewer. But if they still insisted, they were allowed to fill out the questionnaire themselves. This proved quite unsatisfactory. If the individual did not have the time to be interviewed, he most certainly did not have the time to interview himself. Of the five who insisted on handling the interview in this way, only one completed the questionnaire satisfactorily.

Many of the introductory letters were sent after early experience had shown that the interview could be completed in less than an hour, and this reassurance about the time required was added to the letter.

Number of Attempts Required to Secure an Appointment

With only one-fifth of the respondents were the interviewers able to secure an appointment for an interview at the first attempted contact. In

27 percent of the cases where interviews were eventually obtained, the interviewer had to make five or more calls before getting an appointment. The distribution of cases by the number of attempts required to secure an interview was as follows:

Number of attempts required	*Percent of completed interviews*
One	21
Two	22
Three	17
Four	13
Five through eight	21
Nine or more	6
Total	100
Number of interviews[1]	1,051

The number of attempts required to secure interviews with medical doctors was calculated separately. Even though the proportion of medical doctors in the final set of interviews was probably smaller than that in the original sample, those doctors who agreed to be interviewed generally required fewer attempted contacts than did the other respondents. The distribution of doctors by the number of contacts required to secure an interview was as follows:

Number of attempts required	*Percent of completed interviews with doctors*
One or two	52
Three or four	26
Five or more	22
Total	100
Number of interviews	72

There was little difference in the number of attempts required to secure interviews with female as opposed to male respondents.

The size of place where the respondent lived did make some difference in the number of contacts needed. Interviewers found generally that more attempts had to be made in metropolitan areas than in smaller communities. The percentage distribution of completed interviews was as follows:

[1] Including the 94 cases with incomes under $10,000.

Number of attempts required	Twelve largest metropolitan areas	Other metropolitan areas	Nonmetropolitan areas
One or two	37	46	52
Three or four	32	26	33
Five or more	31	28	15
Total	100	100	100
Number of interviews[2]	388	457	206

Reasons for Nonresponse

Of the 1,696 individuals originally selected, 645 could not be interviewed. Sixty percent of these nonresponse cases, classed as "refusals," declined because they were either too busy or simply not interested. Another 6 percent declined because of ill health. Ten percent could not be interviewed because for various reasons they were unavailable through the duration of the study. Another 10 percent were deceased or minors. Fourteen percent could not be located in any public directory.

About half of those who finally refused were sent one or more of the special letters mentioned earlier. The letters were sent only if both the interviewer and the Ann Arbor staff thought that such action would be helpful.

Many of those who eventually refused were very difficult to contact in the first place, either by phone or personal visit. Often, owing to distance from the individual, the interviewer was unable to assess the situation before attempting the first contact. Hence, she was unable to determine whether a telephone call or a face-to-face contact would be more advantageous for getting an interview. It was generally thought to be more businesslike to contact these individuals by phone during office hours since most were so busy that they would feel the intrusion on their personal time more acutely if contacted at home. Of all the refusals, 88 percent were contacted exclusively by phone. In 1 percent of the refusal cases the interviewer made only a personal visit to try to secure an appointment. In 11 percent of the refusal cases, the interviewer attempted to make contacts both by phone and by personal visit.

For 10 percent of those who refused, only one contact was attempted. Their refusals were so firm that a second attempt was thought inadvisable. However, for 46 percent of the refusals, the interviewer made five or more attempts to contact the individual before accepting

[2] Including the 94 cases with incomes under $10,000.

the refusal as final. For 15 percent of the refusals, the interviewer attempted to contact the person nine or more times. It should be noted that these were attempted contacts, and not always was the interviewer actually able to talk with the individual.

In many of the instances of ill health, the interviewer was not even allowed to speak with the designated respondent. Women accounted for 40 percent of the ill-health cases, but for only 13 percent of all nonresponse cases.

Ten percent of the nonrespondents were simply unavailable for the duration of the study. All of these individuals were verified as residing at a particular address, but were never available at that address or any other address we might have had for them. Many of these individuals were out of the country for the entire duration of the study—some on business and some taking extensive winter vacations. A few were in the armed services. In a few other cases, the interviewer simply was not able to catch the individual at the right time.

Another 10 percent of the nonrespondents were either deceased or minors. Since the list of names from which the sample was drawn was two years old and the median age was higher than that of adults in the population as a whole, it is not surprising that so many were deceased. The number of deceased individuals is probably understated since some of those who could not be verified may actually have been deceased. A very small fraction of the sample were minors.

The names and addresses of 14 percent of the nonrespondents could not be verified. Since we were pledged not to reveal the source of our sample to the respondents, no attempt was made to contact anyone unless his name and address could be verified in some recent public directory. The most common source for verifying a name was the local telephone book, but extensive use was also made of *Standard and Poor's Directory of Executives* and even *Who's Who in America.*

Forty percent of those who could not be verified were individuals with addresses "in care of" a bank or another individual, usually a lawyer or an accountant. Since we did not wish to make any personal contact with the individual's banker or lawyer, we had to find some other address that we were certain was his in a public directory. Many of those whose other addresses could not be identified in this way were females. Twenty-seven percent of those whose addresses were in care of a bank or another individual and whose other addresses could not be identified in a public directory were females, whereas only 13 percent of all the nonrespondents were females.

About half of the unverified individuals had moved from the addresses available to us. In these cases, numerous attempts were made to locate the individuals in telephone books and city directories of nearby communities.

Eleven percent of the unverified addresses were so vague that the right individual could not be found with certainty. Often these addresses consisted only of a Post Office box number. In these cases, it was surmised that the individual did not live in the town where he held a Post Office box or perhaps only lived there for part of the year. Another small group of unverified individuals had addresses that were invalid—that is, there was no such street, the address was that of a vacant lot, etc.

Characteristics of Nonrespondents Who Returned a Mail Questionnaire

To determine any differences between respondents and the eligible and verified nonrespondents, the latter were sent a two-page mail questionnaire. Not all of the bias possibly existing in the final set of interviews could be detected in this way, since these mail questionnaires obviously could not be sent to those nonrespondents with unverified names or bad addresses. There may also be undetected and important differences between those who did and those who did not return the mail questionnaire. Seventy-four percent of all nonrespondents were sent the mail questionnaire, and 113 completed and returned them, for a response rate of 24 percent.

Both personal-interview respondents and those to whom mail questionnaires were sent were asked to state the degree of importance of each of four investment objectives—a high rate of return, liquidity, safety, and capital gains. Personal-interview respondents were asked: "How important is each one of these things to you?" Their answers were coded into a five-point scale. Mail-questionnaire respondents were asked to check a box placing themselves on a five-point scale for each of the four objectives from "very important" to "not important at all." The mail-questionnaire respondents tended to rank each item higher in importance than those interviewed personally, as is shown in the following table:

Investment objectives	*Some degree of importance*		*Some degree of unimportance*	
	Personal interview	*Mail questionnaire*	*Personal interview*	*Mail questionnaire*
High rate of return	52%	78%	48%	22%
Safety	89	92	11	8
Liquidity	68	80	32	20
Capital gains	85	93	15	7

This tendency may have resulted from the technique of questioning rather than from a real difference in attitudes.

It is also interesting that quite similar proportions of both types of respondents said that a high rate of return, safety, and liquidity were "very important." But in the case of capital gains, a higher percentage of personal-interview respondents (55 percent) than of mail-questionnaire respondents (36 percent) called the objective "very important."

The largest difference in ranking occurred with respect to the high-rate-of-return objective. Seventy-eight percent of those who answered the mail questionnaire thought it had some importance, while only 52 percent of the personal-interview respondents ranked it as having some degree of importance, although it was ranked the lowest of the four objectives for both groups. Indeed, the implied rankings that the two groups gave for the four objectives were quite similar.

Those answering the mail questionnaire were asked an additional question to determine what type of asset they were putting the bulk of their savings into at the time. The percentage distribution was as follows:

Type of asset in which individual has invested the most in the past five years	*Mail-questionnaire respondents*
Variable-yield assets	68%
Fixed-yield assets	28
About the same in both types	4
Total	100

Slightly more of the mail-questionnaire respondents were putting the bulk of their new savings into fixed-yield assets than currently had the bulk of their savings in such assets.

Table C-1 summarizes replies on various other characteristics where a comparison between personal-interview and mail-questionnaire respondents was made.

There were interesting occupational differences between the personal-interview and the mail-questionnaire respondents. Fifty-four percent of the former said that they were self-employed, compared with only 39 percent of the mail-questionnaire respondents. This is consistent with the fact that a larger percentage of personal-interview respondents than of mail-questionnaire respondents had their largest investments in unincorporated businesses. However, the percentages for the two groups are not directly comparable since those personal-interview respondents who denied being self-employed but were nevertheless corporation presidents or chairmen of boards of directors were later classified as being self-em-

TABLE C-1. Comparison of Personal-Interview and Mail-Questionnaire Respondents on Various Characteristics

Characteristics	Type of respondent[a]	
	Personal-interview	*Mail-questionnaire*
1961 income $75,000 or higher	33%	43%
1961 income less than $10,000	9	9
Aged 65 or older	17	30
Female	4	6
All management of assets delegated	3	10
Investment concentrated in one or more of the variable-yield assets	76	76
Self-employed	54	39
Retired or rentiers	11	16
Investment concentrated in real estate, unincorporated businesses, or farms	24	13

[a] Both sets of percentages are unweighted.

ployed. This adjustment was not made in the case of the mail-questionnaire respondents.

Among the seven characteristics on which the two groups were compared (importance of investment objectives, delegation of asset management, portfolio composition, income, sex, age, and occupational group), four pointed to noticeable differences between the two groups. The personal-interview group was biased in the direction of containing too few with the highest incomes, too few who were aged sixty-five or older, too few who were concerned about current yield as distinct from other investment objectives, and too many whose investments were concentrated in their own unincorporated businesses or real estate. A correction for the income bias was automatically included in the weighting procedure, but the other biases remain uncorrected.

Characteristics of All Nonrespondents

Very little information was available on the nonrespondents who did not fill out the mail questionnaire. In about half of these cases, however, it was possible to determine the individual's occupation through city directories, *Standard and Poor's Directory of Executives,* or *Who's Who in America.* All nonrespondent females not completing the questionnaire were assumed to be housewives or rentiers unless there was evidence to the contrary. The paragraphs below refer to all nonrespondents—those who did and those who did not fill out the mail questionnaire.

It appears that the proportion of medical doctors in the personal-interview sample was probably lower than that in the original sample. Of those from whom interviews were not obtained, about 13 percent were medical doctors; but of those from whom we did obtain personal interviews, only 7 percent were doctors. It is also probably true that there is a higher percentage of rentiers and retired individuals in the sample as a whole than among the personal-interview respondents, especially when account is taken of the deceased. It is difficult to speculate on any other occupational bias since, apart from the case of medical doctors, it proved impossible to render the occupational categories reported by respondents comparable to those used in the public directories.

The personal-interview respondents were generally younger than the nonrespondents. Seventeen percent of the former were sixty-five or older, compared with 30 percent of the mail-questionnaire respondents. The remaining individuals in the original sample may also have had a high average since this group contained those who refused to be interviewed on account of illness and those who were too secluded to be reached.

The personal-interview respondents also contained a slightly smaller proportion of females than did the sample as a whole. Only 4 percent of the personal-interview respondents were females, compared with 13 percent of the nonrespondents. They too were generally more secluded and more difficult to contact. Most were widows.

In addition to the biases revealed by the mail questionnaire, the analysis of the remaining noninterview cases therefore showed that the personal-interview sample contained too few women and too few medical doctors.

Nevertheless, the overall response rate was not so low, nor (probably) were the differences between personal-interview respondents and the rest so great that there is large error in the results presented for the entire population on the basis of what was reported by the personal-interview respondents alone. For example, one of the biggest differences between those who were interviewed and the remainder appeared to lie in the proportions aged sixty-five or older. But even if it is assumed that the high proportion reported by the mail-questionnaire respondents (30 percent) applied also to the remaining noninterview cases, then the proportion for the entire original sample would become 22 percent, a figure that differs only moderately from the 17 percent derived from the personal-interview respondents alone.

APPENDIX D

Misreporting of Income

THERE WAS EVIDENCE OF widespread understating of income by respondents. Assuming that the sampling and sub-selecting were done properly, we can estimate the income distribution of the total sample sent to the field interviewers. It is given in the first column of Table D-1. The frequency distribution of the 1,051 completed interviews by actual 1961 income is shown in the second column of Table D-1.

Comparison of the first and second columns indicates that there is a somewhat smaller proportion of completed interviews from the higher

TABLE D-1. 1961 Income Comparisons for High-Income Sample

1961 income	*Actual income distribution for total sample sent out for interviewing*	*Actual income distribution for completed interviews*	*Distribution of interviews by income reported by respondents*
Under $10,000	89	47	94
10,000– 14,999	237	171	169
15,000– 24,999	313	222	215
25,000– 49,999	239	160	225
50,000– 99,999	347	220	184
100,000–149,999	80	48	74
150,000–499,999	280	138	67
500,000 and over	111	45	23
Total	1,696	1,051	1,051

TABLE D-2. Adjustments for Understating of Income by Respondents

Income brackets	Distribution of cases by actual 1961 income	Distribution of cases by 1961 income indicated by respondents	Number in each SRC bracket whose actual income was in a higher bracket[a]	Assuming that the misclassified cases shown in Column (3) had the lowest incomes in the next higher bracket[b]: Estimated actual bracket for each SRC group	Implied degree of understating at lowest income in each estimated bracket	Median income for estimated actual SRC brackets: Detailed	Median income for estimated actual SRC brackets: Rounded	Percentage distribution of aggregate income: Between actual brackets[c]	Percentage distribution of aggregate income: Between estimated actual SRC brackets
	(1)	(2)	(3)	(4)	(5)	(6)	(7)	(8)	(9)
Under $10,000	47	94	47	Under $10,740	. . .	. . .	. . .	. . .	. . .
10,000– 14,999	171	169	45	10,740– 16,420	6.9%	$12,270	$12,000	47.8%	44.1%
15,000– 24,999	222	215	38	16,420– 30,940	8.6	19,544	20,000	22.8	24.1
25,000– 49,999	160	225	103	30,940– 73,400	19.2	41,770	40,000	16.3	19.5
50,000– 99,999	220	184	67	73,400–164,680	31.9	90,850	100,000	7.1	7.9
100,000–149,999	48	74	74	164,680–314,700	39.3	192,980	200,000	2.0	1.4
150,000–499,999	138	67	22	314,700–843,000	52.3	441,400	400,000	2.6	2.1
500,000 and over	45	23	0	843,000 and over	40.7			1.4	1.0
Total	1,051	1,051	396					100.0	100.0

Source for cols. (4)–(9): U. S. Treasury Department, Internal Revenue Service, *Statistics of Income, 1961*, p. 32. An even distribution of returns within each of the detailed income brackets used in the source was assumed.

[a] Estimated as column 2 *plus* column 3 for the preceding line *minus* column 1. This assumes that (a) no case indicated too high a bracket to SRC and (b) all cases indicating too low a bracket indicated the bracket next below their actual bracket. The procedure yielded consistent results except for the $100,000–149,999 bracket, where there were too few cases to permit the assumption that all of the 67 cases misclassified in the $50,000–99,999 bracket should actually have been in the $100,000–149,999 bracket. It was therefore assumed that 19 of these 67 cases were wrong by *two* brackets instead of one and should have been in the $150,000–499,999 bracket.

[b] For example, the 45 cases who indicated incomes of $10,000–14,999 to SRC but who should have been in the $15,000–24,999 bracket are assumed to have had the lowest incomes among the 222 cases actually in the $15,000–24,999 bracket. See note [a] for the exception applying to the 67 cases misclassified in the $50,000–99,999 bracket.

[c] Differential weights were assigned to the 1,051 cases on the basis of the reported brackets so that the weighted distribution of the cases was the same as this column.

income groups than from the lower income groups, the proportion of completed interviews within each group varying from 72 to 41 percent.

The third column of Table D-1 gives the distribution of the completed interviews according to the 1961 incomes *actually reported* by the respondents during the interviews. It is clear from this table that substantial understating occurred. Since the weights did not vary much from one income group to the adjacent one, the misclassifications did little damage to the weighting system described in Appendix B. But to describe realistically the characteristics of the high-income respondents, it was necessary to adjust somewhat their stated income figures.

Despite the unavailability of data on the actual income of each respondent, it was still possible to make a reasonably correct income bracket for those in each *indicated* bracket. Revised descriptions of the income brackets are shown in column 4 of Table D-2.

Table D-2 shows the procedure used in estimating the revised brackets. One illustration of the computations may be helpful. Forty-seven of the 94 respondents stating that their incomes were under $10,000 actually had incomes above that level. These 47 cases were assumed to have actual incomes in the next higher bracket ($10,000-$14,999) and, moreover, were assumed to have the lowest incomes among the 171 cases actually in the $10,000-$14,999 bracket. From *Statistics of Income, 1961,* it is seen that 27.5 percent (47/171) of the returns in the $10,000-$14,999 bracket had incomes below $10,740. Thus those respondents reporting themselves in the $10,000-$14,999 bracket are assumed to be actually in a bracket that begins at $10,740. This implies that those at the lower end of this bracket understated their income by 6.9 percent ($740/$10,740). The implied degree of understating tended to increase with income, as is shown in column 5. This tendency seems plausible.

Since understating apparently occurred at all income levels, the actual distribution of aggregate income (received by those with actual incomes over $10,740) between the seven "new" brackets was similar to the actual distribution of aggregate income (received by those with actual incomes over $10,000) between the seven *original* brackets. Details are shown in columns 8 and 9.

The question also arises as to whether 1963 income was as seriously understated as 1961 income. If not, the original brackets describing 1963 income could have been retained in the analysis. Median reported income for the 1,051 cases rose from $30,000 to $34,000 between 1961 and 1963, or by an average annual rate of about 6 percent. This rate seems close to what actually occurred. It was concluded that understating was about as extensive for 1963 income as for 1961 income and that the revised brackets should be used in describing the income of both years. These revised brackets (expressed in rounded form as shown in Table D-3) have been used throughout the text.[1]

TABLE D-3. Derived Income Brackets Used in Text Compared with Income Indicated by Respondents

Derived income brackets used in text	*Median of bracket used in text*	*Income reported by respondents*
Under $10,000	...	Under $10,000
10,000– 14,999	12,000	10,000– 14,999
15,000– 29,999	20,000	15,000– 24,999
30,000– 74,999	40,000	25,000– 49,999
75,000– 149,999	100,000	50,000– 99,999
150,000–299,999	200,000	100,000–149,999
300,000 and over	400,000	150,000 and over

This evidence of understating of income should not be generalized to other studies, even of high-income people. It should be remembered that the present survey asked in early 1964 a single question about 1961 income (after first asking the respondent to exclude tax-exempt interest and the nontaxable part of capital gains). And later there was a single question about 1963 income. There was also an extensive effort to interview as large a proportion of the sample as possible, including some who were quite reluctant.

A study of high-income people in one midwestern city, the substantive findings of which have been published previously, found less error in the stating of income and also much less bias since the errors were in both directions.[2] Fewer than one-fourth of the cases, all of whom had incomes over $15,000, had discrepancies amounting to more than 15 percent of income. Nearly 40 percent of the discrepancies were within $1,000. Even at incomes over $50,000, only a third were in error by more than $8,000, and in most of these cases the personal-interview report was *higher*. It is likely that the detailed attention given to income in the interview mainly accounts for the higher precision obtained in the midwestern city study.

[1] Understating of income rendered useless the 94 cases who reported a 1961 income under $10,000. It had been hoped to use that group for comparing the "high-income" individuals with the rest of the population. But fully half of the 94 cases actually had income over $10,000.

[2] For the substantive findings see George Katona and John B. Lansing, "The Wealth of the Wealthy," *Review of Economics and Statistics* (February 1964), pp. 1-13.

APPENDIX E

Questionnaire and Distribution of Responses[1]

THE ANSWERS TO ALL the questions asked in the interview are given in this appendix in the order in which the questions were asked. Two distributions are given of (a) the aggregate income received by those giving particular replies and (b) high-income "individuals." The first distribution required the use of weights for each response according to the amount of income it represented. The second required the use of weights for each response according to the number of high-income individuals it represented. A comparison of the two distributions for any question will show how the frequency of the different replies varied with income. If the percentage of aggregate income associated with a particular reply exceeded the percentage of individuals associated with that reply, then it can be concluded that the reply tended to become more frequent as income rose, and vice versa.

Some questions were asked only of an appropriate subgroup, but the percentages given are always of the total high-income sample.

[1] For cases with 1961 adjusted gross incomes of $10,000 and over.

Section 1. Saving Objectives and Investment Policies

	Percentage of aggregate income	*Percentage of individuals*
Different people have different reasons for saving. In your case, what are the purposes for saving? Anything else?		
Retirement, old age	50	53
Children's education	29	31
Buy house; pay off mortgage; make house additions	2	3
To make gifts to charitable organizations	2	1
Travel, vacations, personal pleasures	10	11
To invest it; earn a return on it	11	10
To bequeath money (no mention of charities)	26	23
For security, emergencies	34	35
To buy consumption items	9	10
Other reasons	14	13
Not ascertained	0	0
Total	[2]	[2]
What kinds of things do you consider when deciding where to put money you don't plan to spend right away?		
Tax considerations	6	4
High rate of return	30	32
Safety; diversification	37	37
Liquidity	11	12
Capital gains	22	21
Convenience; avoid bother	1	1
Protect family interests	0	0
Other reasons	8	8
Not ascertained; or respondent answer in terms of types of assets (for example, common stock)		
Total	[2]	[2]
Do you (and your immediate family) have any savings, investments, or reserve funds?		
Yes	97	97
No	3	3
Total	100	100
Would they be worth $1,000 or more, all together?		
Yes	94	92
No	3	5
No savings, investments, or reserve funds	3	3
Total	100	100

[2] Adds to more than 100 percent because some respondents gave more than one reason.

	Percentage of aggregate income	*Percentage of individuals*
Some people are not fully satisfied with the way their funds are distributed among the various investments. Are you fully satisfied or not?		
Yes	71	70
No	22	21
Not ascertained	1	1
Savings, investments, or reserve funds under $1,000	6	8
Total	100	100
How is this—could you tell me about it?		
Should take better advantage of tax laws	1	1
Too much in risky assets; not diversified enough	2	2
Not enough income	3	3
Too illiquid	1	1
Too much in fixed-yield assets	2	3
Too much in common stock	1	0
Too much in real estate or business	1	1
Too much in other assets	1	1
Wants more of a specific type of asset	2	3
Restrained by things beyond own control	1	1
Generally dissatisfied; bothered by frequent changes that have to be made in investment portfolio	5	5
Other reasons	1	1
Not ascertained	2	2
Total	[3]	[3]
How frequently do you review where your savings are invested to determine if you would like to make any changes?		
Every day; continuously	20	16
Every few days	3	3
Once a month	8	8
Every few months	19	18
Every year	13	13
Every few years	11	11
Never	12	14
Regularly, but no time period given	1	1
Not ascertained	7	8
Savings, investments, or reserve funds under $1,000	6	8
Total	100	100

[3] This question was asked only of those who were not fully satisfied with their investments, but some of these respondents gave more than one reason.

	Percentage of aggregate income	*Percentage of individuals*
Here [listed on card] are some of the things people tell us are important to them in managing their investments. How important is each one of these things to you?		
How about high rate of return (rent, interest, dividends, profits)?		
Very important	18	19
Important	20	21
Somewhat important	13	14
Not very important	21	20
Not important at all	17	14
Not ascertained	5	4
Savings, investments, or reserve funds under $1,000	6	8
Total	100	100
How about safety (absence of risk)?		
Very important	45	46
Important	25	24
Somewhat important	12	10
Not very important	4	4
Not important at all	4	4
Not ascertained	4	4
Savings, investments, or reserve funds under $1,000	6	8
Total	100	100
How about liquidity (ease in cashing)?		
Very important	19	18
Important	27	26
Somewhat important	15	16
Not very important	14	15
Not important at all	15	13
Not ascertained	4	4
Savings, investments, or reserve funds under $1,000	6	8
Total	100	100
How about capital gains (things that will increase in value)?		
Very important	46	42
Important	20	20
Somewhat important	7	7
Not very important	7	8
Not important at all	9	10
Not ascertained	5	5
Savings, investments, or reserve funds under $1,000	6	8
Total	100	100

	Percentage of aggregate income	*Percentage of individuals*
Is there anything else important to you in managing your investments?		
Yes	31	26
No	63	66
Savings, investments, or reserve funds under $1,000	6	8
Total	100	100
What is it?		
Lower taxes	4	3
Stable current cash income	1	1
Freedom from having to manage things	1	1
Ethical considerations	1	1
Diversification	3	2
Good management of company; desire for personal control over where funds are invested; desire for something he is interested in; other	19	16
Not ascertained	2	2
Nothing else important to respondent in making investments; or savings, investment, or reserve funds under $1,000	69	74
Total	100	100
Do you have some funds which you have set aside just to take advantage of opportunities that may come along, even if they are a bit speculative?		
Yes	40	37
No	54	55
Savings, investments, or reserve funds under $1,000	6	8
Total	100	100

Section 2. Trust Funds and Joint Ownership

Do you or any of your immediate family have a beneficial interest in a trust fund?		
Yes	24	19
No	70	73
Savings, investments, or reserve funds under $1,000	6	8
Total	100	100

	Percentage of aggregate income	Percentage of individuals
Do you have any control over how it is invested?		
Yes, complete control	3	2
Yes, some control	2	2
Yes, degree of control not ascertained	9	6
No	10	9
No beneficial interest in trust fund; or savings, investments, or reserve funds under $1,000	76	81
Total	100	100
Do you have some things that are jointly owned with friends or with relatives who do not live with you?		
Yes	29	27
No	65	65
Savings, investments, or reserve funds under $1,000	6	8
Total	100	100
What kinds of investments are these? Anything else?		
Fixed-yield assets	2	2
Real estate, farm, or unincorporated business	16	14
Common stock	7	7
Fixed-yield assets and real estate, farm, or unincorporated business	0	0
Fixed-yield assets and common stock	1	1
Real estate, farm, or unincorporated business and common stock	3	1
Fixed-yield assets and real estate, farm, or unincorporated business and common stock	0	1
No jointly owned assets; or savings, investments, or reserve funds under $1,000	71	73
Total	100	100
With whom are they owned—your parents, your children, a friend, or whom?		
Related adults	15	16
Children	2	1
Friends or business associates	9	8
Related adults and friends or business associates	2	2
Children and friends or business associates	1	0
No jointly owned assets; or savings, investments, or reserve funds under $1,000	71	73
Total	100	100

	Percentage of aggregate income	*Percentage of individuals*
What are the reasons why these investments are jointly owned?		
Avoid taxes; lower taxes	1	1
Investments were inherited or otherwise received in that form	9	9
Business partnership	9	7
Other	12	10
Not ascertained	1	1
Total	[4]	[4]
Who would be responsible for deciding what to do with those things—whether to sell them and invest the money somewhere else, for instance?		
Respondent	7	7
Other owner	2	2
Respondent and other owner	16	15
Other responses	3	2
Not ascertained	1	1
No jointly owned assets; or savings, investments, or reserve funds under $1,000	71	73
Total	100	100

Section 3. Family Structure

Now in the remainder of this interview, I want to talk about all the investments you and your immediate family own and control the disposition of. "Immediate family" includes your wife and children and other dependents.

Are you single, married, widowed, divorced, or separated?		
Single	3	3
Married	87	86
Widowed	3	2
Divorced	1	1
Separated	0	0
Savings, investments, or reserve funds under $1,000	6	8
Total	100	100

[4] This question was asked only of those who had jointly owned assets, but some of them gave more than one reason.

	Percentage of aggregate income	Percentage of individuals
Do you have any children who are still dependent on you?		
Yes	55	55
No	39	37
Savings, investments, or reserve funds under $1,000	6	8
Total	100	100
Do you have any other dependents?		
Yes	11	8
No	83	84
Savings, investments, or reserve funds under $1,000	6	8
Total	100	100
Do you have any living children who are no longer your dependents?		
Yes	40	36
No	54	56
Savings, investments, or reserve funds under $1,000	6	8
Total	100	100

Section 4. Delegation and Consultation

Do you (and your immediate family) handle the job of managing your investments, or have you turned over some of your investment decisions to someone else?		
All delegated	2	1
Some delegated	8	6
None delegated	84	85
Savings, investments, or reserve funds under $1,000	6	8
Total	100	100

	Percentage of aggregate income	*Percentage of individuals*
What kind of investments are managed by someone else?		
Fixed-yield assets	0	0
Real estate, farm, or unincorporated business	1	1
Common stock	4	3
Fixed-yield assets and real estate, farm, or unincorporated business	0	0
Fixed-yield assets and common stock	3	2
Real estate, farm, or unincorporated business and common stock	0	0
Fixed-yield assets and real estate, farm, or unincorporated business and common stock	1	0
Not ascertained	1	1
Respondent manages own assets; or savings, investments, or reserve funds under $1,000	90	93
Total	100	100
Is the person who manages them a stockbroker, a bank officer, or what?		
Qualified professional	8	5
Two or more qualified professionals	2	2
Respondent manages own assets; or savings, investments, or reserve funds under $1,000	90	93
Total	100	100
What kind of policy or instructions is he following in handling your investments?		
Tax advantages	0	0
High rate of return	0	0
Safety, stable current income	1	1
Liquidity	0	0
Capital gains	1	1
Follows his own policy	3	2
Manager has no discretion	2	2
Not ascertained	3	2
Total	[5]	[5]

[5] This question was asked only of those who delegated some or all of their investment decisions to someone else, but some of these respondents gave more than one reason.

	Percentage of aggregate income	Percentage of individuals
How frequently does he check with you about your investments—once a month, once a year, or what?		
Every week or more frequently	1	1
Once a month; every few weeks	2	1
Every few months	4	3
Once a year or less frequently	2	1
Whenever there is a problem or something needs to be discussed	1	1
Respondent manages own assets; or savings, investments, or reserve funds under $1,000	90	93
Total	100	100
In handling the investments which you manage yourself (yourselves), do you get advice from other people?		
Yes, always	22	20
Yes, occasionally	43	41
No	26	29
Not ascertained	1	1
Respondent manages none of his own assets; or savings, investments, or reserve funds under $1,000	8	9
Total	100	100
For what kinds of investment decisions do you usually get advice?		
Fixed-yield assets	2	2
Common stock	32	31
Real estate, farm, or unincorporated business	6	6
Fixed-yield assets and common stock	5	4
Fixed-yield assets and real estate, farm, or unincorporated business	1	1
Common stock and real estate, farm, or unincorporated business	6	5
Fixed-yield assets and common stock and real estate, farm, or unincorporated business	2	1
Other investments (such as home)	1	2
Whether to buy or sell (in general)	4	4
Not ascertained	6	5
Respondent does not get advice from others; or manages none of his own assets; or savings, investments, or reserve funds under $1,000	35	39
Total	100	100

	Percentage of aggregate income	*Percentage of individuals*
Do you get advice from a stockbroker, a business colleague, or whom?		
One person		
Qualified professional	25	25
Not a qualified professional	7	8
Not ascertained whether qualified professional	1	1
Two persons or more		
Qualified professionals	11	9
Not qualified professionals	3	2
Qualified professionals and others	15	13
Not ascertained what either or all persons are	3	3
Respondent does not get advice from others; or manages none of his own assets; or savings, investments, or reserve funds under $1,000	35	39
Total	100	100
What special information are you able to get?		
Tax features of investments	1	1
Other features of specific investments	43	41
General information (trends in industry as a whole, trends in entire economy)	5	5
Tax and other features of specific investments	2	1
Other features of specific investments and general information	1	1
Tax and other features of specific investments and general information	1	1
Not ascertained	12	11
Respondent does not get advice from others; or manages none of his own assets; or savings, investments, or reserve funds under $1,000	35	39
Total	100	100
Do you try to keep informed about various kinds of investments?		
Yes	63	58
No	31	34
Savings, investments, or reserve funds under $1,000	6	8
Total	100	100

	Percentage of aggregate income	*Percentage of individuals*
What would you say are your main sources of information?		
Business colleagues	5	4
Individuals who are not business colleagues	16	15
Newspapers (other than *Wall Street Journal*)	25	25
Periodicals; business magazines; *Wall Street Journal*	38	33
Books	1	1
Financial and other corporation reports	6	5
Publications or agencies specializing in information about investments	23	18
Libraries; government documents (form of publication not specified)	1	1
Other	7	7
Not ascertained	1	0
Total	[6]	[6]

Section 5. Nature of Assets

Now let me ask some questions about the kinds of savings and investments that you and your immediate family have.

Are you covered by Social Security?		
Yes	92	92
No	8	8
Total	100	100
Are you covered by some other retirement or pension program or deferred compensation plan?		
Yes	58	61
No	42	39
Total	100	100
Does this retirement plan have a number of variations, so that you had to make some kind of choice between them?		
Yes	14	14
No	44	47
Respondent not covered by other retirement plan	42	39
Total	100	100

[6] This question was asked only of those who tried to keep informed about various kinds of investments, but some of these respondents mentioned more than one source of information.

	Percentage of aggregate income	*Percentage of individuals*
What choices did you make?		
Variable yield with some risk	1	1
Fixed yield with no risk	0	0
Lump sum payment or fixed series of payments	1	2
Lifetime annuity or pension	3	3
Annuity to cover wife (or other dependent)	3	2
Annuity to cover respondent only	1	1
More than one of above, or other	2	2
Not ascertained	3	3
Respondent could make no choice; or not covered by other retirement plan	86	86
Total	100	100
On what basis did you make your choice?		
Tax considerations	1	1
Need to protect dependents	3	3
Need for income during retirement	3	3
Other	4	4
Not ascertained	3	3
Respondent could make no choice; or not covered by other retirement plan	86	86
Total	100	100
Are payments still being made into it, or are you retired, or what?		
Payments still being made	49	53
Payments not being made, but not retired	3	2
Retired	5	5
Other	1	1
Respondent not covered by other retirement plan	42	39
Total	100	100
Do you have a choice as to the amounts paid into it?		
Yes	8	8
No	42	46
Payments not being made into plan; or respondent not covered by other retirement plan	50	46
Total	100	100

	Percentage of aggregate income	Percentage of individuals
On what basis did you make your choice?		
Tax considerations	0	0
Need to protect dependents	0	0
Need for income in retirement	2	2
Need for income now	1	2
Other considerations	3	3
Not ascertained	2	2
Total	[7]	[7]
Can you still change the amount you pay in?		
Yes	7	7
No	1	1
No choice as to amount paid in; or payments not being made into plan; or not covered by other retirement plan	92	92
Total	100	100
Do you get a pension when you retire or a lump-sum payment, or a choice between the two?		
Pension	25	28
Lump-sum payment	3	3
Choice of pension or lump sum payment	20	21
Not ascertained	2	2
Payments not being made into plan; or respondent not covered by other retirement plan	50	46
Total	100	100
Does the plan have any way of increasing benefits to adjust for price and cost-of-living changes?		
Yes	12	15
No	42	42
Not ascertained	4	4
Respondent not covered by other retirement plan	42	39
Total	100	100
Do you have any group term life insurance that is paid for by a company?		
Yes	55	55
No	44	44
Not ascertained	1	1
Total	100	100

[7] This question was only asked of those who had some choice as to the amount paid into their retirement plan, but some of these respondents gave more than one reason.

	Percentage of aggregate income	Percentage of individuals
Do you have any life insurance that has a cash value, or that you can borrow on if you want to?		
Yes	86	85
No	13	14
Not ascertained	1	1
Total	100	100
What do you think of life insurance as a way of saving money?		
Good, because of tax considerations	1	1
Good, because of other considerations	17	17
Good, not ascertained why	17	18
Both good and bad features	26	24
Bad	28	29
Extremely bad	6	5
Other	0	1
Not ascertained	5	5
Total	100	100
Do you own your own home, or pay rent, or what?		
Owns or is buying	91	89
Rents	7	8
Both owns and rents	1	1
Neither owns nor rents	1	2
Total	100	100

We have talked about retirement programs, insurance, and your home. Beyond these basic things, some people have other financial investments. Here is a list of investments that pay a fixed amount each year. Can you tell me which of these you or someone in your immediate family have.

	Percentage of aggregate income	Percentage of individuals
Whether respondent owns U.S. Savings Bonds[8]		
Yes	50	50
No	44	42
Savings, investments, or reserve funds under $1,000	6	8
Total	100	100

[8] The interviewers obtained the answers to this question by handing the respondent a card which listed the nine types of fixed-yield assets.

	Percentage of aggregate income	Percentage of individuals
Whether respondent owns U.S. bonds that pay interest currently[8]		
Yes	13	9
No	81	83
Savings, investments, or reserve funds under $1,000	6	8
Total	100	100
Whether respondent owns Treasury bills or notes[8]		
Yes	7	5
No	87	87
Savings, investments, or reserve funds under $1,000	6	8
Total	100	100
Whether respondent owns "municipals" (state and local bonds)[8]		
Yes	19	12
No	75	80
Savings, investments, or reserve funds under $1,000	6	8
Total	100	100
Whether respondent owns corporate bonds or debentures[8]		
Yes	19	14
No	75	78
Savings, investments, or reserve funds under $1,000	6	8
Total	100	100
Whether respondent owns savings accounts in banks or savings and loan associations[8]		
Yes	76	75
No	18	17
Savings, investments, or reserve funds under $1,000	6	8
Total	100	100
Whether respondent owns preferred stock[8]		
Yes	24	22
No	70	70
Savings, investments, or reserve funds under $1,000	6	8
Total	100	100

	Percentage of aggregate income	Percentage of individuals
Whether respondent owns credit union deposits[8]		
Yes	15	19
No	79	73
Savings, investments, or reserve funds under $1,000	6	8
Total	100	100
Whether respondent owns mortgages and land contracts[8]		
Yes	18	17
No	76	75
Savings, investments, or reserve funds under $1,000	6	8
Total	100	100
Considering all these investments listed on the card, about how much do you and your immediate family have invested here? Would it be less than $10,000, between $10,000 and $100,000, or more than $100,000?		
Less than $10,000	32	37
Between $10,000 and $100,000	41	42
More than $100,000	16	8
No fixed-yield assets; or savings, investments or reserve funds under $1,000	11	13
Total	100	100
Have the changes in interest rate on savings accounts had any effect on where you keep your money? In what way?		
Yes, keeps more money in savings accounts	6	5
Yes, transferred money in savings accounts from one bank to another, from banks to savings and loan associations, from one kind of financial institution to another	11	11
Yes, other effects	3	3
Yes, but not ascertained what effect	2	2
No	72	71
Savings, investments, or reserve funds under $1,000	6	8
Total	100	100

	Percentage of aggregate income	Percentage of individuals
Have you or your immediate family bought any bonds or preferred stock in the last few years? When was the last time?		
Yes, in 1964	15	13
Yes, in 1963	14	11
Yes, in 1962	6	6
Yes, in 1961	3	3
Yes, in 1960 or earlier	3	3
No	53	56
Savings, investments, or reserve funds under $1,000	6	8
Total	100	100
Have you (or your immediate family) ever sold any bonds or preferred stock? When was the last time?		
Yes, in 1964	4	2
Yes, in 1963	9	8
Yes, in 1962	6	6
Yes, in 1961	3	3
Yes, in 1960 or earlier	18	18
Yes, not ascertained when	1	0
No	52	54
Not ascertained	1	1
Savings, investments, or reserve funds under $1,000	6	8
Total	100	100
What did you do with the money?		
Bought fixed-yield assets	4	3
Bought common stock	10	8
Bought real estate, farm, or unincorporated business	3	3
Bought fixed-yield assets and common stock	1	1
Bought fixed-yield assets and real estate, farm, or unincorporated business	0	1
Bought common stock and real estate, farm, or unincorporated business	0	0
Bought fixed-yield assets, common stock, and real estate, farm, or unincorporated business	0	0
Other purchases only (durable goods, current living expenses)	22	21
Not ascertained	1	0
Never sold bonds or preferred stock; or savings, investments, or reserve funds under $1,000	59	63
Total	100	100

	Percentage of aggregate income	*Percentage of individuals*
Would you say that you keep more money in your checking account now than you did a few years ago, or less, or what? Why is that?		
More in checking account		
Income or assets have increased; more expenses	32	32
Other reasons	15	14
Combination of above reasons	3	3
Same amount in checking account; or sometimes more, sometimes less	30	28
Less in checking account		
Income or assets have decreased; fewer expenses	2	2
Rise in interest rates makes it desirable to put money somewhere else	3	2
Other reasons	6	6
Combination of above reasons	1	1
Not ascertained	0	1
Has no checking account; or savings, investments, or reserve funds under $1,000	8	11
Total	100	100
Do you (or any members of your immediate family) own any common stock?		
Yes	73	65
No	21	27
Savings, investments, or reserve funds under $1,000	6	8
Total	100	100
In about how many different companies do you have common stock?		
One	10	12
Two	7	8
Three	6	6
Four	7	8
Five through nine	13	12
Ten through fourteen	9	8
Fifteen through twenty-four	9	6
Twenty-five or more	11	6
Not ascertained	1	1
Does not own common stock; or savings, investments, or reserve funds under $1,000	27	35
Total	100	100

	Percentage of aggregate income	Percentage of individuals
Do you follow the stock market closely?		
Yes, closely	30	24
Yes, fairly closely	9	8
Sometimes follows the stock market	3	2
Occasionally; not very closely	5	5
Does not follow the stock market at all	24	24
Not ascertained	2	2
Does not own common stock; or savings, investments, or reserve funds under $1,000	27	35
Total	100	100
Do you try to keep stocks with high current dividends, or ones that are likely to increase in price, or what?		
Stocks with high current dividends	5	5
Stocks that are likely to increase in price	44	39
Stocks with other characteristics	3	3
Stocks with high current dividends and those likely to increase in price	11	9
Stocks that are likely to increase in price and with other characteristics	2	1
Stocks with high current dividends and those likely to increase in price and with other characteristics	1	1
Not ascertained	7	7
Does not own common stock; or savings, investments, or reserve funds under $1,000	27	35
Total	100	100
What are the reasons why you do that?		
Tax considerations	17	12
Larger return	9	9
Need for extra income in future	16	13
Need for income now	3	3
Desire for both current income and future growth	5	4
Safety; diversification	15	13
Other reasons	13	13
Not ascertained	8	8
Total	[9]	[9]

[9] This question was asked only of those who owned stock, but some gave more than one reason.

	Percentage of aggregate income	*Percentage of individuals*
Do you work for any company in which you own stock? Are you an executive or director of the company?		
Owns stock in company where works and is executive or director of that company	31	23
Owns stock in company where works but is not executive or director of that company	7	9
Does not work for any company where owns stock	35	33
Does not own common stock; or savings, investments, or reserve funds under $1,000	27	35
Total	100	100
In those companies in which you are active, are most of the earnings reinvested, or most paid out in dividends, or what?		
Most reinvested	19	15
Most paid out in dividends	4	3
About half reinvested, about half paid out	4	3
Other	2	1
Not ascertained	2	1
Not executive or director of company in which he owns stock; or does not own stock; or savings, investments, or reserve funds under $1,000	69	77
Total	100	100
Why is it done that way?		
Tax considerations	2	1
Other considerations	26	20
Both tax and other considerations	1	0
Not ascertained	2	2
Not executive or director of company in which he owns stock; or does not own stock; or savings, investments, or reserve funds under $1,000	69	77
Total	100	100
Do you own shares in a mutual fund or in an investment trust?		
Yes	28	26
No	66	66
Savings, investments, or reserve funds under $1,000	6	8
Total	100	100

	Percentage of aggregate income	*Percentage of individuals*
Is it a diversified fund, or does it invest mainly in growth stocks, or what?		
Fund is diversified	13	11
Fund invests in growth stocks	8	8
Fund has other characteristics	2	2
Any combination of above types	4	4
Not ascertained	1	1
Does not own mutual fund shares; or savings, investments, or reserve funds under $1,000	72	74
Total	100	100
About how much do you (and your immediate family) have invested in common stock and mutual funds? Would your net investment be less than $10,000, between $10,000 and $100,000, or more than $100,000? Would it be worth more than $500,000?		
Less than $10,000	22	27
Between $10,000 and $100,000	31	30
More than $100,000 but less than $500,000	10	6
More than $500,000	9	4
More than $100,000 but not ascertained whether more than $500,000	4	2
Not ascertained	2	2
Owns neither common stock nor mutual fund shares; or savings, investments, or reserve funds under $1,000	22	29
Total	100	100
Have you bought any common stock in the last few years. Was the last purchase made in 1963 or 1964, or was it in 1962 or earlier?		
Yes, in 1963 or 1964	50	41
Yes, in 1962 or earlier	13	14
No	31	37
Savings, investments, or reserve funds under $1,000	6	8
Total	100	100

	Percentage of aggregate income	*Percentage of individuals*
About how frequently do you buy stock on the average—every few weeks, a few times a year, or what?		
Once a month or more frequently	8	6
A few times a year	24	18
About once a year	5	5
Less than once a year	4	5
Regularly (time period not ascertained)	1	1
Whenever there is a good buy (time period not ascertained)	2	1
Occasionally; irregularly	4	3
Not ascertained	2	2
Did not buy stock in 1963 or 1964; or savings, investments, or reserve funds under $1,000	50	59
Total	100	100
Have you sold any common stock in the last few years? When was the last time?		
Yes, in 1964	15	11
Yes, in 1963	20	16
Yes, in 1962	7	6
Yes, in 1961	3	4
Yes, in 1960 or earlier	3	4
Yes, not ascertained when	1	0
No	44	50
Not ascertained whether has sold	1	1
Savings, investments, or reserve funds under $1,000	6	8
Total	100	100
How did you happen to sell at that time?		
Tax considerations	7	5
Profit-taking	10	8
Stock looked like poor prospect	15	12
To transfer funds to other stocks	7	5
To transfer funds to real estate, farm, or unincorporated business	1	1
To use funds for other purposes (buy house, pay bills, etc.)	8	8
Other reasons	9	7
Not ascertained	1	1
Total	[10]	[10]

[10] This question was asked only of those who sold stock in the last few years, but some gave more than one reason.

	Percentage of aggregate income	*Percentage of individuals*
Now, finally, I'd like to ask you about direct investments.		
Do you or your immediate family have money invested in an unincorporated business?		
Yes	25	23
No	69	69
Savings, investments, or reserve funds under $1,000	6	8
Total	100	100
How active are you in running the business?		
Full-time	15	15
More than half-time but not full-time	1	1
Active but not ascertained how active	2	2
Half-time	1	1
Less than half-time	1	0
Not at all active	4	4
Not ascertained	1	0
No investment in unincorporated business; or savings, investments, or reserve funds under $1,000	75	77
Total	100	100
Do you reinvest most of the earnings back into the business, or pay most of them out or what? Why is that?		
Reinvested for tax reasons	1	1
Reinvested for other reasons	11	10
Paid out for tax reasons	1	1
Paid out for other reasons	6	6
Other responses	3	2
Not ascertained	3	3
No investment in unincorporated business; or savings, investments, or reserve funds under $1,000	75	77
Total	100	100
How long do you plan to stay in the business?		
One through five years	2	2
Six through fifteen years	2	2
Sixteen through twenty-five years	2	2
Indefinitely	13	12
Not ascertained	6	5
No investment in unincorporated business; or savings, investments, or reserve funds under $1,000	75	77
Total	100	100

	Percentage of aggregate income	*Percentage of individuals*
What will happen to the business after that?		
Business will be continued: financial interest will be sold or otherwise passed to a relative	6	4
Business will be continued: financial interest will be sold or otherwise passed to someone not related who is already in the business as partner or management	2	2
Business will be continued: financial interest will be sold to someone not related and not already in the business as partner or management	2	2
Business will be continued: financial interest will not be sold; or not ascertained what will happen to financial interest	2	2
Business will be liquidated, discontinued	2	2
Other	3	3
Not ascertained	8	8
No investment in unincorporated business; or no savings, investments, or reserve funds under $1,000	75	77
Total	100	100
Do you or your immediate family own any real estate, land, or a farm (excluding your home)?		
Yes	47	43
No	47	49
Savings, investments, or reserve funds under $1,000	6	8
Total	100	100
Is this something you hold mainly for current income, or mainly for long-term increase in value, or what?		
Current income	15	13
Long-term increase in value	30	26
Tax reasons	0	0
Held because inherited or received as a gift	1	1
Mainly for family reasons	1	1
Present or future family consumption (land for building a home on, land for vacationing)	2	2
"Noneconomic" (sentimental) reasons	2	2
Other reasons	5	5
Not ascertained	2	2
Total	[11]	[11]

[11] This question was asked only of those who owned real estate, land, or a farm, but some respondents gave more than one reason.

	Percentage of aggregate income	Percentage of individuals
Now, considering all your direct investments in unincorporated business, farm, land, or real estate, what would you say your net investment in them was worth? Would it be less than $10,000, between $10,000 and $100,000, or more than $100,000?		
Less than $10,000	8	9
Between $10,000 and $100,000	30	32
More than $100,000	16	9
Not ascertained	1	1
Does not have investments in unincorporated business, real estate, land, or farm; or savings, investments, or reserve funds under $1,000	45	49
Total	100	100
Have you ever considered forming a corporation to hold any of these investments?		
Yes	15	12
No	38	37
Not ascertained	2	2
Does not have investments in unincorporated business, real estate, land, or farm; or savings, investments, or reserve funds under $1,000	45	49
Total	100	100
Why is it that you haven't done so?		
Tax considerations	4	3
Indifference; inertia	2	2
Expenses of incorporation	1	1
Already done so	3	2
Planning to do it, still considering it	2	2
Other reasons	4	3
Not ascertained	1	1
Total	[12]	[12]

[12] This question was asked only of those who had considered forming a corporation to hold their interests, but some respondents gave more than one reason.

	Percentage of aggregate income	*Percentage of individuals*
Have you or your immediate family bought or sold any interest in a business, farm, or real estate in the last few years (excluding your home)? When was the most recent transaction?		
Yes, in 1964	4	3
Yes, in 1963	9	8
Yes, in 1962	5	5
Yes, in 1961	3	3
Yes, in 1960 or earlier	4	3
Yes, not ascertained when	1	0
No	67	69
Not ascertained	1	1
Savings, investments, or reserve funds under $1,000	6	8
Total	100	100
What kind of thing did you buy or sell?		
Bought interest in real estate	8	7
Bought interest in business (unincorporated)	2	2
Bought interest in farm	1	1
Bought interest in more than one of above or some other asset	1	0
Sold interest in real estate	8	7
Sold interest in a business	3	1
Sold interest in a farm	1	2
Sold interest in more than one of above or some other asset	1	1
Bought *and* sold interests in business, farm, or real estate simultaneously	1	1
Did not buy or sell interest in business, farm, or real estate in the last few years; or savings, investments, or reserve funds under $1,000	74	78
Total	100	100

	Percentage of aggregate income	Percentage of individuals
What were your main reasons for doing that?		
Tax considerations	1	0
Bought to extend own control of business or to enlarge business	2	2
Bought to get current income	2	2
Bought to get increase in value	3	2
Bought because looked like a good investment	3	3
Sold because wanted money to buy other earning assets	2	1
Sold because wanted money for other reasons	1	1
Sold because asset was unpromising	3	2
Sold because offered a good price	4	3
Sold because of a clash of personalities among owners	1	0
Sold because someone else wanted to buy the property; property too far away from where lived; did not have enough time to care for it; tired of being a landlord	3	3
Bought or sold for personal or family reasons; sold business because of health reasons; bought property to use in retirement	3	2
Other reasons why bought or sold (sold to increase liquidity; bought or sold to get more safety, security, or stability; condemned for right-of-way)	3	2
Not ascertained	1	1
Total	[13]	[13]
We have talked about three main types of investments—direct business interests, common stocks, and fixed-yield investments, like bonds and bank accounts. Which of these constitutes your biggest investment?		
Real estate, farm, or unincorporated business	22	23
Common stock	41	35
Fixed-yield assets	24	29
Real estate, farm, or unincorporated business and common stock	1	1
Real estate, farm, or unincorporated business and fixed-yield assets	0	0
Common stock and fixed-yield assets	3	2
About the same interest in all 3 types	1	1
Other (life insurance, home)	1	1
Not ascertained	1	0
Savings, investments, or reserve funds under $1,000	6	8
Total	100	100

[13] This question was asked only of those who bought or sold real estate, a farm, or an unincorporated business interest in the last few years, but some respondents gave more than one reason.

	Percentage of aggregate income	*Percentage of individuals*
How does your present distribution among these categories differ from the distribution five years ago?		
More in real estate, farm, or unincorporated business	7	7
More in common stock	15	14
More in fixed-yield assets	8	8
More in real estate, farm, or unincorporated business and common stock	1	1
More in real estate, farm, or unincorporated business and fixed-yield assets	0	0
More in common stock and fixed-yield assets	1	1
More in other assets	1	1
No change in distribution	55	54
Not ascertained	6	6
Savings, investments, or reserve funds under $1,000	6	8
Total	100	100
What are the main reasons for those changes?		
Tax considerations	2	1
Increase in asset values without further investment outlays	3	3
To obtain higher rate of return	2	2
To obtain increase in value	4	4
To obtain more safety; diversification	4	4
To obtain more liquidity	2	2
Because of gifts and inheritances received or given	2	3
To expand own business	2	2
For convenience, less trouble	2	2
Assets sold to finance consumption or housing expenditures	1	1
Because of retirement, advancing age, or ill health	1	1
Less concerned with safety	1	0
Other reasons	1	1
Not ascertained	9	9
Total	[14]	[14]
Are you generally satisfied with the way your money is now distributed among these categories, or are there some changes you have been thinking of making?		
Satisfied	60	58
Satisfied, with qualifications	8	7
Pro-con response	17	17
Dissatisfied, with qualifications	1	1
Dissatisfied	6	6
Not ascertained	2	3
Savings, investments, or reserve funds under $1,000	6	8
Total	100	100

[14] This question was asked only of those whose asset distribution differed from that of five years ago, but some of these respondents gave more than one reason.

	Percentage of aggregate income	Percentage of individuals
What changes have you been thinking of making?		
Increases respondent has been thinking of making		
More in real estate, farm, or unincorporated business	4	4
More in common stock	8	9
More in fixed-yield assets	2	2
More in real estate, farm, or unincorporated business and common stock	1	1
More in real estate, farm, or unincorporated business and fixed-yield assets	0	0
More in common stock and fixed-yield assets	0	0
No increases	7	6
Not ascertained	2	2
Satisfied with present asset distribution; or savings, investments, or reserve funds under $1,000	76	76
Total	100	100
Decreases respondent has been thinking of making		
Less in real estate, farm, or unincorporated business	3	2
Less in common stock	3	2
Less in fixed-yield assets	3	4
No decreases	13	14
Not ascertained	2	2
Satisfied with present asset distribution; or savings, investments, or reserve funds under $1,000	76	76
Total	100	100
Why are you thinking of doing this?		
Tax considerations	3	2
To obtain higher rate of return	6	7
To obtain increases in value	6	6
To obtain more safety; diversification	4	3
To obtain more liquidity	1	1
Other reasons	6	8
Not ascertained	3	3
Total	[15]	[15]

[15] This question was asked only of those who were thinking of making changes in their asset distribution, but some of these respondents gave more than one reason.

Section 6. Gifts and Inheritances Received

	Percentage of aggregate income	*Percentage of individuals*
Would you say that most of your present assets are from gifts or inheritances, or savings out of income, or the result of assets that went up in value, or what?		
Gifts or inheritances	7	6
Savings out of income	44	49
Result of assets that went up in value	10	7
Gifts or inheritances and savings out of income	5	7
Gifts or inheritances and assets that went up in value	4	4
Savings out of income and assets that went up in value	19	15
Gifts or inheritances and savings out of income and assets that went up in value	4	3
Not ascertained	1	1
Savings, investments, or reserve funds under $1,000	6	8
Total	100	100
Did you or your immediate family ever receive any money or property from your parents or other people?		
Yes	50	47
No	44	45
Savings, investments, or reserve funds under $1,000	6	8
Total	100	100
Did you get it as a gift, or as an inheritance, or both?		
Gift	9	9
Inheritance	32	31
Both gift and inheritance	9	7
No gifts or inheritance received; or savings, investments, or reserve funds under $1,000	50	53
Total	100	100
Speaking of the gifts, about what fraction of your total assets do they account for?		
Less than 5 percent	5	4
5 - 14 percent	6	5
15 - 24 percent	2	2
25 - 49 percent	2	2
50 - 74 percent	2	2
75 percent or more	0	0
Not ascertained	1	1
No gifts received; or savings, investments, or reserve funds under $1,000	82	84
Total	100	100

	Percentage of aggregate income	*Percentage of individuals*
In what form did you get them—cash, a home, real estate, business, stocks, or what?		
Cash or fixed-yield assets	6	7
Real estate, farm, or unincorporated business	2	2
Common stock	5	3
Cash or fixed-yield assets and real estate, farm, or unincorporated business	0	0
Cash or fixed-yield assets and common stock	2	1
Real estate, farm, or unincorporated business, and common stock	1	1
Cash or fixed-yield assets and real estate, farm, or unincorporated business, and common stock	1	1
Other assets only (including home)	1	1
No gifts received; or savings, investments, or reserve funds under $1,000	82	84
Total	100	100
When was that?		
1964	0	0
1963	1	1
1962	0	0
1961	1	1
1960	1	2
1955-59	2	2
1950-54	2	2
1949 or earlier	4	3
Two or more of the above periods	6	4
Not ascertained	1	1
No gifts received; or savings, investments, or reserve funds under $1,000	82	84
Total	100	100
Are you free to do what you want with it, or is it in trust for you, or restricted in some way?		
Free (all or part)	16	14
All restricted or in trust	2	2
No gifts received; or savings, investments, or reserve funds under $1,000	82	84
Total	100	100

	Percentage of aggregate income	Percentage of individuals
Have you kept them in the same investments, or have you reinvested them in some other ways since you got them?		
All kept same	6	5
Reinvested some or all	9	8
Not ascertained	1	1
Gifts all restricted or in trust; or no gifts received; or savings, investments, or reserve funds under $1,000	84	86
Total	100	100
Why have you kept them in the same form?		
Tax considerations	0	0
Could get no better investment	4	4
Interested in managing it (e.g., a family business)	1	0
Noneconomic restraints	0	0
Inertia	0	0
Other	1	1
Reinvested gifts; or gifts all restricted or in trust; or no gifts received; or savings, investments, or reserve funds under $1,000	94	95
Total	100	100
In what did you reinvest them?		
Fixed-yield assets	1	0
Real estate, farm, or unincorporated business	1	1
Common stock	3	2
Fixed-yield assets and real estate, farm, or unincorporated business	0	0
Fixed-yield assets and common stock	1	0
Real estate, farm, or unincorporated business and common stock	0	0
Fixed-yield assets and real estate, farm, or unincorporated business, and common stock	0	0
Other investments or expenditures only (such as expenditure for a house, car, travel, etc.)	2	3
Not ascertained	1	1
Gifts kept in same form as received; or gifts all restricted or in trust; or no gifts received; or savings, investments, or reserve funds under $1,000	91	92
Total	100	100

	Percentage of aggregate income	Percentage of individuals
When was that?		
1964	0	0
1963	0	0
1962	0	1
1961	1	0
1960	0	0
1955-59	0	0
1950-54	2	2
1949 or earlier	1	1
Two or more of above periods	3	2
Not ascertained	2	2
Gifts kept in same form as received; or gifts all restricted or in trust; or no gifts received; or savings, investments, or reserve funds under $1,000	91	92
Total	100	100
Why did you make that change then?		
Tax considerations	0	0
To obtain better yield	1	1
To obtain assets with less risk; more diversification	0	0
To secure better prospects of capital gains	1	1
To get better investments (not ascertained why better); favorable opportunity arose; dissatisfied with present investment	2	1
Because wanted to or needed to	2	2
Other	1	1
Not ascertained	2	2
Gifts kept in same form as received; or gifts all restricted or in trust; or no gifts received; or savings, investments, or reserve funds under $1,000	91	92
Total	100	100
Now, speaking about the inheritance, about what fraction of your total assets today does it account for?		
Less than 5 percent	10	7
5-14 percent	10	10
15-24 percent	4	4
25-49 percent	5	5
50-74 percent	6	6
75 percent or more	3	3
Not ascertained	3	3
No inheritance; or savings, investments, or reserve funds under $1,000	59	62
Total	100	100

	Percentage of aggregate income	*Percentage of individuals*
In what form did you get it—cash, a home, real estate, business, stocks, or what?		
Cash or fixed-yield assets	14	15
Real estate, farm, or unincorporated business	7	8
Common stock	5	3
Cash or fixed-yield assets and real estate, farm, or unincorporated business	3	2
Cash or fixed-yield assets and common stock	4	4
Real estate, farm, or unincorporated business and common stock	3	2
Cash or fixed-yield assets and real estate, farm, or unincorporated business, and common stock	3	3
Other assets only (including home)	1	1
Not ascertained	1	0
No inheritance; or savings, investments, or reserve funds under $1,000	59	62
Total	100	100
When was that?		
1964	1	1
1963	2	2
1962	2	3
1961	1	2
1960	2	2
1955-59	8	8
1950-54	5	5
1949 or earlier	14	11
Two or more of the above periods	4	2
Not ascertained	2	2
No inheritance; or savings, investments, or reserve funds under $1,000	59	62
Total	100	100
Are you free to do what you want with it, or is it in trust for you, or restricted in some way?		
Free (all or part)	37	35
All restricted or in trust	3	2
Not ascertained	1	1
No inheritance; or savings, investments, or reserve funds under $1,000	59	62
Total	100	100

	Percentage of aggregate income	*Percentage of individuals*
Have you kept them in the same investments, or have you reinvested them in some other ways since you got them?		
All kept same	11	12
Reinvested some or all	25	22
Not ascertained	1	1
Inheritance all restricted or in trust; or no inheritance; or savings, investments, or reserve funds under $1,000	63	65
Total	100	100
Why have you kept them in the same form?		
Tax considerations	0	0
Could get no better investment	5	5
Interested in managing it (e.g., a family business)	0	0
Noneconomic restraints	1	1
Inertia	1	1
Other	2	2
Not ascertained; thinking of selling right now	2	3
Inheritance reinvested; or inheritance all restricted or in trust; or no inheritance; or savings, investments, or reserve funds under $1,000	89	88
Total	100	100
In what did you reinvest it?		
Fixed-yield assets	3	4
Real estate, farm, or unincorporated business	3	2
Common stock	10	8
Fixed-yield assets and real estate, farm, or unincorporated business	0	0
Fixed-yield assets and common stock	3	2
Real estate, farm, or unincorporated business, and common stock	1	1
Fixed-yield assets and real estate, farm, or unincorporated business, and common stock	0	0
Other investments or expenditures only (such as expenditure for a house, car, travel, etc.)	4	4
Not ascertained	1	1
Inheritance kept in same form as received; or inheritance all restricted or in trust; or no inheritance; or savings, investments, or reserve funds under $1,000	75	78
Total	100	100

	Percentage of aggregate income	Percentage of individuals
When was that?		
1964	0	0
1963	1	1
1962	0	0
1961	3	3
1960	0	0
1955-59	4	4
1950-54	3	3
1949 or earlier	5	3
Two or more of the above periods	6	5
Not ascertained	3	3
Inheritance kept in same form; or inheritance all restricted or in trust; or no inheritance; or savings, investments, or reserve funds under $1,000	75	78
Total	100	100
Why did you make that change then?		
Tax considerations	1	0
To obtain better yield	4	4
To obtain assets with less risk; more diversification	1	1
To secure better prospects of capital gains	3	2
To become more liquid	1	1
To get better investment (not ascertained why better); favorable opportunity arose; dissatisfied with present investment	3	2
Because wanted to or needed to	5	4
Other	1	2
Not ascertained	6	6
Inheritance kept in same form as received; or inheritance all restricted or in trust; or no inheritance; or savings, investments, or reserve funds under $1,000	75	78
Total	100	100

Section 7. Philanthropy and Gifts to Relatives

We're interested in the decisions people make about giving away their assets.

Within the last couple of years, have you (or your immediate family) made any large gifts, in cash or property, either outright or in the form of a trust, or some other way?

	Percentage of aggregate income	Percentage of individuals
Yes	28	19
No	66	73
Savings, investments, or reserve funds under $1,000	6	8
Total	100	100

	Percentage of aggregate income	Percentage of individuals
Were the gifts made to individuals, or to churches or charitable organizations, or what?		
Individuals	10	8
Churches or charitable organizations	10	7
Individuals and churches or charitable organizations	8	4
Made no large gifts in last few years; or savings, investments, or reserve funds under $1,000	72	81
Total	100	100
Within the last couple of years, have you transferred any money or property to your children or other relatives?		
Yes	18	10
No	10	9
Made no large gifts in last few years; or savings, investments, or reserve funds under $1,000	72	81
Total	100	100
To whom have you given these gifts (and transfers)?		
Children	11	7
Grandchildren	1	0
Other relatives	2	2
Children and grandchildren	2	0
Children and other relatives	2	1
Has not transferred money to children or other relatives in the last couple of years; or savings, investments, or reserve funds under $1,000	82	90
Total	100	100
Now about these gifts (and transfers), were they outright gifts or in the form of a trust, or what?		
Gifts	11	7
Trust fund	4	2
Both gifts and trust fund	2	1
Not ascertained	1	0
Has not transferred money to children or other relatives in the last couple of years; or savings, investments, or reserve funds under $1,000	82	90
Total	100	100

	Percentage of aggregate income	*Percentage of individuals*
What was the form of the gifts (to each beneficiary)? Was it cash or common stock, or what?		
Cash or fixed-yield assets	6	4
Real estate, farm, or unincorporated business	1	0
Common stock	6	3
Cash or fixed-yield assets and real estate, farm, or unincorporated business	0	0
Cash or fixed-yield assets and common stock	4	2
Real estate, farm, or unincorporated business, and common stock	0	0
Cash or fixed-yield assets and real estate, farm, or unincorporated business and common stock	0	0
Not ascertained	1	1
Has not transferred money to children or other relatives in the last couple of years; or savings, investments, or reserve funds under $1,000	82	90
Total	100	100
What particular reasons did you have for making the gifts at that time?		
Tax considerations	8	4
Beneficiary needed the gift at the time	3	2
Beneficiary fulfilled some condition	1	1
No particular reason	3	1
Other	5	3
Not ascertained	1	1
Total	[16]	[16]
Have you ever given to church or charity an asset that was worth more than you had originally paid for it?		
Yes	13	7
No	81	85
Savings, investments, or reserve funds under $1,000	6	8
Total	100	100
Have you given some thought to how your estate will be handled when you die?		
Yes	83	78
No	11	14
Savings, investments, or reserve funds under $1,000	6	8
Total	100	100

[16] This question was asked only of those who had transferred money to children or other relatives in the last couple of years, but some of these respondents gave more than one reason.

	Percentage of aggregate income	*Percentage of individuals*
Have you already made any changes in your asset holding because of this?		
Yes	16	12
No	67	66
Has not given thought to how estate will be handled; or savings, investments, or reserve funds under $1,000	17	22
Total	100	100
What have you done?		
Set up trusts or life estates for children	4	3
Set up charitable trust to which assets will be left at his death	0	0
Increased liquidity of assets	2	1
Increased insurance to be paid to beneficiaries	2	1
Distributed property in the form of gifts	3	2
Made a will only	2	2
Other	5	4
Total	[17]	[17]
What reasons did you have for doing that?		
Tax considerations	7	4
To make estate more liquid so as to pay for expenses	1	1
To make estate less risky for heirs	2	2
To make estate easier to manage	2	2
Other	5	4
Total	[17]	[17]

Section 8. Capital Gains and Losses

Looking at the investments which you (and your immediate family) now have—such as your business, or your common stock—are any of them currently worth a great deal more than when you got them (excluding your home)?		
Yes	68	60
No	25	31
Not ascertained	1	1
Savings, investments, or reserve funds under $1,000	6	8
Total	100	100

[17] This question was asked only of those who had made changes in their asset holdings for estate purposes, but some of these respondents gave more than one reason.

	Percentage of aggregate income	*Percentage of individuals*
What kinds of investments are those that are worth more?		
Fixed-yield assets	1	2
Real estate, farm, or unincorporated business	14	15
Common stock	37	30
Fixed-yield assets and real estate, farm, or unincorporated business	0	0
Fixed-yield assets and common stock	1	1
Real estate, farm, or unincorporated business and common stock	13	10
Fixed-yield assets and real estate, farm, or unincorporated business and common stock	1	1
Other	0	1
Not ascertained	1	0
No assets worth a great deal more; or savings, investments, or reserve funds under $1,000	32	40
Total	100	100
Have you considered selling any of those assets that are worth more than when you bought them?		
Yes	24	19
No	43	41
Not ascertained	1	0
No assets worth a great deal more; or savings, investments, or reserve funds under $1,000	32	40
Total	100	100
Why is it that you haven't sold the asset? Why haven't you considered selling it?		
Tax considerations	13	10
Could get no better investment	41	38
Interested in managing it (e.g., a family business)	5	5
Noneconomic restraints	2	2
Inertia	1	0
Difficult to sell; no market; worth more in present form	2	1
Other	7	7
Not ascertained; thinking of selling right now	6	5
Total	[18]	[18]

[18] This question was asked only of those who had assets worth a great deal more, but some respondents gave more than one reason.

	Percentage of aggregate income	*Percentage of individuals*
When did you (or your immediate family) last sell an asset for more than it was when you got it?		
1964	13	9
1963	20	16
1962	8	8
1961	7	6
1960	3	3
1955-59	6	7
1950-54	3	3
1949 or earlier	2	2
Never	31	37
Not ascertained	1	1
Savings, investments, or reserve funds under $1,000	6	8
Total	100	100
What kind of asset was it?		
Fixed-yield assets	3	4
Real estate, farm, or unincorporated business	13	12
Common stock	42	35
Fixed-yield assets and real estate, farm, or unincorporated business	0	0
Fixed-yield assets and common stock	0	0
Real estate, farm, or unincorporated business and common stock	1	0
Fixed-yield assets and real estate, farm, or unincorporated business and common stock	0	0
Other	3	3
Not ascertained	1	1
Never sold asset for more than purchase price; or savings, investments, or reserve funds under $1,000	37	45
Total	100	100
Do you think you did well to sell it when you did?		
Yes	47	40
Pro-con response	3	3
No	12	11
Not ascertained	1	1
Never sold asset for more than purchase price; or savings, investments, or reserve funds under $1,000	37	45
Total	100	100

	Percentage of aggregate income	*Percentage of individuals*
Why is that?		
Tax considerations	3	2
Did well because of the way the market behaved after the sale	14	13
Other reasons why did well	32	27
Did badly because of the way the market behaved after the sale	11	9
Other reasons why did badly	2	2
Had to sell; emergency; needed cash for illness; wanted money for vacation	3	4
Not ascertained	4	3
Total	[19]	[19]
How long had you owned it?		
0-5 months	3	4
6-11 months	4	3
1-1.9 years	6	4
2-4.9 years	19	18
5-9.9 years	11	11
10 years or more	15	13
Not ascertained	5	2
Never sold asset for more than purchase price; or savings, investments, or reserve funds under $1,000	37	45
Total	100	100
Did you reinvest the money, or spend it, or what?		
Reinvested it	45	38
Spent it	8	9
Other dispositions; left the money in the bank	5	4
Reinvested and spent it	3	3
Not ascertained	2	1
Never sold asset for more than purchase price; or savings, investments, or reserve funds under $1,000	37	45
Total	100	100

[19] This question was asked only of those who sold an asset for more than its purchase price, but some of these respondents gave more than one reason.

	Percentage of aggregate income	Percentage of individuals
When did you (or your immediate family) last sell an asset on which you took a loss?		
1964	6	5
1963	21	17
1962	8	7
1961	4	3
1960	3	3
1955-59	5	5
1950-54	1	1
1949 or earlier	2	2
Never	42	47
Not ascertained	2	2
Savings, investments, or reserve funds under $1,000	6	8
Total	100	100
What kind of asset was it?		
Fixed-yield assets	1	1
Real estate, farm, or unincorporated business	5	5
Common stock	40	33
Fixed-yield assets and real estate, farm, or unincorporated business	0	0
Fixed-yield assets and common stock	1	1
Real estate, farm, or unincorporated business and common stock	0	0
Fixed-yield assets and real estate, farm, or unincorporated business and common stock	0	0
Other	3	4
Not ascertained	2	1
Never sold asset for less than purchase price; or savings, investments, or reserve funds under $1,000	48	55
Total	100	100
Do you think you did well to sell it when you did?		
Yes	38	32
Pro-con response	2	2
No	10	9
Not ascertained	2	2
Never sold asset for less than purchase price; or savings, investments, or reserve funds under $1,000	48	55
Total	100	100

	Percentage of aggregate income	Percentage of individuals
Why is that?		
Tax considerations	10	7
Did well because of the way the market behaved after the sale	17	15
Other reasons why did well	14	12
Did badly because of the way the market behaved after the sale	8	7
Other reasons, why did badly	2	2
Had to sell; emergency; needed cash for illness; wanted money for vacation	3	3
Not ascertained	4	4
Total	[20]	[20]

Section 9. Occupation and Work Effort

	Percentage of aggregate income	Percentage of individuals
Are you working now, unemployed, retired, or what?		
Working now	91	93
Unemployed or laid off	0	0
Retired; disabled; not working	7	6
Housewife	2	1
Total	100	100
What is your main occupation? What kind of business is that in? What kind of work do you do when you are employed? What kind of work did you do when you worked?		
Physician, dentist	6	5
Engineer, architect, scientist, technician, other professional	16	19
Lawyer	5	4
Businessman	32	26
Real estate broker, builder, contractor	3	3
Stockbroker, investment counselor, accountant, auditor, banker, insurance man, other financial adviser	11	10
Farmer, rancher	2	2
Other	23	30
Housewife; widow; manages own *financial* investments only; rentier; never worked	2	1
Total	100	100

[20] This question was asked only of those who sold an asset for less than its purchase price, but some respondents gave more than one reason.

	Percentage of aggregate income	Percentage of individuals
Do you work for yourself, or someone else, or what?		
Self-employed; works for privately held corporation of which he is an owner	39	32
Works for someone else	46	55
Both self-employed and works for someone else	6	6
Does not work	9	7
Total	100	100
Do you have more than one kind of work at which you earn money?		
Yes	18	17
No	73	76
Does not work	9	7
Total	100	100
What is your other work?		
Physician, dentist	0	0
Engineer, architect, scientist, technician, other professional	3	3
Lawyer	0	1
Businessman	6	4
Real estate broker, builder, contractor	1	0
Stockbroker, investment counselor, accountant, auditor, banker, insurance man, other financial adviser	2	2
Farmer, rancher	1	1
Other	4	5
Not ascertained	1	1
Does not have second job; or does not work	82	83
Total	100	100
Is that an occupation where you work for yourself, or for someone else, or what?		
Self-employed; works for privately held corporation of which he is an owner	9	8
Works for someone else	7	7
Both self-employed and works for someone else	2	2
Does not have second job; or does not work	82	83
Total	100	100

	Percentage of aggregate income	*Percentage of individuals*
Do you have any choice between fringe benefits and current pay? Did you choose any of the non-money benefits instead of more pay now?		
Yes, has choice; chose non-money benefits	6	6
Yes, has choice; did not choose non-money benefits	1	1
No, does not have choice	83	85
Not ascertained	1	1
Does not work	9	7
Total	100	100
Why did you do that?		
Reasons why chose non-money benefits instead of more pay		
Reduces taxes	1	1
Forces saving	0	0
Will provide more income for retirement	1	1
Protects dependents	1	2
Other	3	3
Reasons why chose more pay instead of non-money benefits		
Needs the cash	0	0
Cash more valuable than fringe benefits; doesn't like the fringe benefits	0	0
Prefers to make own investment decisions	0	0
Other	0	1
Not ascertained	1	1
Total	[21]	[21]
About how many hours a week do you work ordinarily?		
1 - 19	1	1
20 - 34	4	4
35 - 40	27	31
41 - 48	14	14
49 - 59	22	21
60 or more hours	21	20
Not ascertained	2	2
Does not work	9	7
Total	100	100

[21] This question was asked only of those who had some choice between fringe benefits and more pay, but some respondents gave more than one reason.

	Percentage of aggregate income	Percentage of individuals
How many weeks did you work last year?		
13 weeks or less	0	0
14 - 26 weeks	1	1
27 - 39 weeks	3	2
40 - 47 weeks	9	8
48 - 49 weeks	21	23
50 - 52 weeks	55	58
Not ascertained	2	1
Did not work	9	7
Total	100	100
Do you have opportunities to earn additional income by working more or taking on extra work?		
Yes	34	38
No	56	55
Not ascertained	1	0
Does not work	9	7
Total	100	100
How do you decide how much work to do then?		
Tax considerations *limit* the work done	1	1
Need to earn enough to pay taxes	0	0
Need to earn enough to pay other expenses	2	2
Does as much as is necessary	7	8
Works as hard as possible	11	12
Must leave time for leisure	4	5
Works as much as he wants to	6	7
Other	5	5
Not ascertained	3	3
Total	[22]	[22]
Do you spend more time at your work than you did a few years ago, or less, or what?		
Spends more time now	25	25
Spends the same amount of time now	43	46
Spends less time now	22	21
Not ascertained	1	1
Does not work	9	7
Total	100	100

[22] This question was asked only of those who had opportunities to earn additional income, but some respondents gave more than one explanation.

	Percentage of aggregate income	*Percentage of individuals*
What are the main reasons for the change?		
Reasons for working more now		
Wants more money, because of higher taxes	0	0
Wants more money, for other reasons	1	1
Wants business to succeed; trying to expand	2	2
Business is better now; market has grown	6	6
Has more responsibility; increase in work load	13	13
Health has improved	0	0
In a different job now (no other reason stated)	3	3
Other	3	3
Not ascertained	1	2
Total	[23]	[23]
Reasons for working less now		
Taxes too high	1	1
Does not need money so badly any more	1	1
Business is big enough now	1	1
Business is worse now, not so much work available	4	5
Wants more leisure	2	1
Health has deteriorated	2	2
In a different job now (no other reason stated)	2	2
Nearing retirement age (no mention of worsening health); getting older	5	4
Business is better organized now; can get others to assume more responsibility	6	6
Other	1	1
Not ascertained	1	1
Total	[23]	[23]
When did you retire?		
1960 or later	4	4
1955-59	1	1
1950-54	1	1
1949 or earlier	1	0
Not retired (working now, housewife, unemployed, student)	93	94
Total	**100**	**100**

[23] This question was asked only of those who spent more or less time at their work than they did a few years ago, but some respondents gave more than one reason.

	Percentage of aggregate income	Percentage of individuals
How did you happen to retire when you did?		
Taxes too high	0	0
Reached compulsory retirement age	1	1
Bad health	1	1
Wanted leisure time to enjoy other activities	1	1
Had accumulated enough savings	0	0
Others (in business) were ready to take over	1	1
Family considerations	0	1
Other	3	2
Total	[24]	[24]
Have you had opportunities to work for money since your retirement? What opportunities have you had?		
Yes, has had opportunities to work		
Mentions job requiring about as much skill and talent as his job before retirement	2	1
Mentions job requiring less skill	0	0
Mentions job; relative level of skill not ascertained	1	1
No, has had no opportunities to work	4	4
Not retired (working now, housewife, unemployed, student)	93	94
Total	100	100
Have you accepted any of them?		
Yes	2	1
No	1	1
No opportunities to work since retirement; or not retired (working now, housewife, unemployed, student)	97	98
Total	100	100
What were your main reasons for doing (not doing) that?		
Reasons why accepted		
Tax considerations	0	0
Needed money for other reasons	0	0
Congenial colleagues; interesting work; other "positive" attractions	1	1
Was bored; was at loose ends; other "negative" attractions	1	0
Did not accept opportunities to work since retirement; or no opportunities; or not retired (working now, housewife, unemployed, student)	98	99
Total	100	100

[24] This question was asked only of those who were retired, but some respondents gave more than one reason.

	Percentage of aggregate income	Percentage of individuals
Reasons why did not accept		
Tax considerations	0	0
Not enough pay for the effort	0	0
Preferred leisure	1	1
Bad health	0	0
Work would have been uninteresting, irksome	0	0
Dislike of certain individuals	0	0
Family responsibilities	0	0
Working would have reduced Social Security payments	0	0
Accepted opportunities to work since retirement; or no opportunities; or not retired (working now, housewife, unemployed student)	99	99
Total	100	100
Sex and marital status of respondent[25]		
Male and married	92	91
Male and single	4	4
Female	4	5
Total	100	100
In what year was your wife born?		
Wife born in 1914 or later	37	37
Wife born between 1900 and 1913	48	49
Wife born before 1900	7	5
No wife	8	9
Total	100	100
Has she had a job any time in the last ten years, that is, since 1953?		
Yes	36	43
No	49	43
Wife born before 1900; or no wife	15	14
Total	100	100
Did your wife earn any money by her own work during the last year?		
Yes	26	33
No	9	10
Wife has not had job in last 10 years; or wife born before 1900; or no wife	65	57
Total	100	100

[25] This information was recorded by interviewers without asking any questions.

	Percentage of aggregate income	Percentage of individuals
Did she work full-time, part-time, or what?		
Full-time	19	26
Part-time	6	7
Wife did not work last year or in last 10 years; or wife born before 1900; or no wife	75	67
Total	100	100
How long does she plan to keep on working?		
One year or less	1	1
2 - 3 years	1	2
4 - 5 years	2	3
6 years or more	13	17
Depends	1	2
Has already stopped working	2	2
Not ascertained	5	6
Wife did not work last year or in last 10 years; or wife born before 1900; or no wife	75	67
Total	100	100
Why is that?		
Until has enough money to finance children's education	3	4
Until has enough money for retirement or other expenses	2	3
Until husband's income or business make it unnecessary	0	0
Until children are born	0	0
Until the family moves from this location	0	0
Will reach (compulsory) retirement age	3	4
The employment will no longer be available	0	0
Enjoys the work	9	11
Other	8	11
Not ascertained	2	2
Total	[26]	[26]
How did she happen to give up her job?		
Tax considerations	0	0
Not enough pay for the effort	0	0
Preferred leisure	1	1
Bad health	0	1
Work was uninteresting	0	1
Dislike of certain individuals	0	0
Family responsibilities	5	5
Other	3	3
Not ascertained	1	1
Total	[27]	[27]

[26] This question was asked only of those whose wives worked last year, but some of these respondents gave more than one reason.

[27] This question was asked only of those who had wives who worked in the past ten years but not during 1963, but some respondents gave more than one reason.

	Percentage of aggregate income	*Percentage of individuals*
When was that?		
1963 or later	0	0
1960 - 62	4	4
1959 or earlier	5	5
Not ascertained	0	1
Wife worked last year; or wife did not work in last 10 years; or wife born before 1900; or no wife	91	90
Total	100	100
What about the future? Do you think she will go to work for money sometime in the future?		
Yes	7	8
No	29	28
Not ascertained	1	1
Wife born before 1914; or wife worked last year; or no wife	63	63
Total	100	100
Why is that?		
Reasons why she will work		
Tax considerations	0	0
Need the money for other reasons	1	1
Need to keep busy	5	5
Children will be in school	2	2
Other	1	1
Reasons why she will not work		
Tax considerations	0	0
Not necessary	14	12
Prefers leisure	13	12
Bad health	0	0
Other	2	1
Not ascertained why will or will not work	7	7
Total	[28]	[28]

[28] This question was asked only of those whose wives were born in 1914 or later and had not worked in the previous year, but some respondents gave more than one reason.

	Percentage of aggregate income	Percentage of individuals
If you (or your wife) earned any extra money, about what fraction of it would be taken in added income taxes?		
None	2	3
1 - 19 percent	3	3
20 - 29 percent	20	25
30 - 39 percent	20	22
40 - 49 percent	8	8
50 - 59 percent	9	7
60 - 69 percent	6	3
70 - 79 percent	4	1
80 - 89 percent	1	0
90 percent or over	3	2
Does not know; information refused; or no response recorded[29]	24	26
Total	100	100
Has the income tax had any effect on how much work you (or your wife) do? In what way?		
Yes, respondent and/or wife work less	12	10
Yes, respondent and/or wife work more	1	1
Yes, not ascertained which way effect goes	1	0
No	85	88
Not ascertained	1	1
Total	100	100
Would you give me a specific example?		
Gives an example	12	9
Does not	2	2
Taxes have no effect on work effort	86	89
Total	100	100

Section 10. Income Patterns

	Percentage of aggregate income	Percentage of individuals
Did you or your immediate family have any income in 1963 from tax-exempt municipal bonds, that is, state and local, and school bonds?		
Yes	18	10
No	82	90
Total	100	100

[29] For more details on these responses, see Chapter XI.

	Percentage of aggregate income	*Percentage of individuals*
About what proportion of your total income was tax-exempt interest?		
Less than 10 percent	11	7
10 - 24 percent	3	1
25 - 39 percent	1	0
40 - 59 percent	1	1
60 - 69 percent	0	0
70 percent or more	0	0
Not ascertained	2	1
No tax-exempt interest	82	90
Total	100	100
Did you or your immediate family get any money in 1963 from the sale of appreciated assets, that is, from capital gains?		
Yes	33	25
No	67	75
Total	100	100
Were they mostly long-term gains so that only part was taxable, or what?		
Mostly long-term gains	28	20
About half long-term gains, half not long-term gains	1	1
Mostly not long-term gains	2	2
Not ascertained	2	1
Had no capital gains	67	76
Total	100	100
Now, if we leave out the tax-exempt interest, and the non-taxable part of your capital gains,[30] which of these groups would indicate your family's income for 1963?		
Less than $5,000	0	
$5,000 - 9,999	2	43
$10,000 - 14,999	28	
$15,000 - 24,999	33	38
$25,000 - 49,999	22	16
$50,000 - 99,999	9	3
$100,000 - 149,999	2	0
$150,000 - 499,999	3	0
$500,000 - 999,999	1	0
$1,000,000 or more	0	0
Total	100	100

[30] Simpler questions were used if there was no tax-exempt interest, or no long-term capital gains, or neither. The respondent was handed a card on which the income brackets were printed.

	Percentage of aggregate income	Percentage of individuals
Which of the groups would include your family income for the year 1961, for instance (still leaving out income not subject to tax)?[31]		
$10,000 - 14,999	48	69
$15,000 - 24,999	23	21
$25,000 - 49,999	16	8
$50,000 - 99,999	7	2
$100,000 - 149,999	2	0
$150,000 - 499,999	2	0
$500,000 - 999,999	1	0
$1,000,000 or more	1	0
Total	100	100
In the next few years, do you think your family income will go up considerably, stay the same, or what?		
Go up considerably	6	8
Go up some	34	38
Stay the same	44	41
Go down some	3	3
Go down considerably	0	0
Will go down but does not know how much; will retire	7	5
Not ascertained	6	5
Total	100	100

Section 11. Tax Considerations

	Percentage of aggregate income	Percentage of individuals
Do you usually get expert advice in making out your income tax forms? Is it from a professional accountant, or what?		
Yes, accountant	59	54
Yes, lawyer	2	1
Yes, bank	0	0
Yes, investment counselor	0	0
Yes, stockbroker	0	0
Yes, other financial experts or tax experts	1	1
Yes, other persons, not ascertained whether experts or not	2	3
Yes, not ascertained from whom	0	0
No	36	41
Total	100	100

[31] The distributions shown here are for the incomes reported by respondents. There is reason to believe that the respondents understated their incomes. See Appendix D. The disparities between the distributions for 1961 and 1963 arise from the fact that the respondents who, as a result of the sampling method all had 1961 incomes over $10,000, tended to experience rising incomes between 1961 and 1963.

	Percentage of aggregate income	*Percentage of individuals*
How helpful have you found the advice to be?		
Very helpful	48	44
Fairly helpful	10	10
Not very helpful	2	2
Not ascertained	4	3
Respondent gets no advice in making out tax returns	36	41
Total	100	100
Does your wife file a separate income tax return?		
Respondent married; wife and husband file separate income tax returns	2	3
Respondent married and files a joint income tax return	91	90
Respondent not married	7	7
Total	100	100
About what fraction of the family income is hers then?		
1 - 9 percent	0	0
10 - 24 percent	0	0
25 - 39 percent	1	1
40 - 59 percent	1	2
60 percent or more	0	0
Respondent not married or wife does not file separately	98	97
Total	100	100
Do any of your dependent children file separate income tax returns?		
Respondent has dependent children; one or more do file separate income tax returns	17	15
Respondent has dependent children, but none of them files a separate income tax return	42	45
Respondent does not have dependent children	41	40
Total	100	100
About what fraction of the family income is theirs then?		
1 - 9 percent	13	11
10 - 24 percent	2	1
25 - 39 percent	0	0
40 - 59 percent	0	0
60 percent or more	0	0
Not ascertained	2	2
Respondent has no dependent children; or children do not file separately	83	86
Total	100	100

	Percentage of aggregate income	Percentage of individuals
Have you heard about some special income tax advantages of investing in real estate? Have you made any such investments, or have you thought about doing so?		
Yes, and made or has thought about making such investments	19	17
Yes, but has not made or thought about making such investments	27	25
Yes, but not ascertained whether has made or has thought about making such investments	2	2
No	51	55
Not ascertained whether heard about tax advantages	1	1
Total	100	100
Are there other features of the income tax laws that affect the way you invest your savings?		
Yes	32	25
No	68	75
Total	100	100
What are they?		
Favorable treatment of capital gains	22	...
Tax-exempt status of municipal bonds	2	...
Percentage depletion allowances	2	...
Provisions relating to timber and livestock	2	...
Offsetting of capital losses against gains	1	...
Dividend credit and exclusions	1	...
Transfer of income to relatives	1	...
Holding period for long-term gains	1	...
Provisions relating to life insurance	1	...
Other provisions[32]	4	...
Not ascertained	3	...
Total	[33]	

[32] No other tax provision beyond those listed above was mentioned by as many as one-half of one percent of the high-income group. After the provisions relating to life insurance, the next five most commonly mentioned provisions were those relating to state and local income taxes, the timing of income receipts during the fiscal year, the opportunities for treating living expenses as business expenses, the withholding of taxes, and the deductibility of interest on loans.

[33] This question was asked only of those reporting that other features of the income tax law affected their investing, but some of these respondents gave more than one answer.

	Percentage of aggregate income	*Percentage of individuals*
Do you think your state and local taxes are higher where you live than in other places where you might live? Have you thought of moving your residence to another area to save taxes?		
Taxes higher and has thought of moving residence	7	7
Taxes higher but has not thought of moving residence	40	39
Taxes not higher	48	49
Not ascertained whether thinks taxes higher	5	5
Total	100	100
Tell me about it.		
Probably will move	1	1
Might move	2	2
Probably will not move	2	2
Not ascertained whether will move	2	2
Taxes not higher or has not thought of moving residence	93	93
Total	100	100

Section 12. Social Characteristics

Finally, I'd like to ask a few questions about you and your family. Where did you grow up?

	Percentage of aggregate income	Percentage of individuals
Northeast	30	28
North Central	32	33
South	22	23
West	10	10
Other U.S. States (Alaska, Hawaii)	1	1
Foreign countries	4	4
Several	1	1
Total	100	100
Was that on a farm, or in a large city, or small town, or what?		
Farm	13	14
Small town	29	30
Middle-sized city	11	11
Large city, or suburb	44	42
Other; many different places	2	2
Not ascertained	1	1
Total	100	100

	Percentage of aggregate income	*Percentage of individuals*
How many different states have you lived in?		
One	38	38
Two	27	28
Three	13	13
Four or more	21	20
Not ascertained	1	1
Total	100	100
How long have you lived in this locality (within 100 miles of here)?		
Less than 3 years	3	3
3 - 9 years	12	14
10 - 19 years	17	18
20 - 29 years	11	10
30 - 49 years	33	34
50 or more years	23	21
Not ascertained	1	0
Total	100	100

In what year were you born?
(For the relevant information, see Section 14 below.)

	Percentage of aggregate income	*Percentage of individuals*
How many grades of school did you finish? Have you had any other schooling? What other schooling have you had? Do you have a college degree?		
0-8 grades	7	8
9-11 grades	10	11
12 grades	10	12
12 grades plus noncollege training	7	8
College, no degree	19	20
College, bachelor's degree	30	27
College, advanced or professional degree	17	14
Total	100	100

	Percentage of aggregate income	*Percentage of individuals*
Generally speaking, do you usually think of yourself as a Republican, a Democrat, an Independent, or what? Would you call yourself a strong Republican (Democrat) or a not very strong Republican (Democrat)? If Independent, do you think of yourself as closer to the Republican or Democratic party?		
Strong Democrat	11	13
Not very strong Democrat	19	21
Independent closer to Democratic Party	8	9
Independent	7	7
Independent closer to Republican Party	9	7
Not very strong Republican	25	25
Strong Republican	20	16
Not a citizen; a-political; minor party	1	2
Total	100	100
Is your church preference Protestant, Catholic, or Jewish?		
Protestant	68	67
Catholic	15	16
Jewish	14	14
Other	1	1
None	2	2
Total	100	100
If Protestant, what denomination is that?		
Baptist	8	9
Methodist	14	15
Episcopalian	10	8
Presbyterian	13	12
Lutheran	7	8
Congregationalist	6	6
Christian Science; Dutch Reformed; Friends (Quakers); Latter-Day Saints; Mormon; Unitarian; Universalist	4	3
Other Protestants	4	5
Denomination not ascertained	2	1
Respondent is not a Protestant	32	33
Total	100	100

	Percentage of aggregate income	*Percentage of individuals*
About how often do you usually attend religious services?		
More than once a week	11	12
Once a week	30	31
2 - 3 times a month	13	13
Once a month	7	7
A few times a year, or less	31	29
Never	8	8
Total	100	100
Have you ever been an officer or a committee chairman in a church or in a civic group like the United Fund?		
Yes	54	51
No	46	49
Total	100	100

Section 13. Interviewers' Observations

	Percentage of aggregate income	*Percentage of individuals*
Race of respondent		
White	98	97
Negro	1	1
Other (Puerto Rican, Mexican, Filipino)	1	2
Total	100	100
Who was present during the interview?		
Respondent only	73	69
Respondent and spouse	16	19
Respondent and someone else (not spouse)	7	8
Respondent and spouse and someone else	3	3
Not ascertained	1	1
Total	100	100
Where was the interview taken?		
Home	45	52
Office	50	43
Other	4	4
Not ascertained	1	1
Total	100	100

	Percentage of aggregate income	Percentage of individuals
Length of interview		
30 minutes or less	6	7
31 - 60 minutes	56	59
61 - 90 minutes	30	28
91 - 120 minutes	5	4
121 minutes or more	2	1
Not ascertained	1	1
Total	100	100

Section 14. Variables Constructed During Analysis Stage

	Percentage of aggregate income	Percentage of individuals
Occupational group[34]		
Male rentier or retired	7	6
Female rentier	2	1
Business owner-manager in financial sector	7	6
Other business owner-manager	26	22
Self-employed professional	12	10
Professional employee	14	17
Employee in financial sector	4	4
Other employee	28	34
Total	100	100
Estimated marginal tax rate before 1964 tax cut[35]		
20 - 29 percent	27	38
30 - 39 percent	33	39
40 - 49 percent	23	17
50 - 59 percent	10	5
60 - 69 percent	4	1
70 - 79 percent	2	0
80 - 89 percent	1	0
Total	100	100

[34] The "financial sector" consisted of banking, insurance, stockbrokerage, and accountancy. A "professional" was a physician, lawyer, engineer, architect, or scientist. An "owner-manager" held ownership interests in a business where he either was the chairman (or president) or considered himself as "self-employed."

[35] Each respondent's marginal rate under the federal individual income tax was estimated on the basis of (a) his adjusted gross income in 1963, and (b) whether or not a joint return was filed. Estimates are median marginal rates for the appropriate income groups, and are derived from a table of marginal rates by income groups appearing in U.S. Treasury Department, Internal Revenue Service, *Statistics of Income, 1961: Individual Income Tax Returns* (Washington, 1963), pp. 149-54.

	Percentage of aggregate income	Percentage of individuals
Estimated marginal tax rate after 1964 tax cut[36]		
14 - 19 percent	27	38
20 - 29 percent	33	39
30 - 39 percent	23	18
40 - 49 percent (No cases)	0	0
50 - 59 percent	14	5
60 - 69 percent	3	0
70 percent	0	0
Total	100	100
Index of tax consciousness[37]		
Zero: not conscious	55	65
1	20	19
2	11	8
3	7	5
4 - 5	6	3
6 - 7	1	0
8 or over	0	0
Total	100	100
Percentage of assets from gifts and inheritances[38]		
Less than 5 percent; savings, investments, or reserve funds under $1,000	62	63
5 - 14 percent	14	14
15 - 24 percent	5	5
25 - 49 percent	5	5
50 - 100 percent	14	13
Total	100	100
Age of respondent		
34 or less	8	9
35 - 44	23	26
45 - 54	34	36
55 - 64	22	20
65 - 74	10	7
75 or over	3	2
Total	100	100

[36] Each respondent's marginal rate after the tax cut enacted in 1964 was estimated in the same way as his marginal rate before the tax cut, except that the rate schedule designed for 1965 income was applied.

[37] The index describing the respondent's consciousness of tax considerations was compiled by assigning one point to the respondent for each occasion during the questionnaire when he mentioned tax considerations without being specifically asked about them. There were 39 such questions in the interview where taxes could conceivably be mentioned in the respondent's answer. The questions dealt with investment objectives, reasons for buying and selling of assets, motives for making gifts, and working behavior.

[38] The variable was derived from answers to the question, "What fraction of your total assets today do they account for?" Interviewers and editors were instructed to use the ratio of original amounts received to the current value of assets. The estimation involved combining two bracket codes for gifts and inheritances, respectively.

	Percentage of aggregate income	*Percentage of individuals*
Age of respondent's wife		
34 or less	11	13
35 - 44	28	30
45 - 54	30	30
55 - 64	16	13
65 - 74	5	4
75 or over	1	1
Not ascertained	1	0
Respondent is either female or an unmarried male	8	9
Total	100	100
***Number of asset-groups*[39]**		
1	1	8
2	4	6
3	8	10
4	7	8
5	10	12
6 - 9	20	22
10 - 14	14	13
15 - 19	9	7
20 - 24	10	6
25 or more	11	2
Savings, investments, or reserve funds under $1,000	6	6
Total	100	100
***Hours worked in 1963*[40]**		
None (retired, housewives)	9	7
1 - 799 hours	1	1
800 - 1,199 hours	2	2
1,200 - 1,799 hours	8	8
1,800 - 2,199 hours	29	33
2,200 - 2,799 hours	26	25
2,800 - 3,399 hours	18	17
3,400 hours or more	7	7
Total	100	100

[39] The number of asset-groups owned by the respondent was compiled by counting (a) the number of companies in which he owned common stock, and (b) the number of the following fourteen asset-groups held by the respondent: own home, nine types of fixed-yield assets, mutual funds, unincorporated business interests, real estate, and other assets.

[40] Estimated by combining bracket codes for hours worked per week and weeks worked in 1963.

	Percentage of aggregate income	Percentage of individuals
Level of investment information[41]		
Very highly informed	15	11
Highly informed	21	18
Fairly well informed	18	19
Somewhat informed	17	17
Relatively uninformed	11	13
Uninformed	10	13
Delegates all investment management to others	2	1
Savings, investments, or reserve funds under $1,000	6	8
Total	100	100
Portfolio diversification[42]		
Concentrated in stocks and has own corporation	7	5
Concentrated in stocks and does not have own corporation	8	8
Concentrated in real estate or unincorporated business interests	11	12
Concentrated in fixed-yield assets	12	15
Diversified with emphasis on stocks and has own corporation	13	9
Diversified with emphasis on stocks and does not have own corporation	13	12
Diversified with emphasis on real estate or unincorporated business interests	11	11
Diversified with emphasis on fixed-yield assets	13	15
Diversified with emphasis on both types of variable-yield assets (stocks and real estate or unincorporated business interests)	1	1
Diversified with equal emphasis on fixed-yield assets and one or both types of variable-yield assets	4	3
Savings, investments, or reserve funds under $1,000	6	8
Not ascertained	1	1
Total	100	100

[41] A respondent was classified as "very highly informed" if he (a) either worked in the financial sector or always obtained advice from qualified professionals in managing his investments and kept informed by reading investment-related publications, and (b) either had heard of special income tax advantages of investing in real estate or claimed to be affected by other features of the income tax in managing his investments. A respondent was classified as "uninformed" if he did not work in the financial sector, did not obtain advice from other people in managing his investments, did not read investment-related publications, and neither had heard of special income tax advantages of investing in real estate nor claimed to be affected by other features of the income tax in managing his investments. The same criteria were used to classify other types of respondents in the intermediate groups between these two extremes. For further information, see Chapter VI.

[42] "Concentrated" in one type of asset means that the dollar bracket for that asset ($1 - $9,999; $10,000 - $99,999; or $100,000 and over) was higher than the brackets for the other two types. "Diversified" means that two types were in the same bracket, one of which was mentioned in answer to the question in Section 5: "Which of these [main types of investments] constitutes your biggest investment?" Those with "own corporation" were executives or directors of corporations in which they owned stock.

	Percentage of aggregate income	*Percentage of individuals*
Index of investment activity[43]		
Zero; delegates all investment management to others	28	31
1 - 2	20	23
3 - 4	20	19
5 - 6	17	14
7 - 8	6	3
9 - 10	2	1
11 - 12	1	1
13 - 14: highly active	0	0
Savings, investments, or reserve funds under $1,000	6	8
Total	100	100
Portfolio size[44]		
Less than $1,000	6	20
Less than $30,000 ("small")	15	53
$10,000 - $300,000 ("medium-sized")	46	15
More than $100,000 ("large")	23	4
More than $500,000 in common stock ("very large")	10	8
Total	100	100
Preference between capital gains and current yield[45]		
Strong preference for capital gains over current yield	37	32
Moderate preference for capital gains over current yield	12	10
No preference between capital gains and current yield	29	33
Moderate preference for current yield over capital gains	8	8
Strong preference for current yield over capital gains	8	9
Savings, investments, or reserve funds under $1,000	6	8
Total	100	100

[43] The index of investment activity measures the frequency of investment transactions in which the respondent was engaged. The highest index (14) was scored by a respondent who both bought and sold bonds or preferred stock in 1964 (the interviewing took place in March-May 1964), who both bought and sold common stock in 1963 or 1964, who as a general rule bought common stock once a month or more frequently, and who either bought or sold interests in an unincorporated business or real estate in 1964. The lowest index number was scored by a respondent who neither bought nor sold bonds, preferred stock, common stock, or interests in an unincorporated business or real estate in 1963 or 1964, and who as a general rule did not buy common stock more frequently than once a year. The same criteria were used to classify other types of respondents in the intermediate groups between these two extremes. For further details, see Chapter VI.

[44] Included in these amounts are the value of fixed-yield assets, common stock, and interests in real estate and unincorporated businesses. The way in which the information on these values was obtained makes it impossible to avoid overlapping between the brackets describing the value of the total portfolio. See also Table 5.2.

[45] This description of the respondent's preferences was derived not from his behavior but from his concerns stated in answer to questions in Section 1. A "strong" preference means that the desired objective was said to be "very important"; a "moderate" preference means that the desired objective was said to be "important" or "somewhat important."

	Percentage of aggregate income	Percentage of individuals
Marginal tax rate awareness[46]		
Definitely overstates marginal tax rate	7	8
Conceivably correct as to marginal tax rate	66	63
Definitely understates marginal tax rate	3	3
Does not know marginal tax rate; information refused; no response recorded	24	26
Total	100	100
Past and future income changes[47]		
Past income up; future income up	15	19
Past income up; future income the same	13	15
Past income up; future income down	2	2
Past income the same; future income up	23	25
Past income the same; future income the same	32	28
Past income the same; future income down	8	7
Past income down; future income up	2	1
Past income down; future income the same	4	3
Past income down; future income down	1	0
Total	100	100

[46] Respondents who claimed that their marginal income tax rate (under the 1963 federal income tax rate schedule) was less than 20 percent were classified as "definitely understating" the marginal rate. Those who claimed that their marginal rate was above the maximum possible were classified as "definitely overstating." The maximum possible marginal income tax rate (federal and state) for each respondent was computed on the basis of (a) his stated 1963 adjusted gross income bracket, and (b) whether or not a joint return was filed. Further assumptions were made as follows:

1. The respondent's adjusted gross income was at the upper end of the income bracket.
2. Married taxpayers claimed only two personal exemptions, and single taxpayers only one.
3. The taxpayer either took the standard deduction or itemized only his state income taxes.
4. The taxpayer had no net long-term capital gains included in his adjusted gross income.
5. The taxpayer resided in the state (New York) which imposed the largest state income tax burden. The deductibility of state income taxes from income subject to federal tax was allowed for. (New York does not permit mutual deductibility.)

[47] Past income was counted as having changed if the respondent's income bracket changed between 1961 and 1963. Future income changes were derived from answers to the question in Section 10, "In the next few years, do you think your family income will go up considerably, stay the same, or what?"

	Percentage of aggregate income	Percentage of individuals
Size of place from which individual was selected (U.S. Census definition)		
Twelve largest Standard Metropolitan Statistical Areas	41	40
Other Standard Metropolitan Statistical Areas	39	39
Places which are not part of a Standard Metropolitan Statistical Area	20	21
Total	100	100
Region from which individual was selected[48] (U.S. Census definition)		
Northeast	28	25
North Central	29	30
South	25	25
West	18	20
Total	100	100

[48] *Northeast* includes Connecticut, Maine, Massachusetts, New Hampshire, New Jersey, New York, Pennsylvania, Rhode Island, and Vermont.
North Central includes Illinois, Indiana, Iowa, Kansas, Michigan, Minnesota, Missouri, Nebraska, North Dakota, Ohio, South Dakota, and Wisconsin.
South includes Alabama, Arkansas, Delaware, District of Columbia, Florida, Georgia, Kentucky, Louisiana, Maryland, Mississippi, North Carolina, Oklahoma, South Carolina, Tennessee, Texas, Virginia, and West Virginia.
West includes Arizona, California, Colorado, Idaho, Montana, Nevada, New Mexico, Oregon, Utah, Washington, and Wyoming.

APPENDIX F

The Computer Program Used in the Analysis

MOST OF THE MULTIVARIATE analysis reported in this book is based on a new computer program called the Automatic Interaction Detector (AID). It was developed for the IBM 7090 with the help of a grant from the National Science Foundation.[1]

An interaction effect exists where the explanatory or "causal" variables do not act independently and additively. The effect of one factor may depend on the level of another. Sometimes a variable affects only one part of the population, as when tax disincentives affect only those with some freedom to alter their work patterns. Sometimes several explanations are alternatives, as when *any one* of two or three circumstances—such as a small asset portfolio, not being active in investing, or not being concerned about taxes—leads to a low level of investment information.

The new program imposes no restrictions on the data, except that the dependent variable—the thing to be explained—must be a reasonably

[1] For a full explanation of the program with examples, see John Sonquist and James Morgan, *The Detection of Interaction Effects,* Monograph 35 (Survey Research Center, Institute for Social Research, University of Michigan, 1964). An earlier statement by these authors, which is reprinted in the monograph, is "Problems in the Analysis of Survey Data, and a Proposal," *Journal of the American Statistical Association* (June 1963), pp. 415-34.

normally distributed variable or a dichotomy where the proportions do not get too close to zero or to 100 percent. It is really an automated replication of the process researchers have always used in looking for structural relations in a rich set of data with many variables and a large number of cases.

The parallels between the program and the strategy of an exploratory researcher are striking. More often than not, investigators have only a rudimentary theory and must generally let the data speak for themselves. Even if they first subordinate the data to a tight test of a prior hypothesis, they generally proceed to a great deal of secondary searching or revised hypotheses. They often fix attention on a single dependent variable, the aim being to find independent variables whose categories separate the sample into widely differing subgroups, each internally homogeneous. This feature underlies regression models as well as analysis of variance models. But in a less formal way researchers often conduct an intuitive and unsystematic search for homogeneous subgroups without conceptualizing it as such. One of the program's virtues is that it bares this approach. Using it, the researcher must face squarely the exploratory nature of his method. Because it is made explicit, the method is "exposed to fraternal judgment." AID merely formalizes a common strategy and gives it astronomically greater power by harnessing the computer to it.

The program operates sequentially. It first looks at the effect on the whole sample of each explanatory characteristic in turn, finding the best way of using that factor to divide the sample into two groups. By "best," we mean the division that reduces the unexplained sum of squared deviations (or "error variance") the most. Using two subgroup averages instead of one overall average to predict the dependent variable reduces the predictive error, and the process looks for the largest such reduction. The test is a test of importance, not significance. The two groups so formed must not only be different, they must also each contain a substantial number of cases.[2] Within each of the two groups, the individuals are more like one another (homogeneous) than they are like those in the other group.

Where the explanatory characteristic has a natural ordering or rank order, that order can be preserved, but it is also possible to try for the best re-ranking and then the best division of the sample along that new ordering.

[2] If a few cases can be split off and the unexplained variance reduced substantially, the dependent variable clearly contains extreme cases (is heteroscedastic), a highly dangerous situation for any statistical analysis based on least squares. This has not been a problem in the present study.

The program then recalls which predictor's best split is better than that of any of the other predictors, and actually divides the sample into two subgroups on that basis. Each of the two subgroups thus generated is examined in turn in the same way, using all the predictors, and is split again. Each of those new groups is examined in turn and split if possible. The new groups spread out like the roots of a tree, containing fewer cases, each split doing its best to maximize the explained variance (minimize the unexplained variance).

The process stops when no division of a group can reduce the unexplained sum of squares (variance) by as much as some predetermined criterion level, usually 0.5 percent or 1 percent of the original full-sample sum of squares (around the average). Or it stops when one or both of the groups produced would be so small that there would be a serious question as to the sampling stability of the results—that is, we could not be reasonably sure that another sample would show anything similar. Some of the roots end before others, of course, and different predictors are used in different roots.

Since the search process looks at so many possibilities, it cannot be thought of as testing a hypothesis. There are no "degrees of freedom" left and no way to estimate the stability of the results over different samples.[3] This problem exists whenever a number of analyses are made of the same body of data, but the present formalization of the process makes it more obvious.

There is one way in which we can come to a conclusion about the effect of a particular predictor. If it has no apparent effect either over the whole sample, or on any of the major subgroups generated, then one can be reasonably sure it does not matter. (The program prints out the subgroup averages according to each predictor at each stage.)

Even this certainty is reduced where there are two predictors that are correlated with one another. With the sequential approach, once the sample is divided on the basis of the more important predictor, the other is often unable to assume any importance at all. With multiple regression, by comparison, both predictors would show some apparent effect, dividing up the credit, but the sampling errors tend to become large.

The results of the process are independent of the order in which the variables are introduced, but they do depend on which variables are allowed into the analysis, and on the precision with which they are measured. It is always possible that introducing a different variable or

[3] Tests with the program indicate that the first parts of the process remain reasonably stable with different samples, and the groups developed somewhat more stable than the path by which they are generated.

a better measurement of one already used, would produce different results.

The program should not be confused with the large number of multivariate analysis programs for data reduction now in use based on multiple regression, multiple discriminant analysis, or factor analysis. All these other programs assume additivity of effects of different factors in one way or another. They impose various other restrictions to make the problem manageable. In the case of factor analysis, the factors are sets of weights (loadings) assigned to explanatory variables and used to provide a new, smaller set of indexes used as predictors. The weights are based on intercorrelations among the variables, however, not on their relations to the variable to be explained.

The new program is, of course, no substitute for theory, which is involved in the selection of the variables and the interpretation of the results. Nor does it provide the final word, since ultimately the findings need to be tested against other samples and at a later date for stability and persistence. What has been done here is to focus on the factors that seem to matter now.

In a few cases where it was important to assess the effect of one predictor relatively free of spurious effects through other variables, and where a substantial amount of symmetry (additivity) seemed to exist, a multiple regression with dummy variables was used.[4]

On the other hand, previous tests have shown that frequently a predictor that had a significant multiple regression coefficient turned out in the new analysis to be affecting only one subgroup of the population.

[4] For an earlier study making extensive use of this approach, see James N. Morgan, *et al.*, *Income and Welfare in the United States* (McGraw-Hill, 1962).

Index